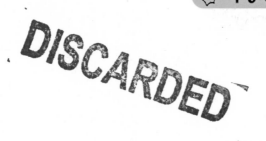

The Human Senses

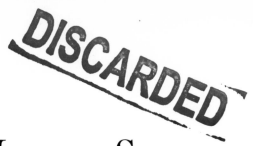
The Human Senses

Second Edition

Frank A. Geldard
Professor of Psychology
Princeton University

John Wiley & Sons, Inc.
New York • London • Sydney • Toronto

Library of Congress Catalogue Card Number: 72-37432

ISBN 0-471-29570-1

Printed in the United States of America.

10 9 8 7 6 5 4 3

To Jeannette and Debby, still good girls

Preface

The trend of the 1950s seems, in the 1970s, to be even more deeply grooved. In the world of sensation, as in many other areas of human thought, we continue to "know more and more about less and less." Sensory specialists abound while sensory generalists are all but extinct.

I have been asked about this phrase, "sensory generalist." Do I really mean "sensory dilettante"? Acquisition of knowledge being what it is in these days of exploding science, how can anyone hope to have more than a nodding acquaintance with all the senses? The charge is not unreasonable, but there is another view. Perhaps the designation I should be using is "sensory impartialist." The distinction is charmingly pointed up in a Croatian toast. Whenever wine glasses are raised, the Yugoslav injunction is to hold the glass deftly by the stem and touch rims ever so gently. "For the little ears," they say as the miniature clang rings out. The eyes see the color, the bouquet is wafted to the nostrils, the lips feel the cool pressure of glass and liquid, and the tongue savors the wine's character. But what about the poor little ears? For them there is nothing. So clink your glasses and be a sensory impartialist.

Specialization, of course, has its recompenses. One of its outcomes, the intensive exploration of the neural foundations of sensory experience, has already changed many facts and opened the avenues to the discovery of many more. This development, proceeding relatively quietly since the vacuum tube was first employed in the interest of recording biological potentials, has raised its pitch almost to that of a frenzy in the age of the transistor. Not only have all sensory pathways succumbed to attack at several stations on their ascent to the highest levels of the central nervous system but also, for certain of them, techniques have become available for obtaining accounts of the most intimate intracellular events. And so neural specialization, forcing concentration on such phenomena as excitation and inhibition, adaptation and accommodation, convergence and divergence, recruitment, spontaneous discharge, orthodromic and anti-dromic conduction—to single out but a few that prove to be common to all channels—achieves the goal of generalization and once again stresses the inevitable unity of the senses.

Comparison of the old and new editions of this book will reveal that the really radical changes have occurred in the electrophysiological sphere, but there have also been notable advances in the realm of psychophysics, and there are many additions to our understanding of the physics of stimuli and the anatomy of the sense organs. Indeed, psychology's hand-maidens have done somewhat better than has psychology.

Many people have been helpful with the second edition, as with the first. Because we engage in an almost continuous colloquium on sensory matters, my thanks must be directed most especially to my friend and colleague, Carl Sherrick. He has read and criticized the entire manuscript. Others who have rallied around with partial readings and comments are, for the vision chapters, John Lott Brown and Robert Boynton; for the auditory chapters, Glen Wever, who also performed a similar service for the first edition. I also acknowledge the influence of Edwin G. Boring, who set nearly all the chapters on the right track by roundly criticizing, in the kind of detail only he could handle, the entire first edition. It is a moral certainty that the revision would never have been brought to com-pletion were it not for the more or less steady sifting process occasioned by my graduate seminar in Sensory Psychophysiology at Princeton. Facts, theories, and their interrelations have been under constant appraisal through several rotations of Cutaneous Senses, Vision, and Chemical Senses. I think especially of Gary Rollman, Jim Craig, and Dick Fay as outstanding contributors to the seminar.

As in the first edition, acknowledgment of permission to reproduce material from other authors, almost exclusively graphs and photographs, has been made in situ. The willingness of so many copyright holders to make their figures available for this purpose is much appreciated.

FRANK A. GELDARD

Princeton, New Jersey

Preface to the First Edition

Once upon a time—not too deeply buried in the moldering past, for it falls within the memory of a generation yet alive and active—the greater portion of psychology was "sense psychology." "Experience" was psychology's proper object of study, and experience comes by way of man's senses.

The same generation has seen changes—some of emphasis, many merely of terminology, but a few of fundamental conception. Psychology has become "the science of behavior." This development has made the role of the human senses no less important, for all behavior is triggered by stimuli, and stimuli must have sense organs on which to operate. But the elaboration of a science of behavior calls for much more than variations on the simple theme provided by the stimulus-response formula. Such rubrics as learning, motive, attitude, and interest—in short, the central adjustive mechanisms generally—have taken on an air of urgency. Preoccupation with these topics naturally results in a relative de-emphasis of others. In the contemporary picture, therefore, sensation seems to have receded somewhat into the background; more "dynamic," if less mature, concepts are crowding the center of the canvas. These trends in psychological fashions partially account for the current rarity of books on sensation. In part, also, the lack is to be attributed to the circumstance that, whereas we have no dearth of specialists in vision and in audition, and even a few experts in each of the other senses, there are not many "sensory generalists" in psychology.

The basic credo underlying this book is that the highroad to the understanding of human nature is by way of an appreciation of man's senses and of the fundamental role they play in the attainment of knowledge and the regulation of behavior. If, through its auspices, students or general readers are set on the path towards such an appreciation; if, so to

ix

speak, they are "brought to their senses," the book will have realized the major aim set for it.

Were I cataloguing all the influences responsible for the genesis and final completion of the book I should certainly have to begin with John Paul Nafe's course in systematic psychology at Clark University in my graduate student days. My appetite for sensory psychology clearly came into being then. It has been whetted, in seminars extending over a score of years, by my own students at Virginia. In the actual preparation of the manuscript there has been the valuable help of several professional colleagues. The chapters on vision were read and criticized, at various stages, by Clarence H. Graham and S. Rains Wallace, Jr. The audition chapters had the benefit of critical readings by E. Glen Wever, Frank W. Finger, and Willard R. Thurlow. The chapters on the chemical senses profited from the suggestions of Carl Pfaffmann. The entire manuscript was appraised, and improved no little, by Professor Herbert S. Langfield. To all these friends I am very grateful; my earnest hope is that they find the finished product not too disappointing.

Finally, my thanks are due Mrs. Jane Watson, accustomed to turning out perfect copy, for a typical performance on the manuscript, thereby lightening the labors of author and publisher alike.

FRANK A. GELDARD

Charlottesville, Virginia
January, 1953

Contents

The Human Senses

1
Introduction

Man has ever been the most engaging object of study for man. In the behavior of his fellows he is confronted with a never-ending source of wonder and perplexity, and in his every new experience he finds a challenge to his understanding. The intricacies of human action are myriad, and it is no accident that psychology, whose business it is to cut through the complexities and disclose the broad principles governing human nature and conduct, should have been among the last subjects to attain the stature of a scientific discipline. Prescientific psychology has a history as long as that of human thought itself.

There is probably no topic in connection with which the average layman is more ready to pronounce a judgment or express an opinion than that of psychology. We may be content to leave the intricacies of physics or chemistry or any other of the fundamental natural sciences to experts in these fields, satisfying ourselves with a few basic ideas about the operation of the complicated world around us. But the business of living and conducting ourselves in a world of human beings is very much the concern of each of us. We are all under the necessity of acquiring and pressing into service a workable set of conceptions of human nature. Moreover, the materials with which psychology attempts to come to grips are immediately available in the form of our own thoughts and feelings and in the actions of others. We come readily to generalize from our experiences and to develop a set of beliefs concerning the operation of the human mind. The demand for working principles is so insistent that it is not surprising that hasty convictions, half-truths, even superstitions become lodged in our mental constitutions and sometimes are modified or expelled only with the greatest difficulty. We feel "from experience" that we are rather good judges of the motives of other people. We have "explanations" for the fact that some persons have good memories while others have not. We acquire beliefs as to the relative influence of nature and nurture in shaping our behavior. We do not hesitate to ascribe the genesis of anomalies we observe in others to temperament and character "types." We have convictions concerning the effects of sleep, the importance of dreams, the influences of age, sex, fatigue, climatic conditions, and a host of other matters. In fact, unless we turn the searchlight of self-criticism upon these beliefs we may go on indefinitely, trusting our crude observations, never pausing to draw into question the processes whereby we form our prejudices and set up our standards.

In all ages there have been thoughtful people who have tried to bring order out of the chaos that is personal experience; the production of various philosophical "systems," of one or another degree of satisfying-ness, attests the success of such ventures. In an earlier day such systematic groupings of personal observations *were* psychology, and there are many acute descriptions and cogent explanations of psychological phenomena in philosophical writings. Indeed, many such accounts have never been surpassed. The chief danger in abiding by such systems lies, of course, in the narrow factual perspective they afford. Bodies of acceptable scientific knowledge represent joint enterprises by many different people united by common purposes and concepts; modern sciences are not compounded exclusively of personal fireside speculations, however shrewd they may be.

The scientific approach to the study of psychology differs not in the least, at the present time, from that which is employed in undertaking the study of any other basic science. The details differ; the point of view is the same. As a modern science psychology employs the method of experiment, the accoutrements of the laboratory, and the procedure of objective observation, just as do all other natural sciences. Taking its cue from the imposing successes of the more mature sciences of nature, psychology adopted the experimental method only a few score years ago in the clear recognition that, while its objects of study might be vastly more complicated and correspondingly more difficult of exact experimental manipulation, knowledge meeting the rigid demands of science could be acquired in no other way. The step taken by physics in the sixteenth century was repeated, at least in all outward characteristics, by psychology in the latter part of the nineteenth.

The beginnings of scientific psychology are peculiarly bound up with our subject—the human senses—and we shall do well, for that reason, to take a brief backward glance at experimental psychology's origins. Through it we may hope to gain a perspective not obtainable in any other way. Though the senses have doubtless been the objects of interest and study since pre-history, their scientific description is a relatively recent product of the laboratory and of the experimental method.

The Origins of Experimental Psychology. We like to date experimental psychology from the establishment of the first laboratory devoted solely to the prosecution of its problems. In 1879, Wilhelm Wundt, one of the great figures of all time in psychology, formally opened at Leipzig a laboratory designed for the experimental investigation of a broad range of psychological processes. There were begun important studies of action, attention, feeling, association, memory, and especially, sensation and perception. All these are still important rubrics in experimental psychology, and the vast influence of Wundt and his students in shaping the future course of the infant science can hardly be overestimated. Of course, experimental psychology did not spring, like Athene, "full-fledged from the forehead of Jove"; Wundt was in no sense entirely and single-handedly responsible for its inception. Even had he been a different sort of person he could not have boasted, as Napoleon is said to have done, that he was his own ancestor. The movement that had its first institutional expression in the Leipzig laboratory had been initiated by a very considerable number of worthy predecessors, chiefly physiologists, physicists, and philosophers. What made Wundt's work a "founding" effort was the fact that it gave clear expression and implementation to several converging influences in nineteenth-century science.

There had been important figures, such as Helmholtz, Fechner, Weber, and Johannes Müller, as well as a host of lesser lights, who had not only set the stage for the advent of a distinct science of experimental psychology but who, through important physiological and physical experiments, had partially determined its ultimate trajectory. Also, there had been a very real and many-sided preparation for coming events within philosophy, particularly on the part of the British empiricists of the eighteenth century and the associationists of the early nineteenth.

It has become apparent, in retrospect, that the first experimental psychology was not so much a borrowing from the more firmly established sciences and philosophy as it was an expression of a real need for a direct frontal attack, by approved scientific methods, on broad problems of human nature. One cannot go far into physics without confronting problems concerning the sensitivity and reliability of instruments, and the most commonly employed "instrument" is, of course, the human observer. Similarly, one takes few steps into physiology, studying the manner of functioning of various bodily organs and tissue systems, without encountering the most general problems of the behavior of the organism as a whole. Further, the most persistent and abiding problems of philosophy, especially those having to do with the question of how knowledge is acquired, find answers possible only when they are made specific and cast in terms of the details of human experience. Thus it is not surprising to find Ernst Mach, a physicist "unconstrained by the conventional barriers of the specialist," publishing a volume on *The Analysis of the Sensations,* Charles Darwin producing a work on *Expression of Emotion in Man and Animals,* and Bishop Berkeley giving to the world, in successive years, his *New Theory of Vision* and the *Principles of Human Knowledge.* Nor are these in any sense isolated instances. Knowledge may be partitioned only through an artifice. The most thoughtful workers in any field will come, sooner or later, to a consideration of the most fascinating of all objects of study, man himself.

The Psychophysical Law.   One development of special significance in the pre-Wundtian days, important not only because it brought measurement into the service of psychology but because it supplied methods and materials destined to dominate much of the later work, was that coming from the pioneer work of Ernst Weber (1795–1878) and G. T. Fechner (1801–1887). Weber, a physiologist greatly interested in problems of sense organ functions, a field to which he made many signal contributions, came in the course of his studies to direct special attention to the then little-understood sensations originating in muscles and their attachments. A discovery which will forever be linked with his name came out of an experiment designed to disclose the role of muscle sensations in the discrimination of weights of different magnitudes. He first found that differences could be detected somewhat more readily when the weights were lifted, thus imposing strains on the muscles of the hand and arm, than when they were simply laid on the resting hand. In true experimental fashion he set out to vary systematically the various factors involved, using initial weights of 4, 7.5, and 32 oz. Adding small weights to these standards and noting the effect on the feelings of strain in the muscles, he soon discovered an interesting relationship. All his results pointed to the generality that discrimination depends, not upon the absolute size of the difference between two weights, but upon the ratio of this size to that of the weight with which one starts. The ratio proved to be a constant one and to be independent of the absolute masses involved; the "just noticeable difference" (j.n.d.) always corresponded to a constant fraction of the standard stimulus. To produce a just perceptibly increased feeling of strain it was necessary to add a weight $\frac{1}{40}$ as large as the amount already in force. Intrigued with this evidence for the relativity of human judgments, Weber tested the applicability of his formula to other kinds of sensations and found that it apparently held. Lines of slightly different length, provided they were presented in succession, could be just discriminated when they differed by a constant small fraction. For the sharpest observers, the difference needed to be only 1–2% of the overall length; for the less discriminating, it might be as high as 4%. It did not matter whether the first line was an inch long, twice that, or a small fraction of an inch. Our estimation of a difference, said Weber, depends not on the absolute magnitude of the difference but on the ratio of this magnitude to the magnitude of the things compared. Other experiments, some less thoroughgoing than might be desired, led him to extend the law to touch and hearing, where he found pressures to be correctly discriminated if they stood in the ratio of 29 to 30, and tonal pitches to sound different to the musically trained ear if they bore the relation of 321 to 322.

Recognition of the wide applicability and basic significance of "Weber's Law" came at the hands of another, Gustav Fechner. For one whose early interests lay in the field of pure physics and whose leanings throughout a long and varied lifetime were broadly philosophical, it is a strange quirk of fate that Fechner should now be best known for the bias he gave to early experimental psychology. Yet Fechner's contribution came out of his philosophy. His general view, first expressed in his *Zend-Avesta* (1851), an odd mixture of oriental mysticism and occidental materialism, and later in his classical *Elements of Psychophysics* (1860), called for the most embracing of beliefs in the essential identity of the mental world and the physical world of matter. The transition from the one to the other would seem to be not impossible if a combining principle, involving a universal relation between the two, could be discovered. This principle Fechner believed he had found in Weber's Law. But, whereas Weber had been content with the "just noticeable difference," Fechner reasoned further that all sensations, perhaps all mental processes, must be measurable in terms of their stimuli, and he came to formulate a more general "psychophysical" law. This law stated that the intensity of sensation is proportional to the intensity of stimulation, but that the relation is not a simple direct one. As sensations increase in equal steps, the stimuli necessary to set them off increase by equal ratios. The mathematical statement is S (sensation intensity) $= k \log I$ (stimulus intensity, ideally energy).

It happens that the Weber-Fechner Law, as a later generation has named it, has been shown not to have anything like the universal applicability its originator claimed for it. Indeed, there is some doubt as to whether it is ever strictly true; certainly there are many instances in which it represents not even a fair approximation to reality. Numerous criticisms have been directed against it on logical and factual grounds, and some critics, such as William James, have attempted to discredit it entirely. Indeed, what James said was, "Fechner's book was the starting point for a new departure in literature, which it would perhaps be impossible to match for the qualities of thoroughness and subtlety, but of which, in the humble opinion of the present writer, the proper psychological outcome is just *nothing*" (*329*, Vol. I, p. 534). S. S. Stevens, with the advantage of a perspective afforded by a full century of psychophysical effort since Fechner's *Elements,* was able to be more charitable but still concluded that the father of psychophysics "led the way as a true pioneer, but it now appears that he may have taken a wrong fork in the road. He was faced with two alternatives. He could have assumed that equal stimulus *ratios* produce equal sensation *differences,* or that equal stimulus *ratios* produce equal sensation *ratios*" (*552*, p. 202). Fechner's selection of sensory differences, despite strong espousal of sensory ratios by some of his contemporaries, notably Plateau, necessarily led to an approach that has turned out to be altogether indirect and, indeed, confusing. Moreover, what might have been a more direct path to the assessment of sensation intensity was discouraged by no less an authority than the founder of experimental psychology himself. Wundt said, in 1863 (see James, op. cit.): "How much stronger or weaker one sensation is than another, we are never able to say. . . . To measure the strength of sensations is . . . impossible; we can only measure the difference of sensations."

What appears now to have been the more obvious truth—that stimulus ratios beget sensation ratios—began to assert itself formally in psychophysics at midtwentieth century. Ever since, there has been a lively pursuit of a program of subjecting all manner of sensory input-output

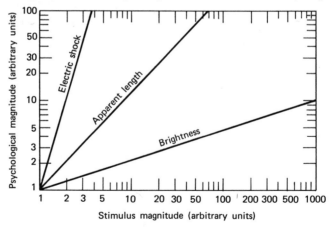

Fig. 1–1. Power functions for electric shock, apparent length, and brightness. Exponents for these three functions are, respectively: 3.5, 1.1, and 0.3. From Stevens (*551*). Copyright 1962 by American Psychological Association, and reproduced by permission.

relations to experimental test, guided by the empirically fortified belief that sensation intensity can be estimated or rated in direct observation.

It is currently found that, when estimates of sensation magnitude, judged on a ratio scale, are plotted against stimulus magnitudes, laid out on a ratio scale, a straight-line function of one or another slope is realized. Figure 1-1 depicts three such functions, one for electric shock, one for apparent length of a line, and one for visual brightness. It is to be noted that both axes of the graph are plotted logarithmically. Whenever two variables are joined linearly in a log-log plot, we have a power function. Stevens' substitute for Fechner's Law is thus commonly called the *power law* of sensory intensity.

We shall be encountering power functions in many different contexts; it is therefore important that we know how they come into being. There are several different ways of getting sensory magnitudes quantized. The simplest approach is to present a sequence of different intensities and ask an observer to assign numbers to them that will indicate their relative strengths. If one seems twice as strong or half as strong as another, a number twice or half the other is assigned to it. This is *magnitude estimation,* and it can make use of a preliminary standard (the modulus) or not; this detail is not as important as one might think. Another approach is to estimate a ratio between two stimuli separated on the scale of physical intensity. Is the weaker of two tones ½, ⅘, or some other fraction of the stronger one? This is the method of *ratio estimation.* A not uncommon device here is to ask the observer to divide 100 points between the two (*constant sum* technique). Still another way of getting the ratios expressed is to put the stimulus under the control of the observer. He is given a cutaneous pressure of a predetermined magnitude, for example, and, with the strength of the sensation as the only cue, he is asked to produce a pressure ⅓ as strong, 4 times as strong, etc. This is the method of *ratio production.* There are good reasons for combining the two procedures, fractionation and multiplication, in a single experiment; such an approach tends to cancel out certain biases that creep into this method. A final procedure, know as *magnitude production,* is really the obverse of the simple magnitude estimation method. Instead of assigning numbers to sensory intensities, the experimenter supplies the observer with a number and requires that the stimulus intensity be adjusted to the corresponding sensory magnitude.

Whatever the method used to get a direct indication of sensory intensity, it appears that sensation magnitude may grow rapidly or slowly, depending on what particular kind of sensation is involved. In Fig. 1-1 we saw power functions having radically different slopes, that for electric shock being very steep, that for brightness being quite gentle. The slope is given by the exponent of the independent variable, β, in the expression

$$\Psi = k(\phi - \phi_0)^\beta$$

where Ψ is the psychological magnitude (sensory intensity), ϕ is the intensity of the physical stimulus, ϕ_0 is threshold intensity, and k is a constant determined by the choice of unit selected for measurement. The exponent, β, varies with the sense modality involved and apparently also with some of the experimental parameters entering into the measurement. A great many sensory continua have been studied by now, and it is clear that, whereas exponents may vary over a wide range (3.5 for electric shock and 0.3 for the brightness of a white light target, e.g.), the full meaning of the power function slope is not yet evident. One clear significance has to do with the "dynamic range" of the modality. Thus, in the instance of the exposure of the skin to 60-Hz (hertz, cycles per second) electric shock, it is only a relatively short distance from threshold "tingle" to a disagreeable "pounding" so intolerable as to bring the experiment to an abrupt stop. Figure 1-2 shows power functions of nine continua with as many slopes and dynamic ranges.

Figure 1-2 serves another purpose for us, however. It will be noted that the ordinate is labeled "force of hand grip in pounds." This legend reveals another interesting departure in experiments done under the

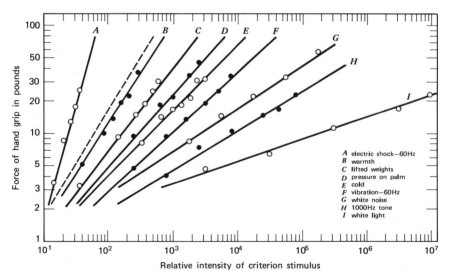

Fig. 1–2. A family of power functions obtained by letting force of hand grip indicate sensation intensity. The dashed line shows where an exponent of 1.0 lies on these coordinates. From Stevens (*551*). Copyright 1962 by American Psychological Association, and reproduced by permission.

aegis of power-law thinking. Instead of asking the observer to indicate strength of sensation, he may be asked to squeeze a hand dynamometer to the degree necessary to indicate the apparent strength of sensation. Such intermodal matches can be made with great reliability and, after some practice at it, also with a fair degree of assurance. Loudness of white noise has been manipulated in the same way. And there are other possibilities of cutting across modalities or comparing intensities of different qualities within the same modality: matching white noise to vibration imparted to the fingertip or matching the loudness of two differently pitched tones, for example. It has long been the practice in measuring light intensities involving two different colors to make a straightforward brightness match of the two, disregarding the hue difference between them. This is a kind of "cross-modal" matching.

This little excursion into modern psychophysics will prepare us, at several points, to interpret facts of sensory operations. But let us now return to our historical approach. It was not psychophysics alone that was responsible for experimental psychology having developed to the point where it was ready to join the family of sciences, though psychophysical experiments loomed large in the total effort, and its preoccupation with the topic of our immediate concern—the human senses—makes it of special interest to us.

The Influence of Experimental Physiology.   Any inventory of the influences leading to experimental psychology's founding must include the very considerable one exerted by studies of nervous functions. From the beginning, psychologists have been intensely interested in the workings of the nervous system, and with good reason. It is truly the "organ of mind," and, presumably, no fact concerning its operation is without some value or interest in aiding the interpretation of psychological data.

The years that were formative for experimental psychology were also those of significant and spectacular discovery for its older brother, experimental physiology. The first years of the nineteenth century had seen revealed the most basic principles of operation of the nervous system, especially Sir Charles Bell's discovery that the spinal nerves were arranged in accordance with function, sensory fibers entering the posterior and motor fibers the anterior portions of the spinal cord. His "law of forward direction" in the nervous system has been considered to be as fundamental as Harvey's discovery of the circulation of the blood. Just at the time when Weber was doing his lifted weight experiments there was being disclosed the essential difference between the kinds of nervous pathways involved in voluntary actions and those responsible for purely automatic or "reflex" activities. Also, Johannes Müller was marshalling his arguments for his famous doctrine of "specific energies of nerves," an idea so basic and far-reaching that it forms the crux of many of our current disputes in sensory theory, to say nothing of its profound influence in shaping early experimental problems. The battle between "specificity" and "nonspecificity" has filled many a psychological day.

While Fechner was devising his psychophysical law and performing somewhat tedious experiments in support of it, Helmholtz' brilliant measurements of the speed of nervous conduction were being made. Helmholtz' teacher, Johannes Müller, had supposed such measures to be impossible, regarding nerve impulsion to be of the order of the speed of light! The middle of the century saw also the beginnings of modern nerve cell theory and the development of techniques for staining nerves, thus permitting their more exact anatomical study. Altogether, it was a happy combination of circumstances that joined neurological discovery and interest in psychological phenomena in such a way as to provide mutual impetus to the two fields. To this day their contents, if not inextricably interwoven, are mutually complementary. Experimental psychology would be pale without the interpretative coloring provided by an expanding knowledge of nervous functions, and, at the same time, experimental neurology may count among its most conspicuous successes discoveries prompted by psychological observations.

Some of the influences responsible for the creation of a separate field of experimental psychology have been pointed out. Once established, its growth was rapid and its frontiers were greatly expanded. Its central topic, sensation, was a natural interest which continued to be prosecuted wherever the young science took root. Over half the studies issuing from Wundt's laboratory and those of his students were concerned with sensation and perception. Of these the large majority were on vision, then as now preeminent among the sense channels as the conveyor of the most detailed and frequently the most urgent messages. Second in popularity as a research topic was the sense of hearing; next came touch and its near relatives in the family of senses and, finally, the chemical senses, smell and taste. This order still represents the relative importance of the various classes of sensation, whether one relies on professional judgment in coming to a conclusion about it or lets the number of technical publications in each of these areas serve as a criterion. It is the order we shall follow in our systematic survey of the senses.

It would be a mistake to suppose, because its origins are so closely bound up with the study of sensation, that experimental psychology thereby has the sole proprietary right to this field. We have already seen that physiology, especially neural physiology, has a legitimate claim to the senses, as do also some other neighboring disciplines. To come to an appreciation of what interests impinge upon the human senses, considered as objects of study, we do well to attempt to get into perspective the world of scientific knowledge and its mode of organization.

The Unity of Knowledge and the Diversity of Human Interests. Scientific knowledge, painstakingly amassed by many devotees over an extended period of human history, is nothing if not unitary when viewed in the large and against the background of superstition, folklore, and rule of thumb over which it has had to triumph. Its unity derives from a commonness of purpose, a rigor of logical planning and observational procedure, and a strict fidelity to the rules governing the use of the experimental method. Science seeks out, with detachment and disinterest, the unvarnished fact. In part, its unity derives also from the circumstance that different particular sciences, all having the same reality to view but doing so from different standpoints, come to describe many of the same objects and thus develop with other sciences a community of content. How this can come about is revealed by a useful figure once suggested by Titchener (575). He pictured the "world of experience as contained in a great circle, and . . . scientific men as viewing this world from various stations on the periphery. There are . . . as many possible sciences as there are distinguishable points of view about the circle . . . no one of them in truth exhausts experience or completely describes the common subject-matter, though each one, if ideally complete, would exhaust some aspects of experience. . . . One and the same item of human experience may enter, as part of their subject-matter, into a large number of sciences; whence it follows that the sciences themselves cannot be distinguished, in any final accounting, by the specific character of the 'objects' with which they deal."

We know, of course, that sciences do not just "happen"; they do not find themselves in position on the circle by accident. Sciences are only slowly and arduously "constructed," and each has a history peculiar to itself. Moreover, the stuff of which sciences are compounded is "mediate," not "immediate" experience. Nevertheless, this view of the way in which the sciences are organized is helpful, not only in stressing the unity of knowledge but also in emphasizing, in the peripheral dimension, the intimacy of relation among the various approaches. One sees that it is, after all, but a step—albeit one that offers at the conclusion of it a new and different vista of reality—from psychology to physiology, say, or from pathology to physics. Nor does any particular harm come from the journeying of the individual scientist if he chooses to traverse the scientific circle. He is under no compunction to remain uncompromisingly at one position on the perimeter. Not only should he be permitted to wander from his own observation post, but, provided only that he preserve his orientation constantly, he should be encouraged to make frequent visits to his scientific neighbors. It is only necessary that he avoid too great a peripheral velocity, for that way lies superficiality, dilettantism, or even, as Boring has termed it, "epistemological vertigo."

Nowhere in science is there a content having more points of impingement on human interests than that provided by the senses of man. All knowledge, as the Sophists of ancient Greece knew, comes only through the senses, and those who would "know how they know" turn quite naturally to the contemplation of the senses as the originators of experience. "The eye," John Locke noted in his *Essay Concerning Human Understanding*, "whilst it makes us see and perceive all other things, takes no notice of itself," and it becomes the special business of the sciences arranged about the circumference of Titchener's great circle, not to mention a variety of artistic and technological concerns representing powerful springs of human action, to furnish the means whereby an understanding of the visual process—and those of the other senses—can be attained.

The range of interests brought to bear on sensation and the senses is of prodigious extent. Consider vision. The study of what and how we see is not alone the business of scientific man, though he is doubtless in the most favored position to supply a full and impartial description. The visual process is also of importance to man considered medically, artistically, economically, educationally, and even politically. Charles II of England, perhaps remembering the price on his own head in Cromwell's time, is said to have derived much amusement from Mariotte's demonstration of the blind spot of the eye (1668) and required his courtiers to repeat the experiment to observe how they would look with their heads off! The mode of operation of the human eye is of practical concern to the physician as he checks the retinal color zones for evidences of disease or malfunction, to the painter in oils as he teases depth out of light and shade, to the advertising expert as he assaults the eye with all manner of suggestions for purchase, and to the professional educator with his modern reliance on visual aids. And these are, of course, in no wise isolated examples. Man viewed militarily or legally or as an engineering or linguistic creature would yield up myriads of instances in which visual sensation is a central consideration and thus itself a natural object of study. The visual implications have to be taken into account whenever there swing into action the illuminating engineer, the stage lighting expert, the designer of aircraft instruments or submarine controls, the railroad signalman, the paper chemist, the fabricator of ceramics or textiles, the manufacturing pharmacist, the designer of automobile bodies, the blender of paints, or the optical instrument maker. The list might go on and on, for it is difficult to think of human skills or technical knowledge or artistic endeavors apart from the visual sensations on which they in such large measure depend.

Nor is the visual channel the sole one of importance in human affairs. The fields of communication, entertainment, and education make almost incessant demands on our hearing apparatus, while the housing and clothing industries are monuments to our cutaneous senses, just as the food technologies are to our chemical senses. Little wonder that philosophers throughout the ages, when they have not been exalting Reason, have been extolling Sensation as the very essence of Truth. Little wonder that the scientific study of sensation and the senses forms today, as it did in Wundt's time, the most fundamental of psychological contents.

The Senses, Human Engineering, and the Limits of Perception. In the chapters that follow we shall be dealing, for the most part, with the senses considered in their fundamental or "pure science" aspect. The treatment accorded them will be systematic, and the aim will be to arrive at descriptive accounts which may be expected to hold good in a variety of settings. However, the impression should not be given that sensory psychology, as presently constituted, has no "applied" or technological side, that it fails to square with the manifold human needs and interests which, we have seen, may be brought to bear on it. Indeed, in evidence of just such a meeting of practical demands there has been witnessed in recent years the very lively growth of what has been variously called "human engineering," "psychotechnology," and "engineering psychology," a central concern of which is sensation and the senses. This development is a significant one and one whose latent possibilities have not even been estimated as yet.

Modern transportation and communication equipment, for example, impose an incredibly heavy burden on man's senses. We think of shipboard radar as a device for dispensing with the masthead lookout and thus of circumventing the limitations of man's sensory endowments. Radar searches where the eye cannot see, through darkness and fog and beyond the acuity limits of human vision. However, what radar and similar devices also do is to substitute one sensory task for another and, while effectively extending the range of exploration, also come to require discriminations that tax the capabilities of sense organs. "This recent war," writes Stevens in evaluation of the role of human engineering in World War II (548, p. 390), "was different from other wars in the peculiar respect that it was fought largely on margin—sensory margin—where the battle hangs on the power of the eyes or the ears to make a fine discrimination, to estimate a distance, to see or hear a signal which is just at the edge of human capacity . . . and the paradox of it is that the faster the engineers and the inventors served up their 'automatic' gadgets to eliminate the human factor the tighter the squeeze became on the powers of the operator. . . ."

Of course, not all human engineering affairs are sensory ones. If equipment, work and living spaces, tools, and control procedures are to be suited to human capacities and limitations, there are important questions of motor abilities, problem-solving and decision-making proclivities, not to mention a whole host of temperamental and other personality characteristics, that have to be brought into the picture. But it was largely a set of problems connected with signals and displays, warning devices, and communication systems that originally brought into being this new scientific effort, mainly on the parts of psychologists and physiologists.

Now, with some maturity attached to it, human engineering (or "human *factors* engineering," as this interdisciplinary movement is coming to be called) ranges broadly across all manner of problems, from design of dials and pointers to urban planning, from selection of symbolic codes for highway signs to procedures for effecting noise abatement, from construction of restraining devices in vehicles to the modus operandi of air-sea rescue operations. And the list could go on and on, for there is scarcely a human concern that fails to interest the human factors engineer. The central concept that has evolved is that of the *man-machine-environment system*, with all three components interacting maximally.

It is clear that the environment contains many "givens" that are unlikely to be controlled, at least outside narrow limits, by either man or machine, though the history of civilization is in part a history of just such encroachment by man and machine on the environment. Of the other two elements, there are obviously some functions that are better performed by man, some by machine. Machines can exert large forces in a controlled, efficient, and repetitive way for long periods of time, store and retrieve errorlessly upon demand vast quantities of coded information, detect prespecified events over extended "observation" periods, sense a range of stimuli that man is powerless to receive directly (X-ray, ultrasonic energy, etc.), and often perform several operations simultaneously and flawlessly. Man, on the other hand, has a facility for handling unexpected contingencies, can cut through to principles and apply them in a variety of novel contexts—he need not be narrowly "programmed"—and can develop new solutions as he goes along. He can draw on seemingly disparate experiences in coming to a decision or in making a choice.

However, it is not a question of dividing up the world's work between men and machines. Rather, it is one of assessing the proper role to be assumed by each in bringing the two into cooperative relation in problems that always involve the total man-machine-environment system. By and large, man's primary contribution is one based on his flexibility, not his consistency; the machine has the latter, but cannot cope with the novel exigency. An optimal integration of the two is what is needed in system design.

Our concern with these questions, naturally, centers around the input end of the system. In more situations than one might imagine, the human receptors are capable of sensing extremely low levels of stimulation, usually lower levels than those to which machines can be attuned. We shall deal with many such instances. At the same time, there are absolute limits that have to be considered. Man's senses are not infinitely acute, and there are barriers, partly arising from without the organism, partly from within, that circumscribe his intake behavior.

However, not all behavioral limitations are those of sense organs; acuity boundaries do not uniquely determine the adequacy of observation and perception. A principle that has been extraordinarily slow to emerge—despite some early glimmerings—is that humans seem to have a built-in restriction with respect to the amounts of information that can be processed. That is, there is such a restriction if one attempts to make judgments, on an absolute basis, about any stimulus that varies on only a single dimension.

Let us be more specific and approach by way of an illustration. Suppose we present a tactual signal to an observer, the signal being in the form of a "buzz" on the back of the hand. The observer is told that sometimes the vibration will be strong, sometimes weak. He is to report on the apparent strength of the stimulus, "two" if strong, "one" if weak. If the two intensities are a fair distance apart, there will be no difficulty whatever; the observer will give the correct report every time. He is transmitting perfectly one *bit* (binary unit) of information.

Suppose, now, we add a middle intensity (also well spaced between the weak and strong buzzes already in use) with the instruction to report "three" for the high, "two" for the middle, and "one" for the low intensity. Again, there will be no errors committed, but more information is being processed by the observer. If we continue in this fashion, spacing four, then five, then six different intensities along the scale, there will come a series—and for this particular judgment, it will be encountered earlier than might be thought, probably at four—where the observer will begin miscalling some of the stimuli. As we say, his *channel capacity* has been exceeded. It is not a matter of the several signals now being too close together. We can take care to give the weakest stimulus the lowest value that can be felt 100% of the time and place the highest at the tolerable upper limit, the strongest that will not produce discomfort, and the result will be the same. Indeed, the separation of any two neighboring intensities can be many "just noticeable differences" apart and the results will not be altered.

If, now, we repeat the experiment, this time keeping all vibratory stimuli at the same intensity but varying the durations of the buzzes by some fractions of seconds, we shall again find that some spacing of stimuli—perhaps by enough to accommodate five different stimuli this time—will bring with it the introduction of error. Channel capacity for vibratory duration will be exceeded. We can do the same thing for stimulus location on the skin and for frequency of vibration (the number of discrete impacts per second). If sufficient categories are introduced, confusion will always result.

This particular series of experiments on cutaneous sensitivity is in no way unique, either for this sense modality or within the family of senses. Many similar experiments have been made in hearing, especially on pitch and loudness of tones. In one experiment (217) loudnesses ranged from just a little above absolute threshold to a value close to the tolerable limit. Stimulus intensities were presented in 4, 5, 6, 7, 10, and 20 equally spaced intervals. Channel capacity proved to be 2.3 bits, on the average (about 5 identifiable steps; bits are expressed as powers of 2). In another experiment (477) tonal frequency was similarly manipulated to yield a wide range of pitches from low to high. With two and three tones there were no errors; with four there were occasional confusions; from five on, misidentifications were common. Channel capacity for pitch turned out to be 2.5 bits.

All modalities have by now received attention along these lines. Not infrequently throughout this book we shall encounter in context this question of channel limitation. A complete enumeration of instances will not be attempted here, but it may be well to note the great diversity of situations in which the principle is known to operate. In addition to the instances already mentioned, they include: visual intensity (brightness); judged area of geometrical figures; length, direction, and amount of curvature of lines; distances of objects; hue and purity of colors; intensity of electric shock; strength of taste of salt solutions; and odor qualities and intensities. G. A. Miller, in a paper rapidly becoming a classic in psychophysical theory (420), draws attention to the ubiquitous number seven (plus or minus two), and notes that there appears to be no exception to the general rule that information processing has this built-in limitation. Channel capacity for a considerable range of performances averages out at 2.6 bits (about 6.5 useful categories) and, while range seems, on the surface, to be great (from 3 to 15 or more steps, depending on the function under test and its manner of testing), the standard deviation of this distribution, in terms of bits, is really quite small, 0.6.

All that has been said about category limitations implies that information processing is thus restricted when judgments about stimuli fall on a single continuum. Let there be simultaneous variation in two or more stimulus dimensions and things improve somewhat. A case in point is provided by the task of identifying the location of dots in a square (*364*). Each dot falls on two coordinates, of course; the judgment is bidimensional. Channel capacity now expands to 4.6 bits, even though there are no aids to location (no grid supplied) and dot exposure is only 30 msec (milliseconds) in duration. Not nearly enough has been done as yet to establish general rules for combining dimensions. Colors in some profusion are recognizable and can be correctly identified by the well-trained observer, but there are available three sets of cues here: hue (color tone); saturation (color purity); and brightness (color value). Presumably, a tridimensional judgment is made on each sample. The rule that seems to be on its way to getting established is that increase in number of dimensions brings with it a net gain in overall information transmission with, however, some loss in accuracy within the individual dimensions. It follows that discriminations made in the several stimulus dimensions are not simply additive. Presumably, the greatest efficiency attends the combining of a very few steps in a large number of variables, and this, of course, approximates the practical situation in the identification of objects. Ordinarily, things and situations are multidimensional; they have a number of different aspects on which they can be judged.

In the light of what we know about information processing, then, we shall be duly cautious in applying to everyday situations what we learn about sense organs and sensations. Sensory systems have their operational limits but, because they can make much finer distinctions than the central processing mechanism can, they rarely put the total behaving organism at a disadvantage in its job of adjusting to a complex world of space and time.

2

The Visual Stimulus
and the Eye

Of the several senses giving us information about things and events in the world around us, none is richer than the visual one. The eye is the most highly developed of our sense organs, being at once the most complex in structure and the mediator of the most elaborate of our experiences. It is because vision yields the most varied sensations, setting the pattern for many analogous phenomena in other departments of sense, that we do well to consider it first.

To appreciate fully the way in which visual sensations are initiated it is necessary to understand not only the manner of functioning of the eye but also the nature of the stimuli that operate upon it. The normal or *adequate* stimulus for vision is, of course, light, but other forms of energy, properly brought to bear upon the visual apparatus, can produce visual sensations. Press upon the eyeball, and diffusely patterned "luminous" patches are seen; apply a sufficiently strong galvanic current to the closed eyelid, completing the circuit through some other part of the body, and a pinkish white or bluish white "glow" is seen at the moment of contact. Thus light is not the only possible stimulus for vision, though nearly all visual experiences are generated through its action.

Physical Conceptions of Light. Light, throughout the history of physical science, has either been conceived as a barrage of emissive particles or as a form of energy propagated by wave motion. Newton's "corpuscular" theory of light and modern quantum theory join hands in the former conception; the undulatory theory that dominated nineteenth and early twentieth century physics embodies the latter. The two conceptions have seemed, until recently, to be inevitably at odds with each other, though both were needed if a wide range of phenomena were to be explained. In general, wave theory seemed necessary to account for

18

the progression of light through optical systems, especially the facts of diffraction, interference, and polarization. Quantum theory has been needed to understand the emission of radiant energy from sources and, especially, the electrical properties of light.

Fresh discoveries about light have been aided by both types of theory, the two having been put to work somewhat indiscriminately as guides to experiment. Indeed, translations from one mode of thinking to the other have now come to be possible, for the present conception of the nature of light is one that necessarily recognizes that light is a quite specific kind of matter made up, as all matter is, of particles (*193*). The particles of light are *photons*. As with other particles of matter—electrons, protons, neutrons, mesons, etc.—photons display all the properties of wave motion as well as those of energy expenditure and momentum.

It can be shown that the wave properties characteristic of light are associated with individual photons, not a beam of them. G. I. Taylor, working at Cambridge University a half-century ago, employed a light source so low in power as to insure that rarely did more than a single photon make its way to the collecting screen at any given instant. An exposure of several months yielded a photographic plate that revealed clear interference patterns. The "wave" properties must have been expressed by single photons! Contemporary experiments with laser beams provide the same kind of proof.

Light sources, then, emit particles of matter, photons. These exhibit a great range of phenomena, and quantum mechanics and wave mechanics join harmoniously in their description.

Light Sources. Sources of light are of two kinds: incandescent bodies ("hot" sources), and luminescent bodies ("cold" sources). Practical sources for experimental purposes have, until recently, been almost exclusively of the incandescent variety. The sun, some kinds of flames, electric arcs, and most electric lamps are incandescent sources. In general, this kind of light generator is highly wasteful of energy because much of the emission is at wavelengths outside the visible spectrum, especially in the infrared region. However, standardization of incandescent lamp equipment has reached a high point of development, and convenience of operation favors its use. Within recent years there have been seen the beginnings of the practical use of luminescent sources but the possibilities of their application to experimental needs have hardly been explored as yet. Light may be obtained from cathode rays (electroluminescence), from crushing and rubbing certain materials (triboluminescence), from the chemical activity basic to certain biological processes, for example, the flashing of fireflies (chemiluminescence), and from the action of short-wave radiation upon "phosphorescent" and "fluorescent" materials. It is this last sort of luminescence that currently is displaying such widespread commercial usefulness. Fluorescent materials are those that glow during activation; phosphorescence is an effect continuing after the cessation of activation.

For many experiments in vision "daylight" is an ideal source. Light from the sun is, of course, a natural standard, but only those observations that can be made relatively quickly can utilize this illuminant. Not only are there likely to be wide intensive variations from moment to moment, when reflected daylight is used, but the wavelength composition changes with the elevation of the sun. Inconstancies may be minimized with "north" light and a moderately overcast sky; the illumination favored by artists is also the best for the laboratory. For extended experiments involving repeated observations, especially those of a quantitative kind, it is better to employ an artificial illuminant, the characteristics of which will remain invariable throughout the experiment. Several such illuminants have become standard and are used in the most careful visual research. They utilize suitably filtered light from a lamp, the "color temperature" of which is specified. However, in most experiments reproducibility is assured if only the type of lamp and the power supplying it are known. One is ordinarily not so much interested in the source as in the illumination yielded by it, and this may be measured with accuracy.

The Visible Spectrum.   Light waves of significance for vision occupy but a relatively short range of the total electromagnetic spectrum (Fig. 2–1).

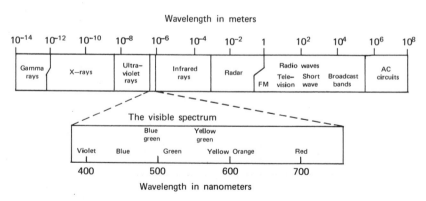

Fig. 2–1. The total electromagnetic spectrum. That portion of it normally affecting the eye, occupying a relatively narrow band of wavelengths, has been enlarged in the lower part of the diagram. After Chapanis, Garner, and Morgan (*114*).

The entire range of radiations extends from the extremely short cosmic rays (10 trillionths of an inch), at one end, to the long radio and power waves (many miles), at the other. Under usual conditions visual stimulation involves less than $\frac{1}{70}$ of this range, waves whose lengths vary from about 380 nm (nanometers, millionths of millimeters) to about 760 nm. Below the shortest visible ("violet") waves lie the highly chemically active ultraviolet ones, and above the longest ("red") are the thermally active infrared waves. Nearly all light sources emit waves belonging to one or the other neighboring region or to both. Actually, under some special conditions, the eye is capable of responding to waves coming from the infrared and ultraviolet regions. Reliable measurements of visible light, involving very high energies, have extended into the ultraviolet to wavelength (λ) 312.5 nm and into the infrared to $\lambda 1050$ nm. The calculation has been made (*593*, p. 129) that $\lambda 310$ nm and $\lambda 1150$ nm represent the approximate theoretical limits of light absorption by the eye, assuming presently available sources of radiation. To see a light of $\lambda 1000$ nm, say, there is required a source 10 billion times as strong as that needed to see a light of $\lambda 562$ nm.

Actually, to say that the visually significant portion of the electromagnetic spectrum is but $\frac{1}{70}$ of the total is perhaps to stress the wrong variable. Wavelength is not the sole feature of interest. The distribution of radiant energy in our general environment has to be taken into account. Radiation from the sun, by the time it penetrates the earth's atmosphere and is received at sea level, has an energy distribution that peaks within the wavebands comprising the visible spectrum (maximum transmission at 480 nm when calculated on an energy basis, 555 nm on a quantum basis). Solar energy is quite sharply cut off by the ozone layer, 15 mi up, at about 290 nm and has only relatively little power above 2000 nm. The net result is that about $\frac{4}{5}$ of the sun's radiation filtering through to the earth lies between 300 nm and 1100 nm, precisely the range to which the human eye has adapted itself over the ages. Other eyes, below the sea's surface, have available to them light that is still further restricted; at 100 fathoms, 90% of the energy falls between 420 nm (violet to humans) and 520 nm (green), with a peak in the neighborhood of 480 nm (greenish blue). It is of interest that fish living below a depth of 100 ft or so have not been found with color vision, whereas shallower dwellers frequently do have excellent discrimination of colors.

Although most visual objects send to the eye an elaborate mixture of waves of various length, it is possible with suitable apparatus to confine the waves to a narrow band and thus produce relatively "pure" stimuli. One way is to mask out all but a narrow wavelength band by the use of an adjustable slit placed over the spread-out spectrum. Spectrometers and monochromators employ this principle. Another method is to utilize filters which, by absorbing a great proportion of light incident to them, pass only a short range of waves. Such filters, made either of dye dissolved in glass or of colored gelatine films (ordinarily protected by optical glass), are said to be "monochromatic," though in any literal sense the term is obviously a misnomer. They are "monochromatic" only in the sense that a single color is seen when looking through them. Filters are available for many specific uses, and a wide range of transmission characteristics may be obtained.

A relatively recent development, one that is beginning to render some older types of filters obsolete, is the *interference filter*. As its name suggests, it relies on the principle of light interference (wave cancellation) achieved by combining thin quartz plates and evaporated metallic films. Interference filters are generally "sharper," that is, transmit a narrower band of wavelengths, than filters based on light absorption by dyes. At the same time, they are more efficient light transmitters than more complex systems involving slits, diaphragms, etc.

Far more common than exposing the eye to light transmitted directly from the source is the practice, in visual experiments, of using reflected light as the stimulus. Light impinging on any object meets one of three fates: it is transmitted, absorbed, or reflected. Whatever is transmitted or reflected produces no change in the object. If the object absorbs *visible* light, it is, by definition, a pigment. Colored papers and other pigmented surfaces, commonly used in visual experiments of a qualitative nature, owe their "color" to the fact that they selectively absorb light, reflecting those waves which, when sensed, yield sensations of color. It is vital that the concept of "color" be reserved for the sensation. Light, physically speaking, has no color; a color is not a color until it is seen. At the stimulus level we are dealing only with light waves which, to be sure, may vary among themselves in important respects, but color is not one of their physical properties.

Light Units. A physical dimension of light stimuli, of the utmost importance for our consideration, is that of intensity. The potential stimulating value of an object reflecting or transmitting light is in large measure determined by its intensity. There are four fundamental concepts concerned here: luminous *flux,* luminous *intensity* or candlepower, *illuminance,* and *luminance.* Luminous flux, measured in units of *lumens,* is the basic concept, and the remaining three are defined in terms of it. Luminous flux is the rate of flow of light energy and is thus analogous to power in other energy systems. Since the rate of flow is constant, for practical purposes, luminuous flux may be regarded as an entity which varies only in amount. The lumen, the unit of flux, is defined as the amount of light emitted in a unit solid angle by a standard candle. Thus the amount of light falling on an area of 1 m² situated 1 m distant from a standard candle (or an area of 1 ft² at a distance of 1 ft), would be 1 lumen. A point source of one candle emits a total flux of 4π lumens.

The intensity of a *source* is measured in candlepower, 1 candlepower being the intensity of the accepted "standard" candle. From time to time there have been in use many variously defined "candles," but current practice is based on the *international candle*, adopted by England, France, and America in 1909 and defined in terms of electrical consumption in a lamp. Secondary standards are readily set up by matching the primary one, and it is convenient to refer to these. Incandescent lamps, calibrated by some certifying agency such as the National Bureau of Standards, constitute our actual "reference" standards, and "working" standards can be reproduced quite simply by the methods of photometry.

The concept of illuminance (illumination intensity) involves the idea of interception of light flux by a surface. Illuminance is measured in terms of the density of flux falling on a surface. There are several available illuminance units of which the *foot-candle* is perhaps the most commonly used. The foot-candle is defined as the illumination received on a surface 1 ft² in area when this surface is supplied by a uniformly distributed flux of 1 lumen. Most illuminometers, portable devices for measuring illuminance, are direct-reading in foot-candles. An important relation, the inverse square law, applies to illuminance. This states that illumination intensity is inversely proportional to the square of the distance from the source, E (ft-candles) $= I$ (candles)$/D^2$ (ft²). Knowing the intensity of the source in candlepower we may compute the illuminance at a given point, or, conversely, illuminance having been measured at a surface, the candlepower of the source may be calculated.

Ordinarily, we are less interested in specifying the intensity of illumination incident to an object than we are in stating the flux proceeding to the eye from a *unit area* of its surface. In the latter case the *luminance* of the surface is determined. Specifications of luminance are made in terms of candles per square centimeter. Numerical conversions into other units of luminance are possible, and there will be found in the literature of vision a veritable plethora of such units, including the lambert (lumens/cm²) and millilambert (0.001 lambert), the foot-lambert or apparent foot-candle, and many others.

A useful scale of luminance is one expressed in terms of millilamberts (mL), the most commonly encountered unit in visual science (Table 2–1). The full range of possible visual exposures is represented, from the absolute threshold (RL), the minimum visible amount of light, to the conceivably damaging luminance entailed in a direct view of the sun's surface at high noon. Later we shall get fuller meaning into the terms "photopic" and "scotopic"; for now, let us read them "daylight" and "twilight."

Table 2–1.   The Range of Luminances Affecting the Human Eye. From Graham (*240*).

	Scale of luminance (millilamberts) ↓	
	10^{10}	
Sun's surface at noon	10^{9}	Damaging
	10^{8}	
	10^{7}	⎫
Tungsten filament	10^{6}	
	10^{5}	
White paper in sunlight	10^{4}	Photopic
	10^{3}	
	10^{2}	
Comfortable reading	10	⎭
	1	Mixed
	10^{-1}	⎫
White paper in moonlight	10^{-2}	
	10^{-3}	
White paper in starlight	10^{-4}	Scotopic
	10^{-5}	
Absolute RL	10^{-6}	⎭

Photometry.   Photometers, the instruments with which light intensity measurements are made, exist in a profusion of designs. However, many of them are basically similar in that they provide two or more neighboring fields of view which permit the direct comparison of two luminances, the unknown and a known standard (Fig. 2–2). The greatest accuracy in light measurement is associated with the use of the Lummer-Brodhun type of photometer, though there are several others only a little less sensitive. The Macbeth Illuminometer, a portable photometer using a Lummer-Brodhun cube, is perhaps the best known of the precision instruments for luminance measurement. Since the development of the generating type of photoelectric cell, there has been a wide application of this device to photometry. In visual photometry the eye can only tell us

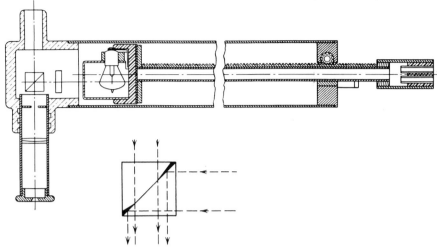

Fig. 2–2. Schematic diagram of the Macbeth Illuminometer. The little carriage housing the standard lamp may be moved back and forth with a rack and pinion, and thus, by utilizing the inverse square law of illuminance, there may be brought about an equation with the unknown light. The standard illuminates the outer field, the unknown the inner one. The Lummer-Brodhun cube, shown in the head of the instrument and enlarged in the lower diagram, makes possible juxtaposition of the two lights to be compared. Reproduced by courtesy of Leeds and Northrup, Philadelphia.

when two adjoining surfaces are equal, or approximately equal, in brightness. It cannot tell us directly *how* bright the surface is. Since the electrical output of a photocell is proportional to the intensity of light falling on it, a meter connected to the cell can be calibrated to read directly in foot-candles (or some other unit) of illuminance. Photoelectric tubes having multiple cathodes, so-called "photomultipliers," are extremely useful in the measurement of very small luminances; indeed, because they rival the human eye in absolute sensitivity, they represent a considerable achievement in light measurement.

The Gross Anatomy of the Eye.   The structure of the eye has been frequently compared to that of a camera, and in a very general way the analogy is a sound one. Like the camera it admits light through an adjustable "diaphragm" and focuses images by means of a lens on a sensitive surface. But the details of the two differ in many important respects, and the human eye appears, upon detailed study, to be much more complex in construction and operation than the most elaborate camera ever conceived.

The main features of the eye's form and its chief components may be seen in Fig. 2–3. It will be noted that, in the main, three layers are present. The outer covering, the *sclera*, forms a tough, fibrous, protective coat for the delicate layers within. The cornea is continuous with the sclerotic coat but, being transparent, forms one of the refracting media of the eye. Loosely attached to the sclera and forming the second of the

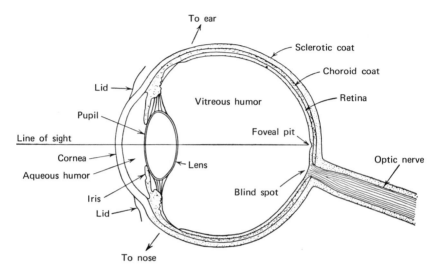

Fig. 2–3. Gross structure of the human eye. From Judd, *Color in business, science, and industry*. New York: Wiley, 1952.

layers is the *choroid*, consisting largely of blood vessels freely interlaced with each other. The choroid is the great nutritive structure of the eyeball, but in addition it contains brownish black pigment cells, probably important in light reception. The choroid becomes modified in the front of the eye to form the iris. The innermost layer, the *retina*, is of utmost importance for our consideration, since it is the retina that contains the terminations of the optic nerve and hence is the locus of light reception. The retina extends nearly as far forward as the ciliary body, the latter composed largely of muscular tissue and situated at the junction of the iris and choroid.

The *crystalline lens* of the eye, a remarkable body whose shape may change and thus have its focal length altered, is attached to the ciliary body by ligaments. The lens is completely encased within a membranous capsule, one that is under some tension in its normal state. This force tends to flatten the capsule and thus accommodate the eye for far vision. If a stimulus for near focus appears, the ciliary muscle fibers go into action, reducing the existing tension and permitting the lens to assume a more rounded shape. The change of curvature of the lens is accomplished chiefly, if not entirely, by its anterior surface.

The space between the front of the lens and the cornea is filled with a dilute salty solution, the aqueous humor ("watery substance,") while the great bulk of the eyeball, the space between the back of the lens and the retina, is composed of transparent vitreous humor ("glassy substance"). The latter gives "body" to the eyeball and preserves its nearly spherical shape.

The *iris* has important properties for vision. The tissue comprising it is largely muscular, one set of muscle cells being arranged circularly to make a "sphincter," the other set forming radial muscles which, when they contract, enlarge the central opening of the iris, the *pupil*. The two sets of muscles are thus mutually opposed in their action and, at any moment, represent a fine balance of forces. The pupil opening determines the amount of light flux that will fall on the retina and is capable of a considerable range of adjustment. Its major response is a reflex one, controlled almost exclusively by the sense cells situated at and near the center of the retina (*101*). When bright light strikes the retina the pupil may be constricted to an opening of less than 2 mm diameter. In the absence of light the pupil may dilate to over 8 mm diameter. Such a change represents about a seventeenfold increase in the area of the opening. The pupil is thus a primary determiner of the effective stimulus at the retina and, since its response is a prompt one, serves as an emergency device to help bring about an adjustment of the organism to fluctuations in light intensity (*492*).

Two other features of the gross anatomy of the eye are important. One is the occurrence of a small indentation at the back of the eye known as the *fovea centralis*. The fovea has special functional properties which we shall have occasion to consider. The other area to be noted is the colliculus or *optic disc*, situated about 4.5 mm to the nasal side and 1 mm above the fovea. Here the nerve fibers from all parts of the retina are collected and leave the eye as a bundle, the second cranial or *optic nerve*. Functionally, the area of exit is known as the "blind spot" because no nerve terminations exist here and there is no way whereby incident light may become effective. Figure 2–4 will aid in the location of the blind spot. It extends roughly between 12° and 18° (center at about 15°) in the temporal part of the visual field, the major portion of it slightly below a meridian cutting horizontally through the foveal fixation point.

Viewed as an optical instrument, the globe of the eye may be thought of as a system possessing an overall refractive power of about 65 diopters.

Fig. 2–4. Demonstration of the blind spot. By looking at the black cross with the right eye at about 20 cm (the left eye being closed), one sees the black circle disappear from the visual field.

Such a system brings parallel light to a focus within a span of 15 mm. (A power of one diopter, D, focuses light in one meter.) About two-thirds of the 65 D present in the eye is represented by the cornea (42 D); the remainder is represented chiefly by the front and back surfaces of the crystalline lens. The latter, by itself, can make adjustments over a 12-diopter range and can thus focus objects on the retina all the way from infinity to a few inches in front of the eye. However marvelously constructed, the human eye is far from being a perfect optical system. Diffraction of light occurs at the edge of the pupil, causing scattering within the globe, and the crystalline lens produces both spherical and chromatic aberrations. A point source of light in space cannot, therefore, ever be represented by a "point" on the retina, but by a tiny "blur circle." When we come to the topic of visual acuity we shall have to ask how the high precision found in human vision is possible in view of the structural defects possessed by the eye.

The Structure of the Retina.   The larger picture of the eye, then, is of three coats or layers: the sclera (protective), the choroid (nutritive), and the retina (sensitive). The retina must now be considered somewhat more intimately. Figure 2–5 shows, in schematic form, the plan of the retina. It is seen to have a somewhat complicated structure, though not an unintelligible one. The first fact to note is that two different types of nerve endings are present, *cones* and *rods,* so named from their conical and cylindrical tips. The next is that they are oriented away from the source of light, the front of the eye, their tips pointing toward the choroid. It is for this reason that the human eye, in common with the

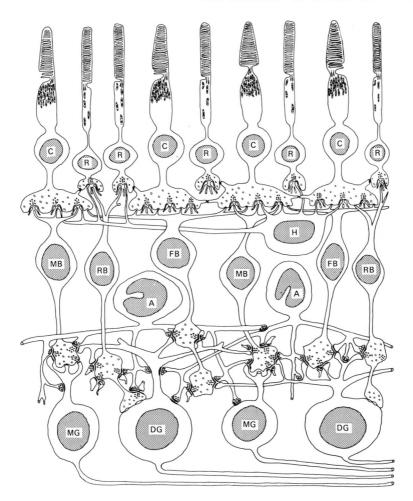

Fig. 2–5. The vertebrate retina. A schematic summary of its known structures and connections. Rods (R) and cones (C), at the top of the diagram, point toward the choroid (not shown) and away from the front of the eye. In general, the retina contains three kinds of elements: (1) the specialized receptors, rods and cones, each with its outer segment (platelets) and inner segment (mitochondria); (2) conducting elements, including three kinds of bipolar cells (RB, rod bipolars; FB, flat bipolars; MB, midget bipolars) and two kinds of ganglion cells (MG, midget ganglia; DG, diffuse ganglia); (3) neural elements having an "association" or cross-connecting function (H, horizontal cells; A, amacrine cells). There are also sustentacular or supporting elements (not shown) as in all other highly organized tissues. From Dowling and Boycott, *Proc. roy. Soc. (Lond.),* 1966, 166B, 80–111. By kind permission of the Royal Society and the authors.

eyes of other vertebrates, is said to have an "inverted" retina. A third general feature concerns the type of connection the cones and rods make with the fibers of the optic nerve. By and large, each cone connects, through a bipolar cell, with its own optic nerve fiber. This seems invariably to be true of foveal cones. In the peripheral parts of the retina, multiple connection of cones with ganglion cells brings about a somewhat different situation, as we shall see later. Rods, on the other hand, are said to be connected molecularly; that is, often several of them impinge upon a single bipolar. The innervation of the cones would thus seem to favor discreteness of response of the single elements, while the lateral connections of the rods make for cooperative action among them. The cones of the human eye vary in length between 0.028 and 0.085 mm, and, over most of the retina, they vary in width between 0.0025 and 0.0075 mm. Rods are 0.040 to 0.060 mm long but have an average width of only 0.002 mm.

Rods and cones are not haphazardly distributed throughout the retina. At the center of the retina, the fovea centralis, there can be found only cones. In that region the cones are tightly packed together and, in consequence, are longer and thinner (0.001 mm) at the fovea than elsewhere. In fact, were there not so many proofs to the contrary, we should suppose from their appearance that they were rods. The fovea itself is of very small area, not larger than 0.3 mm across and subtending a visual angle of about 1°. Anatomically, it consists of a pit or depression in the center of the retina, an area in which several retinal layers are greatly thinned out. Functionally, the fovea may be expected to operate differently from the rest of the retina, not only because it has higher optical efficiency here and is thus the area of clearest definition but also because it is the only place in the retina that is totally rod-free. There should be a homogeneity of performance about it not found in other parts of the retina. As we shall see, such an expectation is confirmed.

Another peculiarity of the central retina is the presence of an apparent "discoloration" of the tissue. This is the *macula lutea* ("yellow spot"), so called because of its appearance when viewed through an ophthalmoscope. The macula subtends about a 6–8° angle. Just outside the foveal depression, rods begin to put in their appearance, and as one goes further into the periphery of the retina the population of rods becomes progressively denser. The concentration of cones falls off rapidly just outside the fovea and, at a distance of about 20° from it, reaches a low value which remains fairly constant throughout the rest of the periphery. There has been only one careful count of retinal rods and cones and that in only a single human eye. In 1935, Østerberg took the tally, examining 164 different sample areas of the retina (*453*). The plot of his findings appears in Fig. 2–6; the shaded area of the inset shows where the counts were made.

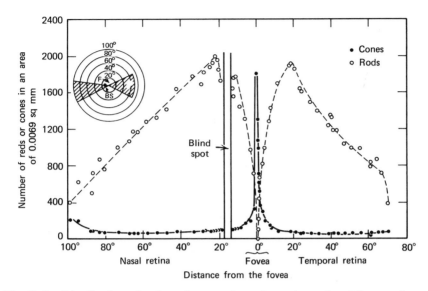

Fig. 2–6. Distribution of rods and cones throughout the retina. The number of of end organs per unit area from the fovea to the extreme periphery has been plotted. Cones are represented by solid, rods by open, circles. The inset shows the regions sampled by Østerberg (*453*) in obtaining the counts. From Chapanis, (*113*). Courtesy of the National Research Council and the author.

In the human retina there are about 6½ million cones and upward of 125 million rods. In any given area of the retina the number of functioning end organs (under a specified set of stimulus conditions) determines the fineness of detail that can be seen, just as in the photographic plate the intimacy of detail in the picture depends on fineness of "grain" in the emulsion. Whereas, on the average, there are 140,000 to 160,000 cones per square millimeter in the human retina, it must be that not all are functioning at one time except under conditions of maximal stimulation. Otherwise variations in light intensity would not bring with them corresponding changes in the acuteness of seeing.

Rods and cones differ from each other not only in anatomy and distribution; chemical differences between them are known to exist. Either contained within them or closely associated with rods is a material known as *rhodopsin* or "visual purple." The characteristics of rhodopsin are by now well known, since it may be extracted from the vertebrate retina and used experimentally. Visual purple is found to be sensitive to all but extremely long-wave red light and will bleach when exposed to light from all other parts of the spectrum. Its absorption curve has been determined, and its bleaching properties correspond well with those predicted from a knowledge of the behavior of rods in the visual process. Rhodopsin has been subjected to a careful chemical analysis and is found to be one of the so-called conjugated carotenoid proteins and, like all similar substances, has a large molecule, with a molecular weight of 30,000 or more.

The material of the cones is not so simply described, for it appears that there is not just one substance present in them but at least three, that is, there are three materials having different spectral properties, each housed in a separate "type" of cone. Later, when we discuss the complications inherent in color theory we shall have to examine carefully the evidences for three different cone photochemicals.

The advent of the electron microscope opened a new era in anatomical research and in our understanding of the ultrastructure of the sense organs. Discoveries concerning the fine structure of the retinal cells have been truly startling and have, for the time being at least, provided us with morphological information for which we have no corresponding functional facts.

The chief novel feature is that the tips of the outer segments of rods and cones are made up of hundreds, perhaps a thousand or more, of tiny discs or platelets stacked up in an orderly array. At least, they look like platelets in photomicrographs (see Fig. 2–7). There is, however, good evidence that in the cone they are continuous with each other at the edges and thus constitute a tremendously long double membrane folded layer on layer, whereas in the rod each platelet is completely separate from its neighbors (502). Either arrangement presents a laminated appearance, and this is found in electron micrographs of rods and cones from a great variety of species. Such arrangements are typical of a basic pattern also known to exist in the myelin sheaths of nerves and in some other tissues concerned with transfers of energy (594).

Whatever the structural arrangement of tissues in the outer segments of rods and cones, whether they be flattened sacs or continuously enfolded membranes, this is the place at which the sensitive photopigments must reside. It is here that light must trigger a complex set of events that leads ultimately to the firing of optic nerve fibers.

The Optic Nerve Pathway.   There remains for consideration the course taken by the optic nerve as it leaves the eyeball and proceeds to the brain. The bundles of fibers from the two eyes converge to join and apparently cross at the *optic chiasma* (from the Greek *chi*, a cross). But the complete crossing is only apparent. At the chiasma there occurs

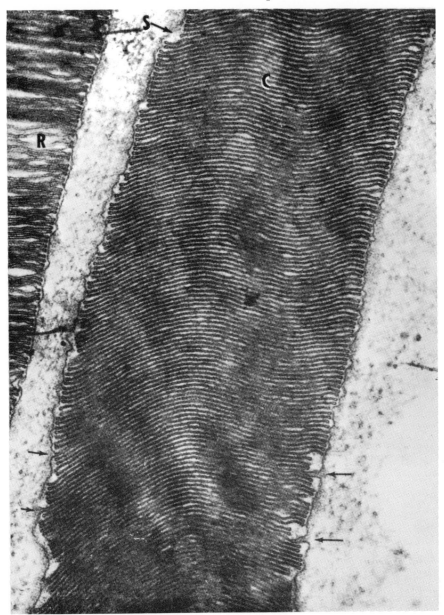

Fig. 2–7. A portion of the outer segment of a cone (C) and an edge of an adjoining rod (R). Both structures are constituted of "piled-up" platelets or sacs, with similar spacing in the two. From Dartnall *(144)*. Courtesy of Academic Press, Inc.

instead a half-crossing, or hemidecussation, one part of the fibers cross-ing to the opposite side of the brain, the other continuing on its own side. The fibers which cross over in each optic nerve are those originating in the nasal half of the retina. The effect of this arrangement is to include in the right optic tract, behind the chiasma, all fibers coming from the right halves of the two retinae. Fibers from the left halves terminate in the left side of the brain. Beyond the chiasma the fibers proceed to the thalamus and terminate chiefly in the lateral geniculate body of that center. Other fibers, arising at this point convey impulses to the occipital lobes of the cerebrum.

In the main, there is a preservation of an anatomical point-to-point conduction in the entire pathway. Pathological studies and especially nerve degeneration experiments on animals (375) prove this to be the case. Distinctly favored, in the entire scheme, are the fibers coming from the central portions of the two retinae. It appears that the macular region either has special representation in the brain or it sends fibers to both hemispheres. The point is still disputed, but it is definitely known that, in those brain injuries where an entire occipital lobe is put out of commission, the resulting damage to the visual field, oftener than not, spares the macula.

The consequences of this arrangement of fibers for interpretation of visual phenomena are many. The design of the optic pathways must be kept in mind in the setting of visual experiments. Light stimuli impinging on corresponding points of the two eyes must release optic nerve impulses that find a common path, while those from opposite sides of the retinae presumably cannot do so.

Specification of the Visual Stimulus.   Having now seen something of the nature of light and of the tissue systems implicated when light strikes the eye, we are in a better position to ask a fundamental *psychophysical* question: In attempting to determine the relations existing between the visual stimulus and the behavior of the sensory system it excites to action, how shall we specify the salient features of the stimulus?

Since the organism is constantly making adjustments to the external environment, it is best not to look toward events remote from the body in defining the responsible stimuli. Ideally, the stimulus for vision should be specified at the receptor cells themselves, at the rods and cones of the retina—better still, within these cells and in terms of the energetic changes standing in the most immediate relation to nervous action. But this is a large order. About the best that can be done is to state the illuminance falling on the eyeball and further to indicate any alterations imposed during the passage of light from the cornea to the retinal cells.

The most important single influence will be the pupil of the eye which, as we have seen, can change its size to produce an areal variation of about 17:1. Since all light rays from a given point in the viewed object that pass within the confines of the pupil will be focused at approximately a single point in the retinal image (see Fig. 2–8), pupil area will

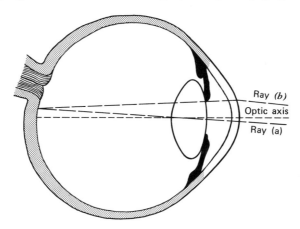

Fig. 2–8. Light paths involved in the Stiles-Crawford effect. Ray *a* passes straight through the center of the cornea and lens, and arrives at the focal point on the retina without any deviation. Ray *b*, the most deviant one, its position dictated by pupil size, also falls on the focal point but after refraction by the cornea and lens. Ray *b* has less stimulating power than *a*. From Stiles and Crawford, *Proc. roy. Soc (Lond.)*, 1933, 112B, 428–450. Courtesy of the Royal Society and the authors.

naturally determine stimulating power of the rays. A light unit devised to specify illuminance of the retinal image is the *troland*, which is defined as a luminance of one candle per square meter passing through a pupil of one square millimeter.

Actually, the troland only approximates to a correct measure of retinal illuminance, for there are several complicating factors at work. To begin with, there is the important *Stiles-Crawford effect* (see Figure 2–9). The rays passing straight through the center of the pupil are more effective than any other. A small beam, projected from a given point in front of the eye, may be directed to the center of the cornea (and of the pupil) or it may enter the eye at any point as far out as the margin of the pupil opening. Its luminous efficiency will vary with the entrance angle in accordance with the curve of Figure 2–9, an empirical one obtained by systematically varying the entrance beam angle and determining threshold intensities. A marginal beam, it will be noted, has only one-fifth the stimulating power of one striking the retina "head on," so to speak.

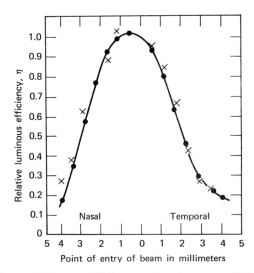

Fig. 2–9. Luminous efficiency of light entering the eye at different points along a horizontal meridian through the center of the pupil. A beam making its entry at the edge of a fully dilated pupil has about 20% the stimulating power of one coming straight through the center of the eye. From Stiles and Crawford, *Proc. roy. Soc (Lond.)*, 1933, 112B, 428–450. Courtesy of the Royal Society and the authors.

Another difficulty, in specifying retinal illuminance, is the fact that the pupil opening is never quite constant in size, even under unvarying illumination conditions. The pupil response is mediated by the autonomic nervous system and, like other organs under autonomic control, may sometimes be influenced by quite remote bodily events. Your dentist knows this and is likely to pay some attention to your pupil diameter when drilling near a nerve. Your doctor knows it and often lets pupillary data enter his diagnostic procedures when identifying an illness.

There are two standard devices, in visual research, for contending with the inconstancy of the pupil opening. The first is to employ a so-called *artificial pupil*. There is arranged an aperture smaller in diameter than the smallest one the natural pupil will attain in the course of the experiment. This is placed close to the cornea and concentric with the real pupil. The latter provision is difficult to comply with, since strict registration of the two "pupils" relative to each other must be maintained. This implies the use of head holders or, more uncomfortably, a "biting board" (a rigidly positioned wax dental impression, gripped by the teeth). The second means of rendering pupil fluctuations inconsequential is to provide in the optical system a *Maxwellian view*. This is accomplished by inserting a spherical lens in front of the eye, one of such curvature that all light from the stimulus will be brought to a focus in the plane of the pupil, then allowed to diverge again within the eye. Since all light now enters the eye near the center of the pupil, fluctuations of its rim have no influence on illuminance. See (*627*).

3

Basic Visual Phenomena

The Absolute Threshold. Light may be thrown into the eye at such a low level of energy as to produce no detectable response on the part of the visual apparatus. A general phenomenon, encountered in all sense departments, is that of the threshold; a certain minimum amount of energy must be delivered to the sense organ before sensation can be aroused. This value is known as the *absolute* or *stimulus threshold.*

Of what order is the minimum energy necessary to elicit a visual sensation? This question has been raised experimentally many times, and several answers are available. However, a set of determinations by Hecht and his co-workers *(286)* is superior to earlier ones, with respect to both technique of measurement and control of the several complicating factors encountered in such experiments. Moreover, its results have, in general, been confirmed by a succession of well-designed experiments made in repetition of this significant piece of work (see *472* and *34*).

A small patch of light, of variable intensity but of constant wavelength composition, was thrown into the eye so as to fall on a small area, containing perhaps 500 rods, situated outside the macula. The exposure time was held constant at 0.001 second (1 msec). In successive trials the intensity was varied with an optical wedge, and the observer's task was simply that of reporting whether or not the light flash was seen. Over a large series of trials the average intensity necessary to produce a just visible flash was determined. From the intensive measurement the liminal energy was calculated. This value varied from 21 to 57 hundred billionths of an erg in different observers, extremely small values indeed. Not all the light emitted by the test patch was effective, of course, and a series of corrections had to be applied. A small amount, about 4%, was lost through reflection back from the surface of the cornea and another 50% was lost by scattering through the optic media of the eyeball, while perhaps 80% of the remainder failed to be absorbed by the rhodopsin of the rods. Cones, as we shall see later, presumably did not participate in such low-intensity reactions. Allowance being made for all these, it turns out that the effective light energy at the threshold is of the order of a few hundred billionths of an erg. Stated otherwise and in terms of quantum calculations, it appears that between 5 and 14 light quanta (average of 7) are necessary to stimulate the visual organ. Assuming each rod to act when a single quantum is absorbed, it must require the release of but 1 molecule of rhodopsin in each of only 7 rods to initiate a visual effect. From these measurements an important conclusion may be reached. The visual apparatus is apparently tuned to the highest possible degree consistent with the nature of light energy. If man's eyes were much more sensitive to light than they are the "shot effect" in photon emission would be perceived, and "steady" light would no longer appear steady! A similar state of affairs obtains in hearing, as we shall see: if man's ears were any better attuned they would be assailed by noises coming from the "dance of the molecules" in the very air in which he lives.

Cast in terms of luminance, rather than energy units, the absolute threshold for vision in the peripheral part of the field is about 0.000001 millilamberts. The precise value varies with the size of the stimulus and the location of the retinal area on which it falls. It also varies with the duration of the stimulus, but for the present we are considering relatively long exposures rather than short flashes. A light spot projected on the macula and filling it would require a luminance ten thousand times as great, or about 0.01 millilambert, to reach threshold.

The influence of stimulus size on the absolute threshold is not simple. For very small areas of the retina, entailing visual angles of 10′ or less, *Ricco's Law* holds with some precision. This generality states that the product of retinal area and luminance is a constant for threshold stimulation ($A \cdot L = C$). For somewhat larger retinal areas and in regions several degrees out from the fovea, a second formulation obtains. This is *Piper's Law* ($\sqrt{A} \cdot L = C$). Finally, for relatively large fields, area need not be taken into account; threshold is a simple, direct function of luminance ($L = C$). Such "laws" obviously possess undesirable limitations of range and suggest that broader, if perhaps more complex, relations are at the heart of the matter. In Chapter 5 we shall confront them in the problem of "retinal interaction."

The influence of location of the test object on absolute threshold is also not simple. Obviously, the fact that rods and cones are distributed throughout the retina in the way we have seen them to be will have a bearing on expectations concerning thresholds. Where the receptive population consists of cones, thresholds should be high; where rods are present, thresholds should be much lower. In general, this is true as regards fovea-periphery comparisons, but the details are not quite as anticipated. Figure 3–1, which presents a plot of absolute thresholds

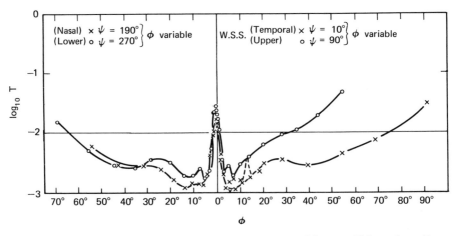

Fig. 3–1. Absolute thresholds of one observer to a white test light subtending about 4′ of arc and presented in 50-msec flashes. Deviation from the fovea, ϕ, is given in degrees along the abscissa. Azimuth angles, Ψ, were held constant while ϕ was varied. Nasal and temporal azimuthal angles (190 degrees and 10 degrees, respectively) were selected so as to avoid the blind spot. After Stiles and Crawford, *Proc. roy. Soc. (Lond.)*, 1937, **122B**, 255–280. By kind permission of the Royal Society and the authors.

for one subject, the measurements running all the way from the fovea out to the extreme limit of the visual field, reveals local variations in sensitivity that are not to be accounted for simply by reference to rod and cone populations counts (compare Fig. 2–6). Apparently, absolute sensitivity of the retina is not entirely dependent on the presence of either a certain density or absolute number of receptors at the spot where the test image falls. Rod-cone density, for example, is greatest about 4 mm (somewhat over 13°) from the fovea; light sensitivity reaches its peak (threshold is lowest) somewhat nearer the fovea, in the neighborhood of 10° (a little less than 3 mm out). And there are other noncorrespondences of this kind.

Duration of the test flash is an interesting determinant of threshold. Just as there is a kind of reciprocity between luminance and area for small visual fields (Ricco's and Piper's Laws), there is a similar "trading relation" between time and luminance for brief flashes of light. Below a certain *critical duration*, t_c, the product of time and luminance is constant $(Lt = C)$. This relation, when encountered in photochemistry, is known as the *Bunsen-Roscoe Law*; in visual science it is known as *Bloch's Law*.

The durations involved are very short, less than $\frac{1}{10}$ sec, a value that is usually taken as the critical duration, though it is not an immutable quantity, varying as it does with the state of the retina left by prior stimulation. The stimulus may be presented as a single flash or as a train of them, so long as the critical duration is not exceeded, and the reciprocal relation between amount of energy and the time period over which it is delivered will hold firm. Bloch's Law has been shown to hold for pure cone vision in the fovea, for mixed cone and rod populations in the periphery, and for a variety of field sizes and modes of stimulus composition.

The Differential Threshold. If we begin with an illumination just sufficient to stimulate, i.e., with threshold intensity, and determine the increment of intensity (ΔI) necessary to increase the seen brightness by the least perceptible amount, we shall have passed through a distance on the intensive scale corresponding to a "just noticeable difference" (j.n.d.). The experiment is performed by the use of a divided light field, the two parts of which are capable of independent manipulation. Either a field presenting a bisected disc or two concentric fields (a so-called disc-annulus arrangement) may be used. Obviously any other intensity, except that yielding maximum brightness, may be taken as a starting point and ΔI determined. If the initial intensity on one side of the field is designated I and the just noticeably different intensity on the other is called $I + \Delta I$, we should find that the ratio $\Delta I/I$ would vary in a systematic way over the range of visible intensities. The Weber fraction, $\Delta I/I$, was originally thought to be a constant one ("Weber's Law"). It is roughly so for the middle ranges of illuminations but deviates very considerably at the two ends of the scale. At the lowest intensities the fraction is nearly $\frac{1}{1}$, while at the highest intensities is decreases to as little as $\frac{1}{167}$ under some viewing conditions.

The first extensive determinations of the relation of $\Delta I/I$ to I were made over a century ago. Since that time there have been many remeasurements of ΔI, and several factors influencing the function in one direction or another have been isolated and studied.

The classic data are those of König and Brodhun, dating from 1888–1889. They explored the full observational range of visual intensities, measuring ΔI in a bipartite field, the two halves of which were disposed one above the other. Not only was white light presented at all intensity levels but six different "monochromatic" stimuli were tried as well. There was substantial agreement among the general outcomes of all experiments.

Figure 3–2 combines König's and Brodhun's observations for white light in what, at first glance, appears to be a continuous function. There is a sharp decline in the Weber fraction ($\Delta I/I$) throughout the low luminances, then a roughly constant middle portion, and finally a slight rise at the highest intensities. A disjunction midway of the curve should pique our curiosity, however, for it is no accident that the facts are better satisfied

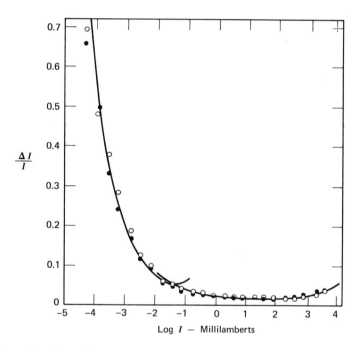

Fig. 3–2. The data of Koenig (open circles) and Brodhun (solid circles) for differential sensitivity to white light. From Hecht (*280*).

by drawing two curves through the array of points than a single, continuous one. The next section will explain why.

We saw that absolute visual sensitivity is influenced in its measurement by such factors as field size, location of the test patch on the retina, and duration of the test flash, among others. It should not surprise us to learn that differential sensitivity is a function of these same variables. To the above three there may be added, for both absolute and differential thresholds: the level of illumination to which the eye has previously been exposed, the particular psychophysical measurement technique in use, the wavelength composition of the test light, the shape of the test field and its sharpness of focus on the retina, to mention only the most obvious physical determinants. (See *98.*) And there are many so-called "subject" variables, factors having to do with the past experience of the observer, attitudes and predispositions, attentional matters, and many others. It must never be forgotten in dealing with psychological experiments, whether one is designing them or interpreting their results, that such apparently simple and straightforward indices of sensitivity as absolute and differential thresholds are themselves sensitive to a multitude of variables that have to be rigorously controlled in measuring them.

Duality of the Receptive Process. A distinction, based upon anatomical differences and distribution, has already been made between rods and cones. That the two types of end organs actually subserve different visual functions as well seems certain. On the basis of studies made by him on the vertebrate retina, Max Shultze in 1866 came to the important conclusion that the eye is not one sense organ, but two. The notion remained neglected for some years but was found useful by Parinaud (1881) to account for certain pathological phenomena of vision, notably night blindness. He restated at that time the "theory of the double retina." The idea gained wide currency only when von Kries, in 1895, brought together a variety of evidences pointing to duality of the receptive process. Since his time we have spoken of the "duplicity" or "duplexity" theory of vision. Rods function differentially at low intensities only and initiate colorless sensations; cones operate at higher intensities and are responsible for sensations of color.

It is interesting that the evidence first advanced for a duplex visual sense, the anatomical, should now be the least convincing proof we have. Indeed, further histological examination of the retina reveals a diversity of structure not originally suspected. Because there are to be found in the retina sense cells that are "rodlike" but not true rods and others that are merely "conelike," some scientists have gone so far as to deny the validity of the duplicity theory. However, the distinction between rods and cones is commonly supported by histologists, and there are well-known characteristic differences between the two.

But, even if anatomy did not clearly demand a duplex retina, there can be no doubt that other considerations definitely do. Perhaps the most convincing evidence is that, at different levels of illumination, the retina possesses two distinct sets of absorption characteristics. These are revealed in *luminosity curves* of which there are two separate ones for the normal human eye. The curve obtained for a high-intensity spectrum is known as the *photopic* or "daylight" curve, that for a very dim spectrum as the *scotopic* or "twilight" curve. A high-intensity spectrum appears to the eye colored; if the intensity is lowered beyond a certain point the spectrum is still seen, but as colorless. A landscape viewed at dusk presents the same appearance. As twilight pervades the scene colored objects first lose their brilliance, then become hueless. As a folk saying has it, "At night all cats are gray."

Photopic luminosity curves may be obtained by measuring the relative energy in different spectral regions needed to produce a match with a standard high luminance. The spectrum is gone through step by step, each narrow band being matched with its neighbor for luminosity. If the point requiring the least energy is now taken as unity and for all other spectral positions there is calculated a *luminosity coefficient* that expresses their luminous efficiency relative to this point, it is possible to erect a curve describing the photopic response of the eye to a high intensity spectrum. Such a curve is the one labeled V in Figure 3–3. Its inflection point (lumi-

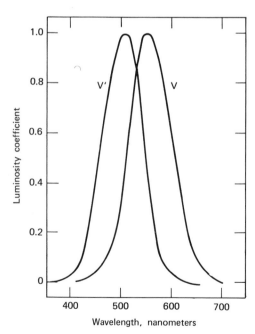

Fig. 3–3. The standard CIE curves of relative spectral luminosity. From Wright (*658*).

nosity coefficient of 1.0) is at λ = 555 nm in what appears to the normal eye as the yellow-green part of the spectrum.

The same procedure can be repeated at very low illumination, so low that the spectrum is without apparent hue, and shows only gradations of dim gray. Again, there will be an optimal point, this time at λ = 505 nm, in a region which, brightened up, would normally be called green. The curve V' of Figure 3–3 is this low-luminance function, the so-called scotopic or "twilight" luminosity curve.

Such functions as those displayed in Figure 3–3 can be arrived at in a number of ways. It should not surprise us by now to find that such factors as field size, shape and location, previous light exposure of the eye, stimulus duration, the presence of a surrounding or background light (to list only a few variables) make a difference. Moreover, color sensitivity is known to vary significantly from one observer to another; there are even instances of differences between the two eyes of a single observer in color sensitivity. It is important, therefore, that some standards be established to make possible specification of such deviations. The two curves of Figure 3–3 constitute such a standard, for they were derived from the measurement of a large number of reliable observers and it is their average that is being plotted. Indeed, these two particular curves constitute an international visual standard, for they were adopted as such by the Commission Internationale de l'Eclairage, the curve V (photopic) in 1924, curve V' (scotopic) in 1951.

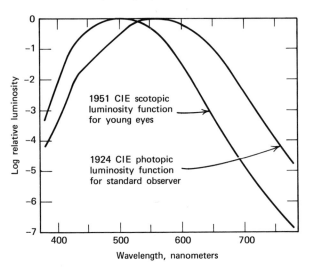

Fig. 3–4. The CIE curves of relative spectral luminosity plotted on logarithmic ordinates. Compare Fig. 3–3. From Graham *(239)*. Used with permission of McGraw-Hill Book Co.

The same data are often displayed with their ordinates put over into logarithmic units, thus spreading them and making some minor "bumps" obvious (see Figure 3–4). Actually, as we shall discover later, these deviations from regularity are quite real and signal some interesting color phenomena. For now, it is only important that we note that the two curves are clearly separated. Indeed, had we compared scotopic and photopic thresholds with each other throughout the spectrum, we should have found that, whereas the two would have nearly coincided in the long wavelength part of the spectrum, at the short end it would have required a thousandfold increase of luminous energy to get from the scotopic to the photopic absolute threshold. (Cf. Figure 3–5.)

Thus far it has only been demonstrated that there are two luminosity

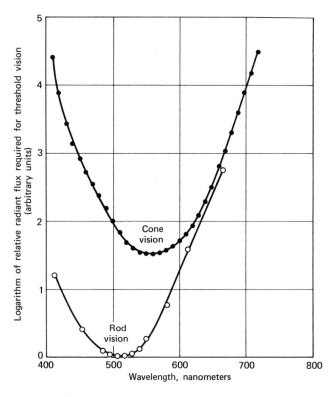

Fig. 3–5. Photopic (cone) and scotopic (rod) visibility curves compared. The relative amounts of energy needed to reach absolute threshold as a function of wavelength. The cone curve is derived from the data of Gibson and Tyndall (*231*), the rod curve from those of Hecht and Williams (*287*). From Chapanis (*113*). Courtesy of the National Research Council and the author.

functions. But, fortunately, identification of one with the operation of the rods can be made. As we have seen, rhodopsin can be extracted and its absorption determined. Many such measurements have been made, and the best of them demonstrate unequivocally that the scotopic curve is that belonging to the rods.

There are several other facts that fit into the picture of photopic and scotopic vision. Since twilight vision involves only the rods, it should be true that the central part of the retina is incapable of being stimulated by very dim light. Such proves to be the case; a *central scotoma* or blind fovea is present in dim illumination of the retina. A simple way to test for its presence is to attempt to search out a very dim star at night. If one looks at it directly, that is, with its image falling on the fovea, it will disappear from view. The French physicist, Arago, gave this advice: *"Pour apercevoir un objet très peu lumineux, it faut ne pas le regarder."*

Another phenomenon, known for over a century, demands the rod-cone distinction. If two quite different colors are matched for luminance at high intensity, then are compared under low illumination, it will be found that the match no longer holds. The same is true for an intensity change in the reverse direction. Colors at the red end of the spectrum drop precipitously to black, as light energy is reduced, while those at the violet end lose brilliance more gradually. This effect is known as the *Purkinje phenomenon*. It is, of course, entirely consistent with the direction of shift of the luminosity curves in passing from daylight to twilight vision. Moreover, the Purkinje phenomenon cannot be demonstrated within the rod-free portion of the retina. In all other parts of the eye a "colored" light is seen at the absolute threshold as colorless; then as the intensity is gradually raised and the light appears brighter, a point is finally reached where color is seen. This happens when the cone threshold has been passed. The point of acquisition of color differs for various wavelengths and retinal areas; for white light the abrupt change to cone vision occurs at a luminance of about 0.003 candle/ft.^{2} When colored light is used, the intensity range over which only gray is seen, i.e., the distance between the rod and cone thresholds, is known as the *photochromatic interval*. As would be predicted from photopic and scotopic threshold data, the photochromatic interval is small in the red part of the spectrum and relatively large in the violet.

Evidences from comparative anatomy and the behavior of lower organisms also support the idea of duplexity. In general, it is the case that nocturnal animals, such as rats and mice, bats, certain lizards (e.g., the gecko), and birds that migrate only at night possess either pure rod retinae or have a great preponderance of rods. Those animals which have only cones, such as the pigeon, hen, and other "day birds," as well as the turtle, and the majority of other reptiles, have strictly diurnal habits. Forms of vertebrates which, like man, possess a double retina show two visibility curves, one for low illuminations, another for high. Fish are known to have both rods and cones, and in them the Purkinje shift has been demonstrated.

A final line of proof comes from abnormalities of vision. Hemeralopia or "night blindness" is a condition in which, under dim illuminations, vision is poor. It may be so incapacitating as to prevent its sufferer from getting about at night. Apparently there are two different forms, one congenital and permanent, the other temporary and due to vitamin A deficiency. Measurements of spectral visibility on night-blind individuals reveal their eyes to have lost one-half their dual function. The remaining one yields the typical high-intensity cone visibility curve. "Day blindness" also exists, though it is of rare occurrence. The symptom most obviously present is total color blindness, and it is in connection with the latter diffi-culty that such cases are usually investigated. The visibility curves of a few totally color-blind individuals have been determined, and even though the measurements be made at relatively high brightness, the function is clearly that belonging to the rods. In fact, the agreement with the scotopic visibility curve of Hecht and Williams is extremely close (see Fig. 4–14).

A backward glance at the origins and development of the idea of the dual function of the retina makes one wonder why we should now speak of the *theory* of duplicity. It was a "theory" at the turn of the century; now we should do well to treat it as established fact. In the light of it a number of things become explicable. For one, there is the peculiar "break" in the intensity discrimination data, already noted. Obviously there are two branches of the curve, a low-intensity rod portion mediating the lowest 30 j.n.d.'s, and a high-intensity cone section covering upwards of 500 such steps. For areas involving more than the pure cone macula it would be surprising if the transition from one to the other did not occur. And there are other phenomena demanding similar interpretation, as we shall see.

Adaptation.   It was noted earlier that the pupil serves as an emergency device, reflexly controlling to a considerable degree the amount of light striking the retina. But there is another, slower-acting but fully as important, means of bringing the retina into equilibrium with the environment. Under stimulation by light the retina progressively loses its sensitivity and in the absence of light recovers it. The process occurring in the presence of light is known as *light adaptation*; the reverse change is called *dark adaptation*. The range of response due to adaptation is very extensive. After a stay in the dark of a half-hour's duration the retina may become responsive to light of only 1/100,000 the intensity originally necessary to stimulate it.

Dark adaptation has been known since its first description by Aubert in 1865. The earliest measurements were those of Piper, in 1903, who set the pattern for such experiments by determining the absolute threshold after various periods in the dark. Piper spoke of the "two phases" of dark adaptation, an initial rapid stage followed by a slower one, but incorrectly ascribed the entire process to the rods. Considering the eye as a whole, it is true that the most extended sensitivity change is due to rod adaptation. The cones do adapt, however, though they do so relatively rapidly and their range of adjustment (as measured by threshold shift) is not nearly as extensive as that of the rods. Excellent modern measurements of dark adaptation are available. Figure 3–6 shows a set of measures obtained with

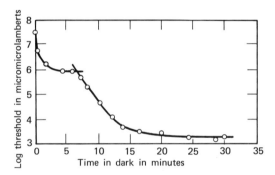

Fig. 3–6. The course of dark adaptation following a high level of light adaptation. The first section of the curve is for the cones, the second for the rods. The test light was restricted to the short waves, below λ460 nm, and appeared violet to the cones. Threshold values are in micromicrolamberts ($\mu\mu$l). From Hecht and Shlaer (285). By permission of the editor, *Journal of the Optical Society of America,* and Dr. Shlaer.

the "adaptometer." The first section of the curve is for the cones. The test light was restricted by a filter to waves below λ460 nm and appeared violet. The larger segment results from rod adaptation, and, though the same test light was used in procuring it, no color could be seen. Moreover, the test object appeared fuzzy in outline; form vision is a specialty of the cones, not of the rods. Again we have the fact of the dual retina evidenced.

The shape of any curve representing the course of dark adaptation is determined by several different variables, and any particular curve is the result of a group of specific conditions. The important variables are: (1) *Size and location of the retinal area tested.* A small field (1–2°) situated centrally can obviously possess only the cone section, while the larger or more peripheral the test field, the more will the rods be involved. A large field, the center of which is fixated, will naturally show both branches. But, the smaller the test field, in any part of the retina, the more rod-cone differences tend to disappear. Arden and Weale (24) reduced the test field in a dark adaptation experiment to a tiny 2.7' of subtended arc. Initially, projection of the test spot into the fovea gave lower thresholds than the same stimulus falling on a region 8° out in the periphery—in the light-adapted eye, cones always do better than rods, at first—but by the end of 20 min in the dark there was no difference in sensitivity as between the two regions. Had a large field been used, the peripheral rods would have had a decided advantage at the end of the dark adaptation process. (2) *The wavelength composition of the test light.* Figure 3–7 shows the effect

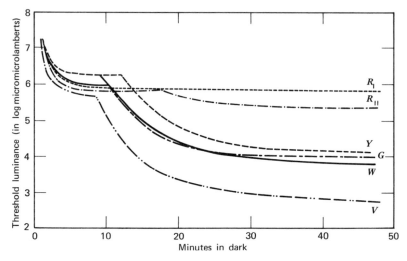

Fig. 3–7. Dark-adaptaton curves as a function of test-flash wavelength. R_I is an extreme red with a lower wavelength cutoff at 680 nm, while R_{II} is a band running from 620 to 700. Y is a yellow with a dominant wavelength of 573, G is a green peaking at 520, and V is a violet falling lower than 485 nm. W is mixed white light. From Chapanis, *Journal of General Physiology,* 1947, **30,** 5, 423–437, by kind permission of the Rockefeller University Press; Fig. 9, p. 434.

of systematically varying wavelength. Rods and cones, when dark-adapted, are not far apart in their sensitivity to long waves, though the rods have a little the better of it, at least when relatively large fields are used. Hence, when extreme red light is used to find threshold (R_1 in the figure) the overall dark adaptation curve appears to be but a continuation of the cone curve. As the wavelength is shifted toward the violet the rod section becomes increasingly more prominent and appears earlier. (3) *Wavelength of the preadapting light.* Despite what was said in (2) above about rod-cone similarities in response to different spectral regions, there is enough disparity between the two to make a practical difference. Reference to Figure 3–5 reveals that, for a given relative luminosity, cones are affected more by extreme red light than are rods. Consequently, if it is important to effect a rapid dark adaptation in the rods following the extinguishing of general illumination, lighting should be confined to the very long waves. This principle was taken advantage of in World War II aviation. Pilots preparing to take off on night sorties wore red goggles when in the ready-room or in the cockpit when it had to be illuminated for map-reading, etc. This gave rods a "head start" toward more acute peripheral vision to spot other aircraft and dimly lit ground targets (*548*). (4) The *intensity of the preadapting light.* If the eye has been previously adapted to a very bright light the cone section will be extensive, and the rod por-tion may not appear as a separate branch for a considerable time in the dark. The less bright the preadapting light, the sooner does the rod branch appear. If the preadapting light is dim enough the cone section may be suppressed entirely. In all determinations of dark adaptation curves the preexposure luminance must, therefore, be specific. (5) *The duration of the preexposure.* The longer the preexposure, within limits, the greater will be the "fatigue" and, therefore, the more prominent will be the cone segment. (6) *The duration of the test light.* As we have already seen (p. 41), thresholds are joint products of intensity and time under some conditions (Bloch's Law). But the value, 0.1 sec, usually taken as that of the critical duration, is not an immutable one. The critical duration becomes longer with increased dark adaptation, shorter with light adaptation; the state of adaptation will obviously, then, have much to say about the effectiveness of a very short-duration test light.

Some evidence exists for dual rates of dark adaptation, quite apart from the typically different properties of the rods and cones in this respect. Data obtained by Wald and Clark (*597*) show that exposure of the eye to a brief, intense, preadapting light is followed by a rapid dark adaptation process, whereas long preexposure results in a relatively slow rate of dark adaptation. This phenomenon suggests that rhodopsin, which presumably is broken down during light adaptation and restored during dark adaptation, may be synthesized in two different ways. Photochem-ical studies tell us that this is indeed the case. Rhodopsin is rapidly resynthesized from retinene, into which it is changed when light acts on it, but is only slowly formed from vitamin A, a reduction product of retinene. The details of the preexposure influence are nicely shown by Fig. 3–8, which summarizes the beautifully systematic experiments of Mote and Riopelle (430). Four different preexposure luminances comprising a logarithmic series were combined with four durations, likewise divided into logarithmic steps. The test light was a 3° patch of violet situated 7° from the fovea and exposed for a 200-msec flash. The field was

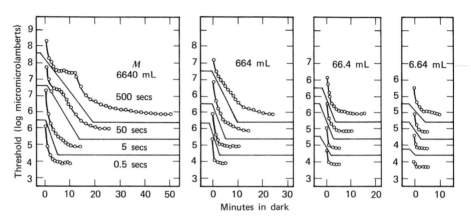

Fig. 3–8. The Mote-Riopelle experiments on peripheral dark adaptation. For all four sets of curves, durations of preexposure decrease (top to bottom) from 500 to 0.5 sec. From left to right, luminances decrease from 6640 mL to 6.64 mL. From Graham (240), after Mote and Riopelle (430). Copyright 1953 by the American Psychological Association, and reproduced by permission.

viewed through a 2-mm artificial pupil to maintain constancy. The 16 resulting dark adaptation curves reveal the same overall relation as that demonstrated by Wald and Clark, that is, steeper functions from low luminances and short times, more gentle paths to the ultimate dark adaptation level from high luminances and long times. At the highest luminance-time combinations, that is, when energy being delivered to the eye was greatest, a "knee" appears in the curve, signaling the transition from cone to rod function.

The broad relations in dark adaptation seem clear. Given a sudden change from light to darkness, the retinal receptors, both rods and cones, begin a fairly rapid drift to higher sensiti●ity, and this is consummated over a generally negatively accelerated course, its exact form being dependent on how rapidly and to what extent prior light adaptation was induced. But the simplicity of the process proves to be illusory to a degree, for attention to events transpiring over a shorter time period, at the very beginning of dark adaptation, reveals complications to be present. The initial changes, those taking place in the first few seconds after the removal of the preadapting light, are somewhat surprising.

The classical study here is that of Crawford (*129*), who followed the changes in threshold prior to, during, and after exposing the eye to a briefly lighted field. Baker (*31*) has obtained a more intimate picture, using much the same procedure and sampling thresholds from 0.4 sec before to 2.0 sec after the termination of a preadapting light. His findings are summarized in Figure 3–9. The sharp rise at "time zero" (where the adapting lights was put out), far from revealing a rapid onset of the dark adaptation process, shows the eye to lose in sensitivity temporarily. Then

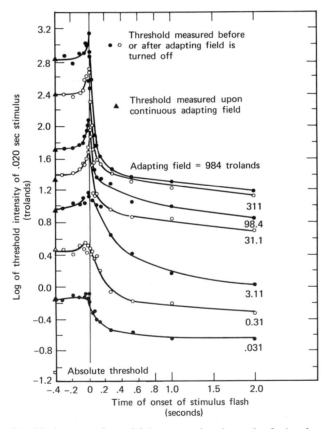

Fig. 3–9. Rapid changes of sensitivity occurring in early dark adaptation. The measurements are for a test field situated 5° from the fovea. In all instances the light-adapting field is extinguished at time 0. From Baker (*31*).

there is a rapid rebound, thresholds dropping precipitously, before leveling off to the dark adaptation rates we see in the conventional curves, such
as Figure 3–6. One can only guess as to what these initial rapid oscillations in sensitivity are about. They are quite transient and spend themselves in an instant. It seems improbable that they are photochemical, at
least exclusively so; indeed, there is presumptive evidence that the fast
initial dark adaptation transient has an origin beyond the retina, in
neural processes. Dowling (174), who has made extensive recordings of
the electrical changes taking place in the retina of the rat (perhaps a
pure-rod retina), is convinced that the neural contribution is considerable
and that the seat of the adaptation process is the bipolar-cell layer of the
retina, its action being one of neural inhibition.

There has been evinced much interest in dark adaptation data as a
result of the discovery that variations in the curves may be associated
with deficiencies of vitamin A. Some people put on a diet deficient in this
necessary food element show a rise in threshold at all points of both the
cone and rod portions of the curve. Some of the changes are quite
extreme and result in *hemeralopia,* "night blindness." Figure 3–10 shows

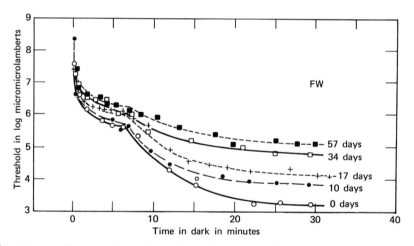

Fig. 3–10. Effect on dark adaptation of avitaminosis A of various durations.
From Hecht and Mandelbaum *(283).* Courtesy of the American Physiological
Society.

the progressive raising of thresholds at all levels of dark adaptation for
one subject having experimental avitaminosis A. This subject showed
the most severe alteration of 17 people studied by Hecht and Mandelbaum *(283).* That the effect was specific to vitamin A is attested by the

fact that the daily diet was supplemented by plentiful quantities of all other vitamins. In some starved subjects, a single large dose of vitamin A was sufficient to lower thresholds measurably.

But, from the beginning of the study of night blindness as it relates to vitamin A deficiency it has been apparent that individual differences are of some magnitude. Many people show no effect whatever when subjected to prolonged avitaminosis A. Also, of those affected, some are completely unresponsive to vitamin A feeding, even though it is kept up regularly over a period of many months. Clearly, some additional factors are at work. The ultimate solution of the problem came with the discovery that vitamin A is stored in the liver in highly variable amounts. Some people have large reserves that may be called upon during vitamin starvation; they may therefore go for months without any alteration of visual sensitivity or other obvious impairment. Those having no such stored supply show a prompt deficiency that reflects itself in dark-adaptation changes, among other symptoms.

What about those who, having suffered a visual setback from vitamin A starvation, fail to be cured by massive administration of the lacking material? It appears that vitamin A is so essential to the body economy that, when it is lacking in the blood stream, there are dire consequences to cell nutrition. The retinal cells, at least the fragile rods, are readily affected and undergo degenerative changes. Having once degenerated

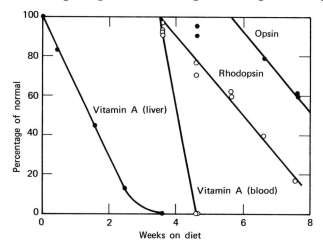

Fig. 3–11. Progressive avitaminosis A and the consequent bodily changes. Vitamin A stored in the liver was first called upon, the amounts present in the blood and eye remaining normal. Then there was rapid depletion of both of these. From "Night Blindness", by J. E. Dowling. Copyright 1966 by Scientific American, Inc. All rights reserved.

beyond a certain point, they cannot be regenerated. Severe avitaminosis A thus causes permanent retinal damage. Figure 3–11 shows the succession of changes occurring in the rat retina, a preponderantly rod structure, during weeks of vitamin A starvation (173). There is at first depletion of the liver reserve, then rapid reduction of the remaining supply of vitamin A in the blood, soon leading to disappearance of the sensitive rod pigment, rhodopsin, and finally a tearing down of opsin, the protein molecule linked to the pigment (in the aldehyde form of vitamin A called retinene). Records of electrical activity in the rat's eye showed the animal to have become totally blind by the tenth month, never to recover sensitivity, though such recovery would have been a possibility within two months or less of the onset of such treatment.

Until only a few years ago it was conventional to cast an account of the dark adaptation process exclusively in photochemical terms. Retinal pigments broken down by the action of light were repaired in its absence. Light falling on the retina dissociated rod rhodopsin and the several photochemicals of the cones, causing them to seek a new, lower level of equilibrium; darkness permitted their resynthesis, perhaps supplemented during restoration by nutritive processes in the choroid, with which the outer segments were in contact. Dark and light adaptation involved simple reversible reactions. There is a well-known set of equations by Hecht (282) that seemed, for many years, to cover the situation. Now we know, from a variety of different attacks on the adaptation mechanism, that this was an over-simplification, since the story of adaptation is not even approximately told by the Hecht equations. Moreover, we have evidence that the complementary processes of light and dark adaptation are not exclusively photochemical ones. Important neural changes are brought about in the course of adaptation, and these make a vast difference in the capacity of the visual system to report on retinal events. When we come, in Chapter 5, to the intriguing question of how the state of affairs in one part of the retina may alter occurrences in another portion, we shall have to recall the adaptation phenomenon, for the facts of retinal interaction amplify our understanding of both light and dark adaptation in a significant manner.

The course of *light* adaptation can be ascertained by any of several techniques. The obverse of the method used in measuring dark adaptations is one possibility. After varying periods of exposure to light and with a return to complete dark adaptation between trials, the absolute threshold can be determined and the decline in sensitivity charted. This is the technique used originally by Lohmann (291, p. 324) and by many others since. The drop in sensitivity, as revealed by such measures, is most rapid in the first few seconds, then progressively slower for many minutes.

This method possesses one inherent defect. To measure the absolute threshold it is, of course, necessary to extinguish the adapting stimulus. Then, some time is required to make the threshold determination; meanwhile, the light-adapted retinal area has undergone some dark adaptation. Since dark adaptation is most rapid at the onset of the process, the error of measurement introduced by this circumstance may be very considerable.

Another, and somewhat more direct, approach to the problem can be made by "fatiguing" one area of the retina with a known intensity of light for a definite period, then quickly effecting a brightness match by means of a comparison light falling in an unfatigued area. The selection of a suitable array of adaptation times will reveal the course of the process for the intensity used. Such measures were made by von Kries, with the crude apparatus then available, as early as 1877. More extensive determinations have been made by the author (*219*), and these, in turn, have been repeated by Wallace (*600, 601, 602*). Representative results for macular cone adaptation, taken from Wallace's work, are shown in Figure

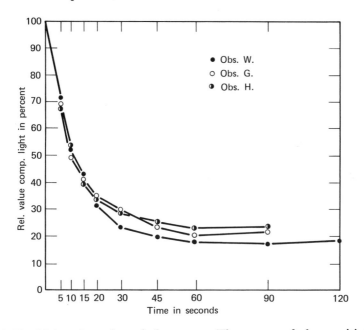

Fig. 3–12. Light adaptation of the cones. The course of the sensitivity loss resulting from steady illumination of the macula has been charted with the aid of the comparison light technique, the measuring light being thrown into the unfatigued eye. The three observers are obviously in close agreement. From Wallace (*600*). Permission of the Journal Press.

3–12. As the adapting light continues to act, the retinal area under stimulation loses more and more sensitivity until, after perhaps a minute's fatigue, an equilibrium point is reached. The amount of loss, while very considerable under all conditions of stimulation, is found to be a function of the intensity of the adapting light; the higher the intensity, the greater the relative loss in brilliance. It is noteworthy that the course of light adaptation, as revealed by the comparison light technique, seems to have run to completion within a relatively short period of time. Over a substantial range of initial light intensities, a 3-min interval would appear to be sufficient to accommodate the process. This result contrasts sharply with that obtained by the "instantaneous threshold" method, which may require a much longer period of time to reach a final equilibrium state (*281*).

To complicate matters, a third and more recently devised technique, that exemplified by the work of Baker (*30*), yields a somewhat different kind of result. This method utilizes ΔI as a measure of sensitivity. As light adaptation proceeds, a small increment of luminance is periodically flashed into the adapting area. The size of the intensity increment is systematically varied until ΔI has been determined for a long series of adaptation times. It is found that sensitivity improves (ΔI gets smaller!) throughout the first 3 min of light adaptation, then declines slowly to a

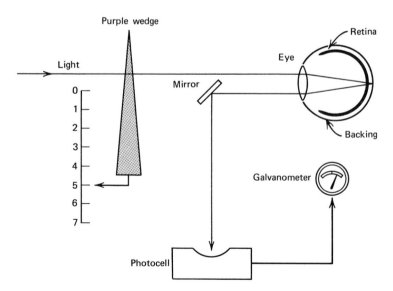

Fig. 3–13. Rushton's technique for measuring the bleaching of visual pigments. From "Visual Pigments in Man", by W. A. H. Rushton. Copyright 1962 by Scientific American, Inc. All rights reserved.

level intermediate between this and that of the original dark-adapted state. It is clear that different measures of sensitivity give different pictures of the adaptation process. Just as there are many dark adaptation curves, each representing a particular combination of experimental conditions, there are many curves of light adaptation, each having clear meaning only insofar as the operations performed in establishing it have been defined unambiguously.

One of the most direct approaches to the study of light adaptation is to be found in the "bleaching" experiments carried out with great ingenuity by Rushton and his colleagues at Cambridge University (*509*). They were able to follow the course taken by rod adaptation in the human eye by passing a weak pencil of light through one portion of the dilated pupil, letting it traverse the retina, reflect back from the choroid coat and, after leaving the eye over a disparate path, fall onto a highly sensitive photocell where its intensity could be measured (see Figure 3–13). En route, the beam passes twice through the retinal layers where the material of the rods, rhodopsin, absorbs some of the light, the exact amount depending on how much of the pigment is in an unbleached state. An

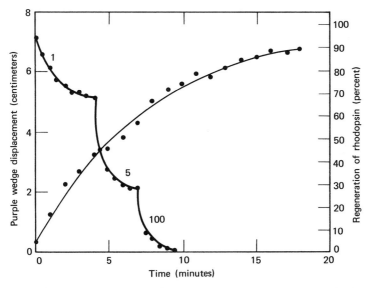

Fig. 3–14. Light and dark adaptation measured by Rushton's method (see Fig. 3–13). The scalloped curve shows bleaching of rhodopsin by light standing in the intensitive relation, 1:5:100. The ascending, negatively accelerated curve represents the course of rhodopsin regeneration during dark adaptation. From "Visual Pigments in Man", by W. A. H. Rushton. Copyright 1962 by Scientific American, Inc. All rights reserved.

optical wedge inserted in the light path permits the photocell output to be brought always to a standard balance point; the wedge thickness (density) thus becomes a substitute in the system for the former unbleached rhodopsin and is a direct measure of it. By this straightforward technique it is possible to ascertain what proportion of the photosensitive pigment is bleached during light adaptation. It is only necessary to add a "bleaching" (adapting) light of known intensity and follow the course of rhodopsin decomposition.

The "scalloped" curve of Figure 3–14 shows what happened with a moderately bright light (value of 1), then when intensity was stepped up by a factor of five (5), and finally when a 20-fold increase was introduced (100). There is, in each instance, a precipitous reduction immediately upon introduction of the new stimulus. The change follows a negatively accelerated course, however, and levels off within a few minutes. It is obviously not a matter of light continuing to tear down visual pigment so long as there remains available any on which to act. The retina comes into balance with the light stimulus either by regenerating rhodopsin to create an equilibrium or possibly by putting into play an as yet undisclosed protective mechanism.

It would be difficult to conceive of a process of greater fundamental importance to sensory psychophysiology than is adaptation. The phenomenon is a very general one, occurring in all the sense departments. Moreover, it reveals the basic mode of action of the sense organ. It is not surprising, therefore, that the interpretation put upon adaptation determines, in large measure, the direction any theory of vision will take. We cannot, at this point, review the many conflicting conceptions, but we shall have to bear in mind that adaptation must be accounted for in a satisfactory manner if visual theory is not to remain pale and incomplete.

Hue Discrimination. We have seen that the eye is capable not only of utilizing very small physical energies but of making fine distinctions between intensities. Another aspect of the physical stimulus calling for discriminatory response on the part of the eye is that of wavelength.

At the extremely long wave end of the spectrum the normal eye sees red (in photopic vision). Progressing through the spectrum there is seen successively orange (about λ600 nm), yellow (λ580 nm), green (λ510 nm), blue (λ470 nm), and violet (λ420 nm), as well as a large number of intermediate hues. Some of these we name, such as yellow-green and blue-green; for others, occurring less familiarly, we have no adequate common designations.

It should be said straightway that the correspondence between wavelength and visible hue is not an entirely constant one. Hue is partially determined by intensity. Except for certain invariant points in the spectrum, all colors seen by the normal eye, upon being brightened, shift slightly toward either yellow or blue. This phenomenon is known as the *Bezold-Brücke effect*. According to the careful determinations of Purdy *(484)*, if the illuminance of a red of λ660 nm is reduced from 2000 to 100 trolands it becomes necessary to decrease wavelength by 34 nm to maintain the original hue. A green of λ525 nm calls for an increase of 21 nm under the same conditions. These are extreme examples, but some such adjustment is needed for most colors. Three spectral points, λ572 nm (yellow), λ503 nm (green), and λ478 nm (blue), are "invariant" ones, displaying no apparent alteration at all. In addition, there is a specific mixture of long and short waves (purple, lying outside the spectrum) which is likewise uninfluenced by intensity change *(483, 484)*. Figure 3–15 shows a set of constant hue contours.

The shifts enumerated above are for relatively moderate alterations of intensity. They are cited more to show what can happen in individual instances than to describe what happens generally, since the Purdy experiment involved measurements on only a single observer. Figure 3–16 displays a set of Bezold-Brücke shifts under somewhat stricter but

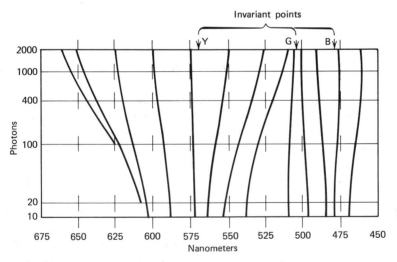

Fig. 3–15. Contours of constant hue. All combinations of intensity (photons = trolands) and wavelength lying along a given contour appear to be of the same hue. Three spectral points, λ572 nm (yellow), λ503 nm (green), and λ478 nm (blue) yield constant hue regardless of intensity. All other points are subject to variations in accordance with the Bezold-Brücke phenomenon. After Purdy *(484)*. Courtesy of the *American Journal of Psychology*.

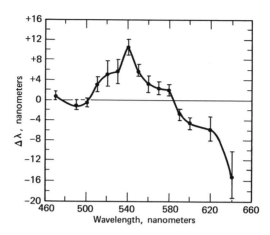

Fig. 3–16. The Bezold-Brücke shift. Average values for a total of 72 subjects are plotted. With a tenfold reduction of luminance, there are required small or relatively large adjustments of wavelength to retain the original hue at all except three spectral points. From Jacobs and Wascher (*328*).

roughly parallel measurement operations and on a population of 72 subjects. A tenfold decrease in luminance at a considerably higher level (from 3200 to 320 trolands) produced the hue change and required a suitable adjustment of wavelength to preserve the hue match between the two fields. These were presented alternately and for short exposures (300 msec). Whereas the general form of the curve does not differ greatly from Purdy's and the invariant points are at substantially the same places in the spectrum, the newer measurements possess the virtue of expressing the variance in a representative population. Individual differences are obviously of substantial size.

In a few experiments on hue changes, really extreme retinal stimulation has been involved. Thus Auerbach and Wald (*29*) let the filtered light from a 1000-watt projection lamp fall on the retina in Maxwellian view, and found the normally orange-red appearance of a certain color filter (Wratten No. 26) to have changed to a momentary pink, followed within 10 to 15 sec by orange, then yellow, then bright green, which it remained throughout the viewing period! Cornsweet and his colleagues (*128, 126*) have done systematic experiments at extraordinary intensities. They found long-wave stimuli (at 620 nm) first appearing orange, then yellow, then green. By the end of a minute or so there was a change back to yellow and, ultimately, to orange. Green below 560 nm, used as an initial stimulus, seems to undergo no hue shift; it merely becomes paler and grayer. Stimuli of short wavelength have given mixed results among those who have tried them, though there are reports of blue appearing white at first, then pink, and finally bright red (29). Participation in experiments of this kind needs to be approached with circumspection; there are records of permanent damage from what amounts to training a burning glass on the retina!

What is the capacity of the eye to detect small changes in wavelength? In raising the same question for intensity discrimination we were interested in seeing the size of ΔI and in determining in what systematic way the size of ΔI varied. Now we need to know the magnitude of $\Delta\lambda$.

If we throw into both sides of a bisected field red light of $\lambda 700$ nm, then change one side by gradually shifting the wavelength downward, we shall arrive at a point where the two hues, the original red and the new slightly orange-red, can be distinguished in hue. As with intensive changes, we shall have passed through one j.n.d., in this case equivalent to $\Delta\lambda$. The first step, according to the determinations of Jones (333), will be 22 nm in length. If the two sides of the field are again equated (at $\lambda 678$ nm) and the next j.n.d. measured, it will this time cover a distance of but 13 nm. In the passage through the spectrum in this manner, it will be found that 128 j.n.d.'s will be traversed, some discriminable differences being but 1 nm and most of them less than 3 nm in length. The size of $\Delta\lambda$ in various parts of the spectrum can be read from Figure 3–17. The function is seen

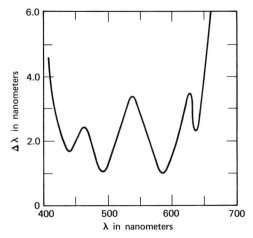

Fig. 3–17. Wavelength discrimination by the human eye. The change in wavelength which can be just detected ($\Delta\lambda$) is plotted as a function of wavelength (λ). The data are from Jones (333).

to be a complex one and to have several inversions in it. It should be added that, whereas these measures represent excellent technique, other sets of data, equally good (*376, 539*), show relatively large individual differences among observers possessing normal color vision. Judd (*337*) has brought together in a single graph the measurements of eight different investigators. All are in agreement about the slight augmentation of $\Delta\lambda$ in the middle portion of the spectrum (near $\lambda550$ nm) but there are some uncertainties concerning the minor deflections in the long and short waves.

An interesting thing happens at the extremely long wavelength end of the spectrum. Beyond 700 nm reds again become somewhat yellower. Brindley (*91*) has been able to identify *pairs* of wavelengths in the extreme red having identical chromaticities. All discriminably different hues between them are redder. The following wavelengths have been found to be paired in this way: 711 nm and 688 nm; 749 and 679; 786 and 674; 850 and 652; 887 and 641. These and other such pairings have come to be called *Brindley isochromes* (see *660*).

Saturation Discrimination.   Besides intensity and wavelength, still a third aspect of spectral light can be discriminated. This is the *purity* or *saturation* of the color yielded by it. We commonly speak of spectral red and blue as saturated colors and orange, yellow, and yellow-green as unsaturated. Saturation has been defined as "that attribute of all colors possessing a hue which determines their degree of difference from a gray of the same brightness." Saturation is thus a third variable in color experience; it may be thought of as the relative absence of grayness in colors. The most direct measurements are those of Jones and Lowry (*334*), who stepped off j.n.d.'s of saturation along eight different hue lines, all intersecting at a gray of the same brightness. The least saturation was found in yellow ($\lambda575$ nm), where but 16 j.n.d.'s could be found. Red of $\lambda680$ nm and violet of $\lambda440$ nm each gave 23 steps, and other colors were intermediate.

Much the same relation between wavelength and the number of saturation steps comes from the less direct but more detailed study of "colorimetric purity" by Priest and Brickwedde (*481*). Poorest spectral saturation, as measured by the luminance of the spectral sample that has to be added to white to make color identifiable, occurs at $\lambda570$. Least chromatic addition is required in the violet and blue, and an intermediate amount is needed in the red. If we think of saturation as the reciprocal of "least colorimetric purity," best spectral saturation is obviously in the short waves, next best in the long, while poorest saturation occurs in midspectrum.

Electrical Signs of Visual Activity.   Our world of visual objects is describable in several dimensions, as we have seen. The phenomena thus far considered are, for the most part, concerned with the more fundamental of them, such dimensions as brightness, hue, and saturation. The data on these are available to direct observation, and we obtain them directly, or at least only as indirectly as the rules of laboratory experimentation require.

There are other ways of obtaining valuable basic information about visual processes, however. Instead of dealing directly with the end product of the visual mechanism's action, the visual perception, we may study the various physiological and neural events underlying it. By taking successive cross sections, so to speak, of the retinal and nervous precursors to central excitation we may hope to gain some insights as to how the direct observational data come into being.

Nerves, during the passage of impulses along their lengths, give evidences of the changes occurring within them. The optic fibers responsible for reporting the state of affairs in the rods and cones are no exception. Nerve impulses consist in progressive local disturbances of fibers and display several interesting chemical and physical properties. Oxygen is used up and carbon dioxide is given off, detectable quantities of heat are emitted, and measurable electric currents are generated. It is this last effect that has proved to be of the greatest service in providing a picture of nervous functioning. The electrical change promptly signals the passage of the impulse; its magnitude is a true reflection of the extent of the alteration within the fiber; and, especially since the development of electronic amplification and the perfection of electrical recording methods, it may be measured with considerable precision. The technique consists in placing one electrode on the nerve tissue at the point from which the record is desired and connecting another, so-called "neutral" electrode to an inactive region. A difference of electrical potential between the two is created as the impulse passes, and it is this small voltage, the "action potential," which is picked up, amplified, and recorded. Placement of the electrodes is, of course, the primary determiner of what changes will be registered. In animal preparations, if they are attached to the front and back of the eyeball itself there is obtained a record of the complex events in the retina, known as the *electroretinogram* (ERG). If they are spaced along the optic nerve bundle, its summed activity is represented in the record. If the "active" electrode is inserted into the tissue of the occipital cortex of the brain, the most elaborate of all visual responses are recorded. And there are intermediate stations, notably at several points within the retinal layers themselves and within various of the subcortical brain centers, from which significant recordings can be obtained.

But, before sampling the electrical changes encountered as the optical tract is ascended, we should pay some attention to the *polarity potential* of the eyeball itself. If electrical contact is made with the cornea, most effectively with a silver electrode embedded in a fitted plastic contact lens according to the technique devised by Riggs (*497*), and an "inactive" electrode is attached to the forehead or the skin at some other neutral point, there will be found, in the absence of eye movements or other activity, a steady "resting" potential having a magnitude of several millivolts. The corneal electrode will be positive with respect to the inactive one. If the eye turns in its socket, there is an abrupt change of potential. This effect may be put to work to record eye movements. A graphic record of such changes is known as an *electro-oculogram*. If four active electrodes are used and are placed above and below the eyeball and at the inner and outer "corners" of the eye, suitable steps being taken to minimize skin resistance at the points of attachment of the electrodes, the resulting record gives such an accurate picture of eye movements as to permit judgment of direction of regard with an accuracy of 1.5° of angle in the horizontal direction and about 2.0° in the vertical. The exact region of origin of the polarity potential is still only a matter of surmise. A cell boundary potential seems clearly to be involved, but it is not obvious as yet which of the interfaces between ocular structures are responsible.

The ERG is of considerably more interest because of its obvious connection with the stimulation process. Whereas it is known that it does

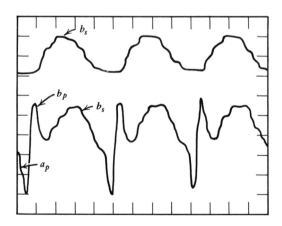

Fig. 3–18. ERG records to lights flashing at a rate of 4 per second. The top tracing was elicited by a violet light of 410 nm, the lower one by an orange-red light of 610 nm. See text for the meanings of the letter designations. From Riggs (*497*).

not reveal directly any purely photochemical events in rods and cones, it is clear that it does mirror changes in neural tissue very closely associated with the photochemical changes, presumably in bipolar and ganglion cells of the retina. Recorded by the corneal electrode method, the ERG shows a complex set of electrical changes, more complex at high stimulus intensities than at low. Figure 3–18 shows (top) a response curve to violet light of 410 nm and involving chiefly rods and (bottom) a more elaborate curve resulting from stimulation by red at 610 nm, which doubtless brought in both rods and cones. These records were obtained from light flashes occurring at a frequency of 4 per second.

The currently accepted analysis of the larger, more complex ERG curve pictures both rods and cones as contributing to it; there are, then, both scotopic and photopic components. Moreover, there appear to be two temporally separated phases connected with both, an early a-wave and a later b-wave. There are thus four contributors to the overall shape of the ERG curve: a photopic a-wave (small, negative deflection), a_p; a photopic b-wave (small, positive), b_p; a scotopic a-wave (small, negative), a_s; and a scotopic b-wave (large, positive), b_s. The relative roles played by the four are suggested by the analysis shown in Figure 3–19. The temporal peaks of the four processes follow in the order: a_p, a_s, b_p, b_s. It is obvious that a_p and a_s are not readily separated and, indeed, it may be

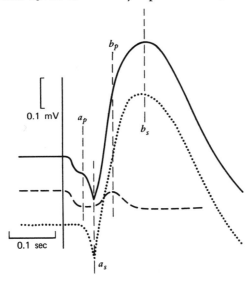

Fig. 3–19. Analysis of the ERG. The solid line is the summation of the dashed line (photopic component) and the dotted line (scotopic component). Both the a-wave and the b-wave have photopic and scotopic components. From **Riggs** (*497*). Courtesy of the Journal of Physiology.

that the second downward deflection in the a-wave is only a further complication in the process responsible for a_p. This point has not yet been settled.

One thing that is clear is that the main constituent of the ERG is b_s. This reflects the intensity of the stimulus creating it. It also changes its magnitude with state of dark adaptation, becoming progressively larger in the dark and thus paralleling the rods' dark adaptation performance. If the retina is light-adapted, the b-wave is markedly reduced, and at high field luminances may drop out altogether. One sure way to eliminate the rods' contribution to the total ERG curve is to deliver the light stimulus to the eye in a series of rapidly repeated short flashes (20 to 30 per second). The scotopic b-wave cannot "follow" under these conditions and the recorded changes are solely those initiated by a_p and b_p.

Differential effects of wavelength are not easy to see in ERG records mainly because other variables—intensity, state of adaptation, etc.—tend to obscure them. However, a technique used by Riggs and his colleagues (499) partials out the influence of wavelength. This is accomplished by alternating in rapid succession (10 per second) two sets of stripes of differing wavelength. The field is a large one subtending 19° at the eye, and each of many stripes covers an angle of a little over one degree. The two colors, red and green, say, having been equated for stimulating power in terms of electrical response of the retina under stationary conditions, the stripes are now rapidly interchanged and the ERG is recorded. The net result is a response curve that expresses the differential effect of the wavelength variation. If one stimulus in the stripe pattern is chosen from the extreme red at 675 nm and is alternated with a second one selected progressively further toward the short waves, there results the family of ERG curves shown in Figure 3–20. Clearly, wavelength is an important determinant of ERG magnitude.

Somewhat elaborate analyses of the ERG, prompted by recordings from subhuman forms, have been made, notably by Granit (243) and K. T. Brown (99). The former was able to bring out the interaction of three "processes" (PI, PII, and PIII, enumerated in the order of their resistance to anesthesia), and their separate existences were demonstrated through the effects of ether and asphyxia. The overall ERG was thought to be the summed effect of the two positive potentials, PI and PII, and the negative (inhibitory?) one, PIII. Brown's analysis is based on an extensive accumulation of facts about the predominantly rod retinas of cats and night monkeys, the pure-cone retinas of diurnal squirrels, and the mixed-type retinas of monkeys having eyes more nearly comparable to the human. An especially intimate approach to the array of retinal potentials has been afforded through the use of microelectrodes whose 0.5-μ

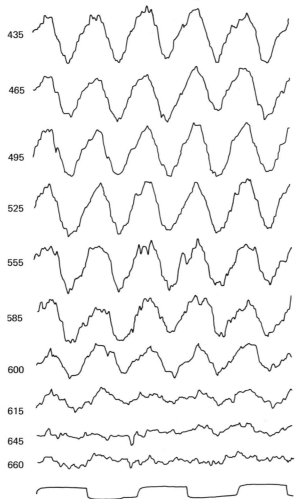

Fig. 3–20. ERG records showing the effect of wavelength on the size of the retinal response. At a 10-per-second rate, stripes of different wavelength are alternated with a constant red of λ675 nm. From top to bottom, the λ difference is thus reduced from 240 to 15 nm. The bottom record is a calibration curve (5.35 Hz, 1 μV photocell response to λ alternation). From Riggs, Johnson, and Schick (*499*).

tips could pick up changes at known distances away from and into the various retinal layers. Also, by such sensitive methods, it was possible to assess the role of the ever-present stray light inside the eye.

It appears that rod and cone systems yield ERGs that are more alike than different. While a light stimulus is present the overall response, in all types of eyes, is much the same, the small *a*-wave and prominent *b*-wave showing up strongly. There is also a steady d.c. potential that lasts as long as the stimulus continues to act. The difference is that the rod system also has a *c*-wave, which appears to be associated with the presence of pigment epithelium since the *c*-wave is never found in the pure-cone retina, whatever its state of adaptation, nor in a retinal preparation isolated from its pigment layer. Another difference, which leads especially to characteristic appearances of the "off-response" of the ERG, concerns the rate at which the rod and cone potentials decay. Cone potentials do so rapidly, those of rods slowly.

The Retina as a Nervous Center.   Until now, we have not paid much attention to the details of retinal anatomy beyond noting that cones, at least foveal ones, connect more or less discretely through their bipolars with fibers of the optic nerve bundle while rods do so molecularly, that is, many rods impinge on a single fiber. But we know that there are both convergence and divergence at work in the retina. A single end organ may connect with several ganglion cells and a single ganglion receives collateral connections from several, sometimes many, receptor cells. The neural provisions for lateral interaction are present in some profusion in the vertebrate eye. A simple count of end organs and optic nerve fibers suggest that the main relations are those of convergence. In the periphery, for example, the ratio of rods to bipolar cells to ganglia is 100:17:1. There are something like one million myelinated fibers in the optic nerve bundle—how many more unmyelinated, far more fragile fibers there are is still a guess—but these have to carry the information output from about 125 million rods and 6 to 7 million cones. Both rods and cones are known to connect, through their bipolar cells, with the same ganglion (*244*, p. 550). It is obvious that the first three nerve cells in the optic nerve chain, all having their cell bodies in the retina itself—end organs, bipolars, ganglia—must do a masterful job of organizing the visual response; even before impulses leave the retina on their way to the brain, they get patterned in a most interesting way.

The basic phenomenon is that described by Kuffler in 1953 (*371*). Recording electrical activity in the retinal ganglia of the light-adapted cat's eye, he found that a whole series of retinal points would produce effects in a given ganglion cell when a tiny light spot was moved back and forth on the retina. However, the effects were not uniform. The discharge of a ganglion might be enhanced or depressed, depending on the spot stimulated. The whole retinal area from which changes could be evoked, known as the ganglion's *receptive field*, became patterned in accordance with one of two plans. For some ganglia, there was a small area of the retina (perhaps subtending only a few minutes of arc) that would discharge while the light was on and would subside promptly when it was extinguished. Surrounding this disclike area, as a roughly circular annulus, there was another larger region that behaved in a quite different way. Throwing the light spot into it tended to suppress spontaneous activity in the ganglion so long as the light was on but set up a train of impulses the moment the light was removed. Obviously, in such a system, the center of the receptive field is excitatory and the periphery is inhibitory. Kuffler dubbed such an arrangement an "on"-center field.

The second plan is the reverse of the first one. Some ganglia have "off"-center fields, that is, stimulation of the middle of the receptive field generates impulses only when the light goes off, whereas the annular surrounding area yields discharges only when the light falls on it. An "off"-center cell is inhibited when the light stimulus is present and returns to its normal spontaneous activity when the light goes out. Thus there appears always to be a "center-surround" mode of retinal organization.

Later, when we come to consider interaction phenomena of some complexity (Chapter 5), we shall have to ask what the full meaning of such events is and also what happens in this regard higher up in the visual system. There have been investigations of similar changes taking place at the levels of the lateral geniculate body of the optic thalamus and the visual cortex (314). Since here is a mechanism involving both excitatory and inhibitory effects, it presumably needs to be looked at in conjunction with such phenomena as facilitation, sensory suppression, and visual contrast. Meanwhile, we need to note that much elaboration of visual response must be introduced no higher in the system than within the retina itself.

With such radical changes taking place at the lowest centers of the visual system, in the retinal ganglia, and with echoes of these changes present in the higher reaches of the visual pathways, it is little wonder that there are many commonly recurring phenomena of vision that cannot be accounted for in terms of a simple reversible photochemical reaction at the level of the most peripheral cells, the rods and cones.

Higher Order Neurons.   The optic nerve in some animal preparations may be "shredded," thus making possible the isolation of a single fiber for test. The first such records were obtained in 1932 by Hartline and Graham (275). They singled out individual fibers still attached to functioning receptor cells, in the eye of the horseshoe crab Limulus, and recorded the impulses generated by light flashes. As had been found a

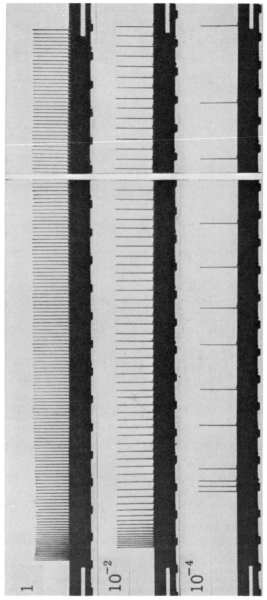

Fig. 3–21. Impulses in a single fiber of the optic nerve. Action potentials from the eye of Limulus, the horeshoe crab, in response to steady illumination. Records for three different intensities varying in the ratio 1.0:0.01:0.0001 are shown. Time is marked off in ⅕-sec intervals. From Hartline (274). Courtesy of the editor, *Journal of the Optical Society of America,* and the author.

few years earlier for single tactile fibers (*11*), the response to steady stimulation consists of a succession of spaced electrical discharges. The responses are uniform with respect to size, in accordance with the "all-or-nothing" principle. The only variation is one of rate of firing (see Figure 3–21); the greater the intensity of the stimulus light, the higher the frequency. A decline in rate of discharge with a continuation of the stimulus is to be noted also. This is, of course, the accompaniment of light adaptation and presumably is the correlate of reduced brightness following steady exposure.

The crab's eye is of relatively simple construction. It was originally selected as experimental material because it was supposed that it contained only a single kind of photosensitive cell attached to a single, uncom-

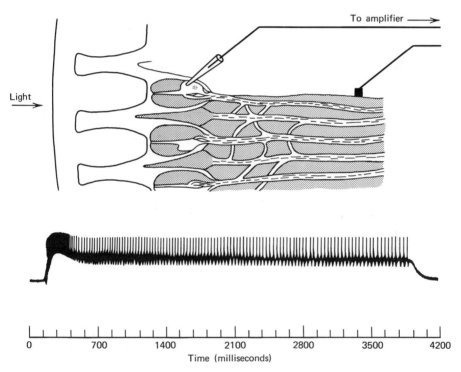

Fig. 3–22. A record from a single ommatidium of the eye of the horseshoe crab. The upper diagram shows the method of recording, the tip of a microelectrode being inserted in the region of the eccentric cell. The lower part of the figure reproduces a record of the generator potential (wavy baseline) and the nerve spikes that follow. From "How Cells Receive Stimuli", by W. H. Miller, F. Ratliff, and H. K. Hartline. Copyright 1961 by Scientific American, Inc. All rights reserved.

plicated nerve fiber. Presumably there were no lateral connections such as are found in the vertebrate eye. The functional picture should be correspondingly simple. Actually, however, some fairly complex effects are producible in even so comparatively simple a retina. Thus Hartline has been able to demonstrate spatial interaction phenomena in which neighboring units of the horseshoe crab's eye mutually suppress each other. And, when techniques had been refined to the point where a microelectrode could be plunged into the tip of a single ommatidium of Limulus, it became possible to get a record of the very genesis of nerve message production. Hartline and his colleagues were able to record at this point true "generator potentials," the initial electrode imbalances that trigger the nerve message (423). In the impulse activity displayed in Figure 3–22, it will be seen that spike frequency follows the generator potential with some fidelity. The generator potential, the magnitude of which is represented in the wavy baseline, proved to be approximately proportional to the logarithm of light intensity.

When a more complex, vertebrate eye is investigated the electrical effects become more elaborate. Three kinds of responses found in indi-

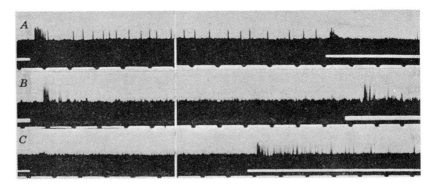

Fig. 3–23. Responses of three types of fibers in a vertebrate eye (frog). The presence of a light stimulus is signaled by the disappearance of the white line just above the time record. Time units are $\frac{1}{5}$ sec. (*A*) response of a fiber of the type found in the crab's eye (Fig. 3–21). This shows regular discharge in the presence of light. (*B*) an "on-off" type fiber. Only the onset or cessation of the stimulus produces a response. (*C*) the "off" type fiber, which discharges only when the light goes out. From Hartline (274). What appears to be an "off" response in the *A* record is in reality the normal response of the fiber, a single spike which happened nearly to coincide with the cessation of the stimulus, combined with several smaller spikes from a nearby fiber of the "off" variety. This was clearly explained by Dr. Hartline in his original description of the record but has not always since been understood. Courtesy of the editor, *Journal of the Optical Society of America,* and the author.

vidual fibers of the frog's optic nerve are displayed in Figure 3–23, taken from the work of Hartline (274). Some fibers respond very much as do those of the crab's optic nerve, maintaining periodic discharges so long as the stimulus light is falling on their attached receptor cells. Others respond only briefly at the onset and cessation of the stimulus (or whenever the light is abruptly increased or diminished in intensity). The third variety of fiber does an even stranger thing; it bursts into activity for a second or two when the light is cut off. Reilluminating the retina immediately suppresses activity in these fibers.

Again, as with the ERG, it would be convenient if clear meaning could be attached to these findings for the optic nerve, but as yet they are extremely perplexing. Recordings from large numbers of samples reveal that only one-fifth of the fibers are concerned with the maintained type of discharge. Apparently the optic nerve is better organized for reporting the disappearance of a stimulus than for registering its presence!

Hartline's findings were subsequently confirmed and extended by Barlow (33) and spectacularly elaborated by a team of MIT investigators (380) who developed an interesting interpretation of the messages "told to the frog's brain by the frog's eye." Recording from individual fibers of the optic nerve and from four anatomically distinct "sheets" of nerve terminals in the frog's brain and determining, from a wide range of choices, the kinds of stimuli that would produce optimal responses in both places, they came to the conclusion that the organization of the frog's visual system is not so much one devoted to handling a mosaic of light intensities and geometrical patterns as it is one subserving certain operations in the life of the frog. To be sure, they confirmed the existence of "on," "off," and "on-off" fibers but, perhaps more significantly, they were able to show that special functions are associated with each.

There seem to be four kinds of operations or functions, each carried on by a different type of nerve fiber and projection layer in the brain. These single out: (a) local sharp edges and contrast, (b) edge curvature of a dark object, (c) progressive movement of linear edges in the visual field, and (d) local dimming caused by movement or general darkening of the field. Unmyelinated fibers of the optic nerve mediate the first two; myelinated fibers take care of the last two. The four "sheets" of endings in the brain also have quite definite allocations. Each group of fibers and brain terminations serves the entire retina and provides a map of it, and the four maps are in registration with each other. Moreover, if the pathways are interrupted by cutting and are allowed to regenerate, the original functional maps, with their four different operations, are restored to their original efficacy.

The "receptive fields" of the four functions are not coextensive, even though they are concentric. The contrast detector field [(a) above] is the smallest (about 2°) but in that area it notes the presence of sharp boundaries, be they moving or still. The convexity detector (b) picks up any object other than a straight edge, providing it has a subtense of 3° or less, whether it is moving or stationary once it has entered the field. They function well at both high and low intensity. The receptive field for the moving edge detectors (c) is quite large, as much as 12°. The only requirement is that the edge be moving; responses die out otherwise. Speed of movement is important, light intensity much less so. The dimming detector (d) has the largest receptive field, 15°. If the dimming occurs in the center of the receptive field, the response is large; as the locus of the dimmed spot is moved toward the periphery of the receptive field, the effect diminishes. Again, absolute light intensity is relatively unimportant.

Clearly, there is much that is already "interpreted" in the bare data that come from the frog's eye. In line with the classical distinction, we should have to say that the frog's eye, "perceives" rather than just "sees" its environment. Analysis of the environment by the frog's visual system is in terms of patterned information vital to the frog, especially information about nearby moving shapes.

In the more elaborate visual system of the higher vertebrates, the optic nerve enters the brain proper at the lateral geniculate body of the optic thalamus. At this level the axons of third-order neurons carry the visual message. Unlike the electrical changes at the receptor, which are graded responses, those at the thalamus are of an all-or-nothing variety; their magnitudes and temporal features depend exclusively on the intrinsic properties of the axon. Yet the optic nerve message must be preserving information coded at the receptor site—data on shapes and contours, colors, and brightnesses, movements, temporal and spatial continuities and discontinuities. A complex set of excitatory and inhibitory influences, intensive changes, and shifting states of adaptation must make the coding itself a truly kaleidoscopic process.

Nor are interactions and complications over with at this point; there is nothing inert about the thalamus. Incoming fibers from the optic nerve may impinge on several different fourth-order neurons arising in the lateral geniculate body, and apparently there also occurs the reverse (several third-order neurons connecting with a single fourth-order nerve cell). There is considerable "spontaneous" activity in the thalamus and much variability of response. The belief is that further recording of the visual message must be brought about at this point in the chain.

"Final" projection is onto the cortex of the brain, in the striate area of the occipital lobe. Lately much information about activity in the visual cortex has been gathered through the somewhat gross technique of implanted electrodes and the much more refined one of cortical exploration with microelectrodes. There have also been important technical developments in amplification methods and, especially, in the application of computers that make possible the cumulation or averaging of responses. These possess the virtue of maximizing the electrical record of nerve response while at the same time minimizing, through a canceling procedure, background "noise" in the recording system. Thus a weak signal, perhaps possessing only a fraction of the strength of the ambient noise level, may be "pulled out" of its background as the stimulus is repeated and trials mount.

If the electrical events in the retina and way stations seem intricate, they are simplicity itself compared to those obtained when leads are taken off the cortex of the brain. The higher cortical centers, in their very construction, provide maximal opportunity for free interplay of excitations. It is therefore not surprising that electrodes placed in this region, particularly if their area is large, pick up many interacting impulses and reveal, in the final record, only summed activity difficult of detailed analysis.

Records of electrical activity in the brain (*electroencephalograms,* EEG) may be obtained in humans without the necessity of contacting the cortical tissue directly. Electrodes collodioned or otherwise attached to the scalp will detect the presence of rather large disturbances, so-called alpha-waves, having an average frequency of 10 per second. Smaller ones, occurring at rates as high as 30 or more per second (beta-waves), and very slow but large undulations (delta-waves), as low as 4 per second in frequency, are also present in the complex. Whatever the exact mode of origin of these rhythms (and this question is as yet unsettled) it is clear that they are, in large part, spontaneous on the part of the brain, more particularly, of the optical brain. The interesting thing about them, for our immediate concern, is their sudden diminution or even complete abolition with the onset of visual stimulation. Many other sensory stimuli have the same result, but excitation of the visual centers seems to be most effective in producing the depression.

To get a more intimate picture of electrical events in the visual cortex, it is obviously necessary to limit the amount of tissue contributing to the record. This is a job for high impedance electrodes of the miniature variety and high amplification of the voltage changes; alternatively, it means the use of rather more gross electrodes in conjunction with the averaging computer to suppress competition from ambient noise. The two attacks will not, of course, provide the same kinds of data, but each has its role to play in revealing the cortical contribution.

It will be recalled that important interactions occur at the retinal level with the consequence that the receptive field for a given ganglion cell is relatively extensive and shows a "center-surround" type of organization. Similar relations are known to persist as the optic tract is ascended; any individual cell in the lateral geniculate body also has its concentric fields. What about the cortex? Are such arrangements preserved all the way to the highest projection areas?

In a general way, it appears that they are, but there are important differences between cortical and subcortical types of organization (*314, 315*). Whereas, in the retina and geniculate body, excitatory and inhibitory portions of the receptive field take their place in concentric disc-annulus arrangements, in the cortex the two functions are likely to be sharply separated from each other by something approaching a straight line. Several different patterns are seen (Figure 3–24) but in many of them there is a clearly defined axis. Indeed, this proves to be a feature of great interest, since a particular cortical cell is likely to be stimulated maximally only when a suitably oriented slit of light, edge, or contour falls on the retina. Other orientations give weak responses or none at all (see Figure 3–25). Shining a diffuse light on the retina, at least the central portion of it, is bound to have little or no effect on most cortical cells,

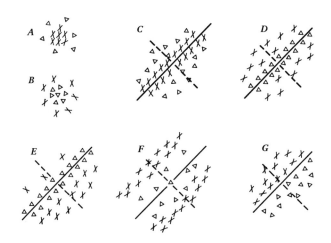

Fig. 3–24. Patterns of response in geniculate and cortical receptive fields. In all instances crosses indicate areas yielding excitatory ("on-") responses; triangles indicate areas giving inhibitory ("off-") responses. In the lateral geniculate body (*A* and *B*), as in the retina, the organization is of the disc-annulus variety; at the cortex *(C-G)*, the two functions are arranged on either side of a receptive-field "axis." From Hubel and Wiesel (*318*). Courtesy of the Journal of Physiology.

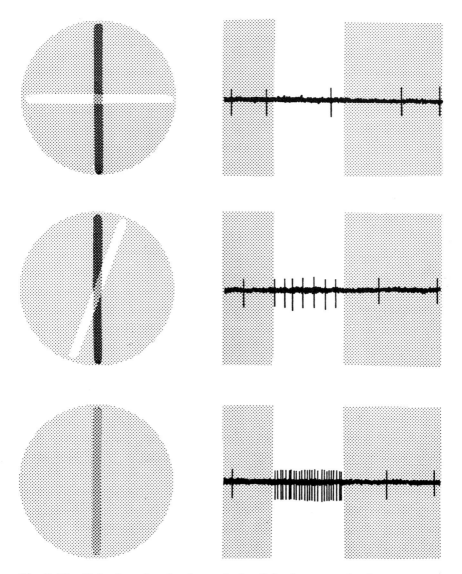

Fig. 3–25. Behavior of a simple cortical cell having a maximal response to a vertically oriented stimulus. From "The Visual Cortex of the Brain," by D. H. Hubel. Copyright 1963 by Scientific American, Inc. All rights reserved.

for this is tantamount to activating simultaneously both the excitatory and inhibitory elements of the cell's receptive field, and the net effect is likely to be complete cancellation of the opposing forces.

Several types of cortical cell are recognized, according to the analysis of Hubel and Wiesel (*318, 319*), who have adduced much striking evidence concerning their behavior. A cell may be *simple, complex,* or *hypercomplex.* Of the latter there are at least two levels of performance, lower order and higher order. The distinctions here are primarily functional, not anatomical, although simple cells seem to be found only in the striate region of the visual cortex (Brodmann's area 17), not in visual projection area II (area 18, anterior to 17) nor in the newly discovered visual III (area 19, lateral to 17). See Figure 3–26 for the orientation of these centers.

Simple cells respond to slits and bars, contours, and "edges" in their own receptive field, providing that the orientation is right, both as to direction and position. Complex cells are less specific in their response;

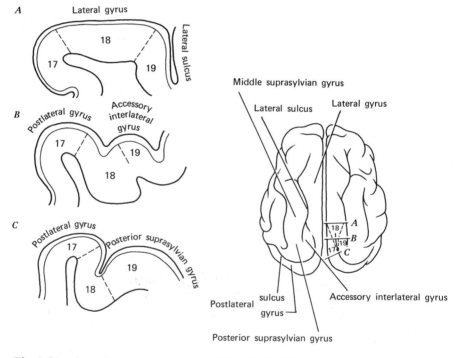

Fig 3–26. Location of visual areas I, II, and III (Brodmann's areas 17, 18, and 19). *A, B,* and *C* depict three antero-posterior cuts. From David H. Hubel and Torsten N. Wiesel. Receptive fields and functional architecture in two nonstriate visual areas (18 and 19) of the cat. *J. Neurophysiol.,* **28**; 229–289, 1965.

they will report such lines and contours in many retinal positions provided the stimulus is of a given spatial orientation. Moreover, cells of the complex variety will respond with a sustained discharge when a stimulus in its receptive field is moved. Nor is there a clear antagonism between "on" and "off" properties in complex cells. Everything points to the interpretation that the complex cell is a "collector" of messages from a number of subservient simple cells. Hypercomplex cells are most easily understood as further processing agents for the output of complex cells. The receptive field of a hypercomplex cell does not summate its responses throughout its entire length or width in the way that a complex cell does. The more elaborate cell apparently has two regions within it, an "activating" element and an "antagonistic" or inhibitory element, since it turns out that a dark edge must definitely be limited in extent to produce a strong response. These are, so to speak, "stopped edge" cells, and slits and narrow tongues of shadows are more effective as stimuli for them. Some of the hypercomplex cells (higher order) have even more elaborate properties; they answer best to limited lengths of line that form dark corners in the receptive field. Such cells thus behave as if they combined the features of two lower-order cells with orientation axes at 90° to each other.

Fibers radiating upward from the geniculate body must contact simple cells and these, in turn, must deliver their messages to complex ones. The latter, having already introduced some degree of generality, pass their data on to hypercomplex cells, and these extract other qualities inherent in original stimulation. The details of coding will doubtlessly continue to unfold, both as new psychophysiological data come to hand and as the functional facts become correlated with anatomical ones. By plunging microelectrodes into the cortex at a variety of depths and angles and recording from their tips, it has been learned that the main organization is a radial one involving projection upward from the lowest laminations of the cortex, bordering the white matter of the cerebrum. It is as if the cortex were organized into a mosaic of little columns, each about 2.5 mm high (the combined thickness of the several cortical layers) and about 0.5 mm wide, each representing a small segment of the retina and each composed of simple and complex cells (in area 17; complex and hypercomplex in areas 18 and 19). The simple cells in a column all seem to have identical axis orientations and each reports on a particular retinal spot. Taking all cells as an aggregate, no single orientation is favored. As has been noted, it is apparently up to the complex and hypercomplex cells (or, possibly, structures beyond) to perform the abstracting or generalizing function. One such task is that of synthesizing broad movements; perhaps another is to build shape or form from its elements.

The end of the story is not with us, despite recent giant strides in electrophysiology of the central nervous system. The important thing is that adequate techniques are now at hand, and one may confidently predict not only a gradual filling in of the details but also newer interpretations of the larger picture.

4
Color Vision and
Color Blindness

Visual Quality. We saw in Chapter 3 the manner in which three different dimensions of the physical stimuli for vision can be separately discriminated. It would be very convenient if there could be found a strictly analogous set of dimensions of visual experience corresponding to the stimulus properties of intensity, wavelength, and colorimetric purity. But to claim such correspondence would be to oversimplify things considerably. It is better to drop our *psychophysical* attack on the problems of vision for the time and assume a *phenomenal* viewpoint. What kind of order comes into the picture if we forget what we know about the physical dimensions of light and attempt a direct description of visual experience?

If the largest possible range of visible objects were to be examined we should see that certain uniformities of light and shade, color tone, and resemblance to gray run through them. There would be textural variations and differences of shape also, but we have raised no question of the geometry of physical objects, and we shall do well here to sidestep the somewhat vexing problem of form perception. The precipitous growth of the literature of visual perception in the last decade attests to both the importance and the intricacy of the problems created when overall human behavior in relation to the world of space becomes the center of interest.

One way of representing the variations in visual sensation is to make use of the *color spindle* (Figure 4–1). Visual qualities occupy its entire surface, while a multitude of intensive series radiate out in all directions from the middle point, neutral gray. The central rim represents all the different hues found in the spectrum and, in addition, a series of hues compounded of red and violet—the purples. White and black are also obviously distinct qualities and are represented at the tips of the spindle.

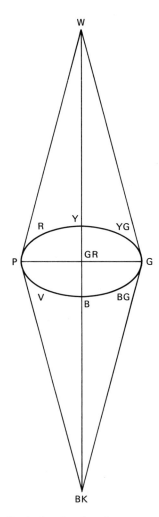

Fig. 4–1. The color spindle in its simplest form.

From each noticeably different hue there runs a series of qualities terminating in white; similarly, a series exists between black and each point on the hue circle. Integrating the entire surface we have a qualitative "shell," all possible colors having positions on its surface.

It is clear also that various series exist within the spindle, but the points on these lines seem to be *intensitively* rather than *qualitatively* different. There is such a series between neutral gray and white and another between gray and black. It is well to note that this makes black a positive sensation which can vary in degree. There has been a good deal of controversy on this point, since the naive view would make black the simple accompaniment of lack of stimulation. But the experience in looking at physical "blackness" is not black, nor is black the lack of sensation! Perhaps owing to autonomous processes working in the brain one gets, in the dark room, not black but gray or purplish gray. This is sometimes called "brain gray" or the *self-light* or *intrinsic light of the retina*. It appears that gray may be a constant background process and that all stimulation must "break through" it, or perhaps "modulate" it, for visual quality to be experienced. One viewpoint is that the intrinsic light is the expression of a more or less ubiquitous "noise" in the visual message system, a background disturbance which, on occasions, augments to such a level as to produce deterioration in or even efface incoming signals.

Other intensitive series radiating from neutral gray to the surface of the spindle must, of course, terminate at colors. These are lines of increasing saturation, and it is perhaps clearer now why saturation is defined in terms of lack of grayness. The outside boundaries of the spindle are not determined by the saturations experienced in viewing the spectrum; under special conditions of observation colors may appear even better saturated than do spectral ones.

There are other ways of representing color sensations and other interpretations to be put on the spindle. Some have stressed the unique character of certain salient hues and have made of the hue circle a square. The figure thus becomes a double pyramid, bases joined, with psychologically "unique" red, yellow, green, and blue at the corners (*163, 164*). The point is well taken; there does seem to be something special about these particular hues. Orange resembles red and yellow, but yellow does not resemble red and green. The question is an old one and long debated (*84*, pp. 145 ff.), but too often the location of special "primary" hues at the corners of the pyramid have provided the impetus for commitment to some special theory of color vision which, in our present state of knowledge, may not be entirely healthy.

If attention is paid to the actual number of observable stages of hue, saturation, and brightness, that is, to the number of just perceptible differences of all kinds within the world of color, one does not come out with a neat geometrical arrangement like the spindle or double pyramid. There results the irregular figure illustrated in Figure 4–2 (*447*). From the measurements that went into the construction of this model there

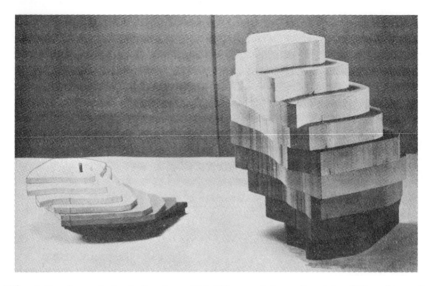

Fig. 4–2. A psychological color solid. The model on the right differs from that on the left in having its vertical dimension increased by a factor of 4. The two models have the same horizontal dimensions. From Nickerson and Newhall, *(447)*. Photograph by courtesy of Dr. Nickerson and the U.S. Department of Agriculture.

may be made a simple computation of the total number of distinguishable colors. The number is a surprisingly large one—7,500,000!

Both the spindle and pyramid are conceived by many to be "qualitative solids" in the sense that all points within the figure, as well as on the surface, are *qualitatively* distinct from each other. It has remained for Boring *(82,* Chap. 2) to show that the figure is, in fact, a solid, but qualitative only on its outer surface; within, it is representative of a host of intensive differences. This view appears to be more in line with present trends of theory in that it unites qualitative and quantitative concepts. But whatever the form of color solid adopted and whatever the details of its interpretation, it represents a useful conception. Observed color is clearly describable in the three dimensions of the figure: brightness, hue, and saturation. An additional step is obviously necessary to get from this purely *psychological* position to the *psychophysical* one, where stimulus properties come to be linked to those of sensation. Then we have a set of major dependencies (though not, of course, exclusive ones) of brightness on luminance, hue on wavelength, and saturation on colorimetric purity.

Color Nomenclature and Specification. The names given colors are notoriously arbitrary. Color vocabularies we acquire in the course of a multitude of varied experiences with colored objects are pretty much fortuitous affairs. It is not only the layman who uses color names inaccurately. A study of the color designations used by chemists and druggists revealed the greatest variety of names for description of a single fluid. But we cannot give up our color names; they are too useful. It is better to attempt standardization of them and thus bring order out of relative chaos. A method of color designation which has been carefully worked out with a view to practical usefulness as well as to theoretical correctness is the system devised by the Inter-Society Color Council, an organization serving as a clearinghouse for color problems of all sorts. The ISCC system is built on ten basic hue names (red, orange, yellow, green, blue, violet, purple, brown, pink, and olive) coupled with modifiers, such as light, vivid, weak, very, deep, etc. By joining one or more modifiers with hue names, 267 separate designations of color are possible. The system has the advantage that common color names are used, but used in such an unambiguous manner that reference to some external standard becomes unnecessary. This set of color names now has the official sanction of several influential organizations concerned with color and vision, including the U.S. National Bureau of Standards, and there is every expectation that it will come into more common use.

Another way to specify colors is to utilize the principle, long known, that any color may be matched by three suitably chosen spectral colors. Such a "tristimulus specification" represents the most exact procedure we now possess. An analysis of any color into three components can be made quickly and accurately with the reflection spectrophotometer. We shall return later to some of the details of tristimulus color specification, after we have learned something of the color mixing process upon which the method is based.

Still a third method of making color specifications is to set up acceptable material standards. This is a practical "must" in such diverse industrial fields as those dealing with textiles, soils and agricultural products, paper, ceramics, dyestuffs and paints, stone and other building materials, plastics, and geological samples. Moreover, there are many scientific, artistic, and recreational activities that impinge upon color, among them pharmacological and dermatological descriptions, specifications of signal lights and of the elements of interior decoration, philatelic identifications and those of birds and flowers. In the search for standards, various sets of solutions, pigmented or dyed surfaces, and filters have been used in conjunction with a known illuminant. The advantage in such a system is its great convenience. The best known of these systems are the

Ostwald color atlas, the Maerz and Paul "color dictionary" containing 7000 color samples keyed to 4000 color names, and the Munsell system. The last is of special interest in that it has been so constructed as to conform as nearly as possible with the basic idea of the "color spindle." Moreover, perhaps because of the extreme care used in its manufacture and replication, it has tended to be the rallying point for practical color systems of all kinds. A somewhat similar construction, one widely used in central Europe, is the DIN color system. This is based, like the Munsell system, on the three principal dimensions of color appearance.

Color Mixture.   If the light reflected from the surface of a colored paper were to be analyzed with a spectrometer there would be found present a great variety of waves, probably extending over the entire spectrum, though having a strong maximum in some one region. Yet the surface appears, upon direct viewing, to have only a single "color." A unitary effect is thus being produced from a complex stimulus. Most of the colors we see are produced in this way; only under very special circumstances are "pure" colors encountered. Obviously, color mixture plays a very important role in everyday seeing.

Color mixtures are produced by two distinct processes, color *subtraction* and color *addition*. The subtraction process is the less common, though it accounts for the results found in mixing paints and other pigments. We all know, from blending water colors, that green can be produced by a suitable mixture of yellow and blue, and, because it is a derived color, green is not regarded as an artistic "primary." It is surprising to learn, therefore, that green (but not yellow) is regarded as a primary in visual science. The confusion disappears when it is disclosed that the production of green by mixing yellow and blue is an accident of the subtractive process. The yellow pigment absorbs all but yellow and green light, reflecting these. Similarly, the blue pigment reflects blue and green, absorbing all other waves. From the incident white light, itself a mixture of all visible waves, a double subtraction has been made. The remainder is green, the only color reflected in common by the two originals. Precisely the same results would be obtained in passing white light successively through color filters having transmission characteristics like the reflectance values of these pigments. Color filters, then, also operate on the subtractive principle.

However, the majority of color mixtures are additive. Especially is this true of color mixing in the laboratory. Combine, by superimposing them on a single screen, two spectral samples such as red and green, and an intermediate hue, yellow, will be seen. Blend green and blue in the same way, and an intermediate green-blue is the result. The experiment may be done systematically for all possible color combinations. If so, it will be found that there is nothing fortuitous about color mixtures but, on the contrary, that they are entirely regular and lawful in operation.

If we select from the long-wave end of the spectrum a red and combine with it green in different proportions, the resulting mixtures will vary continuously through orange, yellow, and yellow-green. A particular red (lithium) of λ671 nm, when mixed with green (thallium) of λ536 nm, yields a yellow indistinguishable from λ589 nm. This is the so-called Rayleigh equation, often used for testing color vision. If the color to be mixed with the initial red is selected further down in the wavelength series, still other intermediates are possible, though the more remote in the spectrum the two components, the less saturated, that is, the whiter or grayer, the mixture will be. If the second component is taken as far down as λ493 nm there will be no hue at all; if intensities are properly chosen this mixture will appear white. The two components in this case are said to be *complementary* colors. This pairing of red (λ671 nm) and blue-green (λ493 nm) is but one instance among a great many such complementary combinations. The data gathered from several independent determinations of complementary pairs are shown in Figure 4–3. The

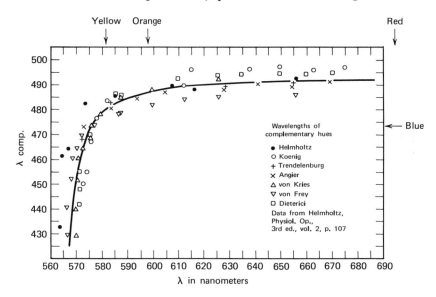

Fig. 4–3. Complementary color pairs. The data of seven different investigators have been combined in a single plot. The curve, one branch of an equilateral hyperbola, is the locus of a large number of pairs of complementary wavelengths. From Priest (*480*) after Helmholtz (*291*). Courtesy of the editor, *Journal of the Optical Society of America.*

curve best fitting the points is one branch of an equilateral hyperbola.

If, in the selection of a second component to be combined with lithium red, one goes beyond λ493 nm to the shorter waves, he finds another series of hues. This is the group of colors made up of non-spectral purples and the purplish reds. It has been determined that this series of hues contains 28 j.n.d.'s, which, added to the 128 found in the spectrum, brings to 156 the total number of discriminable hue steps (536). Thus one may complete the "hue circle," already familiar from the color spindle. The details of this circle are shown in Figure 4–4. Here complementary

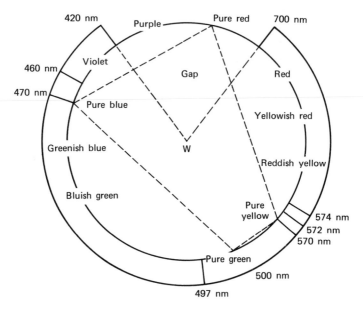

Fig. 4–4. The hue circle. Spectral stimuli from λ420 nm to λ700 nm are arranged in sequence about the circumference. Complementary colors lie at opposite ends of diagonals. The positions of psychologically "pure" yellow, green, and blue in the series are noted, as is also that of "pure" red, which lies in the gap beyond spectral red. From Southall (537). By permission of the Oxford University Press and the author.

pairs lie at opposite ends of each diameter. It will be noted that psychologically "pure" red lies in the gap between the two ends of the spectrum; all spectral reds are judged to be somewhat yellowish.

If one were devising a system for reproducing all possible hues as well as white, three basic components would be necessary. It has long been known that all hues can be obtained through the suitable mixture of "primaries" selected from the long-wave, medium-wave, and short-wave parts of the spectrum. The primaries in question are red, green, and violet. A general color equation can be written: $C = xR + yG + zV$, where x, y, and z are coefficients varying in size for different colors, C. For two-component mixtures, one of the coefficients becomes 0. For white or gray, x, y, and z are equal.

The sizes of the coefficients necessary to reproduce all the colors of the spectrum are shown in Figure 4–5. Here the primaries have been selected

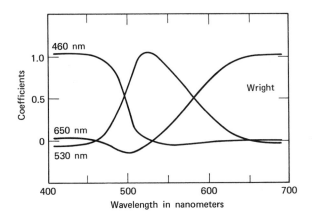

Fig. 4–5. Reproduction of spectral colors by three primaries. The curves represent the average readings for 10 observers and show the sizes of coefficients necessary to reproduce all spectral points when the primaries selected are: λ650 nm, red; λ530 nm, green; λ460 nm, violet. A considerably more extended treatment is called for if the details of calculation of the color coefficients are to be fully appreciated. [See (240), Chap. 13 or (127), Chaps. 8–10]. After Wright, (657). By permission of the Howe Laboratory of Ophthalmology, Harvard University.

as follows: red, λ650 nm; green, λ530 nm; violet, λ460 nm. So long as only the hue relations among different color sensations are being considered there are many sets of primary wavelengths that will answer quite well (537, pp. 313–337). When other aspects of color (e.g., saturation) are also taken into account, however, the number of possibilities becomes definitely limited (278).

Color mixtures, as additions of excitations, have been discussed as though there were but a single means of producing them, that is, the combining of spectral samples. There is little doubt that for the most exact results this method is the best. A high point of instrumentation was reached in the Helmholtz color mixer, which uses this method (537,

p. 314). There are also many excellent colorimeters and spectrophotometers that obtain their color compounds in this way. See *658*, Chapter 5. But there are more convenient ways of seeing the qualitative relations between colors in mixtures. One is to make use of Lambert's method. Two sources, such as colored paper squares, are placed at right angles to each other. A piece of clear glass, bisecting the angle between the papers, now transmit one color to the eye and, through partial reflection, "mixes" the second with the first. Changing the direction and amount of light incident to the papers makes possible a wide range of mixtures.

The most commonly used device for color mixing is the sectored disc or color wheel. Two or more interjoined colored papers, the relative proportions of which can be varied, are rapidly rotated at speeds sufficient to eliminate flicker. A single mixed color results. The effect depends upon the property of the retina whereby an impression, once being set up, requires an appreciable time of "decay" to be eliminated. Two rapidly successive impressions thus "fuse" to yield a unitary one. It is interesting that this mode of color combination, used more uncritically than any other, involves the most elaborate retinal and cortical events and, for its strict interpretation, would require the most complicated account.

A third procedure in color mixing is to take advantage of the fact that we have two retinae, independent in their action, and to present two different colors to the two eyes. Binocular mixtures thus arrived at are notoriously unstable, and yet some facts important for theory can be gained through this method. Two colors very similar in wavelength composition and luminance can be made to combine quite readily; they yield a single fused impression intermediate to the originals in hue. However, two colors from quite separate regions on the hue circle will show only transient mixtures. Steadily viewed, they struggle in *rivalry*, first one and then the other having the upper hand in the conflict. Hecht has questioned a large number of observers on the "mixture" obtained by viewing a bright source through Wratten filter 29 (red), in front of one eye, and filter 58 (green) before the other. Yellow was quite uniformly reported, and from this experiment it seems possible to dispense with yellow as a primary. It appears to be a "brain" mixture, since only in the brain could the two excitations come together. Hecht's account (*277*) leaves out a description of the more obvious action occurring under these conditions, the intense rivalry between red and green, but Hecht's contention was that if yellow is even momentarily and unstably formed in this way it can be regarded as a derived rather than a primary color. Much the same kind of result comes from the binocular mixture of blue and yellow; "brain" white is transiently produced in the struggle.

There has been much debate about the Hecht binocular mixture experiment. Critics have protested that the yellow produced is not a true "spectral" yellow and that it is an artifact of the employment of filters whose transmissions overlap to a degree in the yellow spectral region (438). Others have claimed to have gotten a similar result from combining in rivalry two different reds (175). It remained for Prentice (479) to perform what seemed to be the crucial experiment, once color filters had been developed to the point where absolute separation of the red and green were possible. Deriving his colors from narrow-transmission Farrand interference filters, with provision for equating luminances and adjusting for saturation, Prentice found a good, well-saturated yellow to be produced which, moreover, matched spectral yellow adequately.

Eventually, Hurvich and Jameson (322) examined more closely the logic of the Hecht experiment (and subsequent modifications) and pointed out that, whereas there was no doubting the empirical findings of both Hecht and his successors in this experiment, it could not be assumed that delivery of even a very narrow band of waves from the red and green portions of the spectrum provided a guarantee that the retinae initiated chains of signals that necessarily said "red" and "green" at the brain. Indeed, as we already know from the color circle (p. 90), psychologically pure red does not lie in the spectrum at all, at least at ordinary luminances, but is made up of a mixture of red and blue in suitable proportions—671 nm tempered by a small amount of 440 nm will do it—and, moreover, psychologically pure green does not lie in a central position of transmission for the filters either Hecht or Prentice used. In other words, no matter how narrow the spectral samples are, what is going to be *seen* is yellowish red in one eye and yellowish green in the other. The combining of the two binocularly leaves a residue of yellow, and this obviously need not be something created by the common projection area in the brain.

There is a natural corollary of all this. What would happen if pure red (neither yellowish nor bluish red) and pure green (neither yellowish nor bluish green) were the two colors entering into the binocular mixture? Hurvich and Jameson have done the experiment (322, p. 202) with the perhaps not unexpected result that there is no residue of yellowish hue; pure red and pure green combine binocularly to yield colorless white.

Now, with the chief facts of color mixture before us, we may return to the question of the specification of colors. It has been seen that the additive combination of three lights—any three, so long as no one of them can be formed by a mixture of the other two—is sufficient to produce a match with any color whatever. This being the case, given (1) the specification of the spectrum in terms of three suitably selected primaries, and (2) a spectral analysis of an unknown light, it should be a relatively simple matter to arrive at a "tristimulus specification" of that unknown.

The exact specification of the various parts of the spectrum in terms of three primaries is no longer an arbitrary matter. An important step was taken by the International Commission on Illumination in 1931 in settling on the color mixture data already carefully compiled by Wright and Guild, working independently in England, to form the basis of a standard tristimulus spectral analysis (267). The data, as adopted, are based on the color matches of a sufficient number of subjects whose settings were in excellent agreement. These data have been given the designation "the I.C.I. standard observer"; they are displayed in Figure 4–6. The values of $\bar{x}$, $\bar{y}$, and $\bar{z}$ indicate the amount of each of the I.C.I.

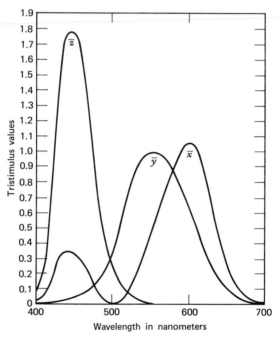

Fig. 4–6. The "standard observer," according to the agreements of the International Commission on Illumination in 1931. The values of $\bar{x}$, $\bar{y}$, and $\bar{z}$ have been so selected as to match, for the average observer, a unit amount of radiant energy at each wavelength. The $\bar{y}$ curve is of special interest, since its values have been chosen to duplicate the photopic luminosity curve for the normal eye. After Hardy (267). By permission of the Technology Press, Massachusetts Institute of Technology.

primaries needed to match a unit amount of radiant energy at each spectral wavelength. The curve labeled $\bar{x}$ represents a reddish purple primary, $\bar{y}$ is a green resembling a spectral green of λ520 nm but more saturated, and $\bar{z}$ is a blue of somewhat greater colorimetric purity than a spectral blue of λ477 nm. Obviously, the primaries have no real physical existence; they are the products of mathematical transformations. At each wavelength the amounts of the three primaries needed, in additive combination, to match the spectral band at that wavelength may be found by simply adding the ordinates of all three curves at that spectral position. Thus, at λ578 nm, there are required approximately equal amounts of reddish purple ($\bar{x}$) and green ($\bar{y}$) to match the yellow seen by the normal observer. In the region of λ475 nm, a large component of blue ($\bar{z}$) joins with small, roughly equal amounts of $\bar{x}$ and $\bar{y}$ to match the particular blue seen there. Other combinations suggest themselves.

The green primary curve ($\bar{y}$) is of special interest in that in selecting the characteristics of the primaries, $\bar{y}$ has been made equivalent to the photopic luminosity curve for the normal eye. This has been done with a view to permitting one of the primaries to specify completely the luminous aspect (brightness) of the color quite apart from its chromatic aspects (hue and saturation). Luminosity of a color is thus known if Y (a particular value of $\bar{y}$) is known.

The chromatic features may also be specified exactly, but a little less directly. This is done by reference to the so-called "chromaticity diagram," a useful construction which tells us a great deal about a color and its relations with all other colors. A typical chromaticity diagram is shown in Figure 4–7. The axes, x and y, are called "chromaticity coordinates," and the following relations define them: $x = X/(X + Y + Z)$; $y = Y/(X + Y + Z)$. Because $x + y + z$ must necessarily equal unity, it is sufficient to specify a color in terms of two of these coordinates, usually x and y. The solid curved line of Figure 4–7 is the locus of the colors of the spectrum between its "practical" limits, λ400 nm to λ700 nm. All colors possible with real stimuli are represented by points within the area bounded by this line and the lower straight line connecting extreme violet and extreme red (the purple series). The point C, near the center of the diagram, shows the location of "daylight," the light supplied by I.C.I. Illuminant C.

The points G and P are nonspectral color samples such as might be encountered in paints. Sample G may not only be specified in terms of its coordinates, x and y (and, by subtraction of the sum of these from 1.00, z as well), but its position on the diagram permits two other things to be said about it. Its "dominant wavelength" and its "purity" may also be specified. A line drawn from the illuminant, through the sample, to the spec-

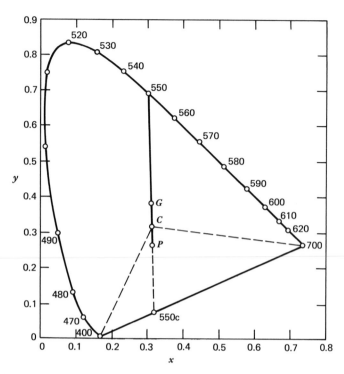

Fig. 4–7. A chromaticity diagram. The sample, *G*, lies on the line between the illuminant, *C* "daylight"), and λ550 nm. This identifies its color as yellowish green and as highly unsaturated (since it lies about 17% of the distance from *C* to the spectral curve). Sample *P* may be specified, as to dominant wavelength, as the complement of λ550 nm, hence "550c." Its purity may be judged to be about 20%, since its position is about ⅕ of the distance between Illuminant *C* and the line connecting λ400 nm and λ700 nm (the purple series). From Hardy (*267*). By permission of the Technology Press, Massachusetts Institute of Technology.

tral locus (the vertical line of the diagram) intersects the boundary of the color area at λ550 nm. This is the sample's dominant wavelength. Since λ550 nm lies in the yellowish green part of the spectrum, this reveals that the sample will appear yellowish green in daylight. Moreover, a numerical specification for the purity of the sample can be arrived at by determining, on the chromaticity diagram, the relative distances of the sample and the corresponding spectral point from the point at which the illuminant is situated. Our sample *G* lies about 17% of the distance from *C* ("white") to spectral green, and it therefore has a purity of 17%. Similarly, sample P is a purple whose specifications can be given exactly in terms of x, y, and z. However, purples lie outside the spectrum, and an artifice has to be resorted to in defining dominant wavelength and purity of all purples. The convention is to specify the wavelength of the exact complement of the purple sample, in this case $\lambda550$ nm, and to write it "550c." Perfectly saturated purples are regarded as occupying the straight line connecting the ends of the spectrum. This particular purple sample is situated about one-fifth of the way from the illuminant to the purple line; its purity turns out to be 21%.

What has been said thus far about color specification suggests that here, unlike all other situations involving measurements dependent ultimately on human observation, a point is a point and no variability surrounding it need be considered. This would be patently absurd. It is a commonplace that judgments about color matches often lead to disagreements, sometimes extreme ones. It is desirable, then, not only to set up color standards but to have some way of expressing allowable tolerances in deviations from those standards. This matter has been extensively investigated, chiefly by MacAdam (398), who has given us a set of *tolerance ellipses* that express on the tristimulus chromaticity diagram the variations in x and y that are encountered in typical color matching operations (see Figure 4–8). For each of 25 color samples, widely distributed throughout "color space," there were determined just noticeable differences of chromaticity along several diagonals of the x–y chart. D of Fig. 4–8 is a representative one. The standard deviations of these measures (multiplied by 10 to produce a more visible scale on the chart) were laid off from the color points. These distances, when connected with a continuous line, yield an ellipsoid contour the smoothed form of which is shown in Fig. 4–8. It is obvious that there are distortions of size and shifts of orientation, and for some purposes it would be preferable to have them more nearly commensurate with each other and also circular in shape. There have been ingenious efforts to bring this about and thus to arrive at a "uniform chromaticity scale diagram," but the major difficulty is that it is mathematically impossible to represent colors with equal spacing either on a plane or a uniformly curved surface. Moreover, the scaling has been done for local differences and their extrapolation to global ones is questionable.

Afterimages.   When light is allowed to fall but briefly on the retina, the excitation does not cease abruptly with the termination of the stimulus. Indeed, we have seen that this phenomenon may be put to work and that it is basic to one of the common color mixing methods (not to mention that it is basic to the entire motion picture industry!). The sensation

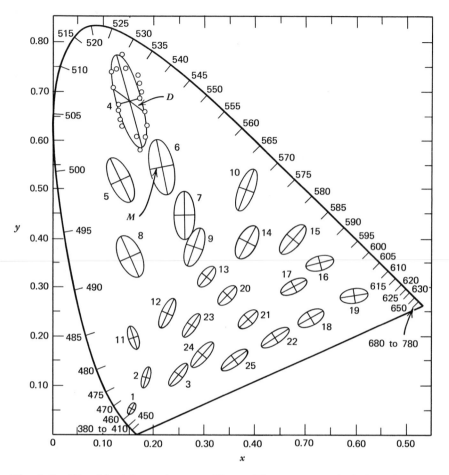

Fig. 4–8. The MacAdam tolerance ellipses. These express deviations from the standard found in typical color-matching operations. Each ellipse has been artificially increased in size by multiplying the standard deviation of the distribution of measures by a factor of 10. Courtesy of Prof. Yves LeGrand.

invariably lags behind the stimulus, sometimes not even noticeably, but under some special conditions it may persist for a matter of minutes. This means that, as a discriminator of rapid changes through time, the eye does badly. Certainly, as contrasted with the ear, which handles time superbly, the eye is an inferior organ. Its forte is the discrimination of spatial extents, and this it does with sufficient persistence to insure that spatial information will register with some precision.

Afterimages are usually classed as *positive* and *negative,* the terms being used very much as they are in photography. A positive afterimage has the same qualitative characteristics as the sensation of which it is an outgrowth. A negative afterimage, developing as a final stage of the same process, is of antagonistic quality. Sometimes afterimages are additionally classed as *homochromatic* and *complementary,* a distinction based on the hue relations observed in them rather than the brightness relations, which the "positive-negative" classification stresses. However, if black and white are thought of as antagonistic or complementary in the same way that blue and yellow or green and purple are, there is little need for the additional categorization. Moreover, homochromatic images are surely "positive" in these days of color photography and also there is considerable doubt about "complementary" afterimages really being complementary. It has been demonstrated that afterimages induced from short-wave stimuli are too red, whereas those from long-wave stimuli are displaced toward the violet, as compared with the relations existing in additive mixtures of complementary colors (*642*).

Positive images are best observed after brief intense stimulation of the dark-adapted eye. Thus, switching on and off a colored light after a prolonged stay in the dark will yield a brief image of the same hue as the light. A quick glance at the setting sun will often result in a good positive image, so intense is the stimulation. One of the best ways to observe positive afterimages is to expose the eye repeatedly to a well-lighted landscape through a fast-acting camera shutter. Here the details of differently colored and variously shaded parts of the view are seen to fade at different rates.

Negative images are not as fleeting as positive ones and thus are easy to obtain under a wide variety of conditions. However, for their favorable observation a sufficient period of initial stimulation must be given; that is, light adaptation to the stimulus is a prerequisite to the appearance of the negative afterimage. In an experiment designed to produce a negative image it is well to think of two sets of stimuli, the primary one fatiguing or "tuning" the retina, and a secondary one giving the conditions essential to its appearance. Ordinarily, one looks first at a colored light or surface, then after a half-minute or so substitutes a gray or white background on which the complementary image will develop. The secondary stimulus is obviously important. If it is identical with the primary one there is only a continuation of light adaptation, and no afterimage can appear. If it is complementary in hue to the primary stimulus high saturations of the complement are experienced. The most vivid colors possible are obtained by projecting the afterimage of one spectral color on its complement. Thus an eye previously adapted to purple light will see "supersaturated" spectral green on looking at the middle of the spectrum. It was this situation to which reference was made when, in considering the dimensions of the color spindle, it was said that the spectrum does not define saturation limits. Spectral colors, therefore, really lie inside the hue rim of the spindle.

The phenomena observed against darkness after a brief intense flash of white light are elaborate and not easy to explain as yet. The afterimage of such a stimulus is made up of a sequence of many colors, dark intervals being interspersed in the series. This is known as the "flight of colors" and may consist of successive images of purple, blue, yellow, green, red, and bluish green. This series is merely a commonly reported one, and there is no guarantee that it will be reproduced by all observers under all conditions. In fact, it is known that the number of phases observed in the flight as well as the total duration of the flight is determined by the intensity of the initial flash. Berry and Imus (68), conducting a systematic experiment on the two variables of flash intensity and flash duration, were able to show that as log $I \times t$ of the flash varies arithmetically both flight duration and the number of color changes observed vary geometrically. Others have found somewhat different empirical relations to obtain. See J. L. Brown's summary (240, p. 493). Bright flashes of colored lights yield sequences somewhat similar to those yielded by white light, and it is not at all clear why this should be so. In particular, well-saturated purples show up in the "flight." Why this color should be favored above others is likewise not clear.

The early part of the "flight" has been studied intensively and through a variety of attacks. Because so many things happen so quickly following a brilliant flash of light against darkness, the expedient has frequently been adopted of "spreading out" the successive images by employing an illuminated slit traveling in a circular path. The pulsating character of the aftereffects immediately become evident, for there are then, trailing behind the slit, various images separated by dark or, at least, relatively dark areas. Three images, distinct in time, may put in an appearance: (1) a positive image having a very short latency (about 50 msec) and duration (also about 50 msec), known as the *Hering image;* an image with a latency of 200 msec or so and of about the same duration, variously known as the *Purkinje image* and *Bidwell's ghost;* and (3) the *Hess image,* a relatively slowly developing one that may last for several seconds under optimal conditions. For most observational situations, the Hering image is more pronounced than the Purkinje, which in turn is brighter than the Hess image. Indeed, the latter is difficult to observe and has occasioned some uncertainty of description in the literature. These events are sufficiently elaborate as to warrant the suspicion that there have been too many arbitrary decisions by experimenters with respect to observational conditions. Not all features of the "flight" are equally observable in a fixed situation. Obvious variables that would make a difference are: luminance of the primary image, its duration, its wavelength composition, its area and shape, its angular subtense and rotary speed, the observer's state of adaptation, whether an adjacent viewing field is present, and so forth. One sees that a rigid classification of afterimages as to "type" performs no service.

A certain "objectivity" inheres in afterimages. Since the effect is due to adaptation of a local area of the retina, the image moves with change in direction of regard. It is a "stabilized image." Also, its apparent size varies with fixation distance. Look at a small colored square at reading distance sufficiently long to develop a negative image, then change fixation to a distant wall. The colored square now assumes huge proportions. Shift back to short focus, and the square becomes tiny.

Afterimages, both positive and negative ones, even contain within them the cues to tridimensionality. This was apparently first noted by Sir Charles Wheatstone, the inventor of the earliest device for synthesizing the visual third dimension, the mirror stereoscope. Observing afterimages derived from broad, colored lines superposed on backgrounds of their complements, he reported that he could perceive depth in the fused images from the two eyes. Recently, by a somewhat more elegant method involving the use of gas discharge tubes viewed against darkness, Ogle and Reiher (452) have shown that quite accurate localizations in the third dimension can be based on amounts of retinal disparity between two afterimages separately "branded" on the two eyes.

In the fading process an image tends to have its form changed. The corners of a square become rounded, and a complex outline is smoothed in the direction of simpler shape. This is a general tendency in unstable

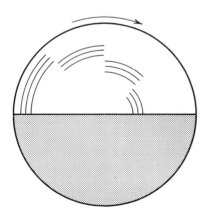

Fig. 4–9. Benham's top. Though providing only black and white stimuli in various temporal sequences colors, notably reddish yellow and blue, are seen upon rotating the disc at the proper speed. From Southall (537). By permission of the Oxford University Press and the author.

forms throughout nature, as the Gestalt psychologists have correctly noted.

Some especially curious effects may be obtained if spatial variations of the stimulus are allowed to complicate the arousal of after-images. In viewing "Benham's top" (Figure 4–9) the innermost rings take on a yellow-ish or reddish appearance, while the outer ones are seen as bluish, and yet there is given only alternate black and white stimulation. A reversal in direction of spinning moves red to the outer and blue to the inner rings. The speed of rotation is critical; above and below an optimal range of speeds the effect disappears. Another phenomenon, also revealing an undulating process to underlie the afterimage, is that known as "Char-pentier's bands." An illuminated radial slit, rotated against darkness at the rate of 2 rpm has the appearance illustrated in Figure 4–10. The pulsating nature of the afterimage, which here trails after the excitation

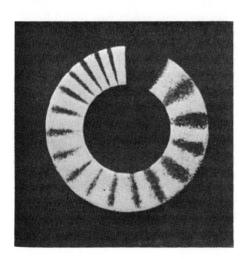

Fig. 4–10. Charpentier's bands. An illuminated slit, moving in a clock-wise direction at a rate of 2 rpm and viewed against darkness, has a reported appearance somewhat like this. The dark bands and progres-sive dimming of the trailing after-image attest the undulating char-acter of visual excitation. After McDougall (*401*).

proper like the tail of a comet, is clearly revealed by the presence of the dark bands. The size and prominence of the bands change with variations in speed, intensity, and slit width. McDougall has gathered similar evidence, from a study of stationary images, of an undulating decay of the sensation (*401*).

Peripheral Color Vision. Not only are images falling on the extreme peripheral retina vague in outline and lacking in detail, but they are likely to appear colorless as well. In fact, the peripheral retina may be said to be normally relatively color blind.

A small colored test object, brought into the visual field from its peripheral limits and moved steadily toward the point of fixation, will at first be seen as gray. At a certain visual angle it will take on hue, though not necessarily the "correct" one. Finally, approaching the center of the field, it will be clearly and correctly recognized. Different colors behave differently in this regard. Red and green are likely to appear yellowish before assuming their proper hue, while blue is rarely misidentified. The exact point of correct identification varies with a number of stimulus characteristics: wavelength, intensity, wavelength composition (saturation), size, exposure time, and contrast between test object and background, as well as conditions of retinal adaptation. The last-named factor, adaptation, is an influence of some importance. Color sensitivity of the peripheral retina is relatively greatly affected by the state of light and dark adaptation. This is particularly true of sensitivity to the short spectral waves; light adaptation brings with it a disproportionate enhancement of blue, a phenomenon not unconnected with the belief on the part of some that rods are responsible for blue vision.

It would be surprising indeed if there were no differences between the central and peripheral portions of the retina in the reception of color. The anatomical differences between the two are great enough. In addition to what we know about structural and topographical contrasts between rods and cones and their neurological connections in the retina, there are the additional facts that (1) the macular region is pigmented in such a way as to absorb short-wave energy (blue and green) more readily than the periphery does, and (2) the final projections of the two portions on the optical brain are quite different. Whereas the fovea is a relatively tiny area—the depression itself subtends an angle of less than 1°—its representation in the brain is quite large. Contrariwise, the periphery lays claim to only a relatively meager projection area in the occipital cortex.

One of the clearest ways of seeing what happens to colors as they are moved into the periphery is to note the radical shift of spectral locus occurring when a set of wavelengths is compared, at the fovea and at different positions in the periphery. Figure 4–11 shows the great shrinkage of "colorfulness" of the spectrum, expressed in terms of the relative amounts of the red, green, and blue of the colorimeter needed in foveal viewing to match colors seen at different peripheral positions (loci 15, 25, and 30 degrees out from the fovea). Clearly, the trichromatic mixture at an angle of 30 degrees into the periphery is but a pale analog of the rich color display seen in direct vision. The withdrawal of the spectrum locus curve from the axes indicates the occurrence of extreme desaturation of all colors. As the retinal test site becomes more peripheral, hue discrimination becomes progressively more difficult. The subjects on whom these curves were determined tended to call all samples either pale green or pale blue. Finally, in the region of 40 to 50 degrees from the line of sight, color confusion is complete; the dark-adapted observer reports no color distinctions at all.

There has been much speculation as to whether the color failure is one of altered photochemistry in the peripheral retina, an effect attributable

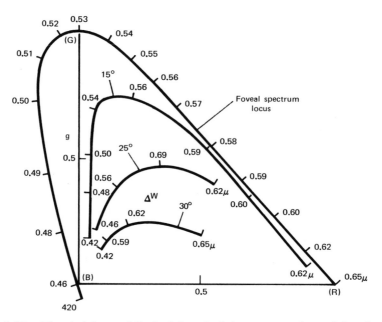

Fig. 4–11.   The shrinkage of "colorfulness" of the spectrum in peripheral vision. As colors are moved from the fovea to loci 15, 25, and 30 degrees away from it, there is a typical contraction in colorimetric locus. From Wright (*659*), utilizing the data of Moreland and Cruz (*429*). Courtesy of Pergamon Press.

to the intrusion of the rods into the color process, or a neural mechanism involving some kind of synaptic disengagement or inhibition (*429*). It is not possible, with our present dearth of information about color in the periphery, to decide among these or other possibilities. Nor are the crucial data likely to come readily to hand. There is probably no situation in sensory experimentation more fraught with observational difficulties, problems of control of variables, and, at the same time, recognition of so many variables to control.

Color Blindness.   The inability to distinguish between simple colors has long been a matter of curious interest. As early as 1777 an account was given of a certain Mr. Harris of Cumberland, England, who at the age of four, "having by accident found in the street a child's stocking, he carried it to a neighboring house to inquire for the owner; he observed that the people called it a red stocking, though he did not understand why they gave it that denomination, as he himself thought it completely described by being called a stocking" (*320*). In his later life there was abundant proof that he was indeed color-blind, and this appears to be the first recorded instance of the defect. A score of years later the anomaly was being called "Daltonism" after the famous English chemist who was himself "red blind" and who gave a remarkably accurate description of the defect. Dalton said, in 1798: "I found that persons in general distinguish six kinds of colour in the solar image. . . . To me it is quite otherwise. I see only two, or at most three, distinctions. These I should call yellow and blue, or yellow, blue and purple. My yellow comprehends the red, orange, yellow, and green of others; and my blue and purple coincides with theirs. . . . Woolen yarn, dyed crimson, or dark blue is the same to me." The English-speaking world has long since given up the intimate association of color blindness with the name of John Dalton, preferring to remember him for his part in the establishment of the atomic theory of matter, but the French name for color blindness is still "daltonisme."

There are several different kinds of color defect, ranging from simple color "weakness" to the complete incapacity to detect hue differences. The common classification of the various forms, originated by von Kries, comes out of considerations due to color theory (the trichromatic theory of Young and Helmholtz) and is, therefore, not free from prejudice. However, it accommodates well the most frequently encountered forms. The von Kries classification is as follows:

    I. Anomalous trichromia (color "weakness")
       A. Protanomaly (red weakness)
       B. Deuteranomaly (green weakness)
   II. Dichromia
       A. Red-green blindness
         1. Protanopia (red blindness)
         2. Deuteranopia (green blindness)
       B. Blue-yellow blindness
         1. Tritanopia
  III. Monochromia (total color blindness)

Concerning the first class of color disturbances, the "weaknesses," it is difficult to make general statements; too little is known about individual differences in "normal" hue sensitivity. We have already seen that different observers characteristically get different results in the spectral hue discrimination experiment. However, some people have extraordinarily high $\Delta\lambda$ values in either the red or the green region and, especially in dim illuminations, may confuse reds and greens. If low discriminability is in the red they are said to be *protanomalous,* if in the green *deuteranomalous.* There is in these cases no absolute absence of red or green sensitivity; the loss is merely a relative one, and hence higher intensities are needed to permit correct color recognition. Instances of anomalous trichromia are encountered fairly commonly, though with what frequency and to what degree it occurs in the general population we cannot know until a comprehensive program of careful color testing has been launched. The practical urge to settle the question is not as great as with the true color blindnesses, and an adequate survey has never been made. Perhaps color weakness exists in all gradations; perhaps it exists in distinct "types."

In the case of *dichromia* we can be more definite. The two forms of "red-green" blindness, *protanopia* and *deuteranopia,* occur quite commonly. Some surveys place the incidence as high as 8% of the male population, but such a figure must include many anomalous cases. Deuteranopia is the more common of the two. Red-green blindness appears to be one of those sex-linked biological traits which, like hemophilia and several others, is transmitted by the plan of alternation of generations. In successive generations it is transmitted from the male, through the female (who, however, is not likely to be afflicted with it), to the male. Thus, if one is red-green blind he has his maternal grandfather to hold responsible. Theoretically, a female may be red-green blind if both her father and her maternal grandfather are afflicted. There is still considerable disagreement among geneticists as to whether red-green dichromia involves one or two genes on the X chromosome. There may even be three. The facts of inheritance are difficult to establish, of course, in the absence of comparable sensitivity measurements over several generations, and the techniques of assessment have not remained unchanged through the years.

In a general way the two forms of red-green blindness are alike. Both protanopes and deuteranopes confuse red and green, seeing both as poorly saturated yellow. They have, then, only two colors remaining in their spectrum, yellow and blue, and hence they are "dichromats." However, each type can detect errors of matching on the part of the other, for there are important detailed differences between them. Protanopes have a "foreshortened" spectrum at the long wave end; much higher than normal intensities are required for "red" to be seen. Contrariwise, deuteranopes are able to see hue (yellow, to be sure) out to the normal limit of the red. The brightest part of the spectrum is, for the protanope, shifted about 15 nm towards the violet, as compared with the normal. Some deuteranopes appear to have their peaks of sensitivity shifted in the opposite direction, slightly toward the long wavelengths, but the majority of them do not. Their luminosity function is entirely normal. Indeed, this difference, though a slight one, has been made the basis for a further classification of deuteranopes into Type I (normal sensitivity distribution) and Type II (some short-wave loss). In the spectral region where yellow fades out and blue begins, for the majority of deuteranopes near 497 nm, there is seen a "neutral point" or narrow gray band that can be matched with white light. A similar neutral point exists for the protanope (at λ493 nm), but it is barely noticeable in the spread-out spectrum. The position of the neutral band varies a little with the method of measurement. Some "whites" used as matching stimuli are a little blue, others a little yellow, and the exact point of match will vary accordingly. These differences between the two forms, though minor, are definite and measurable and must be taken into account in any final theory of color vision. One clear way of representing them is to chart the color confusions involved on a chromaticity diagram. Figure 4–12 compares the

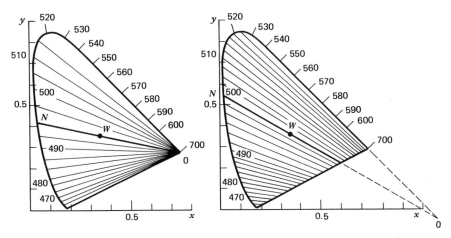

Fig. 4–12. Lines of chromaticity confusion. *N* is the neutral point, *W* the locus of the white illuminant. *O* is the "copunctal point." From LeGrand, Y. *Light, colour and vision.* New York: Wiley, 1957. (After Pitt).

chromaticity confusions of protanopes and deuteranopes. As we have previously seen, the curved line is the locus of all spectral lights as seen by the color-normal. The straight lines radiating out from 0, the *copunctal point,* are the loci of colors appearing indistinguishable in hue to these two categories of dichromats. The amount of separation of the converging lines is determined by the size of $\Delta\lambda$. As may be seen, there are 17 such steps for the protanope in these measurements and 27 for the deuteranope.

The question may fairly be asked as to how one knows what colors are seen by a color-blind individual. Mental content is reputed to be private, and color names, after all, are used by the color deficient very much as they are by those with normal color sensibility. The protanope sees a muddy yellow on looking at a red brick building, but, since the word "red" seems to be used quite universally by other people in describing bricks, the muddy yellow is for him "red" and so he calls it. Similarly with green, the particular yellow he sees on looking at the lawn is for him "green." It is because color-blinds ordinarily possess a good color vocabulary (and also because many color-normals have a poor color education!) that tests of color vision cannot be based on color naming if they are to separate successfully the color defective from the normal. The one way to be sure what colors are seen by the color-blind is to find instances of unilateral color defect, people with one normal and one color-defective eye. Such cases do exist, and a few have been competently studied (534). One of these, the case described by Graham and his associates (241), is of special interest for the wealth of exact data it yielded. These were collected over a three-year period.

Graham's uniocular dichromat, a young woman, had a normal right eye and a dichromatic left one. The normality of her right eye was established beyond doubt by color-naming and color-mixing procedures and by measures of spectral luminosity and $\Delta\lambda$ (see Figure 4–13). In all respects, save certain details of hue discrimination in the short waves, her color deficiency was identifiable as the commoner of the forms of red-green blindness, deuteranopia. To her, the spread-out spectrum appeared yellow in the long waves and blue in the short but with saturation variations in both regions. Separating the two special portions was a narrow segment, centering on 502 nm, that appeared colorless.

Quantitative experiments bore out the qualitative observations. The young lady's color-mixing requirements were simple; all spectral hues could be reproduced by some mixture of a blue of 460 nm and a red of 650 nm. The addition of a green primary gave less satisfactory settings. Color matching, carried out binocularly with what amounted to a stereoscopic colorimeter, permitted her to find a spectral equivalent with her normal eye for any color sample presented to the defective one. Since all long-wave samples appeared to be yellow of identical hue (in some saturation or other) and all short-wave samples looked blue, it is of more than ordinary interest to ask what yellow and blue they are. The answer

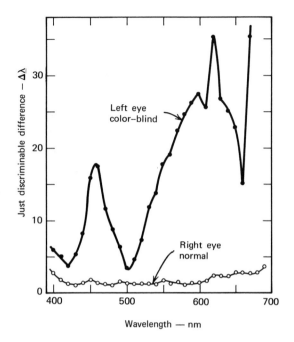

Fig. 4–13. Wavelength discrimination in color blindness. The just discriminable hue difference, $\Delta\lambda$, is plotted for the two eyes, separately, of Graham's uniocular dichromat. The right eye (normal) gave typically small values; the left eye (deuteranopic) yielded huge values, especially in the yellow, orange, and red. From Graham, Sperling, Hsia, and Coulson (*241*). Permission of the Journal Press.

was unequivocal. In this case the "yellow" end of the spectrum could be matched by λ565 nm and the "blue" end by λ470 nm. For the average "normal" observer the yellow would be a somewhat greenish one, while the blue would be well within the range selected as "pure blue" (*105*, p. 57).

An important feature of red-green blindness is the retention, despite the color defect, of normal visual acuity. Details of objects can be detected as well by protanopes and deuteranopes as by the normal. This is of the utmost significance and must mean that there are no nonfunctioning end organs in these eyes. Attempts to account for red-green color blindness on the grounds of the lack of some set of receptors should be immediately discouraged. Obviously protanopes and deuteranopes have a full complement of sense cells, as otherwise their acuity would be cut down by some constant large fraction.

The other form of dichromia, *yellow-blue blindness,* occurs rarely. Few cases have been available for careful study and measurement. However, an intensive search throughout England some years ago yielded 29 allegedly congenital tritanopes. Of these 17 proved genuine in laboratory tests and it was possible to study 7 of them intensively. The average luminosity function did not differ significantly from the normal. A neutral transition appears in the spectrum of the tritanope, as in other forms of dichromia. In those cases successfully measured in this regard there is fair agreement that the gray band occurs in the neighborhood of $\lambda570$ nm, longer waves appearing red, shorter ones green or bluish green.

Acquired color deficiencies have received a fair amount of attention (586), though it is not easy to find a valid generalization about them beyond the simple statement that disease or tissue degeneration of some kind is invariably present. Color defects can take the form of slight red-green or blue-yellow inadequacies or they can be so severe as to terminate in loss of all color discrimination. The underlying pathology can range from slight vascular insufficiencies of the retina and incipient glaucoma to retinal detachment and serious atrophy of the optic nerve.

A final form is monochromia, in which there is no hue discrimination whatever. Cases of total color blindness are rarities, only a relatively few ever having been studied with any thoroughness. The monochromat sees the entire spectrum as varying shades of gray; objects can be discriminated only on the basis of brightness differences. Total color blindness of the more frequently encountered variety is inevitably complicated by other symptoms, some of them quite incapacitating. One such accompaniment, greatly reduced acuity in normal illuminations, either forces the monochromat to seek the protection of dark glasses or requires that he adopt half closure of the lids to prevent being dazzled. More or less constant nystagmic movements, rapid sidewise and vertical oscillations of the eyeballs, vastly complicate seeing and suggest that the central retinal region is being avoided in fixation. Pupil reactions are sluggish and greatly diminished in extent.

All these characteristics of monochromia concur in pointing toward the simple explanation that the entire visual function is here mediated exclusively by the rods. All behavior is in line with the supposition that cones are either missing or failing in function. There is, of course, one way of settling the question. That is to make spectral visibility determinations on the eye of a totally color-blind individual. One such set of measurements has been made by the author (220). The visibility curve is reproduced in Figure 4–14. It will be seen that it coincides almost perfectly with the accepted scotopic curve. Thus there seems to be no doubt that vision in the monochromat is entirely the concern of rods; cones, at least

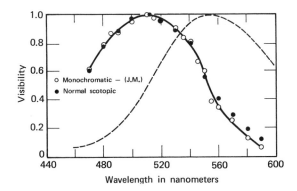

Fig. 4–14. Spectral visibility in total color blindness. The visibility curve for a monochromat is shown as a solid line. The black dots are scotopic visibility values as determined by Hecht and Williams (*287*). The normal photopic visibility curve is shown as a dotted line. From Geldard (*220*).

functional ones, are completely missing from the picture. Whether the cone structures are present is not known. Not enough eyes of this type have been subjected to postmortem histological examination, and the findings are still uncertain.

As the search for monochromats has continued, there have emerged several variations on the main theme. Indeed, there have even come to light a few cases answering to quite bizarre descriptions. Certain cases have shown symptoms, particularly peculiarities of dark adaptation, suggestive of an appreciable remnant of cone function (*533*). Others behave like true rod achromats in all details save the absence of the typical nystagmus, while some seem to have retained blue sensitivity at high luminance levels (*73*). It follows that monochromats still in possession of some degree of photopic discriminability are far less seriously inconvenienced than those who show the classical picture of photophobia, central scotoma (blind fovea), nystagmus, and generally reduced acuity.

The foregoing account of color blindnesses represents something of an oversimplification in that several additional forms, all of them rare, have been encountered since the von Kries classification was devised. Thus, there has been recognized since about 1925 a third kind of anomalous trichromacy, the "tritanomalous" type. Just as the protanomalous may be described as those who require too much red, in a red-green mixture, to match yellow, and the deuteranomalous as those needing too much green in the same circumstance, the tritanomalous use too much blue in creating standard blue-green mixtures. Tritanomaly thus lies between normal trichromacy and tritanopia and, like its partners, exists in various degrees.

Another form of yellow-blue blindness has been distinguished, a variety known as *tetartanopia*. To the tetartanope the spectrum appears red at the long wavelength end, green in the middle region, and red again in the short wavelengths. Two neutral bands separate the three segments, one at λ580 nm and the other at λ470 nm. This type contrasts with tritanopia as classically described. The tritanope has a red-green spectrum also, but typically he has a single neutral band, near λ570 nm.

If we now bring together the salient features of all kinds of color weakness and color blindness discussed we have the condensation provided by Table 4–1.

Table 4–1. Salient Features of the Various Color Defects

Type	Hue Disturbance	Approximate Spectral Peak[a]	Position of "Gray Band"
		(nm)	(nm)
Anomalous Trichromia			
Protanomaly	R-G weak	545	None
Deuteranomaly	R-G weak	560	None
Tritanomaly	Y-B weak	560	None
Dichromia			
Protanopia	Only Y-B seen	545	493
Deuteranopia	Only Y-B seen	560	497
Tritanopia	Only R-G seen	560	570
Tetartanopia	Only R-G seen	560	470, 580
Monochromia			
Rod-type	No hues seen	510	All
Cone-type	No hues seen (?)	Various	All (?)

[a] The values are necessarily approximate and modal ones; individual differences are relatively large. More detailed specifications are given by Judd *(338)*, Wald and Brown *(596)*, and Wyszecki and Stiles *(660)*.

Theories of Color Vision. In approaching the matter of suitable theories of color vision it is well to raise the more fundamental question of what can reasonably be expected of theories in general. A theory does not pretend to be a set of facts. We can only ask of a theory that it provide the possibility of interpreting in a satisfactory manner the facts already in existence and that, in addition, it be sufficiently embracing to point the way to the discovery of new facts. The color theories most actively discussed at the present time meet these criteria very inadequately, though each has its virtues and defects.

The most profitable line of thought in color theory stems from Thomas Young (1807). Beginning with the fact that all colors may be reproduced by the suitable mixture of but three primaries, Young supposed that there existed three distinct sets of nervous fibers, one set sensitive to red, one to green, and the other to violet. The expansion of the theory at the hands of Helmholtz and his followers is classic. Figure 4–15, taken from

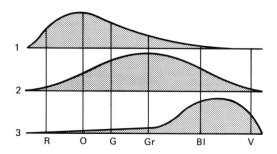

Fig. 4–15. The original excitation curves of Helmholtz. These three diagrams, entirely imaginary in their construction, "indicate something like the degree of excitation of the three kinds of fibres, No. 1 for the red-sensitive fibres, No. 2 for the green-sensitive fibres, and No. 3 for the violet-sensitive fibres" *(291,* p. 143). In the baseline designations, G is for the German "gelb" (yellow), Gr for "Grün" (green).

Helmholtz' great *Physiological Optics,* represents the degree of excitation assumed to occur in each of the three kinds of nerve fibers when stimulated by light from various parts of the spectrum. It will be noted that all fibers are responsive in some measure to all waves, though the "red" fibers (those that report "red" when stimulated) are excited most by long waves, "green" fibers respond best to those of medium length, and "violet" fibers are maximally stimulable by short waves. It should be noted that the peak of the "violet" curve is in a spectral region that may as well be called "blue." The designations "blue" and "violet" are therefore used indiscriminately in discussions of the trichromatic theory. All sensations of color result from these three simultaneous excitations, and one need only know the relative strengths of the components in the stimulus light to predict what color will be seen. Thus yellow, for example, involves approximately equal responses on the parts of the red and green fibers, a small violet component slightly desaturating the mixture. Greenish blue results from equal excitations of the green and violet fibers, a little red "graying" it. White consists of simultaneous and equal activity by all three sets of fibers.

Nowadays we know the mechanism to be three different sets of cones, each with its own light-sensitive material and its own absorption characteristics, but Young's basic idea of three additive processes is retained in the modern statement of the theory. Not all theorists have agreed, over the years, that there are three kinds of cones. Some have argued for three different photochemicals in each cone, while others hypothesize only two sets of cones (for red and green), the blue function being taken over by the rods. The principal argument for the latter position is to be found in the considerations surrounding a curious phenomenon, the so-called "dichromatism of the fovea." When tiny color patches are thrown into the fovea, providing their angular subtense is not over 20 to 30' of arc and the observer maintains rigid fixation, it is found that all colors may be accurately matched with two primaries. A third is not needed. Figure 4–16 gives the essential facts. The fovea appears to be partially color-

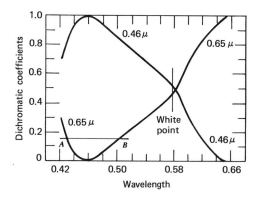

Fig. 4–16. Color sensitivity of the fovea. Relative amounts of red (650 nm) and blue (460 nm) needed by one observer to match various wavelengths when the viewing field subtends only 20' of arc. *A* and *B* are spectral colors that match each other under these conditions. A "white point" is found at 578 nm. From Brindley (*92*), after Willmer and Wright, *Nature (Lond.)*, 1945, *156B*, 119–121.

blind, blue-blind. There is a possibility that this is not strictly a condition limited to the fovea; the claim has been made that dichromatism is generally encountered whenever tiny test fields are employed, in whatever part of the retina. There are other arguments for the "blue rod," but none of them decisive. Moreover, there are many facts that fail to square with this idea, including the imposing evidence, recently acquired—and which we must confront later—that a "blue-receiving substance" is actually found to be present in some cones.

Nevertheless, the case for "small field dichromatism" (specifically, tritanopia; see above) is strengthened by experiments in which colored test patches not only confined in space but in time as well are used to assess foveal color sensitivity. Reduction of exposure time to short flashes (20 msec) and restriction to tiny fields (21′ subtense) brings about a situation where observers fully normal in color sensitivity report green to be seen as blue or blue-green, yellow and orange to look red, and yellow-green to appear to be without hue. Increase in either size or duration, or both, brings about a return of normal appearances. As in fully developed tritanopia, a red-green confusion never occurs in small-field dichromatism (619). Wald (595) has adduced evidence that foveal blue blindness is attributable to topographic rather than functional properties of the central retina. Restricting a test patch to a 7-min field that could be projected anywhere within the central 1° region of the retina, he found only the highly confined area immediately surrounding the center to be lacking in blue sensitivity. Moving the stimulus only 26 min from the fixation point brought blue vision back.

Three kinds of color-receiving elements having been assumed to exist in the retina, it would be very convenient if we could stimulate one set of cones independently of the others. As Maxwell has said (408, p. 448), "This would be truly a primary colour, whether the nerve were excited by pure or by compound light, or even by the action of pressure or disease." But the cones are so small and, especially in the center of the retina, so closely packed together and, moreover, there is so much light scattered throughout the ocular media, that it has never been found possible, in normal human vision, to direct a beam of light, however finely adjusted, on a single element. Were this possible it is still highly probable that the threshold of sensation would never be passed by so meager a stimulus. One would suppose that microscopical study of retinal tissue might reveal peculiarities of the three types of cones, but there is no "tag" whereby one set may be judged to "say red," another "green," and a third "violet" when excited. Presumably the differences are photochemical and neural, not anatomical.

However, important new measurements of the light absorption properties of retinal cones seem to settle the matter. Two independent but similar attacks on the problem have been made: (1) that by MacNichol and his associates at Johns Hopkins (404), and (2) that by Wald and Brown at Harvard (100). Although there are small differences between the two sets of findings, presumably traceable to relatively slight variations in technique, the main conclusions from the two are in agreement.

In each study, single parafoveal cones of the human eye were isolated *in vitro* and, by means of a microspectrophotometer, the relative light absorption for different spectral wavelengths was determined. The results are clear. There are at least three kinds of cones in the retina, one type maximally sensitive in the yellow (570 nm—MacNichol; 555—Wald), one peaking in the green (535, 525), and one with its high point well below the region of maximal absorption for the rods, in the blue (445, 450). The last finding is of great significance, of course. These two researchers were the first to unearth in such a positive manner a "blue cone"; the evidence goes a considerable distance to discourage the notion of "the blue vision of the rods." Moreover, such results go a long way to support the main tenet of the trichromatic theory. There seem to

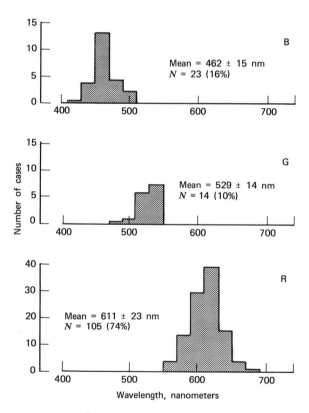

Fig. 4–17. Three types of cones in fish retina. Distributions of peak wavelengths in 142 cone receptors of the carp. From Riggs (*498*), utilizing the data of Tomita. The average red receptor responds most readily at 611 nm, the green at 529 nm, and the blue at 462 nm. Courtesy of *Perception and Psychophysics.*

be "red" cones, "green" cones, and "blue" cones, or at least three definitely differentiated receptors that could mediate these functions.

Even more direct evidence in support of the trichromatic idea comes from the ingenious work of the Japanese investigators. Tomita and his colleagues (see Riggs, *498*) have succeeded in inserting the tiniest of micro-electrodes (0.1μ diam) into individual cones of fishes, such as the carp, that are known to have color vision. Figure 4–17 displays a set of three histograms, each being a frequency distribution of peak wavelengths for an individual type of cone. In the carp, at least, it appears that the average red receptor responds best at 611 nm, the green at 529 nm, and the blue at 462 nm. Whether there is significance in the great preponderance of red cones encountered in this species it is perhaps too early to conclude.

A fourth line of study, concurring generally with all three of the foregoing but having the great advantage of being performed directly on the human eye, is represented by the bleaching experiments of Rushton and his colleagues. They employed much the same methods as those brought to bear on the adaptation phenomenon (see Chapter 3). Selective bleaching, in normal subjects, of the red and green cone substances and comparable isolation of these materials in color-blind eyes permitted measurement of the relative density of the photopigments

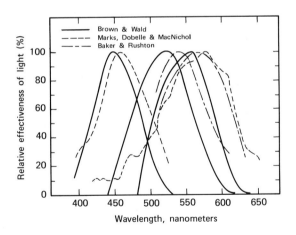

Fig. 4–18. Types of cones in the human retina. Curves derived from three experiments on absorption spectra for cones of the human eye. The bleaching experiments of Baker and Rushton (*32*) are compared with the microspectrographic experiments of Brown and Wald (*100*) and Marks, Dobelle, and MacNichol (*404*). Reproduced, by kind permission of Prof. L. A. Riggs, from *Invest. Ophthalmol.*, 1967, *6* 1–17. Copyright by The Association for Research in Ophthalmology.

throughout the spectrum. Thus, absorption curves for red and green cones were obtained (*32*), and these may be compared with those derived by other techniques (see Figure 4–18).

Despite its many advantages the trichromatic theory of Young and Helmholtz has not always had a clear field, nor have its fundamental tenets remained undisputed. Two other theories, that of Ewald Hering and that of Christine Ladd-Franklin, have contended for prominence, and the weight of opinion, especially in psychological circles, has sometimes favored one or the other. The chief objection of both Hering and Ladd-Franklin to the trichromatic theory is that it fails to recognize the cardinal fact that yellow and white are as elementary and simple in experience as are red, green, and blue. Ladd-Franklin complained that "the Young-Helmholtz theory is at most three-fifths of a colour theory." This point has been encountered before, and we have seen that it has been met, at least formally, by the demonstration that yellow and white may be "brain" processes, since they may be synthesized through binocular mixture.

Whereas the principal facts prompting the trichromatic theory were those of color mixture, it was a purely psychological consideration, the apparent unitariness of the six sensations, white, black, red, green, yellow, and blue, that served as the inspiration for Hering's theory of color vision. He supposed the primaries to be arranged in pairs and thus also arrived at the idea of a three-component mechanism. There are for Hering three complex substances, one mediating white-black vision, another accounting for red and green, and a third responsible for yellow and blue. Each substance, in its unstimulated condition, is in a state of equilibrium and yields gray (the "self-light of the retina"). The white-black material is more plentifully supplied and is more readily excitable than the others. When activated it gives purely achromatic brilliance and can be depressed in the direction of black only through light adaptation and contrast. The other two substances behave somewhat differently, having their activity either depressed (catabolism or "dissimilation") or augmented (anabolism or "assimilation") by the action of light. The red-green substance yields red when "torn down" by light, and green when "built up." In a similar fashion, dissimilation produces yellow in the yellow-blue substance, while assimilation results in blue. Any light, whatever its spectral composition, will necessarily excite all three of the compound substances in varying degree, and the single sensation elicited will be the resultant of the three processes acting jointly, as in the trichromatic theory.

Hering was little concerned about the location of his metabolic substances, always referring vaguely to the *Netzhaut*, the entire optical nervous apparatus, as responsible for light reception and processing. It remained for others to develop thinking along these lines. The first was Troland (583), who made a valiant attempt to deal realistically with the metabolic substances by housing them in cones and trying to square their operation with the main facts of color vision; then Hurvich and Jameson (323) expended unremitting energy over the years in a masterful effort to quantify the phenomena most crucial for the opponent-process type of theory. They succeeded remarkably well, so well that a spate of "zone" or "stage" theories (*vide infra*) has been created, many of them assuming the existence of a "balanced-opposites" mechanism at some level of the visual pathway, if not in the receptors themselves.

Since the components of Hering's three color processes are arranged in antagonistic pairs, it is possible to employ a null method in ascertaining their basic spectral properties. How much bluish green has to be added to primary (bluish) red, at each of the long-wave positions in the spectrum, to eliminate all hue? Similarly, how much blue is required to counteract each of the yellows? Systematic exploration of the spectrum with such cancellation stimuli yields "chromatic valence" curves. Suitably treated, these agree tolerably well with the CIE "standard observer" (see Figure 4–6). The Hurvich-Jameson treatment also provides a basis for the facts of spectral luminosity, wavelength and saturation discrimination, the photochromatic interval, details of the Bezold-Brücke effect, and even the blue blindness of the central fovea. Moreover, the theory has been given a plausible underlying neurology by linking it to "receptive field" and lateral inhibition phenomena.

For many years, Hering's theory was under the cloud of seeming to demand something that was physiologically improbable—the anabolism of a visual substance through direct action of an external stimulus. But Hering was not primarily interested in the receptor materials (*Empfangs-stoffe*); he cut through to the neural visual response process (*Sehsubstanz*) energized by the photosensitive material. It seems clear that Hering was thinking well ahead of his generation in this respect, for now we know with certainty that there can be and are two opposed modes of neural response often linked in the same system. Under some conditions, excitation occurs in some fibers, inhibition in others. Indeed, the two opposed processes may occur in one and the same fiber under different conditions. This is the interpretation that follows if we allow ourselves to think of any increase in spike discharge frequency (over the resting or "spontaneous" rate) as excitation and any reduction below that level as inhibition.

The Ladd-Franklin theory represents in a sense a compromise, being trichromatic for mixture purposes but tetrachromatic in its insistence on the primacy of yellow. The distinctive feature of this theory is the stress it lays upon the possible development of the color sense; it is therefore sometimes spoken of as a "genetic" theory of color vision.

It is supposed that our present capacity to discern colors has evolved from a primitive mode of seeing in which only blacks, whites, and grays could be discriminated. Vision was mediated exclusively by a white "mother substance" which, in two subsequent cleavages, has first split into blue and yellow materials, and then the yellow has further differentiated into red and green substances. The end products of this evolution are thus the components of the trichromatic theory: red, green, and blue. It should not surprise us if the theory is able to interpret color mixture data adequately.

The greatest appeal of the Ladd-Franklin theory lies in its apparent ease of interpretation of the facts of color blindness and those of the retinal color zones. Red-green color blindness would appear to be an atavistic phenomenon, a "throwback" to a more primitive stage of color vision in which only blue and yellow are present. But why, then, the distinct differences between protanopia and deuteranopia? Are there two atavistic paths—and leading to what variations of the yellow substance?

The color "zones" might reasonably represent the present state of evolution of the color sense. The primitive white substance is present throughout the entire retina, and hence brightness discrimination occurs out to the limits of the visual field. The blue and yellow substances, being the first decomposition products, have not yet invaded the extreme periphery but are more extensively distributed than the red and green, which, being relatively recent acquisitions, are restricted to the inner zone. It would be convenient for the theory if the red and green fields were more nearly coincident and if the limits for blue and yellow similarly fell together.

A more serious difficulty arises from the failure to "house" the sensitive substances. The theory does not lend itself to the picture of discrete types of cones. This in itself is not necessarily bad, but the alternative is to suppose that three or more different kinds of messages may be conveyed over identical nerve fibers. This does violence to some very well-established neurological ideas which, until we are in possession of better ones, we would do well not to discard.

Certain color phenomena are not handled at all adequately by any existing theory. The satisfactory explanation of the common varieties of color blindness has, in particular, been a stumbling block. It will not do to assume, as some proponents of the Hering theory have done, that R-G blindness represents simply the absence of the R-G substance. Again, why protanopia and deuteranopia? The R-G substance cannot be "missing" now one way and now another. Acuity, we have noted, is normal; presumably nothing is missing.

If an explanation of color blindness is to be based on a purely photo-chemical mechanism the most nearly adequate one would appear to be that of Fick (195). Reasoning within the framework of the Young-Helmholtz theory, he supposed protanopia to result from the substitution in the "red" cones of the green receiving substance with, however, a retention by the fibers attached to the red cones of their normal capacity to report "red." There would then be a shortening of the spectrum at the long-wave end, and the red cones would respond simultaneously with, and to the same extent as, the normal green cones. Neither "red" nor "green" could be reported in isolation, and all spectral lights down to about λ500 nm would appear yellowish. Similarly, deuteranopia involves the substitution in the "green" cones of the red receiving material. No shortening of the spectrum would be occasioned, and, owing to the manner of crossing of the red and blue curves, an appreciable "gray band" should appear in the deuteranopic spectrum in the region of λ500 nm. As with the protanope, all visible waves longer than this should yield yellow, since there is no way in which the "green" and "red" could be elicited singly.

This special modification of the trichromatic theory explains the two forms of R-G blindness tolerably well and is clearly in advance of all other color theories in this regard. A difficulty appears, however, when one attempts to relate it to the quantitative facts of spectral luminosity in red-green blindness. There is no trouble with deuteranopia, at least the classical Type I. The protanope, however, sees the spectrum as too bright in the blue and violet and too dim in the long waves to accommo-date the theory precisely, however ingenious it may be. Of course, the facts have been changing since Fick interpreted them. Indeed, the facts of spectral luminosity have changed significantly enough to make a differ-ence to theory. Graham and his colleagues (240, pp. 408–420; 241), by relieving the measurement problem of relative luminosity coefficients and dealing directly with absolute losses of sensitivity, have shown that some deuteranopes, at least, do lose luminosity in the green and blue. To account for the quantitative variations found in such cases they have made good use of the Fick type of substitution theory. With its aid they are able to explain sensitivity fluctuations in the two common kinds of dichromia and keep the overall interpretation consistent with trichromatic theory.

There is no necessity for adhering to the idea of a strictly retinal mechanism in attempting to account for color phenomena. It is perhaps short-sighted of the classical theories of color vision that they have so little to do with the optical pathway and optical brain. It is as though these organs were not participants in the visual response. One theory, which is reasonably adequate to the facts of color blindness, takes some account of processes other than the photochemical ones of the retinal receptors. This is the formulation of G. E. Müller (338). It is made up of the chief elements of the Young-Helmholtz and Hering theories and is sometimes spoken of as a "zone" or "stage" theory of color vision. The first stage is the photochemical one of light reception by the cones. For this initial step Müller supposes the primaries of the Young-Helmholtz theory (red, green, violet) to be present. A second stage is chemical and involves two pairs of antagonistic processes, the red-green and yellow-blue balanced reactions of the Hering theory. The final stage is that of excitation of the optic nerve; here may be aroused the six "psychological primaries": red, yellow, green, blue, black, and white.

Stage theories, until quite recently, have more nearly represented exercises in logic than collections of testable hypotheses. Now, overnight, so to speak, neurophysiological and photochemical facts have come flooding in upon us, and many ideas that formerly would have remained in the realm of conjecture may be weighed for their probable correctness.

What are the facts that have such an important bearing on theory? Chiefly, those concerning the three retinal photochemicals—it is now certain that the trichromatic theory was essentially correct about the materials in the cones—and those concerning responses of retinal bipolar and ganglion cells and other nerve cells higher in the optical pathway. Let us examine some of the findings about the nervous connections to the cones.

When, in Chapter 3, we were considering the basic electrical phenomena of the eye, it was observed that a "generator potential" was created in the receptor and that this triggered a whole catenary series of changes in the afferent pathway. As early as 1953 the Swedish investigator, Svaetichin, obtained graded direct current potentials from the retina that were maintained steadily so long as a light stimulus continued to act. These he got with tiny pipette electrodes plunged into the fish retina, contacting, as he thought, the end organs themselves. Although it is now believed that this was an error—he must have been recording from cells just proximal to the cones—some very interesting records were forthcoming, and the validity of these has been confirmed by many different investigators in subsequent experiments (576; 490, Chapter 4). The direction of electrical change (whether depolarization or hyperpolarization) and its amount proved to be a function of the wavelength of the stimulating light. Some electrode placements very close to the cones showed a hyperpolarization to light from any part of the spectrum but with a maximal response in the middle wavelengths, around 575 nm. This suggests the luminosity function, of course. Other cells situated a little deeper—bipolars, perhaps—gave wavelength-specific responses, and it is these that have the greatest significance for color theory. Some cells shifted electrically in one direction to red light and in the opposite to green. Some gave positive shifts to yellow and negative shifts to blue.

It is not only the retinae of lower forms, like fish, frogs, and turtles, that display these properties. Some work has been done on the monkey retina and, more especially, on individual fibers of the ascending tracts. In particular, there has been careful work on the lateral geniculate nucleus, the optic nerve's great relay station. DeValois and his co-workers (*159*, *2*) have studied assiduously the macaque monkey and not only have found fibers there that respond with spikes very much as Svaetichin's retinal cells did with slow potentials but they were also able to classify different cells of the lateral geniculate nucleus on the basis of their responses to spectral colors. As with the fish retina, there are cells that apparently report only brightness, for they respond with an increase of spike frequency to all wavelengths, most to the center of the spectrum. These so-called "nonopponent" cells have a response that agrees well both with the CIE photopic luminosity function and, from behavioral tests, with the animal's own spectral brightness curve.

There are four kinds of "opponent" cells: $+R-G$ (red excitatory, green inhibitory), $+G-R$, $+Y-B$, and $+B-Y$. These four obviously constitute the color system of the macaque monkey at a point close to the final reporting station and, because the relations involved are those of a tetrachromatic opponent-type theory, it has to be assumed that what started out in the receptor organ as a trichromatic system has become tetrachromatic on its way up the visual afferent tract. Indeed, it apparently became tetrachromatic immediately upon leaving the cones.

There are some data (and much more conjecture) available on this point. Abramov (*2*) has demonstrated how each of the four spectrally opponent cells must be connected with two of the three kinds of cones. The $+R-G$ and $+G-R$ cells receive their inputs from the "red" ($\lambda570$ nm peak) and "green" ($\lambda535$ nm peak) cones. The former is excitatory to the $+R-G$ cell and inhibitory to the $+G-R$; the latter excites the $+G-R$ but inhibits the $+R-G$. The relative contributions of the two materials will decide the balance struck by the two kinds of cells which, in turn, make their summed contribution to the overall sensory response. An analogous set of relations holds for the "blue" ($\lambda445$ nm peak) and "red" ($\lambda570$ nm peak) as they affect differentially the $+Y-B$ and $+B-Y$ cells.

With the wealth of visual data at hand and the complexity of some of the phenomena of color, there is naturally much yet to be worked out in such a scheme. Nor is there anything like complete agreement as yet about some of the details discussed above. But the significant thing is that two "classical" theories of color vision appear to have come together mutually to aid and abet each other. Even a very short time ago it could hardly have been predicted that the trichromatic theory and the tetrachromatic theory, both of which had a long history of having laid exclusive claim to the color domain, would quite abruptly find themselves to be compatible with each other and to have become harmonious neighbors in a single stage theory of color vision. As Riggs has appropriately observed (*498*, p. 8), ". . . Helmholtz and Hering rule separate regions that are only a fraction of a millimeter apart."

5
Visual Acuity and Contrast

Spatial Visual Acuity. Under usual conditions of illumination an object may be seen with the greatest distinctness if we "turn our eyes" toward it, that is, if the image is made to fall on the fovea. Peripheral regions of the retina have little power to discriminate particulars of form. The appearance of the whole visual field has been likened to a "picture the details of which are finely etched in the center as in a steel engraving while the outlying parts are only roughly sketched in as in a charcoal drawing."

Visual acuity, the capacity of the eye to resolve details, thus normally varies greatly in different regions of the retina. The precise definition of acuity is given in terms of the reciprocal of the angular distance separating two contours when they are just distinguishable as two. Because it conveniently represents average performance of the "good" eye, the standard subtense on which the unit is based is taken to be one minute of arc. A person with normal acuity would be able to discern as distinct two points separated by as little as 1' of arc and, if this represented his best performance, his acuity would be 1.0. Actually, some eyes have a resolving power of as much as 2.0 or even 3.0.

Test objects most commonly used for determining visual acuity are the Snellen letters (the familiar letter chart of the oculist's office), Landolt rings (broken circles), ruled gratings, and variations of these. The convention is to employ as a standard an object subtending a 5' angle, the detail to be discriminated being 1' in width. Ideally, the 5:1 ratio should be maintained throughout a set of different-sized test objects. With block letters, such as those of the Snellen series, this requirement can only be approximated, since only a circular form could meet it rigidly. The Landolt "broken circles" (or the Ferree-Rand "double broken circles") are superior and should in time supplant the Snellen letters. Gratings consist of glass plates having equidistant parallel lines ruled on them; their great advantage lies in the fact that transmitted rather than reflected light may be used readily with them. Grids and checkerboard designs have been employed by some. Acuity measurements have also been made with single fine wires suspended in a uniformly illuminated field, the thinnest wire to be resolved determining the acuity level. Clearly, the concept of acuity has here been given a different definition, there being no interspace to be discriminated, and we should not expect exact agreement between results gained by the two methods. Indeed, experiment proves the results to differ in the two cases. Measures of the *minimum visible* (single-fine-line technique) typically show the least width of line that can be detected to subtend an angle of the order of 1″. Acuity as measured by the *minimum separable* (interspace between contours) requires an angle of the order of 1′, as we have seen.

Still other kinds of visual tasks may be used as a basis for measuring acuity. *Vernier acuity* involves the detection of a break in a single vertical line, the displacement being a lateral one. The smallest "jog" in the line that can be seen thus establishes the magnitude of vernier acuity. Acuteness of vision measured in this way is more nearly related to the minimum visible than to the minimum separable, giving optimal values around 5 to 10″ of arc. *Stereoscopic acuity* brings in the binocular relation. It is defined in terms of the least perceptible depth displacement of two objects. The objects may be presented separately to the two eyes, as in the stereoscope, or real distance separations may be effected, as in the "two-rod" (Howard-Dolman) test, familiar as a test for depth perception in the armed services. Visual acuity determined stereoscopically gives optimal values close to those for monocular vernier acuity (5 to 10″ of arc), though the psychophysiological processes concerned in the two are patently different. In a well-controlled experiment employing a stereoscope to present a stationary vertical line to the left eye and a movable one to the right, Mueller and Lloyd (*435*) found stereoscopic acuity to vary systematically with intensity of illumination, averaging around 10″ of arc for high intensities and about 25″ for low.

It is clear that "acuity" is a name for a general concept, rather than for a specific procedural process. Test stimuli may be of almost any shape, may consist of bright objects viewed against dark surrounds, the reverse, or some brightness arrangement between (e.g., two grays providing low contrast). The stimulus object may be supplemented by instructions to the observer that call for *resolution,* discriminating two or more parts from each other, or *recognition,* naming the object, or simple *detection,* merely indicating whether an object is present, or *localization,* reporting where in the field the object appears. Thus the specification of acuity must necessarily contain both a statement concerning the physical conditions of the test and one denoting the observer's task.

Acuity, however measured, varies with illumination in an interesting way. We know from everyday experience that small print, difficult to discern in dim light, may be read with ease under higher illumination. The relation has been worked out systematically, and the data gathered by Koenig, at the turn of the last century, are still standard. They are reproduced in Figure 5–1. The S-shaped curve should by now be sug-

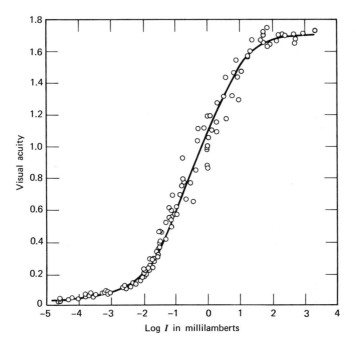

Fig. 5–1. Relation between visual acuity and illumination intensity, according to the data of Koenig (1897). The observer's task was to recognize a hook-shaped test object and report its orientation. From Hecht (*279*). By permission of the Howe Laboratory of Ophthalmology, Harvard University.

gestive. As suspected, the function is really compounded of two. The lower branch is representative of rod mediation; above an acuity of about 0.1 the cones take over the task.

One interpretation that accords well with other phases of visual theory requires us to suppose that both rods and cones vary among themselves with respect to threshold. At the lowest illuminations only a few rods are stimulated. Since they presumably have a "chance" distribution (with respect to threshold), this amounts to a sparse functional population. If the active elements are far apart the resolving power must be poor, just as in a "grainy" photographic film in which the elements are relatively far apart. As light intensity is increased, more and more rods have their thresholds passed, bringing a greater number into play and thus reducing the average distance between functioning receptors. At a certain point (acuity of 0.1, approximately) the cones enter the picture and shortly are exclusively mediating the visual differential response. Vision is now best foveally, and it improves steadily with continued increase in illumination. Only when the thresholds of all cones have been passed will a further intensity increase be ineffective. If illumination is extremely high, reflectance from all objects, "black" and "white" alike, will be great. Receptors can no longer function differentially, all will be stimulated maximally, and "glare" will be the result. The inability to discern any objects when subjected to the dazzling light of a snow field in the full sun is a case in point.

The mechanism assumed by this account is, of course, identical with that postulated for intensity discrimination. And why not? Visual acuity may be thought of as a special case of intensity discrimination. To test the resolving power of the eye one sets up a situation which requires the subject to make a darkness-lightness judgment: to detect the light interspace between two dark contours, to distinguish a dark line against a bright background, to tell when two points of light, seen in the dark, fuse into one or break apart, etc. Any interpretation of visual acuity, to be acceptable, must be in full accord with one's basic account of intensity discrimination.

The above account makes a basic assumption that gets less and less tenable, to be sure, as we learn more about the chain of neural events between receptor and cortex. In settling upon variation of "grain" of the retinal mosaic as the mechanism by which the essential change takes place, there is the implication that something like a one-for-one relation obtains in the afferent pathway, that the nervous pathway is simply an inert conductor. We cannot stop to examine this assumption in detail at this point; it is a question of some generality, and we shall directly encounter it in the field of cutaneous sensitivity. But let us note that nowadays the facts are amassing rapidly in support of the contention that the afferent paths are remarkable, first, for the amount of convergence of signals that takes place at successive relay stations en route to the cortex and, second, for the interactions, both facilitatory and inhibitory, that are possible at any nervous center.

If only the convergence principle were invoked, the explanation of varying visual acuity with changes of illumination would also take a form that relies upon the probability principle. Assuming that all receptors are equal in sensitivity and may be discharged whenever they "catch" a quantum of light, the probability would be that, at low luminance levels, sufficient excitation to activate a center could only come from receptors dispersed over a relatively wide retinal area. At higher luminance levels, there is a greater density of quantum catch, and a more circumscribed peripheral area would trigger the central response. Acuity would be better. This theory, of course, really substitutes a variable "neural grain" for a peripheral one.

There has been much speculation concerning the anatomical basis of visual acuity (*603, 516*). Measurements of the diameter of foveal cones yield suggestive values. According to Polyak's determinations (*478*) the average cone in the center of the fovea centralis is of such size as to subtend a visual angle of 24″, though some are even a little smaller. This value includes the sheath separating adjacent cones. For the minimum separable such a value would serve. It need only be assumed that between two groups of stimulated cones there are two or three unstimulated rows. For the minimum visible, however, the cone diameters are too great to permit of an explanation in terms of end-organ separation.

As matters now stand this kind of thinking about visual acuity proves to be quite unprofitable. One need only recall the many events transpiring between the entrance of light rays into the eye and their final representation in the brain to see that the geometrical features of a test object are unlikely to be preserved without change throughout this elaborate process. To begin with, there is not even complete preservation of the optical image within the eyeball itself. A variety of influences operate to blur it. The eye, in common with most optical instruments, is subject to both chromatic and spherical aberration. Neither of these is of great consequence under ordinary conditions of seeing. But in dim illuminations or in night vision, especially, when the pupil is greatly dilated and rays passing through the peripheral portions of the lens and cornea fail to be screened out, spherical aberration may produce some blurring of the retinal image. Chromatic aberration, in accordance with which lights of different wavelength get focused at different depths in the ocular media, is less serious in the eye than in some other optical instruments by reason of the fact that the yellow macular pigment tends to block the most disturbing rays, those from the blue and violet.

A far more serious source of image distortion than either spherical or chromatic aberration is *diffraction*. For self-luminous points of light in the visual field it is inevitable that an appreciable portion of the beam will deviate from the geometrical path as the eye is traversed. A point of light is always represented at the retina by a series of concentric rings. Figure 5-2 shows how a thin luminous line, subtending at the eye an

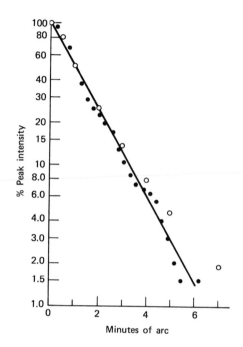

Fig. 5–2. The line-spread function of the eye. Note that the ordinate is plotted as a logarithmic series. From Westheimer, G. *Journal of the Optical Society of America,* 1963, *53,* 91; after Flament (circles) and Westheimer and Campbell (dots).

angle of 1.5′, distributes its energy over a retinal area subtending more than 6′. This graph is known as the *line-spread function,* a logarithmic relation, in ocular diffraction. The consequence of the operation of this principle is that all small luminous stimuli (from about 10″ of arc down) are about 1.5′ in size. There are no smaller visual objects. This fact again renders irrelevant the question of whether the fineness of the retinal mosaic can determine, in an absolute manner, the level of acuity. The thinnest foveal cones have an estimated subtense in the neighborhood of 20 to 30″ (2.0 to 2.3 μ diam), according to reliable calculations (*497*), and at least three closely packed cones must be covered by the smallest diffraction pattern.

As though these factors making for indistinctness of the image were not enough, the entire eyeball, it turns out, is only unstably held in position. The line of regard, in fixating an object, actually dances about slightly. Careful measurements of the eye's fixational movements ("physiological nystagmus," it is sometimes called) have been made by Riggs (491), using an ingenious technique in which a plane mirror mounted on a contact lens is the main element in a sensitive optical lever. Four different kinds of motion are found to be going on when the eyes are being "held still." There are: (1) very rapid movements occurring at frequencies ranging from 30 to 70 per second. These rarely embrace excursions of as much as 1' of arc, having an average extent of 17.5", but may occasionally be as large as 2' of arc; (2) relatively slow motions, highly variable from moment to moment and from one subject to another, occurring generally 2 to 5 times a second and ranging from 1' to 5' in extent; (3) slow drifts extending as much as 5' in any direction and on which both of the above described motions are superposed; and (4) irregular rapid jerks, ranging from 2.2' to 25.8' of arc (average of 5.6'). These jerky motions often seem to be compensatory for the slow drifts. If all these movements of the eye are now combined it is seen that "fixation" of the eye is a very lively event and must be thought of in dynamic, rather than static, terms. In fact, it would appear that the eye is never really motionless. Over a period of 3 to 4 sec, even though their owner is making every effort to maintain steady fixation, the eyes are

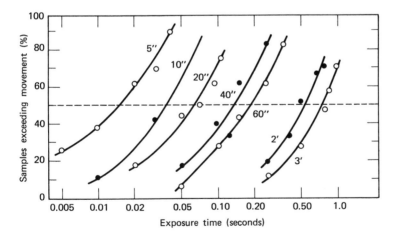

Fig. 5–3.   Relative proportions of eye-movement records revealing a given amount of motion as a function of the duration of the record. Each point represents 50 samples. From Riggs, Armington, and Ratliff, *Journal of the Optical Society of America*, 1954, 44, 321.

totaling up movement that amounts to 10 to 20′ of arc. In all this activity light from any given point of an object being "fixated" must be impinging successively on 25 to 50 different receptor cells and can be expected to remain on one cone for only a few hundredths of a second, at most. Another way of depicting the eye movements of physiological nystagmus is through the family of curves in Figure 5–3, which shows the magnitudes of typical excursions of the retinal image, for exposure periods of different duration, when the observer is making every effort to hold his eyes steady.

Since all this "jitter" in the viewing situation would seem to be highly detrimental to acuity, it would be interesting to know what would happen if the eyeball could be immobilized and the line of regard fixed on a single point in the visual field. Nothing short of paralysis of all six external eye muscles could bring this about, of course, but there are ways of rendering motionless the image of the retina, which amounts to the same thing optically. Two major techniques have been developed: (1) the "optical stalk" approach, devised in the laboratory of the British

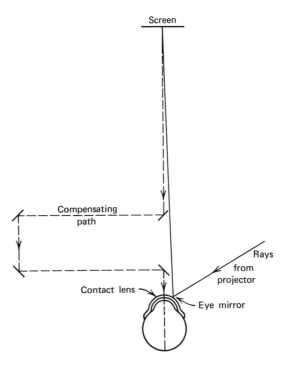

Fig. 5–4. One system for stabilizing the retinal image. From Riggs et al. (*500*). Courtesy of *The Journal of the Optical Society of America*.

physicist, Ditchburn, and (2) the "compensated optical path" procedure of the American psychologist, Riggs.

Ditchburn's technique is straightforward and simple in conception (*166*). A fitted plastic contact lens has protruding from it, at a point opposite to the corneal-scleral junction, a plastic stalk that supports a reticle or other test object that is seen directly through the contact lens. The entire apparatus, being made as a single rigid unit of very light materials and adhering through good fitting to the contours of the cornea and sclera, moves with the eye. The retinal image is thus always fixed in one place. The test object may be elaborate; it may consist even of a tiny projection system replete with lamp.

The Riggs method is a bit more complicated in principle but achieves the same result. Additionally, because somewhat less weight is involved in the contact lens, the apparatus is less subject to slippage. The scheme is diagrammed in Figure 5–4. A plane mirror is built into a contact lens, and this reflects to a screen the projected image of a test object. Through the same contact lens the screen is viewed over a compensating path that effectively doubles the distance from eye to screen. The geometry of the situation is such—doubling of the angle of beam rotations at the mirror—that the compensating path exactly cancels image deviations resulting from eye movements and thus renders motionless the retinal image, whatever the eyeball may do. With such a system it is also possible, of course, to exaggerate retinal movements as well as diminish or cancel them.

Experiments with the stopped image technique show that, for detec-

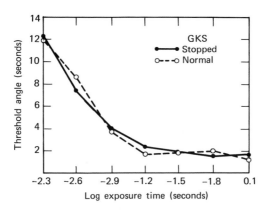

Fig. 5–5. Minimal subtense of a dark line viewed against a luminous field for threshold detection by a single observer. The stopped-image condition is compared with that involving normal eye movements. From Riggs (*497*) after Keesey, *Journal of the Optical Society of America*, 1960, 50, 769–774.

tion of a thin line, for resolution or localization of a test object, or even for stereoscopic discrimination, movement neither enhances nor impairs acuity, providing the observer's judgment is rendered promptly (0.2 sec or less) upon presentation of the test object. Ordinarily it is, of course. Figure 5–5 shows a pair of threshold curves for a single observer in an experiment in which the task was to detect the presence of a single black line against a luminous field. Whether the image was stopped by the Riggs compensation technique or the test object was viewed with the complications of normal eye movements, the results proved to be the same.

There is one important difference between the stopped and unstopped views. After a short period of exposure has elapsed, the motionless image begins to fade precipitously. After 3 to 6 sec it may disappear altogether, especially if the field is simple in organization. The constitution of the field is important, as has been demonstrated in many different ways (482). Colored portions are likely to fade more rapidly than hueless ones. Whole networks of contours are likely to drop out and others remain. Deterioration of complex figures seems to follow rules strongly suggestive of those governing Gestalt "unit formation." Nor does a field simply become obliterated and remain so. Portions may reappear and alternate with other components in a manner not unlike that occurring in the binocular "rivalry" situation.

The fading and revival phenomena characterizing stopped images is perhaps best likened to the similar appearances observable in the periphery of the eye when fixation is maintained as rigidly as possible while viewing linoleum and wallpaper patterns. Peripheral "blanking out" in these instances is a familiar effect and one that has been known in the scientific literature since its description by Troxler in 1804 (see 121). Indeed, it has been suggested that we are dealing, in the stopped foveal image, with a special case of the general conditions responsible for the Troxler effect. In the periphery gross receptor distribution simply renders physiological nystagmus incapable of bringing about renewal of fresh stimulation, as it normally does at the eye's center, where even such tiny movements sweep the image over many consecutive end organs.

Temporal Acuity; Flicker. When a series of equally spaced flashes strikes the retina, flicker is likely to result. Whether flicker will be seen and what its appearance will be are primarily determined by the flash frequency. When it is low the contrast between darkness and the flash is great. As frequency is increased there is an apparent reduction in contrast, and at a sufficiently high rate of repetition the individual flashes will not be sensed at all. The point at which flicker just disappears is known as the *critical fusion frequency* (CFF). It is convenient to provide the flashes by interrupting a steady light with a sectored disc and, by convention, one having equal open and closed sectors. In making a critical fusion frequency determination it is necessary only to increase disc speed until the last vestige of flicker has just been eliminated, leaving a smooth and steady field, and express frequency in terms of the number of flashes (or cycles of light and dark) per second.

Critical fusion frequency proves to be a variable quantity, though precisely measurable for a given set of conditions. It depends upon the intensity of the stimulus, the waveform of the flickering light cycle (whether rectangular, sawtooth, clipped, etc.), the "light-time fraction" (the relative durations of light and darkness in a cycle), overall duration of the flickering stimulus, wavelength composition, stimulus size, the state of adaptation of the eye, the retinal locus of the image, whether or not there is excitation of neighboring retinal areas, and probably other factors. If all but one of these variables is held constant and the effect of the remaining one is systematically investigated, accurately reproducible curves may be obtained. The relation between fusion frequency and intensity of illumination is of special interest and has been determined

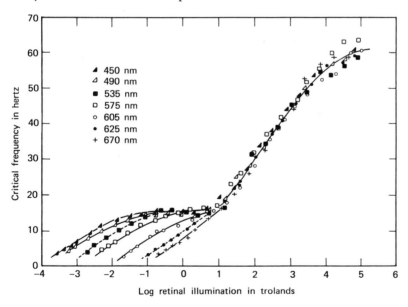

Fig. 5–6. The relation between critical frequency of fusion, in hertz (flashes), and intensity of illumination, in trolands, for seven different spectral regions. From Hecht and Shlaer *(284)*. By permission of the Rockefeller Institute for Research and Dr. Shlaer.

many times. Figure 5–6 gives some typical results. This graph has the additional advantages of showing the dependence on wavelength and the now familiar characteristic break between the rod and cone segments of the function. The main relationship, however, is that between intensity (log I) and fusion frequency. From about 15 flashes per second, the practical lower limit at which fusion may be maintained with the dimmest foveal light, to about 60 flashes per second, above which flicker ordinarily is not detected even in the brightest test patch, there is an approximately linear relation with log I. A series of such lines obtains for lower intensities visible in the periphery, ranging upwards from about 3 flashes. It was originally thought that the relation was a strictly logarithmic one, and the Ferry-Porter law, formulated in 1892, stated this to be the case. We now see that this relation, like that for $\Delta I/I$, has a curvilinear form.

There is an impressive history of research on the parameters surrounding flicker fusion, a story so involved as to be well beyond our present purposes to narrate. See the excellent systematic resume by J. L. Brown (*240*, Chapter 10). Despite the intricacy of relations between variables, it is nevertheless possible to arrive at some generalities; we shall look at the chief conclusions about certain of the major influences affecting CFF.

Stimulus size and retinal locus are conveniently considered together. Obviously, change in size implies concomitant change in place, and it is doubtless the familiar local differences in retinal structure and function that prevent CFF and image size from being related in a simple manner. As it is, there is ample evidence that CFF is, in part, determined by stimulus size. For a considerable range of distances outward from the fovea and over a range of luminances embracing at least a 1000:1 ratio, CFF is proportional to the logarithm of the area. Whether this is exclusively a matter of increasingly enhancing the excitation process as more reacting units are brought into play (*spatial summation*) or a question of expanding contours having more to say about the result is not yet certain. Interestingly, it is possible to darken large portions of the central part of a test field, as much as two-thirds of it, without reducing CFF (*503*).

Any generalization about the dependence of CFF on the retinal location of the flickering test light is difficult to acquire, for absolute stimulus area becomes a consideration immediately. According to the "classic" study of Creed and Ruch (*130*), CFF is always higher at the fovea than in the periphery for *small* fields—they explored with a relatively tiny 12′ test field—whereas the relation may be reversed for *large* ones (at least above 2°). The reason for this perhaps becomes obvious when one considers the enhancement of sensitivity occasioned by increasing amounts of spatial summation in the peripheral part of the retina. A review of the host of flicker experiments performed over the past forty years fails to yield a clear consensus on the CFF-retinal locus problem, chiefly because of the great variety of arbitrary conditions imposed by experimenters in this complex research area. One of the chief faults has been the failure to control the pupil; the pupillary reflex is regulated far less by the outer retina than by the macular region. Another seemingly accidentally applied variable is the surround, sometimes used to control adaptation, at other times to investigate lateral interaction effects.

Whereas, as has been noted, the convention in making CFF measurements is to have regularly spaced "square-wave" (abrupt onset and offset) pulses with a light-time fraction of 0.5, both stimulus features are capable of considerable variation. The flash need be neither abrupt nor exactly half the light-dark cycle in duration. One of the earliest discoveries connected with intermittent light stimulation concerned the light-time fraction. The *Talbot-Plateau Law* states that a periodically flickering light, when the flashes are repeated at a sufficiently high rate as to fuse, yields an impression that is the mean of the periodic impressions. Thus, equally long light and dark phases, joined sequentially at a rate beyond CFF, give a luminance one-half that of the light phase. For any other relative durations of the two phases the time-average luminance will similarly be realized. The fused luminance is commonly called the *Talbot brightness*. There is apparently no limit to the operation of this principle. T. E. Gilmer (*234*), taking advantage of the tremendously high rotational speeds obtainable with the Beams "air-cushion" turbine, has demonstrated that the Talbot relation holds for fused flashes with durations ranging downward from 0.1 sec to 8×10^{-9} sec and for repetition frequencies as high as 1500 per second!

In assessing the effect of varying light-time fraction on the size of CFF, a decision obviously has to be made about luminance. Is it to be held constant, absolutely, or should Talbot brightness be held constant as the relative proportions of light and dark intervals are manipulated? On the reasonable assumption that the latter represents the more solid experimental operation, the facts then become univocal—with average luminance held constant, CFF decreases as the proportion of light in the cycle is increased. The longer the flashes and the shorter the dark periods between them, the less frequently must the flashes be repeated to preserve continuity. However, the exact relation between flash duration and fusion point is not altogether simple. See Brown's discussion (*240*, pp. 271–281).

The consequence of presenting other than rectangular light pulses— waveforms that are sinusoidal, sawtooth, "peak-clipped," or of irregular shape—is less notable than one might suppose. Any consistent difference here would be of significance for the question of how the retina and the optical nervous system utilize available light energy. But there is much experimental evidence, both neurophysiological and observational, that the changes involved are too rapid and transient to be picked up by the relatively sluggish visual system. We shall see later that the ear and even the skin, in some circumstances, have the capacity for following the extremely minute variations associated with waveform changes. The eye is pedestrian by comparison. It is able to follow with fidelity the basic component (the "fundamental") in subfusion flicker but only this relatively slow variation. Hence, all waveforms yield very much the same set of messages, and they appear to be essentially sinusoidal in their waxing and waning.

What of wavelength as a possible determinant of CFF? The question has something of a history by now, but a definite conclusion is not yet possible. The difficulty stems from the fact that the contribution of wavelength is relatively small as compared with the large influence of luminance, and individual differences in sensitivity to flicker tend to swallow hue effects, if they are real. The fact is that, at least for the photopic mechanism, wavelength makes so little difference that, in Figure 5–6, a single line was drawn through the points for the seven different colors represented. To be sure, that work was done some years ago and before narrow passband filters were available. The colors are not sharply defined. A more recent determination by Georgi (*228*), accomplished with the aid of interference filters having transmissions only 10 nm wide, does show a small differential effect of wavelength on the magnitude of CFF. A slightly steeper slope of the log I-CFF function is found for the blue end of the spectrum than for the red end.

Shifts of CFF with changes of retinal sensitivity coming from dark and light adaptation have been studied, though here again sweeping generalities have not resulted. Generally, CFF is numerically reduced as dark adaptation proceeds and increases with continuing light adaptation. This seems to be invariably true for small fields falling in the foveal region. However, the relation between CFF and state of adaptation is complicated by a host of variables. Size of field matters, and test spot location on the retina is very important. Figure 5–7, taken from the basic retinal exploration by Lythgoe and Tansley (*397*), reveals how time in the dark changes CFF for different loci in the periphery as contrasted with the central retina. It seems probable that the "mix" of excitation and inhibition varies with changing structure and neural interconnections, and that this accounts for the reversals of function as overall sensitivity changes.

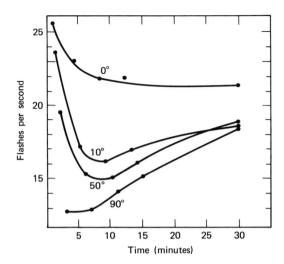

Fig. 5–7. Critical flicker frequency changes in dark adaptation; the classical data of Lythgoe and Tansley, 1929. The eye was initially light-adapted to a level of 24.35 mL for 15 min. Test fields during dark adaptation were: (top) foveal, and (three lower curves) at progressively greater eccentricities. By kind permission of the Royal Society.

It is not necessary to look to adaptation of long duration to get evidences that flicker is a delicate indicator of retinal sensitivity. An eye previously exposed to darkness, then given a series of spaced flashes, undergoes immediate rapid light adaptation, and we have already seen (p. 53) that "initial" light adaptation can create some extreme sensitivity alterations. Normally, for the first tenth of a second or so flicker is not seen, whatever the flicker rate, since multiple flashes below the critical duration simply fuse. But from that point on, for approximately the next full second of time, CFF rises precipitously, then settles down if luminance is held steady. Naturally, the higher the luminance level, the steeper is the CFF gain during the first second of exposure.

To return to the basic relation between flicker and illumination, it is not immediately clear why the fusion point-log I curve should run in the direction it does. One might suppose that a bright flash, arousing a more vigorous response on the part of the retina, would "carry over" farther into the dark interval and thus require a lower flash rate to produce continuity. The positive after-image of a dim light would not persist as long and would seem to require a high critical fusion frequency. The mystery is dispelled when one comes to think of flicker in terms of successive brightness discriminations (Figure 5–8). Flicker can be seen only when excitation level fluctuates outside the limits of one j.n.d. of luminance. An intense flash precipitously raises the excitation level to a high point, but its decline is also sharp. A series of dim flashes yields a more gradually changing excitation curve, and a new flash is not required so promptly to maintain the undiminished level.

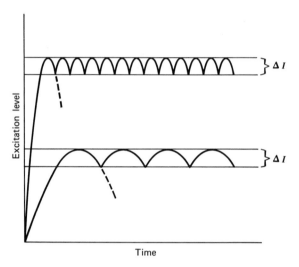

Fig. 5–8. The theoretical course of flicker. The lower curve represents the fluctuations in brightness evoked by a dim light at the critical fusion frequency. The upper curve similarly represents the effect created by a bright light. For the more intense stimulus the rise in excitation is quite abrupt, but so is the decline. The stimulus flashes must be repeated more frequently to maintain excitation within the limits of ΔI and render the flickering light "steady" in appearance.

Because fusion frequency is accurately determinable and because it varies regularly with such a large number of influences affecting visual sensitivity, it may itself be used as an index of sensitivity. The author has elsewhere urged (221) that in the critical fusion point we have a measure of visual *temporal* acuity, analogous to visual *spatial* acuity measures, already discussed.

One of the puzzling features of the critical flash rate is the manner in which it varies, under standard conditions, from one individual to another. For a given moderate illumination it is possible to find values ranging between 35 and 45 flashes per second among a dozen different observers. For a single individual this would correspond to an illumination change of 1:100, a very considerable one indeed. It is not a matter of unreliable measurement. Ten successive settings from the same subject will show a very narrow range of values; as has been said, great precision attaches to such determinations. An extensive study by Tice (574) involving large numbers of measures, not only of fusion points but also of other timed visual phenomena, has failed to provide any correlations suggesting an adequate answer to this question. See also (227).

Another curious effect associated with flicker is that appearing when rotation speed is reduced below the fusion point and the successive flashes begin to be seen as somewhat discrete. Under these conditions there is a great enhancement of brightness, that of the individual flashes increasing far above the level they would reach with steady light of the same intensity. This is variously known as the *Brücke effect* and the *Broca-Sulzer effect* and has been extensively investigated by Bartley (35).

Actually, if priority of observation were the controlling factor, the phenomenon should more appropriately be called the *Brewster effect*, for it was Sir David Brewster, at least 75 years before Broca and Sulzer (94) and fully 30 years before Brücke (102) who seems to have been its discoverer. In an 1834 report (90, p. 245) Brewster says: "In a former paper I had occasion to mention a very remarkable fact, which I had long ago discovered, that the intensity of a given light may be increased physiologically by causing it to act upon the retina by successive impulses of a given duration." He goes on to specify the conditions of disc rotation for obtain-

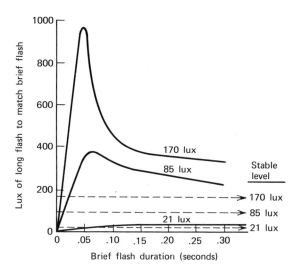

Fig. 5–9. The classical data of Broca and Sulzer (94) on the apparent luminance of brief light flashes. From Katz (345). Courtesy of Pergamon Press.

ing the "maximum physiological intensity." However, both the Brücke and Broca-Sulzer experiments were much more systematic in design and execution, and their descriptions have therefore eclipsed the earlier one. A summary of the Broca-Sulzer experiments, which carefully traced the rise and fall of the brightnesses of a series of short flashes by a comparison field technique—the illuminance of a relatively long, steady flash was adjusted to match the brightness of the short one—is provided in Figure 5-9. A modern repetition of the experiment, by Katz *(345)*, in which the two fields were thrown onto different retinae, thus presumably insuring greater independence of test and measuring fields, failed to alter the original Broca-Sulzer findings in any substantial way.

There is considerable evidence to show that subjective flicker rate is not "locked" to objective flash rate, especially at low frequencies of the latter. Autonomous brain processes, revealed by electrical brain waves, apparently enter the picture to modify flicker phenomena.

Brightness Contrast. Uniform excitation of the retina never happens, though there are approaches to it. The unaccented visual field observed when light shines through the closed eyelids is perhaps the nearest thing to uniformity. Also, in the so-called *Ganzfeld* experiments, in which the eye is covered by a translucent screen formed by half a ping-pong ball, there is the impression of relatively homogeneous stimulation except at the extremes of the visual field. Moreover, if observation is maintained steadily for several minutes, there is much evidence of inhomogeneities, the most prominent feature being a series of filmy, swirling appearances generally encroaching upon the center of the field from the periphery.

Actually, in most of our activities, we are subjected to a vast medley of variegated fields—lights and shades, contours and textures, colors in complex kaleidoscopic patterns. It is natural to think that the objects of our visual perceptions are stimulus-bound, that if we knew the chronology, geometry, photometry, and spectral analyses of all we looked at we should be able to reconstruct with some precision the whole of visual experience.

But, there are many known noncorrespondences, both temporal and spatial, between what is presented to the eye and what is experienced. Illusion is the perceptual rule, not the exception. There are also non-correspondences of considerable magnitude in the luminance-brightness and wavelength-hue domains, some of which we have encountered already in other contexts but the most important of which we have not specifically considered. Now we must face up to the important generalization that wherever two luminances border each other or two hues come into juxtaposition in the visual field there will inevitably be some alterations of brightness or hue, or both, that would not have occurred in a homogeneous field. The former situation, contiguous luminances, leads to *brightness contrast*; the latter, adjoining hues, results in *color contrast*.

Let us consider the two related phenomena separately, at least at first. Place two gray squares side by side and whatever difference between them

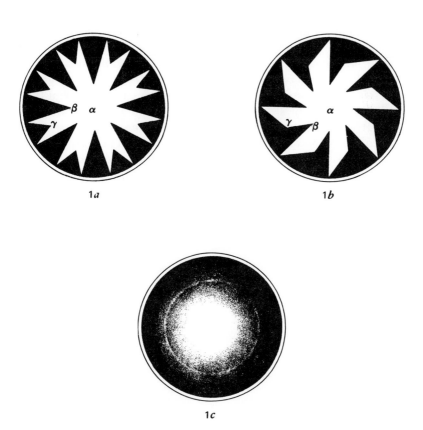

Fig. 5–10. Mach bands. Rotating the disc in either 1*a* or 1*b* results in an appearance illustrated in 1*c*. Where the black centers end or inflect, bright bands appear. The actual distribution of luminance, according to the Talbot-Plateau Law, is shown in Fig. 5–11*a*. From Ernst Mach, *Sitzungsberichte Akad. Wissenschaft, Wien,* 1865.

was apparent initially becomes augmented immediately. Brightness contrast invariably works in the direction of increasing brightness differences; it therefore always serves the function in observation of sharpening any real discrepancies that exist between luminances.

Whereas brightness contrast is, for the most part, a broad effect, not confined to regions near contours but affecting the whole observable field, there are situations in which a most striking contrast effect appears as a relatively narrowly localized one. Such an instance is that found in connection with so-called *Mach bands* or *rings (490)*, named thus because one of the most astute observers of all time, the German physicist, Ernst Mach, discovered the phenomenon.

Figure 5–10, taken from Mach's original 1865 paper, shows two discs having systematic variations, from center to periphery, in the amounts of black and white exposed. When rotated rapidly both discs (1*a* and 1*b*) should yield, according to the predictions of the Talbot-Plateau Law, a uniform white in the center (from α to β), increasingly darker gray (from β to γ), and a more rapidly darkening gray (from γ to the edge of the disc). What is actually seen is depicted in 1*c*. A bright ring appears at β and another at γ, and for these there are no objective counterparts. They are the Mach bands, induced by brightness contrast. The abrupt transition from high to lower luminance is responsible; the transition border becomes "sharpened up" into a contour. Additionally, broad areas of

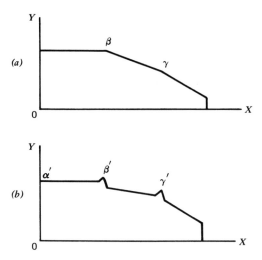

Fig. 5–11. Mach bands. The difference between what the eye sees (*b*) and what is presented to it by way of luminance (*a*) is immediately obvious. From Ernst Mach, *Sitzungsberichte Akad. Wissenschaft, Wien,* 1865.

constantly decreasing luminance, such as that between β and γ, appear more uniform in brightness than their luminance gradient warrants. The discrepancy between what is presented to the eye and what the visual system sees is illustrated in Figure 5–11, also taken from Mach's original paper.

It must be clear that the principle operating so vividly in Mach bands is a very general one. Innumerable sets of special conditions can give rise to similar apparent displacements of luminance. Gentler transitions in illumination than those producing obvious Mach bands yield brightening and darkening effects that are easy to observe, once one knows where to search them out—in shadows falling sharply across bright surfaces, in the printed page and the photographic negative, in a rooftop seen against an overcast sky. Wherever a luminance gradient changes its slope, the possibility of inducing a noticeable contrast effect also exists. As Mach himself generalized, brightness perception depends on the second derivative of the spatial luminance distribution; if the rate of change of gradient slope is sufficient, brightness contrast will ensue (see *324*, Chapter 5).

The more general phenomenon, ordinarily called "simultaneous brightness contrast," may be approached experimentally in many different ways. As has been stressed already, all differential intensitive stimulation in the visual field provides the basic condition for interaction between parts of it. Naturally, with such a general basis, there must be a multitude of variables that affect the degree of contrast that will be evoked. Certain of these are obvious—field luminance and size, proximity or remoteness of the interacting light patches, the time relations of the stimuli, presence or absence of contours, prior adaptation, and so forth. Let us look at some of the more vital factors dictating the extent of brightness contrast.

All contrast experiments involve one or more "inducing" fields (I) and one or more "test" fields (T). In some of them there is a third kind of field, often presented to an otherwise unstimulated eye; it is a "measuring" or "matching" field (M). Several good experiments have put luminance of I under systematic investigation. In one, Diamond's 1953 work (*161*), I and T were adjacent square light patches, each subtending 33' of arc, and were presented slightly eccentrically (21' to the right of the fixation point), one above the other, to the right eye. M appeared only to the left eye, was of the same dimensions as T, and was located 21' to the left of the fixation point. In stereoscopic viewing, the two fixation points were fused. The left eye thus saw one square (M) to the left of center, and the right eye saw two contiguous squares (I and T) to the right of center. By matching M to T in the presence (and absence) of I, it could be ascertained how much reduction of apparent luminance was induced in the neighboring test field by illumination of the inducing field. The effect of varying the luminance of I could also be assessed.

The results were quite definite. Reduction in brightness of T did not occur at a significant level until I was at least as intense as T. Then, as I was further increased, T was depressed in brightness in proportion to the luminance of I. The entire function representing the brightness of T in relation to luminance of I thus consists of a straight line parallel to the abscissa when $I < T$, a bend downward near the equality point, and a steady decline when $I > T$.

Diamond (*162*) subsequently studied the effect of varying the spatial arrangements. This time T was a rectangle situated generally as before but having a vertical dimension only half (16.5′) the width (33′). I was a rectangle of variable height, thus making possible systematic manipulation of area. The dimensions of M were the same as those of T.

As the area of I was increased from zero to twice that of T, something of the same general relation obtained as with variations of luminance, that is, T was depressed only for areas of I equal to or larger than T. It was also found that vertical separation of I and T decreased the contrast effect, a not unexpected result.

The latter factor, field separation, can be studied in a variety of ways. One interesting experiment undertook to vary systematically the spatial separation between I and T while maintaining M constant as a "reference" field (*377*). The arrangements were not too different from those of the experiments described above. I and T, disposed vertically and presented to the right eye, could be separated by 0′, 10′, 30′, 60′, 180′, or 540′ at their closest edges. M, the "reference" field, was identical with T and symmetrically placed with respect to it, but was seen only by the left eye. It was maintained steadily at a luminance of 1.0 mL.

The results were similar to those in the earlier Diamond experiment— no appreciable effect up to the point of equal luminance between I and T, then a proportionally increasing inhibition as intensity was raised— but the effect of field separation was clearer. Maximal contrast occurred at zero separation of the interacting fields, and the effect subsided with increasing distance between them. Nor does the amount of separation have to be great; all separations above 10′ showed about the same amount of induced contrast effect.

Color Contrast. In distinguishing "color" contrast from "brightness" contrast, it is clearly the narrower definition of "color" that is implied, "color" in the sense of "hue." The basic principle we once more encounter here is that of complementariness. Red induces blue-green, its complement, in its surroundings; yellow induces blue, and green induces purple.

But, beyond being able to predict what hues will be seen in the contrast situation, it is also possible to arrive at a few considerably embracing generalities about the working of color contrast, for the phenomenon has been known for a long time. Da Vinci was clear about the effects of juxtaposing hues, and a long line of artists since then has drawn attention to the colors induced in shadows. M. E. Chevreul became an early authority on color contrast effects and, in 1839, published a monograph of over 700 pages on the subject. So well was he known in this context that he was frequently brought in to settle disputes about colors in textiles. The Gobelin tapestry dyers were able to extricate themselves from potential ruin only through Chevreul's proofs that their "off-color" wools owed their "defects" to retinal induction effects (490, pp. 217–225).

Near the end of the last century the general principles governing color contrast were brought together by Kirschmann (362). His "laws of contrast" reduce to the following statements: (a) the smaller the test area and the larger the inducing area, the greater the contrast effect; (b) contrast decreases in proportion to the separation of the two interacting fields; (c) color contrast is maximal when brightness contrast is minimal; (d) if brightnesses are equal, contrast is greater with increasing saturation of the inducing color.

Certain of these generalizations have not gone unchallenged over the years. From time to time, for example, what is generally known as "Kirschmann's third law"—color contrast is best when brightness contrast is lacking or minimized—has seemed to be incorrect. At least, there are apparently valid results that controvert it. And experimental investigation of this point has recently turned up a converse of the "third law"—that brightness contrast is greatest when color contrast is minimal (16). Questions have also arisen concerning the area effects. Thus, Jameson and Hurvich (331) have evidence that the role of stimulus size, both that of the test patch and that of the inducing field, may be much more complex than Kirschmann believed. Also, they find that contrast reaches its maximum for *average* degrees of saturation, rather than getting progressively greater as saturation is increased. But we are talking about empirically generated "laws"; their modification or even outright controversion is no more surprising in this context that in many another in science.

Very vivid contrast effects can be produced by the "colored shadow" technique. If general illumination is supplied to a surface by a colored lamp and an opaque object, such as a rod, is held so as to cast a shadow on the surface, the area on which the shadow falls will be found to possess the hue of the complement of the light. If, now, accessory white general illumination is made to fall on the surface, the contrast color in the shadow will be quite vivid. It is a general rule of color contrast that it is at a maximum when unaccompanied by brightness contrast, and the white light here tends to equalize luminance. The elimination of contours between two contrasting areas also favors maximal color effects. Perhaps the two things are the same visually.

What amounts to a variant of the colored shadow technique, the "partial reflection" method generally attributed to Ragona Scina (see *291*, p. 283), also produces amazingly vivid contrast colors. Figure 5–12, repro-

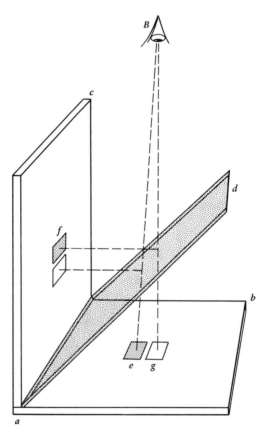

Fig. 5–12. The Ragona Scina method of inducing color contrast. The eye views two patches of light, apparently situated side by side. One of these (on platform) is transmitted through the slanting colored glass plate and so appears in the hue of the glass. The other (vertically disposed) is reflected from the top surface of the glass and, because there is a dark area corresponding to it on the platform, is not colored. However, color contrast induces in the second white patch the complement of the hue of the glass.

duced from Helmholtz's great *Physiological Optics,* illustrates the principle. Surfaces *ab* and *ac* are white, *ad* is a sheet of colored glass (say, green). Spots *e* and *f* are black; *g* is white. An observer stationed at *B* sees *g* as well-saturated green, since its image is not only transmitted through the green glass but also black *f* gives little reflected white light to mix with it. The area optically corresponding to spot *e,* however, now appears bright purple. This is the contrast color of the green by which it is surrounded. Physically, of course, it is colorless, since it consists only of a local patch of mixed white light reflected from the top surface of the green plate.

Color contrast is so undeniable and "real" a phenomenon as to lead to the conviction, on the part of the naive observer of it, that its explanation is to be given in physical terms, that it represents something happening "out there" in the stimulus. The author has seen a student, working in the laboratory on the contrast effect, attempting to recombine, by an ingenious prism arrangement, contrast colors in shadows! Pedagogical principles dictated that the experiment not be interfered with, and the results were instructive if disappointing.

An interesting question that has frequently been raised in connection with color contrast concerns the time relations involved. The phenomenon has often been called "simultaneous" contrast. Is it really instantaneous in its development? Are contrast colors present in the briefest stimulus exposures? The evidences are that not much time is wasted in inducing the contrast effect. There seems to be little doubt that color induction can occur in exposures of only a few milliseconds, times too short to permit eye movements or even too brief to permit the peak of sensation to be reached (*330*). This fact invalidates one of the early arguments, that simultaneous contrast was really "successive" contrast, that eye movements brought about a temporal succession of afterimages.

It is one thing to observe, qualitatively or phenomenally, the altered appearances created by contrast, but quite another to bring them under measurement. Methods of quantifying color contrast effects go back at least to Hering (1887) and some of them are quite ingenious. One way to ascertain how much of the complement has been induced in a gray by a colored surround is to compensate by adding some of the inducing hue to the gray. Thus, in Hering's color disc experiments, a three-component disc (three paper discs interleaved, say black, white, and green) have superposed on them an annular ring, also composed of the same three colors. If the green in the ring is reduced to zero (and a sufficient amount of green is present in the disc) there will be a purplish (or lavender) hue induced in the gray of the ring. The purplish tint may be canceled out by adding a small sector of green to the ring. The amount required just to restore the original gray is, of course, a measure of the contrast effect.

Nowadays, the high degree of sophistication that color specification has attained changes the procedure and, of course, enormously improves the precision. An excellent example of the way in which the CIE tristimulus specification can be employed to quantify contrast phenomena is found in the measurements made by Akita and Graham (12). In these experiments, seven selected spectral colors were first specified in terms of their tristimulus coordinates when viewed against a background of darkness. The specification was then repeated in the presence of one or another of the five colored backgrounds. In different experiments the backgrounds were also systematically varied in luminance, so that ratios between background and test field were 16:4, 4:4, and 1:4. Altogether, there were 126 different conditions realized in the study: 7 test colors × 6 backgrounds (darkness included) × 3 luminance ratios.

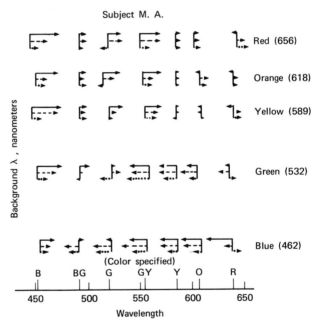

Fig. 5–13. Color contrast effects. Wavelength shifts needed by one observer to maintain a given hue in the presence of differently colored backgrounds. Vertical lines mark the original λ, while horizontal arrows show the direction and amount of shift needed to compensate for background change. In each instance, the top arrow is for a luminance ratio between test color and background of 16:4, the middle arrow for a 4:4 ratio, while the bottom one indicates a ratio of 1:4. From Akita and Graham (12). Courtesy of Pergamon Press.

With so many variables to manipulate, results are not entirely simply represented, but Figure 5–13 succeeds remarkably well, if a little unconventionally, in doing so for one observer. Its legend needs to be studied carefully. It is clear that compensation of the contrast effect is to be achieved, in most instances, by shifting the test field wavelength toward that of the background. Luminance does not have an altogether predictable role to play, but here we ought to recall what we know about the complex wavelength adjustments needed to compensate for luminance changes in the Bezold-Brücke phenomenon.

Many explanations of contrast have been offered. They range from the fantastic suggestion that a rapid "circulation" of decomposed photochemicals goes on in the retina (Ladd-Franklin) to the notion that contrast always represents an "illusion of judgment" (Helmholtz). Neural explanations have not been neglected, either. Many years ago, Allen (13) devised a theory of contrast that made of it a reflex response of the retina. This idea was prompted by the apparent discovery that the optic nerve bundle, like that of the auditory nerve, contains some efferent fibers—a claim still being debated. It seemed improbable then that contrast could be mediated in this way, and the intervening years have only served to make the notion seem more quaint. However, the fact that some neural basis for contrast would emerge has never really been in doubt. Nowadays, we scarcely know whether we are in the realm of theory or fact in appealing to the excitatory-inhibitory relations of the "receptive field" as the inevitable mechanism for both brightness contrast and color contrast.

The basic principle need not be reviewed. We first encountered it in Chapter 3 when we were trying to unravel the complex interconnections between receptor cells and their lowest nervous centers, the retinal ganglia. Again, in Chapter 4, in considering recent developments in the opponent-process type of color theory, we confronted excitatory-inhibitory relations. In both contexts we could not escape the clear implications for the interpretation of both brightness and color contrast.

An old question in connection with contrast concerns its essential "seat." Is it retinal or cortical? Or must some relay station between—the lateral geniculate body has long been suspect—be responsible for introducing the interactions between the inducer and the induced? Many "proofs" that contrast is neither exclusively retinal nor cortical have been adduced. In an earlier edition of this book (1953) the author allowed himself to indulge in such speculation. Now, with the advent of receptive-field theory, the entire question seems to become somewhat academic. At least, the question dissolves into the larger and more general one of how receptor processes get progressively elaborated (or, perhaps, simplified) as the messages they create pass upward to the highest levels of the nervous system. As we have seen, a neural organization in which a sharp juxtaposition of excitatory and inhibitory influences is predominant seems to be evidenced at all levels of the visual afferent system. When the details for human vision become fully known, a satisfactory explanation of contrast will, in all likelihood, be forthcoming.

Meanwhile, it is tempting to extrapolate from what is understood about electrical responses in the visual systems of lower organisms. Receptive-field phenomena have been elucidated in such diverse visual systems as that of the goldfish (*592; 153*), rat (*95*), ground squirrel (*417*), cat (*371; 316*), and spider monkey (*317*), to name only those species that were attacked earliest. Important differences show up when pure-rod, mixed rod-cone, and pure-cone systems are compared. Such functions as differential spectral sensitivity, alterations of field size and responsiveness resulting from dark and light adaptation, and peculiarities of retinal locus vary considerably from one kind of eye to another. Thus, it is too early to attempt a comprehensive account of the neural basis of contrast, either of brightness or color. Still, the simple and direct yet convincing way in which the concentric receptive-field concept can be applied to basic contrast phenomena is itself a strong recommendation for its continued nurture as a theoretical idea. Witness, in Figure 5–14, the application of

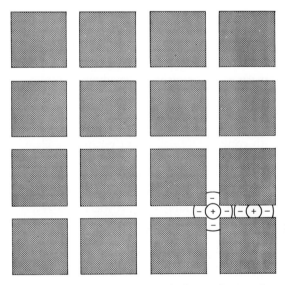

Fig. 5–14. The Hermann grid. Note the dark patches at intersections. The concentric circles at the lower right illustrate one possible mechanism, that proposed by Brown and Mueller (*240*, Chap. 9), for explaining the effect. See text.

the principle to the old puzzle presented by the Hermann grid. Everyone viewing this checkerboard design sees persistent dark spots appearing at the intersections of the grid. Why? One way to answer is to say that, at the intersection, there is twice the amount of white to induce, by brightness contrast, its complementary black. Another way is to point out, as Brown and Mueller (*240*, Chapter 9) have done, the possible role of concentrically organized local receptive fields. At the intersection, there is greater potential inhibition in the white surround than at other loci, thus suppressing the central excitatory field and darkening it. It might just work this way.

6

Sound Energy and the Ear

The procedure was found useful, in studying the visual process, of first becoming acquainted with the characteristics of the stimuli and with the anatomical and physiological features of the receptor organ before considering the various phenomena of seeing. A similar approach to the subject of hearing will prove fruitful. We need to know something of the nature of sound energy and of the manner in which it affects the tissues of the ear before the phenomena of hearing can most profitably be examined.

The Physical Nature of Sound. If uncertainty exists as to what conception of light energy is most useful for experimental purposes there is none concerning sound energy and its manner of propagation. Sound is generated only by vibrating bodies and is transmitted by wave motion of a material medium. Air is usually the medium, though sound may be conducted by other gases and by liquids and solids. Wherever an elastic material exists there are the potentialities for sound transmission. Sound will not travel in a vacuum, as is amply demonstrated by the bell jar demonstration of elementary physics (*419*), first entirely convincingly performed nearly three centuries ago by Robert Boyle. A ringing bell, suspended under a jar, will become inaudible when the air of the container is exhausted by a pump. Readmission of air or any other gas permits the renewal of sound transmission.

The nature of the conducting medium is not a matter of indifference, for the speed with which sound is propagated varies with it. The velocity of sound is a function of the density of the medium and its elasticity. As compared with that of light, the propagation of sound is an extremely slow process. For air at 15° C the rate is 340 m/sec. A convenient figure to keep in mind is the approximate equivalent in the English system, 1100 ft/sec. Sound velocity is about four times as great as this in water and is again approximately quadrupled when such solids as steel, glass, India rubber, and the hardest woods become the medium. It is interesting to note that, whereas the majority of sounds we hear are air-borne over the greater portion of their paths, the final conduction rate we must deal with in audition is that for the liquid filling the inner ear and is thus of the order of about 4500 ft/sec.

When we speak of the velocity of sound it is, of course, the speed of the *wavefront* that is under consideration, for the individual particles of air "conducting" the sound are displaced from their position of rest only slightly and describe to and fro movements of constantly changing acceleration, longitudinal to the direction of propagation. If a sound generator of the simplest sort, such as a tuning fork, is the driving force the motion will be *harmonic* or *sinusoidal*. Figure 6–1 is a representation of such

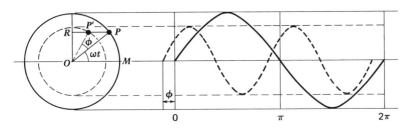

Fig. 6–1. Representation of harmonic (sinusoidal) motion in sound propagation. Besides demonstrating that the sine wave is the projection of uniform circular motion, the diagram shows how two such waves may differ in frequency, amplitude, and phase. From Stevens and Davis (*553*).

motion, spread out on a time axis; it will be seen to be the projection of uniform circular motion. The crests of waves represent points of maximal compression (or, more exactly, points of maximal increase over normal atmospheric pressure), while the troughs are regions of greatest rarefaction of air or reduction of pressure. Sound waves thus consist of successive pressure variations and, in their least complex form, sinusoidal pressure variations.

Frequency, Amplitude, and Phase. The time required for a complete cycle of changes to occur is called the *period* of the wave, and the distance traveled by the wavefront in one period is its *wavelength*. Since, as we have seen, velocity is a function of a number of variables, it has not become conventional, as it has with light, to characterize sound waves by their length but rather by the number of cycles completed per unit of time, that is to say, by their *frequency*. Wavelength and frequency are, of course, related reciprocally. Specifically, wavelength equals propagation speed divided by frequency.

Roughly, the frequencies of importance for human hearing are those between 20 and 20,000 Hz (hertz, cycles per second). For the good ear this wide frequency band represents a region of continuous audibility. There are clear evidences that some animals, cats, dogs, bats, and rats among them, can hear tones higher in frequency than 20,000 Hz (so-called ultrasonic waves), and frequencies below 20 Hz are not without their effect on the human ear, as we shall see.

Another way of designating frequency is by reference to the musical scale. It comprises a range of frequencies extending to nearly 5000 Hz in discrete steps, the latter selected partly on esthetic and partly on practical grounds. The ranges of various orchestral instruments and the human voice are shown in Figure 6–2. It is interesting to observe

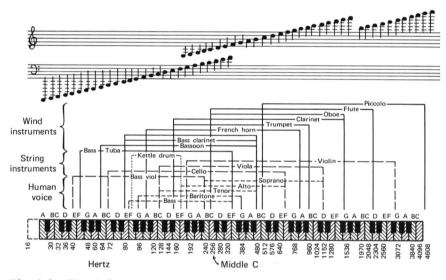

Fig. 6–2. Tonal frequency and the musical scale. After Henney (*294*).

that the lowest frequencies used musically, those generated by the largest organ pipes (16 Hz), extend even below the lower limit of tonal audibility and must make their contribution to musical enjoyment by serving as tactual rather than as auditory stimuli. The largest grand pianos have a range extending from A = 27.4 Hz to c′′′′′ = 4214 Hz (when pitched to a′ = 439 Hz). Orchestral tones encompass the lowest note of the contra bassoon (B♭ = 28.8 Hz) and the b′′′′ of the piccolo

(3951 Hz), but all instruments have *overtones,* some of which are musically effective at least as high as 12,000 Hz.

Certain positions on the frequency scale have come to be of special significance, just as certain spectral points have value for reference. Insofar as there can be said to be any universally accepted scientific standards of frequency they are 256 Hz and 1000 Hz, the former for its coincidence with "middle C" (the nearest power of 2 to musical c') and the latter for its obvious convenience within the decimal system. The musical standard, a', has a long history of fluctuation, having been subject to the caprice of various artistic and practical demands. Ellis, in his remarkable history of musical pitch (*292*, pp. 493–513) has shown that a' has varied from 373.1 to 567.3 Hz, in different times and places and under various influences, the chief of which have been the desire for orchestral "brilliance" (high-pitched a') and the accommodation of the human voice (lower-pitched a'). Attempts to standardize a' include that of the Stuttgart Congress of Physicists in 1834 (a' = 440 Hz, so-called "Stuttgart pitch") and that involving the "diapason normal" (a' = 435 Hz), established by French governmental decree in 1859 and now known as "international pitch." Because that tuning fork which is the prototype of the "diapason normal" has been calculated to have a frequency of 439 Hz at the usual room temperature of 68° F, there has been an attempt to standardize a' at this frequency, despite the numerical inconvenience involved.

Besides differing in wavelength or frequency, sound waves vary in *amplitude,* the amount of displacement of the vibrating particles in either direction from the position of rest. Obviously, amplitude of vibration is related to energy. However, the relation is not a simple, direct one. Energy is proportional to the product of the squares of the amplitude and frequency, or $E = ka^2f^2$. Thus sounds of high frequency possess greater energy than those of equal amplitude but lower frequency.

A third feature of the sound wave is its *phase,* the stage to which vibratory motion has advanced from its starting point or position of rest. Two tuning forks of the same period, struck simultaneously, will move alike at every instant and will be "in phase." If they are struck successively, so as to keep their motions always opposed, they are of "opposite phase." Any other relation is an "out-of-phase" one. Phase differences may be measured in terms of fractions of periods or, more commonly, in phase *angles* (see. Figure 6–1).

Complex Vibrations. Sounds possessing the simple sinusoidal form of vibration are actually of quite rare occurrence in nature, just as "monochromatic" lights are. Only a few sound generators, such as tuning forks and the best electric receivers driven by well-constructed oscillators, yield "pure" tones. All musical instruments emit tones having considerable complexity of waveform. It is, in fact, on the basis of differences in wave complexity that we are able to distinguish the "quality" or *timbre* of instruments. Fortunately for the science of sound, however, complex vibrations are susceptible of exact analysis into simple components. *Fourier's Theorem,* first devised in 1822 in connection with the analysis of heat, states that "a continuous periodic motion of any form can always be represented as the composite of a series of simple harmonic motions of suitable phases and amplitudes." Such motions have periods related to each other in simple mathematical ratio—1:2:3:4:5, etc. Whereas Fourier did not apply the principle to sound, it turns out that it is sufficiently general to permit such application, and the analysis holds exactly for even the most complex of sound vibrations. Figure 6–3 shows

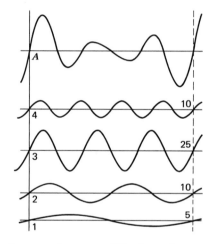

Fig. 6–3. Analysis of a complex wave. The irregular curve at the top may be analyzed into the four regular ones beneath it, each with the relative amplitude given by the number to the right. Viewed synthetically, the top curve is the resultant of the others acting conjointly. From Beasley *(39)*. By permission of Harper and Brothers, publishers.

four simple harmonic components of a complex wave. The diagram may be viewed either analytically or synthetically, for simple harmonic motions may be added together to produce wave forms of any degree of complexity. But the relation is more valuable in its analytic aspect, for it provides the principle on which are based various kinds of tone analyzers. These analyzers are composed of a series of tuned resonators or,

in the case of the electric harmonic analyzer, sharply tuned electric circuits which respond to the individual components of the wave, revealing
not only what frequencies are present but the relative contribution of
each. It is an interesting feature of the ear's action that it behaves as
though it were such an analyzer, and it is possible for the ear to detect, in
a complex tone, many of its harmonic constituents. This fact, that we hear
only pendular vibrations as simple and that all degrees of tonal complexity may be resolved into components falling in the Fourier series, is
known as *Ohm's Acoustic Law.*

The structure of a complex tone, as revealed by the harmonic analyzer,
is illustrated in Figure 6–4. Here the record was obtained from a piano

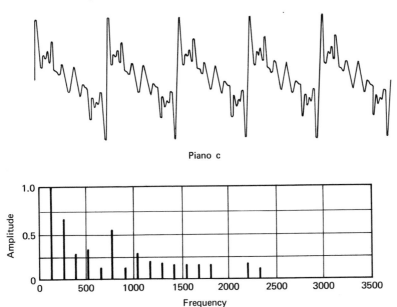

Fig. 6–4. The elaborate waveform produced by a piano playing $c = 128$ Hz. The
relative contribution made by each of the components is shown in the lower
chart. From *Speech and hearing* (revised ed.), H. Fletcher, Bell Telephone Laboratories, Inc., copyright 1952, D. Van Nostrand Company, Inc.

playing C = 128 Hz (one octave below middle c). The components of
the tone, as shown by its *acoustic spectrum,* are seen to extend over a
considerable frequency range. The largest contribution is made by the
fundamental (128 Hz), and, in general, the higher harmonics (overtones)
have smaller and smaller magnitudes as the scale of commensurable
frequencies is ascended. However, it is notable that in this instrument the

sixth harmonic (fifth overtone, $g'' = 768$ Hz) contributes a little more than half the amplitude of the fundamental. Doubtless other keys of the same piano or the same key struck differently would reveal other patterns of harmonics. Almost all other stringed instruments show patterns in which the higher harmonics make relatively greater contributions. Individual instruments vary, and only a small shift of emphasis in the components of the acoustic spectrum may make the difference between a Stradivarius and a run-of-the mine fiddle. The ear is quick to pick up timbre differences, indeed to mediate absolute recognition of tonal quality. Exposures lasting less than one-fifth of a second have been shown to be sufficient to permit quite accurate identifications of orchestral instuments (*119*).

In the process of "knowing thyself," one of the most instructive things one can do is to attempt the analysis of a complex clang, the total tonal mass replete with all its Fourier components. It does more than acquaint one with the structure of tones. The chief reward is that such an exercise teaches an important lesson about attention and its selectivity. Set into vibration a banjo or guitar string—one not too heavily constructed or too tightly stretched—and in the resulting clang listen for the individual components. It is best to pluck or bow the string at a point about one-seventh the distance from its end. This guarantees that the maximum number of partials will be present in the complex gyrations the string will undergo. If one of the overtones is first isolated by stopping the string with a camel's-hair brush at the appropriate point— at midpoint for the second harmonic, one-third the distance from the end for the third harmonic, etc.—thus getting the pitch "in mind," it is then possible to hear that component, to dissect it out attentively from the tonal mass of the freely vibrating whole string. After some practice, it becomes possible to seek out and identify successively as many as six or seven harmonics of the complex clang.

Tones and Noises: Speech Sounds.   Thus far we have been dealing with sustained tones, those having waves repetitive in form and frequency and, for appreciable intervals, unvarying in amplitude. Our ears are also assailed by a variety of other sounds, however—sounds chiefly notable for their lack of sustained frequency and commonly classed as *noise*. A sharp line of demarcation between tones and noises is difficult to draw because noises, like tones, also comprise a large series of components and are thus susceptible of similar analysis. Moreover, most tone generators produce some noise, especially at the moment of being set into operation. Drop a piece of hardwood on a concrete floor, and it may be difficult to judge whether the resulting sound is predominantly noise or tone. It is not entirely facetious to suggest that such a device is, in fact, a musical instrument in embryo—witness the xylophone and marimba. In these instruments resonators strengthening the tonal components throw the balance in the direction of sustained patterns of sound. Other percussion instruments similarly have much of the noise character about them.

Not only have noises a greater conglomeration of frequencies in them, but the components are likely to extend over a wider range. Noises also display more dramatic energy changes. Whereas the sound energy represented in the orchestral rendition of a symphony may vary by a ratio of as much as 100,000 to 1, the moment-to-moment variation in the sound of an explosion may be many times this.

Speech sounds partake of the characteristics of both tones and noises, showing relatively sustained patterns at times and transient irregular waves at others. The characteristic powers ("sensation levels," defined below) and fundamental frequencies of various speech sounds are presented graphically in Figure 6–5, taken from the Bell Telephone Laboratory studies. It will be noted that certain speech sounds appear at several

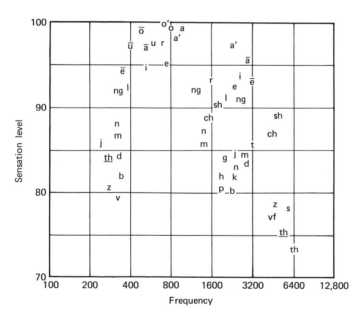

Fig. 6–5. Frequency and intensity characterisics of the fundamental speech sounds. Those elements having more than one principal component appear in two or three different positions on the chart. "Sensation level" is expressed in decibels above absolute threshold (see p. 165). From *Speech and hearing* (revised ed.), H. Fletcher, Bell Telephone Laboratories, Inc., copyright 1952, D. Van Nostrand Company, Inc.

positions on the chart; these have more than one principal frequency component. If the energy distribution throughout the range of audibility is measured for some representative samples of continuous speech, and the resulting values are then averaged, there are obtained curves of the kind shown in Figure 6–6. The greater part of the speech energy lies in

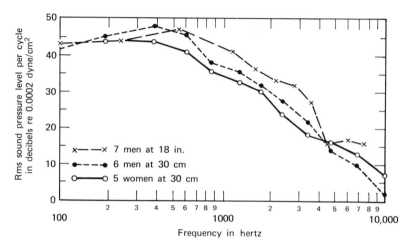

Fig. 6–6. Speech spectra for male and female talkers. The curves are plotted from averages of somewhat protracted sound pressure measurements and thus obscure the known differences in momentary speech patterns. From Licklider and Miller (*388*).

the lower frequencies, below 1000 Hz, whether the speakers are men or women (*388*).

Interference and Reinforcement.   Much of what has been said about the behavior of sound waves is true only when the vibrations are traveling in free space. Most laboratory conditions introduce complications in the control of sound. Walls, ceilings, and articles of furniture provide surfaces which may reflect waves. These return to interfere with the outgoing train and tend thus either to cancel or augment them. Smooth walls are excellent reflectors of sound, and even rough ones, if their irregularities are smaller than the length of the sound wave impinging upon them, behave in this respect as if they were perfectly smooth. It does not do to enclose the sound in tubes, for the opportunities for interference are then augmented. A steady tone released in a room sets up quite promptly an intricate pattern of advancing and returning waves which produce local intensifications and diminutions called *standing waves*. In small enclosed spaces these come to be of extreme importance and, as might be expected, are of common occurrence in musical instruments and other tone generators employing vibrating air columns. It is because interference effects are so intricate and incalculable that their makers use almost entirely empirical knowledge in the construction of most musical instruments, no trustworthy theoretical formulae having been evolved. Not until mid-twentieth century did judicious application of acoustical principles yield violins and cellos rivaling the products of the ancient Cremona craftsmen. Then, interestingly, it was found that the Amatis, Guarneris, and Stradivaris had apparently put together, on purely artistic grounds, the best of such principles in fashioning their intruments. At any rate, meticulous employment of acoustical rules can now lead to the fabrication of stringed instruments that perform in a remarkably similar way to the classic ones (*325*). To a lesser but encouraging degree, this is also true of some of the wind instruments (*125*).

The immediate consequence of these considerations is that it does not suffice, for experimental purposes, to measure the characteristics of a sound generator at the source and assume that they will therefore be known at the ear. Through reinforcement a sound several feet in front of a loud speaker may be more intense than at the instrument itself.

Lately, to be sure, there has been an upsurge in acoustical engineering knowledge, and we appear to have emerged successfully from the age of half-developed ideas when auditoriums were strung with fine wires to "break up" the sound (actually, their effect was negligible) and have begun to use some fairly efficient sound-absorbing materials to reduce reflection. Absorption, changing the rhythmic motions of sound waves into the random motions of heat, is accomplished best by porous materials like sheets of compressed vegetable fiber and acoustical plasters. It appears not to be possible ever to produce complete absorption, and there is little likelihood that rooms will ever be prepared in such a way as to permit their simulating the acoustical properties of free space. However, for all practical purposes, the characteristics of free space are approximated by many so-called *anechoic* chambers (Figure 6–7). Wedges of Fiberglas or porous plastic line the walls, floor, and ceiling; these minimize echoes and thus prevent standing waves for most sound frequencies. Cloth draperies suitably spaced can "trap" waves and have a similar deadening effect.

Sound Intensity. There are several ways of specifying sound intensity, just as a number of alternatives present themselves in the measurement of light intensity. The basic concept for sound is that of pressure variation. We have seen that motions of the vibrating particle are the result

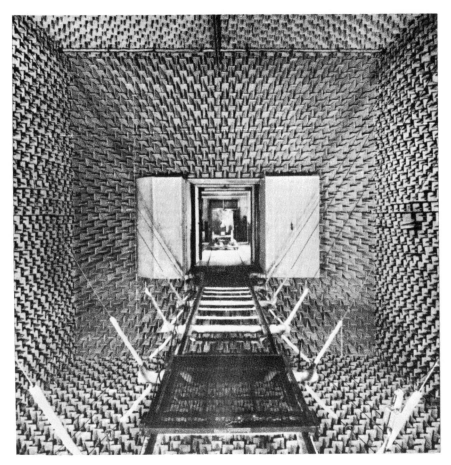

Fig. 6-7. An anechoic chamber. The entire interior of the room is lined with wedges of sound-absorbent material (Fiberglas, covered with muslin). Because there are only inappreciable echoes or standing waves, the chamber simulates the "deadness" of a free acoustic field. From Licklider (*386*).

of alternate increases and decreases of atmospheric pressure. Maximum pressure is realized at the crest of the wave, minimum pressure at the trough. If we were to take a simple average of all pressures throughout the period of the wave we should, of course, arrive simply at the value for atmospheric pressure and should have no indication that energy is being expended in the wave, since there is as much compression as rarefaction of air in the course of the cycle of changes. The difficulty is obviated by taking a root mean square (r.m.s.) value of the pressure variations. The calculation is made in accordance with the formula:

$$\text{r.m.s. pressure (dynes/cm}^2) = \sqrt{(p - p_0)^2/2}$$

where p_0 is normal atmospheric pressure and p is the pressure at the point of maximum displacement in either direction (crest or trough). A short expression is that, for sinusoidal waves, the r.m.s. pressure is equal to the pressure amplitude divided by $\sqrt{2}$.

It is natural that our fundamental unit of intensity should be one of pressure variation, since most practical intensity-measuring devices, such as microphones, have responses directly proportional to r.m.s. pressure of the waves actuating them. These can be calibrated against standard pressures and used as direct-reading instruments. But current practice, growing out of the more or less complete electrification of sound equipment, has dictated that another way of specifying intensity will be preferred. At the present time a newer unit, the *decibel* (dB), has fairly well usurped the field.

The decibel is defined as $\frac{1}{10}$ the common logarithm of the ratio between two energies, the one being measured and some other standard energy or *reference intensity*. Since pressure and energy are related by the square law, the decibel may also be defined as $\frac{1}{20}$ the common logarithm of the ratio between two pressures. Stated as a formula, where N equals the number of decibels:

$$N = 10 \log E_1/E_2 = 20 \log p_1/p_2$$

E_1 and E_2 are the two energies in question, and p_1 and p_2 the pressures. One reference intensity (E_2 or p_2) frequently used, because it is especially meaningful, is the threshold of human hearing—the least energy necessary to produce an auditory sensation. Since this point may be somewhat unstable, another reference intensity has been agreed upon for exact acoustical measurements. This is an intensity represented by a power of 10^{-16} watt/cm²; it corresponds to a r.m.s. pressure of approximately 0.0002 dyne/cm² in a plane progressive sound wave in air. The two commonly used reference intensities are not far apart. The average threshold of hearing for a 1000-Hz tone is very close to the physical reference intensity of 0.0002 dyne/cm².

The physical intensity of sound may be stated either in terms of *intensity level* or *sensation level*. In both cases the unit of measurement is the decibel. The difference between the two lies in the reference intensity used, intensity level being referable to a "zero" of 0.0002 dyne/cm² and sensation level calling for the absolute threshold as the point of zero decibels. Current conventions require that stimulus intensity, when referred to the objective standard of 0.0002 dynes/cm², be designated as *sound pressure level* (SPL), while a specification of stimulus intensity that is referred to threshold be called *sensation level* (SL). Obviously, SL is not the stable measure that SPL is, since with SL the dB value will vary from person to person and will be different for every frequency. However, each has its uses, and in most experimental situations one or the other will be preferred, SPL where absolute intensity values are needed, SL where only a relative measure is indicated. Figure 6–8 will

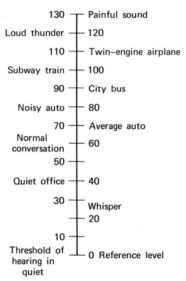

Fig. 6–8. The decibel scale in terms of some familiar sounds. From Chapanis, Garner, and Morgan (*114*).

be of aid in giving concrete meaning to the decibel; the scale shown is one of sensation level, as the definition of zero reveals.

The device most commonly employed in making sound-intensity measurements is a microphone for which a pressure calibration, i.e., the relation between current generated and pressure on the diaphragm, has been obtained for all frequencies to be measured. Since, in the calibration process, the introduction of a microphone to the sound field is likely to distort appreciably the sound waves constituting it (microphones cannot be made infinitely small!), it is necessary to take one additional step. This makes use of a clever device invented by Lord Rayleigh and known as the Rayleigh disc. It consists of a very light plate which will not appreciably alter a sound field in which is is suspended and which will tend to orient itself at right angles to the direction of propagation of the waves flowing past it. The relation between the turning moment of the disc and the velocity of the air particles may be worked out and the device used as a primary standard against which to calibrate a microphone. This so-called "field calibration" of the microphone then permits its use as a secondary standard, provided due consideration is given to the direction in which the microphone diaphragm is oriented with respect to the source of an unknown sound to be measured.

However, measurements of the type described in the foregoing paragraphs are concerned with "ultimates." As has been previously suggested, most modern systems for sound production are electrical, and working standards of intensity are likely to be provided within the control networks of oscillators, resistance boxes, and potentiometers which are already calibrated in decibel units. As with illumination measurements, it is rarely necessary to refer to primary standards.

Anatomy of the Ear.   The mechanism for hearing is divisible, anatomically, into three parts: the external ear, the middle ear, and the inner ear. Functionally, we may think of the external and middle divisions as a

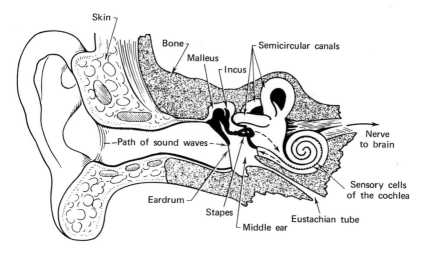

Fig. 6–9. Gross anatomy of the ear. A semischematic drawing showing the main path of sound. Vibrations entering the external auditory canal first affect the eardrum. Oscillations of the drum are transmitted through the middle ear chiefly by bone conduction over the chain of ossicles: malleus, incus, and stapes. The foot of the stapes carries the vibrations to the fluid of the cochlea, in which the hair-like endings of the auditory nerve are immersed. After Davis (*146*). By permission of Rinehart Books, Inc., copyright 1947.

system for collecting and transmitting sounds, by air and bone conduction, to the inner ear where are situated within a fluid medium the sensitive endings of the eighth cranial, or auditory, nerve.

The gross structure of the ear is shown in Figure 6–9. The *pinna* serves to funnel sounds striking it into the external auditory canal, a tube 7 mm in diameter and about 2.5 cm in length. At the terminus of the canal is the eardrum, or *tympanic membrane*. The latter divides the external from the middle ear. The drum serves very much the same function as does the diaphragm of a microphone, not vibrating with a period of its own but forced into oscillation by any and all frequencies of sound impinging upon it. From this point to the terminations of the auditory nerve, vibrations may be conducted: (1) by air conduction through the cavity of the middle ear to the *round window* in the temporal bone, (2) by bone conduction through the walls of the middle ear cavity to the cochlea, and (3) by direct mechanical transmission through the chain of ossicles (hammer, anvil, and stirrup) to the *oval window*, thence by way of the cochlear fluid to the nerve endings. It is by the last route that conduction is mainly effected. The hammer (*malleus*) is securely attached to the tympanic membrane and vibrates with it. The three ossicles, tied together by ligaments, form a remarkable lever system, reducing the extent of the excursions initiated at the drum but preserving in large measure the "thrust" so that the stirrup (*stapes*), driven back and forth in the oval window, moves with an amplitude somewhat less than that of the drum but exerts a correspondingly increased pressure on the fluid of the cochlea. Since the drum (average area of 66 mm²) is about 20 times larger than the foot of the stapes (area of footplate, 3.2 mm²) and the ossicles are pivoted in such a fashion as to provide a small mechanical advantage, there is concentrated on the oval window a very considerable pressure, per unit of area about 25 to 30 times as great as that found at the drum. Some such "impedance matching" is necessary in going from an air to a hydraulic conduction system if efficiency of transmission is to be preserved.

The fact that there is more than one pathway to the cochlea—that sounds can get to the internal ear both by air and bone conduction—leads to an interesting phenomenon. It is a common experience that one's recorded voice, whether speaking or singing, sounds "unnatural." That is, it sounds unnatural to the owner of the voice; if the recording is done with good equipment it does not sound strange to another person. The solution of this puzzle is not hard to find. Normally, one hears one's own voice over two routes—by air conduction through the meatus, as others hear it through theirs, and by bone conduction from the vibrating voice box, chiefly through the jawbone. Indeed, the bone-conduction channel is a very strong one, for the socket of the jaw lies quite close to the temporal bone, and this, of course, houses the cochlea. Many of the low-frequency components of the voice are lost or "thinned" by air conduction, and the rich, dynamic quality of the voice then suffers accordingly.

The way in which the tympanic membrane behaves in response to vibratory pressures is just beginning to be understood. There are difficulties inherent in all the classical approaches to the study of the membrane's action. Direct visual observation with a microscope is difficult by reason of inaccessibility and optical limitations, and fine levers and mirrors attached to the drum membrane are similarly restricted in their application. More has been learned from the use of tiny condenser probes inserted in high-frequency circuits. These may be positioned extremely close to the vibrating tissue where they measure amplitudes quite sensitively. With such a technique Békésy was able to plot, point by point, excursions of the tympanic membrane and show that, for frequencies below 2400 Hz, the membrane vibrates pretty much as a whole, performing as a somewhat stiff but unstressed tissue of more or less uniform elasticity.

As observational methods have become more and more refined it has been possible to achieve greater intimacy of detail. Two techniques have been especially effective, laser interferometry (578) and vibrational holography (579). The latter has yielded systematic measurements down to membrane motions as small as 1.2×10^{-5} cm (roughly, a tenth of a micron). The holographic technique has revealed interesting changes in vibratory patterns as stimulus frequency is shifted. The fundamental pattern displayed by the tympanic membrane seems not to be one suggesting the functioning of a stiff plate, as had formerly been thought, but rather one that comes out of the dynamics of curved membranes. As the schematic drawing of Figure 6–10 shows, there are two areas of peak activity, a strong one posterior to the *manubrium*, the hammer's "handle," and a weaker one anterior to it. With this technique there come to be visible a series of roughly concentric rings or fringes, their number increasing as amplitude of vibration is made greater. The pattern is pretty much the same for all vibratory stimuli up to a frequency of about 1500 Hz. With more rapid impacts a restriction of size occurs and, in the neighborhood of 3000 Hz, the basic pattern begins to break up into subpatterns. At higher frequencies the pattern becomes even more complex. The evidence is that the drum membrane ceases to contribute much to mallear displacements at high frequencies; sound impinging on the system drives the manubrium directly.

The drum and ossicular chain, together with the attachments that

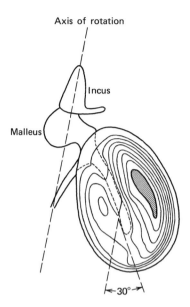

Axis of rotation

Incus

Malleus

|←30°→|

Fig. 6–10. Vibratory patterns of the tympanic membrane. Graphic reconstruction of measures obtained by the method of time-averaged holography. At this frequency (600 Hz) and intensity (111 dB SPL), the membrane has two foci of activity, a strong one anterior, a weak one posterior to the "handle" of the hammer, which rotates about an axis displaced 30 degrees (in cat, nearer 90 degrees in man) from the ossicular axis. Tonndorf and Khanna *(579)*. Courtesy of Annals of Otology, Rhinology, and Laryngology.

keep them in place, form a physical transmission system which, like all such arrangements, is bound to respond more favorably to some vibration frequencies than to others. The middle ear system, taken as a whole, has a "natural period." This has been determined by cementing a tiny chip of mirror to the malleus, reflecting a light beam from it, and setting the system into momentary action by imparting the sound of a click to the eardrum *(61*, p. 1084). The natural frequency revealed by such an optical lever turns out to be in the neighborhood of 1300 Hz. The same experiment tells one about the damping characteristics of the middle ear. The system proves to be highly damped, that is, comes promptly to an equilibrium with the forces acting on it. This permits the middle ear to be a relatively faithful conductor of all manner of tones and noises, however rapidly their wave shapes may change.

Two other features of the middle ear should be noted. The *Eustachian tube,* running from the middle ear cavity to the throat, serves as a pressure-equalizing device. Normally closed, it opens during swallowing and permits air interchanges that keep pressure on the two sides of the tympanic membrane equal. If this were not the case the drum might be painfully bulged or retracted as, indeed, happens when a head cold blocks the Eustachian tube and the drum is subjected to extreme atmospheric pressure variations. Anyone who has traveled by unpressurized plane under such circumstances is vividly aware of the consequences. The other feature of middle ear anatomy concerns the intra-aural muscles, the *tensor tympani* and the *stapedius*. The former is attached to the malleus and by its contraction places the drum under greater tension. The stapedius, the action of which is opposed to that of the tensor tympani, is attached to the stapes. When contracted it changes the articulation between the foot of the stirrup and the oval window. When both muscles contract together, as they normally do, there result more intimate operation of the ossicles and more favorable response to high tones. There is good reason for believing that the two muscles, acting jointly, have an essentially protective function, by reflex contraction reducing possible damaging effects of loud low-pitched sounds by producing a temporary "fixation" of the ossicles.

The *acoustic reflex*, as the combined responses of the tensor tympani and the stapedius are called, could conceivably serve additional functions and several have been suggested (*638*, Chapter 10). A parallel between the acoustic reflex and that of the pupil of the eye is not hard to find. Both belong to the class of consensual reflexes. Just as the arousal of the pupillary response in one eye automatically produces a similar response in the other, stimulation of one ear by sound causes both stapedial and tensor responses in the two ears simultaneously. Also, just as pupil narrowing cannot protect the retina from a sudden bright flash of light, owing to the relatively long latency of the muscle response, a sharp, explosive sound may damage the cochlea before the acoustic reflex can attenuate the sound. Reflex latency depends on intensity—the stronger the stimulus, the shorter the delay—and is preeminently a function of the measurement technique, whether the indicator of muscle contraction is mechanical or electrical, whether the myographic method is isotonic or isometric, or whether the change being observed is optical or one of acoustic impedance. Characteristically, the stapedius is a little faster to respond than the tensor; it also goes into action, especially to low-frequency sounds, at somewhat lower stimulus intensities. In man, reflex latencies ranging from 25 to 150 msec have been reported. Cats typically have faster acoustic reflexes, latencies of about 10 msec being commonly found. But both muscles participating in the acoustic reflex go into action significantly only at relatively high intensities. According to several different experiments in agreement, there is a strong response only when sound intensity is 80 dB or more above absolute threshold (625).

It makes a difference, in measurements of the impedance change brought about by the acoustic reflex, whether the stimulus for the response is introduced in the ipsilateral or the contralateral ear. Even though the reflex is consensual, its threshold is typically several decibels lower if the sound eliciting it enters the ipsilateral ear. There are apparently large individual differences in this regard, just as there are idiosyncracies in the matter of voluntary control of the middle ear muscles. Møller (425) has found regulation of the acoustic reflex varying, in different people, such that ipsilateral exceeded contralateral sensitivity by 2 to 16 dB. Bilateral stimulation is even more effective, a further lowering of the acoustic reflex threshold being realized when both ears are equally stimulated; as with the absolute threshold for the appreciation of sound, the bilateral figure is about 3 dB under that for unilateral stimulation.

Another protective device, demonstrated by von Békésy (61, pp. 1085–1086), consists in a change in the mode of vibration of the stapes in the presence of a very loud sound. The relation of the footplate of the stirrup to the oval window is such that, normally, the stirrup moves about a vertical axis and, in a somewhat hingelike action, compresses the fluid of the cochlea. When overdriven, however, its vibratory pattern changes to one in which most of the motion of the footplate takes place around an axis at 90 degrees to the former one and the large amplitudes brought to the stapes by the malleus and incus are harmlessly expended in rotary motion.

The portion of the auditory mechanism constituting the inner ear begins at the oval window (foot of the stapes) and terminates, as a sound transmission system, at the round window. It occupies a complex cavity, appropriately named the *bony labyrinth,* in the temporal bone (see Figure 6–11). Whereas there are three major divisions of the labyrinth, the *vestibule,* the *cochlea,* and the *semicircular canals,* the last-named structures need not complicate our thinking at this point, for they are not at all concerned with hearing. At one time it was supposed that they were; it is now known that they are exclusively concerned with another class of events, those involved in the maintenance of body equilibrium. Fitting loosely into the bony cavity of the labyrinth and surrounded by a watery fluid, the *perilymph,* is a series of sacs, collectively called the *membranous labyrinth.* All interconnect and are filled with the same fairly viscous fluid, the *endolymph.* That portion of the membranous labyrinth situated in the bony cochlea and following its spiral form is

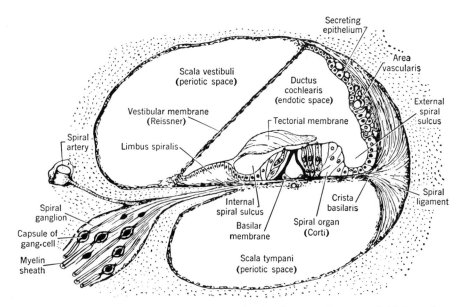

Fig. 6–11. Cross section of the cochlea. The basilar membrane and Reissner's membrane define the limits of the cochlear duct (scala media), within which is located the organ of Corti. The hair cells of the latter are the receptors for hearing. From Rasmussen, by permission of the William C. Brown Co., publishers, and the author.

known as the *cochlear duct.* In it are located all the specialized tissues most intimately concerned with the initiation of impulses in the fibers of the auditory nerve.

Early in embryonic life the cochlea appears as a straight tube, without the coiled "snail-shell" appearance characteristic of full development. About the second month of uterine life the cochlea begins to coil on itself and continues the process until somewhat more than 2½ turns (left to right in the right cochlea and the reverse in the left) have been completed. The cochlea is divided longitudinally by a combination of bony shelf (*spiral osseous lamina*), which extends partway toward the outer wall, and the *basilar membrane,* which completes the division and upon which are situated the highly specialized endings of the auditory nerve. These lie along the inner edge of the basilar membrane and in contact with epithelial hair cells, collectively known as the *organ of Corti.* Movement of these structures is the mechanism whereby impulses are generated in the fibers of the auditory nerve.

The spiral lamina and basilar membrane effectively divide the cochlea into two main chambers, the *scala vestibuli* above and the *scala tympani* below. Both contain perilymph. The oval window, with stapes hinged in it, lies at the base of the upper chamber; the membrane-covered round window is at the lower termination of the scala tympani. Communication between the two is effected by a tiny opening at the apex of the cochlea, the *helicotrema*. This is scarcely larger than a pinhole, being but 0.25 mm² in area. Of course, pressure communication between the two chambers can also be brought about through the basilar membrane itself since, though it is a tough, fibrous structure, it is a flexible one. A further anatomical subdivision is effected by *Reissner's membrane,* a delicate structure running from the spiral lamina to the outer wall of the cochlea and forming an angle with the basilar membrane. The area thus enclosed is the scala media (*cochlear duct*). Still another membrane is to be found in the cochlear duct, the *tectorial membrane*. It is attached to the bony shelf just below Reissner's membrane but, unlike the latter, does not extend entirely across the cochlear canal. However, it is quite firmly attached to the cilia of the hair cells of the organ of Corti, and shearing motions relative to it, created by the basilar membrane, are responsible for bending the cilia and producing changes in the hair cells. This is the final step in the transduction of mechanical force into the series of electrochemical changes that constitutes the nerve discharge, so the tectorial membrane plays a most important role in the generation of auditory messages.

Whereas the bony cochlea necessarily becomes smaller and smaller in cross-sectional area as the apex is approached, the basilar membrane, interestingly enough, becomes progressively wider. At the vestibular end it is about 0.08 mm wide; near the helicotrema it has broadened to 0.52 mm. The hair cells, of which there are about 23,500, according to the best counts, also vary in length from base to apex. At the vestibular end they are of the order of 0.05 mm long, while at the apical end they are 0.085 to 0.1 mm in length. They are spaced quite evenly along the basilar membrane, though not in a single row. About 3500 of them are situated close to the membrane's point of attachment to the bony shelf (*inner* hair cells); the remainder (*outer* hair cells), several of which appear in a single cross section of the cochlear duct, lie further out on the basilar membrane. All hair cells have tiny cilia, or filaments, which extend into the endolymph of the cochlear duct.

Dynamics of the Cochlear Partition. Just how the inner ear works has always been a central concern. Auditory theories of the last century are better differentiated with respect to how they picture the basilar membrane functioning than on any other basis. Clearly, it must respond to incoming sound waves by vibrating in some kind of unison with them. Does it do so as a whole, much as the diaphragm of a telephone receiver does? Some have thought so, and "telephone" and "sound pattern" theories were devised. Does it do so in segments, each portion of its length doing something slightly different from what its neighbors are doing? Others have thought this, and the most influential theory of the last century, Helmholtz's "resonance-place" theory, capitalized on it.

Fortunately, we no longer have to leave to speculation the question of how the basilar membrane and its attachments (the "cochlear partition," in brief) operates in response to sound waves impinging upon them. The main outlines of the action of the cochlear partition were clarified, not too long ago, through the prodigious research efforts of the Hungarian-born Nobel laureate, Georg von Békésy. Over a period of a quarter-century, aided by a long list of ingenious technical innovations of his own devising, he has painstakingly traced the series of dynamic events begun at the eardrum and terminated with the passage of nerve impulses toward the brain. Békésy worked mainly with the cochleas of human cadavers, but he also investigated a wide range of other auditory mechanisms from the frog to the elephant!

The cochlear partition, far from behaving like a stretched membrane or diaphragm, seems not even to be under tension. Tiny cuts made in the basilar membrane do not pull apart, and stiff hairs pressed endwise against it show it to be highly flexible, circular depressions being created near the apex of the cochlea and slightly oval ones near the base, where the membrane is narrower and the tissue is stiffer. When low-frequency sounds are made to drive the cochlear partition, all parts of it respond nearly in unison, with the greatest amplitude of vibration near the apex. At somewhat higher frequencies, say 150 Hz or above, the mode of response is seen to be somewhat different. Not all portions of the partition are in synchrony with the driving force. Békésy discovered in his early work (55, pp. 404–429), chiefly by noting the behavior of finely ground metallic and carbon particles suspended in the cochlear fluid, that streaming effects were visible. He correctly reasoned that these indicated the presence of traveling waves. The waves occasioned by a click delivered to the ear required all of 2.5 msec to travel from base to apex. During tonal stimulation the displacements were regular ones, the wave traveling rapidly at first and gaining amplitude as it ascended the cochlea, then decreasing its velocity and losing strength as it continued (see Figure 6–12). The maximum point, though broad, proved to be located in a characteristic place for a given frequency. The midpoint was represented by a frequency of about 1600 Hz; low frequencies had their greatest bulge toward the apex, high frequencies toward the stapes.

The "traveling wave" has been misunderstood by some. It is not a

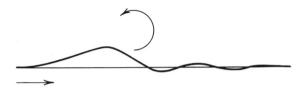

Fig. 6–12. Displacements of the basilar membrane at an instant in time. The wave is traveling from left to right. Eddy currents in the fluid are indicated by the curved arrow. From Wever *(629)* after Békésy.

matter of simple propagation along the length of the partition, like the shaking of a rope. It does not matter where in the system the force is applied; the wave always travels from the stiffer to the broader, more yielding part. In cochlear models, if the "stapes" or driver is made to actuate the wide, instead of the narrow, end of the membrane, the wave travels toward the driver! This fact, incidentally, helps explain why hearing by bone conduction results in sounds that are "natural," indistinguishable from air-conducted sound. "Traveling" of the wave is best thought of in terms of time relations. For a given condition of thrusting force at the stapes, one portion of the cochlear system responds in a slightly different phase from another one.

Many of the factors that might have some effect on vibratory motions within the cochlea have been isolated and systematically explored by Békésy *(629)*: changes of fluid pressure, flexibility of the round window (the terminal "barrier" of the system), tension of the partition components, open versus closed cochlear system, stiffness of the responding tissues and the way they are coupled to each other, overall mass of the vibrating members, internal friction in the mobile parts, especially as this is altered by fluids bathing the cochlear partition. Several of these are important (friction, mass, coupling, and stiffness); several are not (fluid pressure, the round window role, tension, opening of the system). The principle that matters most is tissue elasticity. This factor varies more widely over the length of the partition than any other and thus has most to say about local differentiation of response. In particular, it largely determines the velocity with which the waves travel and accounts for the alignment of frequency maxima along the basilar membrane.

Auditory Nerve Pathways. Nerve fibers, from both the inner and outer hair cells, pass under the spiral lamina and enter the bony central axis of the cochlea, the *modiolus.* Here they assemble to form the *spiral ganglion of Corti,* the beginning of the auditory branch of the eighth cranial nerve. Each of the inner hair cells is supplied with 10 to 20 nerve endings, and each nerve fiber connects with 10 to 20 hair cells. The outer hair cells are differently innervated. Here a single fiber may connect with many hair cells, and a particular outer hair cell may be supplied by many nerve endings. There are at least 35,000 ganglion cells in the twisting auditory nerve of the modiolus, more at the level of the basal and middle turns than near the apex.

Upon leaving the base of the cochlea the auditory nerve enters the medulla of the brain. This organ lies immediately adjacent; in fact, it is only 5 mm away in the human. Here the majority of fibers connect with others which cross to the contralateral side and ascend by way of the lateral lemniscus to the *medial geniculate body* of the thalamus. Radiating fibers from the geniculate body spread, fanlike, to the cortex of the temporal lobe of the cerebrum. A chain of five nerve cells is involved in this devious path from the cochlea to the cortex, and still other nerve cells may be implicated.

The areas of the cortex constituting the sensory projection region have been the subject of intensive research for many years. If answers are not yet definitive it is not the fault of neurophysiologists, neuroanatomists, and behavioral scientists, who have pursued the problem assiduously. There is no difficulty in finding evoked potentials at the cortex, either from electrical stimulation of various loci along the spiral lamina, as was done in the original Woolsey and Walzl study (655) or, as has been done more recently by many investigators, producing sharp airborne clicks in the animal's ear. Indeed, too much happens at the cortex. Well over half of it will give evidence of being involved to some degree in auditory responses. However, not all active areas make equal claims. In particular, not all are capable of displaying frequency specificity, and this perhaps should be a central consideration. Some regions show a quite precise relation between locus and tonal frequency; such areas are said to have a *tonotopic organization*. This feature, probably better than any other functional one, indicates intimacy of connection with the periphery.

The present evidences are that six more or less discrete areas involve auditory projections. Figure 6–13 shows their locations in the cat. AI and AII were the first to be found and are still regarded as primary in that responses to clicks are here strong enough to override fairly deep anesthesia. Moreover, the anatomical evidence shows connections to lower centers to be most obviously joined to this temporal lobe area. Note that, with respect to each other, AI and AII are reversed *en bloc*; the apex (*A*) and the base (*B*) of the cochlea are represented at different ends.

Whether the remaining regions (E_p, the somewhat remote insular area,

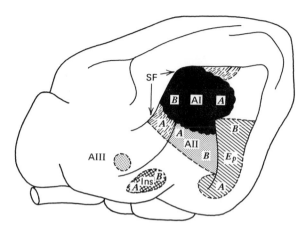

Fig. 6–13. Auditory projection areas of the cat. AI and AII are regarded as the "primary" areas in the temporal cortex. Area E_p ("posterior ectosylvian") is an autonomous center in that it will function in the absence of AI and AII. AIII is a small projection field in a region dominated by somesthesis. There is clear projection to the insular region (Ins) and to the suprasylvian fringe (SF). The letters *B* and *A* in the larger projection fields refer, respectively, to the base and apex of the cochlea where the pathways originate. From Woolsey, C. N. In *Neural mechanisms of the auditory and vestibular systems* (Ed. by Rasmussen and Windle, 1960). Courtesy of Charles C. Thomas, Publisher, Springfield, Ill.

AIII—an apparent interloper in the somesthetic projection system—and the most recently discovered "suprasylvian fringe") will all turn out to be "spares" in the economy of the auditory organization is still in doubt. If so, this must represent Mother Nature at her most conservative. It seems more likely that an overall principle will be found and the six pieces of the puzzle will fall into their proper places. There are already known to be important interactions between various of the six projection areas.

The foregoing has been concerned exclusively with the *afferent* auditory system. There is an *efferent* one as well, though much less elaborately organized and apparently having only a single function to perform, that of imposing inhibitory control over the afferent paths. Anatomically, the presence of the efferent fibers has been known since their identification by Rasmussen in 1946 (*488*); physiologically, it was first discovered by Galambos (*211*) that electrical stimulation of these fibers can reduce normal sound-aroused activity in the eighth nerve.

The fibers in question, only about 400 of them, arise in the superior olivary complex and constitute a well-nigh unique bundle connecting with the hair cells of the cochlea on the opposite side. Another 100 join the bundle from the ipsilateral superior olive. The importance of this discovery is perhaps apparent from the following characterization by Desmedt, who has studied the olivo-cochlear bundle (OCB) extensively: "The OCB offers rather exceptional facilities for the analysis of general physiology and neurochemistry of inhibitory processes. It is apparently the only instance in which an homogeneous bundle of (long) inhibitory axons can be rather selectively activated and brought under control in the mammalian nervous system" (157, p. 1479). As yet we are scarcely above the threshold of knowledge about inhibitory mechanisms in the central nervous system. However, the fact that they are of the utmost importance in regulating the sensory inflow has been demonstrated vividly in conjunction with retinal functioning, as we have seen, and doubtless they have much to say about the nature of messages reaching the brain on stimulation of the ear.

It is still a moot question as to whether there is preserved any neat geometrical arrangement at every point in the complex pathways leading from the basilar membrane to the auditory cortex, and there are many uncertainties about the mode of operation of some of the relay stations en route. This much is certain, however; each cochlea is represented bilaterally in the brain. There are many evidences, anatomical and physiological, that the "projections" of the two ears become completely intermingled in the higher centers. Removal of one cerebral hemisphere of a dog reduces acuity hardly appreciably (414). Of course, the losses observed in behavioral experiments are frequently subject to the caution that more subtle effects, as yet undetected by behavioral methods, may be present. Further removal of the nervous connections, by interruption of the fibers ascending the lateral lemniscus, results in a loss in acuity of about 10 decibels, but it is a matter of no consequence whether crossed or uncrossed tracts, that is, those leading from the contralateral or the homolateral cochlea, are destroyed. The same loss follows either interruption.

A glance at Figure 6–14 will reveal the anatomical provisions for crossing of the pathways. It is obvious that the chief crossover point is at the level where the auditory nerves enter the brain. Upon leaving the cochlear nucleus of the medulla there pass fibers, either directly or by way of the superior olivary body, to the lateral lemniscus on both sides of the brain. Further opportunities for gaining access to the contralateral side are provided at the roof of the midbrain, at the inferior colliculus.

There are, of course, implications for hearing in the fact of bilateral

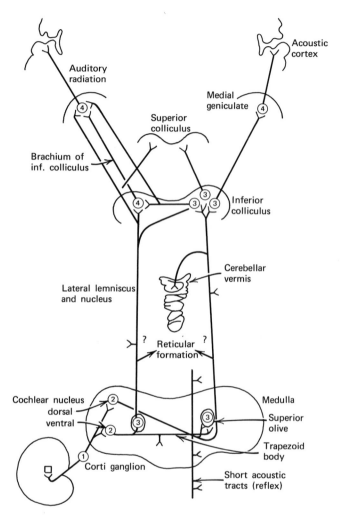

Fig. 6–14. Neurons of the auditory pathway (highly schematic and simplified). From Thompson (*572*) after Davis.

brain representation of the ears—just as for vision—and there are several experimental situations in which the built-in duplication of the pathways has to be kept in mind if results are to be interpreted wisely. One problem that has been explored with some thoroughness concerns auditory localization of external sounds. Space is not a primary dimension for the sense of hearing, yet surprisingly accurate judgments of the direction from which sounds strike the ears can be made in many instances. Such discriminations rest on two kinds of data, *relative intensity* and any appreciable *time difference* in arrival at the two ears. In the final analysis—and this has to be made in terms of the arrival of nerve impulses at the brain—both reduce to temporal discriminations. Which ear makes the prior claim in contributing to the total pool of information? The evidences from both neurophysiological and psychophysical experiments unite in testifying that the time differences need not be great. Temporal separations of clicks at the two ears of less than 0.5 msec are sufficient to insure that the amplitudes of the total evoked electrical changes at the brain will be out of balance, the contralateral temporal lobe showing the larger response (*508*). Similar relations hold for lower centers. Individual nerve cells in the superior olive, the first place at which interactions can occur, have their highest probability of response to clicks delivered to the two ears simultaneously, to decrease that probability markedly if a small time difference (< 0.5 msec) is created, and to lead to complete suppression of response if the time separation falls between 0.5 and 1.0 msec (*214*). In human psychophysical experiments, it has long been known that deviations from the midplane between the ears can be created reliably with clicks separated in time by only a few hundredths of a millisecond.

The physical characteristics of auditory stimuli and the mechanisms for their reception having now been reviewed, we are in a stronger position to examine the phenomena of hearing. At least we may feel some confidence that our interpretations of the phenomena will be realistic in that they are aligned with the known physical and biological facts.

7
Auditory Phenomena

The Intensitive Threshold. We have already had occasion, in considering the "reference intensity" for sound measurements (Chapter 6), to pay some attention to the absolute intensitive threshold of hearing. It will be recalled that "sensation level" is expressed in decibels above that threshold. It remains to ascertain how the threshold value is determined and upon what variables it depends.

Intensitive thresholds may be measured either in terms of minimum audible pressure on the tympanic membrane or intensity of the minimum audible sound field in which an observer is placed. The values obtained by the two methods characteristically differ, and it becomes necessary, in stating the value of the absolute threshold, to specify by what method the result was derived.

In determining the least pressure on the drum necessary to arouse an auditory sensation a sound generator, typically an earphone, is held tightly to the ear, thus enclosing in the external auditory canal a known volume of air. The excursions of the diaphragm of the phone being determined, either optically or by the known electrical response characteristics of the phone, it is then possible to compute with some accuracy the air pressure exerted on the drum. An alternate device is to make use of a "probe tube," an air conductor held very close to the drum, the pressure variations in the end of the tube being regarded as identical with those impinging on the drum. In either case the pressure variations are reduced to the point where the sound becomes just audible (strictly speaking, half of the time just audible, half inaudible), and the pressure is calculated. The ear is so highly sensitive, that is, it will respond to such small pressure variations, that there is no known method whereby direct physical measurement of minimum audible pressures can be made. It is necessary, therefore, to calibrate the sound generator employed at

182

intensities well above threshold and extrapolate downwards. This may be done if the response characteristics of the generator are intimately known.

In measuring thresholds by the "minimum audible field" method there is established a field of sound in "free space" (no disturbing reflected waves), and the effective pressures at a given point in it are determined. An observer is then introduced to the field, his head is placed in the measured area (conventionally, facing the sound), and the intensity is reduced to threshold level. Stimulation may be either monaural or binaural. In the stimulation of two ears the threshold is likely to be about 3 dB lower than for one.

Figure 7–1, which combines the results from several investigations,

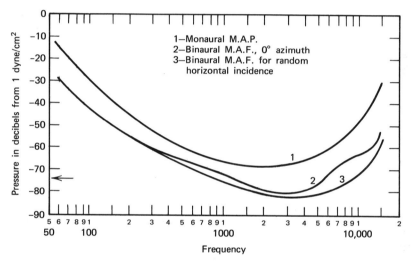

Fig. 7–1. Auditory threshold as a function of frequency. M.A.P. stands for "minimum audible pressure," M.A.F. for "minimum audible field." After Sivian and White (*529*). Courtesy of the editor, *Journal of the Acoustical Society of America.*

shows the size of the threshold (both "minimum audible pressure" and "minimum audible field" measurements) as a function of frequency. Threshold pressure values have been reported in decibels below a reference point of 1 dyne/cm^2. On such a scale the standard "reference intensity" (indicated by the arrow) has a value of -73.8 dB. It is seen from the curves that maximum sensitivity is realized in the region of 2000–4000 Hz and that thresholds are higher in both directions from this region. Thresholds at frequencies below those represented are higher still, being of the order of -20 dB on the same pressure scale for frequencies around 20 Hz, the lower limit of frequency recognition.

To pressures of the magnitude involved in threshold responses the tympanic membrane responds with extremely small excursions. A direct determination of this has been made by Wilska (640), using an ingenious technique. He cemented to the eardrum a light wooden shaft, the other end being attached to a loud-speaker coil. At amplitudes of vibration just arousing tonal sensations the excursions of the rod were measured with a microscope. Whereas such direct measurements could be made only at relatively low frequencies, it was possible to calculate threshold amplitudes for all others in the hearing range. Wilska's data reveal that, for frequencies in the neighborhood of 3000 Hz, the threshold amplitude is of the order of 10^{-9} cm, a value considerably less than that of the wavelength of light. Speculation as to what must be transpiring in the cochlea in response to such slight movements leads to the conclusion (553, p. 56) that the basilar membrane must be capable of initiating auditory sensations with movements smaller in extent than 1% of the diameter of a hydrogen molecule!

Such a figure is surprising enough, but there are indications that Wilska's values may be on the conservative side. It was necessary for him to extrapolate downwards from measurements reaching the limit of visibility near 10^{-4} cm. Also, his system was calibrated at one frequency only. Subsequently, a considerably more sophisticated attack was made on the problem with the use of calibrated vibrators and microphones (577) and, quite recently, with a highly precise laser interferometer (578). For sound intensities known to be approximately at the cat's auditory threshold, the peak displacement amplitude of the tympanic membrane is of the order of 10^{-10} cm in the neighborhood of 1000 Hz and closer to 10^{-11} cm at 5000 Hz. Apparently, the absolute threshold for the cat is at least an order of magnitude smaller than was shown by Wilska's human data. The difference more probably represents sharper measurements than any real difference between the species in absolute sensitivity.

Audiometry.   The measurement of intensive thresholds throughout the range of audible frequencies provides, of course, a means of assessing auditory sensitivity and of detecting any significant impairment of hearing. There has therefore been a large development of testing instruments, known as audiometers, which make possible standardized threshold determinations. The forerunner of the present-day audiometer was the tuning fork. In clinical use it was set in motion in what, hopefully, was a "standard" way; the examinee's task was to say how long the fork's tone could be heard before it died out. Norms of a kind were available but, with such relative lack of stimulus control, they were crude at best and, more often than not, the "standard" came to be the examiner's own hearing performance. With the advent of electronic techniques in the 1920s and 1930s, vast improvement was made in auditory threshold measurement. Telephone receivers were standardized for the purpose, and stable oscillating circuits were devised to drive them. Eight or more fixed frequencies, typically the octaves of C from 64 to 8192 Hz, served as test tones, and well-constructed attenuators, calibrated in what were thought of as "sensation units" (decibels), were varied systematically to assess absolute threshold.

Current practice in audiometry is also the child of electronic technology. Commercial audiometers, of which many designs are available, employ solid-state components, are typically calibrated in a series of frequencies determined by engineering practices (1000-Hz standard) rather than in the musical tradition, employ better constructed and more stable earphones, and are likely to be equipped with either a turntable or a tape deck for testing speech reception as well as the hearing of pure tones. One of the more successful forms is the Békésy audiometer, which slowly sweeps the frequency scale as the examinee "tracks" threshold by an up-and-down method of attenuator control that brackets minimal audibility throughout the major portion of the hearing range.

In the more conventional audiometric procedure, several "crossings" of threshold are made at each test frequency, usually monaurally, and these are averaged. A line connecting these averages, when related to some standard, becomes an *audiogram* (see Figure 7–2). The question of which standard is not a trivial one. Ideally, if individual hearing function is to be related to "normal sensitivity," the latter must be defined. What is "zero level" from which hearing handicap is to be measured? Should sensitivity to pure-tone stimuli or, more practically, to speech sounds be the basis of assessment? Are we interested in the average performance of the entire population or should the standard of normality involve only young ears with no history of hearing impairment?

Of these questions, the one concerning tones versus speech sounds is perhaps most easily answered. For the foreseeable future, largely because audiometry's history has dictated the use of simpler and more readily controlled stimuli, pure-tone audiometry will be the primary procedure. Moreover, the frequency range in which the vast majority of speech sounds fall is fairly adequately covered by three test tones found on the audiometer: 500, 1000, and 2000 Hz. Average results from these three frequencies ordinarily correlate highly with those from the use of recorded speech sounds (typically, lists of two-syllable words—spondees—and "phonetically balanced" single syllables).

The question of the zero-level standard has a long and somewhat

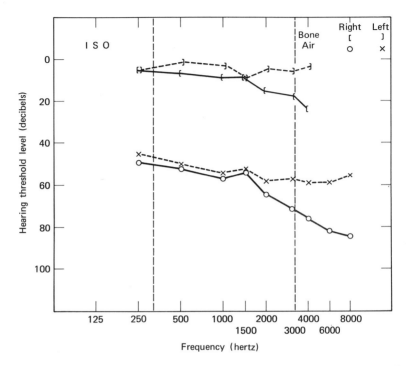

Fig. 7–2. Bone-conduction (top) and air-conduction (bottom) audiograms for a case of symmetrical middle-ear (conduction) deafness. Right-ear loss is more extensive than that in the left ear. Bone-conduction sensitivity, ordinarily measured only over the frequency range shown, is in this case nearly within normal limits but the sensitivity drop in the right ear at high frequencies suggests central (nerve) impairment in the right ear as well. Vertical dashed lines indicate the upper and lower limits of speech frequencies.

vexing history, though a solution seems now at hand. The difficulty arises from the existence of two sets of standards long in common use, not from any disagreement about what ears should be regarded as free from handicap. Tissues of the inner ear, like those of the eye, are subject to various types of atrophy through the ravages of age (and perhaps also those of industrialization!). It is thus obvious that the good, *young* ear should dictate standards of excellence in hearing. However, even confining test populations to relatively young people free of known auditory defect has eventuated in two sets of seriously discrepant standards. American practice, until very recently, has been based on the values adopted by the American Standards Association in 1951 (ASA-1951) and these, in turn, came largely from the first widespread audiometric survey ever conducted, that included in the National Health Survey of 1935–1936. This involved careful testing of over 4600 people (40). British practice, based on later standardization with more adequate equipment (137) found average thresholds in the 20 to 29 age group falling 10 to 20 dB lower than the American standard. Subsequently, there have been many new samples and remeasurements, several modifications in technique, and much rethinking of the problem, especially in its practical aspects. The culmination of all this was the adoption by the International Standards Organization, in 1964, of a set of zero-level values more nearly coinciding with the British norms (and 14 additional reliable studies, some American).

The difference between the old and new standards in use in this country is shown in Figure 7–3. On the average, there is a discrepancy of 11

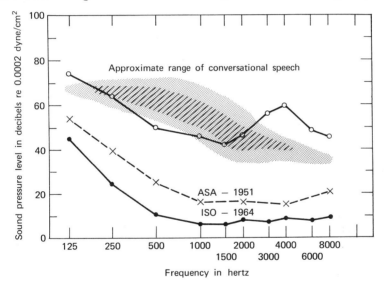

Fig. 7–3. Audiometric standards. The dashed line shows the levels of sound intensity, over a wide range of frequencies, adopted as threshold standards by the American Standards Association in 1951. The more recently (1964) established values are those of the International Standards Organization (lowest curve). From Davis (151).

dB, a really significant amount. Additionally, Figure 7–3 reveals several important features: (1) the widespread use of test frequencies conveniently designated in the decimal system; (2) the specification of hearing levels in dB units referred to the accepted physical intensity standard (SPL);

and (3) a quantitative description of the approximate ranges of both conversational and "fringe" intensities in speech. There is also included in the audiogram, by way of illustration, the record of an individual possessing moderate impairment of hearing.

As with all standards, it is one thing to adopt them, quite another to live up to them. It is common practice to return audiometers to their manufacturers periodically for recalibration. There are evidences that the frequency of return could profitably be increased or, alternatively, that standards need to be built into the audiometers themselves. One study of a sample of 100 instruments used in hearing conservation programs *(571)*, received from only 11 different agencies or individuals and comprising 30 models from eight different manufacturers, revealed that only two were adjusted to be in strict compliance with ISO standards. Of the total sample, 89% failed to provide the correct sound-pressure output of the phones. Some gave excessive harmonic distortion, some failed to preserve their proper frequencies, while some even presented obvious shock hazards!

If there have been difficulties, major and minor, about standards and calibration, there has been little disagreement, either from broad-scale surveys or individual otological practice, about trends in auditory sensi-

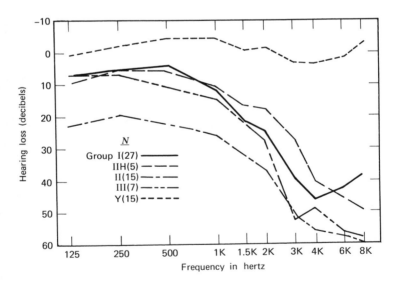

Fig. 7-4. High-frequency hearing impairment in aging people. The amount of hearing loss, for the better ear, in four groups, 65 years of age or older and distinguished on nonauditory clinical bases, compared with a 20-year-old group (top curve.) From Weiss *(616)*.

tivity resulting from the wear and tear induced by age and by exposure to injurious features of the environment such as noise.

The original Public Health Survey (*40*) showed: (1) large and significant losses of auditory sensitivity occurring with advancing years; (2) somewhat larger losses for women than men in the lower frequencies (under 2000 Hz); and (3) considerably greater losses for men than for women in the highest frequencies tested (4096 and 8192 Hz). Indeed, at these two frequencies men over 60 years of age had an average loss of 31 dB as compared with young people.

Subsequent surveys at World Fairs, various State Fairs, in the military, and in industry all point in the same direction. Large losses occur in the high frequencies with advancing age. Figure 7–4 gives comparative audiograms for five groups of male subjects, three of which (I, IIH, and III) can be considered together; the property they possessed in common was age greater than 65 years. Group II had some known severe hearing problems. Group Y were young men of 18 to 30 yrs (Median = 20). The finding is typical, a decline in auditory sensitivity beginning in the neighborhood of high c on the piano, roughly around 1000 Hz, and showing a sharp drop toward the higher pitches.

If shrinking auditory sensitivity traceable to the tissue changes of advancing age is a progressive thing, as it must be, one should expect that the upper frequency limit of hearing would show a steady decline as a function of age. Figure 7–5 reveals that it does and in a systematic manner. Whereas it is probable that the upper frequency cutoff is a quantitative, not a qualitative, matter, doubtless depending to some

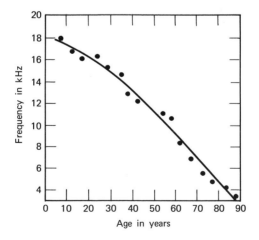

Fig. 7–5. Upper limit of frequency recognition as a function of age. From Hinchcliffe (*309*) after Schober.

degree on the energy with which the test tone is delivered, it is also to be presumed that the resources of the audiometer were exhausted in establishing the readings of Figure 7–5.

Measurement of the impairment of function, temporary or permanent, produced by loud sounds is also a task for audiometry. It has long been known that serious damage to the hearing mechanism can result from sustained or frequently repetitive loud tones and noises. At one end of the range debilitating annoyance and at the other outright auditory deterioration may be produced in many industrial and military situations—the hum and clatter of factory or office, noises created by high-power shop machinery (drop hammers, riveters, punch presses, weaving looms, printing presses, hydraulic rams, lathes and drilling machinery of certain types), shipyard operations (sheet metal and boiler plate fabrications), not to mention those modern champions among noisemakers, the jet engine with after-burner and the .50-caliber machine gun. Clinical otology is replete with case histories of incapacity developed over the years through daily work in the vicinity of trip-hammers and drop forges, so-called "boilermakers' disease."

The question of how best to defend the population in general against

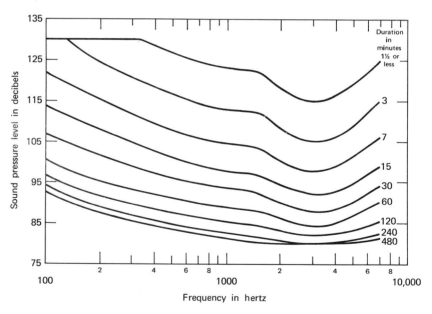

Fig. 7–6. Contours of equal damage risk as a function of exposure duration. All values presuppose an exposure frequency of one per day. From Kryter, Ward, Miller, and Eldredge (*370*).

the injurious noises in its environment is not simple. It is one around which a large literature has centered. The concerns are not all psychophysiological and theoretical; they are economic, legal, and esthetic as well. The same generalities that will serve for steady tones or noises do not obtain where explosive or impulsive noise is concerned. Moreover, as a practical matter, since all of us must withstand attack from generous portions of accidental sound—noise has been defined by the experts as "unwanted sound"!—there is the important question of how much damage risk the individual is willing to take in following the pursuits of his choice. A well-known fact here is that sound pressure level and exposure duration operate conjointly. Figure 7–6 shows contours of "equal damage risk." Provided a person is not going to be exposed to a 300-Hz tone, say, for more than 90 sec he would be safe in listening to one of 130 dB SPL. If, on the other hand, he is to have a continuous 15-min exposure it would be unsafe to listen to one of more than 105 dB. If the tone is one of 3000 Hz, he would do well not to exceed 90 dB (for 15 min), and if he is to spend a full, 8-hour day with the 3000-Hz tone, it should not exceed 80 dB SPL. Other comparable relations can be read from the contours of Figure 7–6. Also, similar charts have been worked out for both broad- and narrow-band noise *(370)*.

In the effort to derive population norms for sound hazards the circumstance should not be overlooked that individuals differ enormously in susceptibility to damage. Also, it is important to note that an ear, once impaired by overstimulation with sound, is thereby rendered more susceptible to further damage in the future.

Intensity Discrimination. In vision we confronted the problem of $\Delta I/I$, or differential intensity discrimination, and found the Weber fraction to vary in an interesting way with changes in intensity. In audition we encounter a strictly analogous problem. Given an initial intensity, I, how much must the energy of the stimulus be increased to produce a just noticeable difference, that is, what is the size of ΔI? A number of determinations have been made, and several variables influencing the magnitude of ΔI have been discovered to exist. It makes a difference whether the starting point is low or high on the intensity scale, at what frequency the measurement is made, whether one or both ears are stimulated, what the durations of the tonal exposures are and whether or not they are separated by a silent interval, whether there is an abrupt or a gradual transition between the two tones to be compared, and whether the observer making the judgments has the exposure sequence under his own control so as to be maximally "set" for change when it occurs. Many of these experimental variables were not encountered in vision. The ear is not essentially a "spatial" organ, as the eye is, and comparison of two intensities simultaneously present is not possible. Successive presentations, which must necessarily be resorted to, introduce complications.

The classic data on $\Delta I/I$ are those of Riesz (*496*). To avoid the production of "transients," unwanted additional sounds which are inevitably involved in presenting successively two discrete tones, he made his measurements by the "beat" method, two tones 3 Hz apart being allowed to sound together. This produced alternate intensifications and diminutions (3 per second) of what was experienced as a single tone. From the energies present at the threshold of the beating complex he arrived at the values presented in the curves of Figure 7–7. The size of ΔI (and of

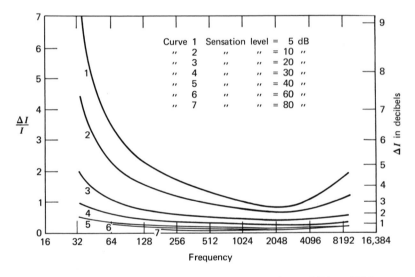

Fig. 7–7. Differential intensity discrimination. The data of Riesz (*496*) at seven different intensities, from 5 to 80 db, and for a wide range of frequencies are plotted. Reference to the ordinates on the right gives the magnitude of ΔI, to the left ordinates, $\Delta I/I$.

$\Delta I/I$) is seen to be minimal, i.e., differential sensitivity is greatest, in the region of 2500 Hz. Thus it appears that the frequency range in which greatest absolute sensitivity occurs is also that to which the ear responds differentially with the greatest efficiency.

The effect of the other major variable, intensity, may be observed by comparing the relative sizes of ΔI in the seven curves, each representative of a different intensity (sensation level). Far from being a constant, as demanded by Weber's Law, $\Delta I/I$ varies roughly between the limits of $\frac{1}{20}$ (2500 Hz at 100 dB) and 7.5 (35 Hz at 5 dB).

Frequency Recognition and Differential Discrimination. The limits of tonal recognition have already been stated to be 20 Hz to 20,000 Hz for the "good" (and young) human ear. These are the approximate limits. Apparently the response system of the ear cannot follow disturbances imposed upon it with frequencies higher than about 20,000 Hz; possibly the mass of the ossicles is too great to be overcome and thus permit threshold energy to be delivered to the cochlea at vibration rates higher than this. The lower limit is not so simply dismissed. If a pure-tone generator is set in operation at the very low frequency of 5 Hz and is raised progressively in vibration rate there are heard, in succession: (1) a "chugging" sound (discrete noises, having prominent high-frequency components); (2) an intermittent flutter; (3) a "thrusting effect" (resembling "piston slap" but complicated at one point in the cycle by high-frequency sound "very like the escape of steam from a jet"); and (4) a "rumbling" tonal effect. In one of the best controlled experiments designed to analyze these phenomena, that of Wever and Bray (*632*), the tonal character entered at 20 Hz, for some observers, and was present for all at 25 Hz with intensities above 15 to 20 dB. The lower limit of tonal recognition depends upon the intensity of the tonal stimulus. If intensity is kept down to 10 dB nothing at all will be heard below 20 Hz; then noises make their entrance, and a tonal character is not present until a frequency of about 60 Hz is reached. Other experiments have placed the lower limit for tone at 18 Hz (*52, 88*), and one of these, that of von Békésy, found "pitch" discrimination to be possible all the way down to 1 Hz, even though fused tones were no longer present below 18 Hz. The great difficulty in establishing the point where tone replaces flutter results from the fact that the transmission system of the middle ear and cochlea responds to even pure sinusoidal waves with a complex spectrum of vibrations. Harmonics thus introduced may serve as the basis of frequency recognition and give a misleading result.

If we begin at the lowest frequency audible as a tone and ascend the frequency scale it is possible to measure the size of successive Δf's and, from such measurements, to determine the differential frequency discrimination of the auditory apparatus, $\Delta f/f$. As with $\Delta I/I$, certain difficulties present themselves. If discrete, successive tones are compared there is encountered the annoying problem of transients, additional harmonics and noises that accompany any abrupt initiation, termination, or change in tone production. If a gradual transition from one frequency to another is resorted to there may be an artificial augmentation of Δf, for it has long been known that continuous changes are less noticeable than abrupt ones. The lesser of the two evils would seem to be to keep the stimuli relatively pure by employing a "sliding" tone. This was done in the classic experiment of Shower and Biddulph (*526*). They found that optimal judgments were made when the two frequencies to be compared were alternated at the rate of two per second, and this comparison frequency was used throughout the range of tones from 31 Hz to 11,700 Hz and for a range of intensities (sensation levels) from 5 dB to the maximum the subjects could "take."

The magnitude of Δf is a function of the absolute frequency at which the measurement is made. It is also a function of intensity. The size of $\Delta f/f$, for each of several frequencies and intensities, may be read from Table 7–1. It may be seen that $\Delta f/f$ is roughly constant for the higher

Table 7–1. The Values of $\Delta f/f$ for a Wide Range of Intensities (Sensation Levels) and Frequencies

The data are those of Shower and Biddulph (526) and represent the performance of five subjects between 20 and 30 years of age. From Stevens and Davis (553). Reproduced by permission of Bell Telephone Laboratories, Inc.

Sensation Level	5	10	15	20	30	40	50	60	70	80	90
Frequency											
31	.1290	.0873	.0702	.0563	.0438	.0406					
62	.0975	.0678	.0546	.0491	.0461	.0426	.0351	.0346			
125	.0608	.0421	.0331	.0300	.0266	.0247	.0270	.0269			
250	.0355	.0212	.0158	.0130	.0109	.0103	.0099	.0098	.0100	.0107	
500	.0163	.0110	.0081	.0067	.0055	.0052	.0042	.0035	.0042		
1,000	.0094	.0061	.0044	.0039	.0036	.0036	.0036	.0034	.0031	.0030	.0026
2,000	.0079	.0036	.0029	.0021	.0019	.0019	.0019	.0018	.0017	.0018	
4,000	.0060	.0044	.0038	.0031	.0027	.0023	.0023	.0020			
8,000	.0063	.0051	.0045	.0038	.0036	.0029	.0025				
11,700	.0069	.0058	.0042	.0038	.0036	.0035	.0030				

frequencies (for a given intensity). For the lower frequencies (below 500 Hz) Δf by itself is roughly constant, though this generality does not pertain to the lowest tones measured.

If the results of Shower and Biddulph may be taken at face value it would appear that there are, between the lowest and the highest audible tones, about 1500 j.n.d.'s. This result contrasts sharply with the older data of Luft (396), which, for many years, were responsible for the common textbook statement that there are 11,000 discriminable frequencies. Boring (83), reviewing the experiments performed on Δf and weighing the many experimental variables that enter into its determination, has concluded, "The 1500 discriminable frequencies given by the results of Shower and Biddulph are thus probably too few to express maximal sensitivity, but the 11,000 tones from Luft's data must be too many—very much too many."

Subsequent empirical studies do indeed demonstrate that the more reasonable figure is one lying between these outside limits. Improvements in stimulus control now permit a procedure that eschews both the frequency modulation device of the Shower and Biddulph experiment and the transient-laden tones of the more abrupt type of presentation. It is common practice, in preparing successive tones for comparison, to "shape" them with an electronic switch that imparts a relatively gradual onset and cutoff to the tonal envelope. Depending on the energy involved, the nature of the ultimate tonal transducer, and some other possible variables, the "attack" may be quite abrupt (perhaps only a few milliseconds) and still permit the minimizing of disturbing transients.

The results of one such study are graphed in Figure 7–8. In this experi-

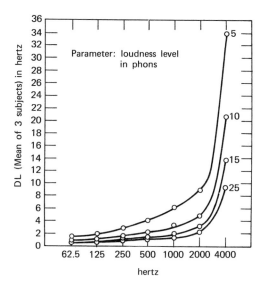

Fig. 7–8. The DL for pitch (Δf) as determined by frequency and intensity variations. From Harris (*273*).

ment (*273*), two successive tone bursts were compared. Each had inaudible transients, and a brief silent interval separated the standard and variable stimuli. A variant of the psychophysical method of constant stimulus differences was employed. The difference limen (DL = Δf) for pitch is shown to be dependent both on absolute tonal frequency and intensity, as in earlier work, but Δf is also appreciably smaller, for the same absolute frequency, than in the Bell Laboratories experiment. Indeed, it is five times smaller for some combinations of frequency and intensity. Unfortunately, the stimulus ranges are considerably more restricted in the more recent experiment, and it would not be possible, without dangerous extrapolation, to answer the earlier question of how many discriminable frequency steps there are in human hearing.

Pitch and Loudness.   Thus far, in dealing with auditory responses, care has been taken to speak always of discriminable features of *physical stimuli*. The sensations aroused by them have dimensions of their own, however, and these are describable from direct observation. *Pitch* and *loudness* are two such dimensions.

Pitch, as a dimension of tonal sensation, is the name given to the highness or lowness of tones. Because low frequencies yield low-pitched tones and high frequencies high-pitched ones it is natural to think of pitch as a simple, direct correlate of frequency. However, pitch is not uniquely determined by frequency, as we shall see.

Loudness is a second dimension, in general determined by the physical intensity of sound, but here again there is no one-to-one relation between the intensity of the sound and the loudness observable in its presence. Loudness is quite complexly related to intensity; also, intensity is by no means the sole determinant of loudness.

The important thing to note, at this point, is that pitch and loudness are names for separate aspects of auditory sensation and that they are not to be identified in our thinking with frequency and intensity of auditory stimuli. The former concepts are psychological, the latter physical. We shall subsequently discover still other psychological dimensions of auditory sensation to exist. It does not follow that, because there are only two dimensions of sound waves, frequency and intensity, there are therefore only two dimensions of the sensations they arouse. The sensation is the final step in a complex chain of events. Modes of variation, arising in the ear and its nervous attachments, may introduce discernible new dimensions.

The history of ideas concerning pitch and loudness is by now a long and involved one. Pitch, especially, has been a central consideration in auditory theory. The way one goes about explaining its mode of operation has everything to do with the form a particular conception of the auditory mechanism will take. We shall be returning to some details of both pitch and loudness when, in Chapter 8, we raise both general and specific questions about the way the inner ear must work. Meanwhile, we shall not be avoiding either dimension; they are completely ubiquitous.

Pitch as a Function of Intensity. A phenomenon reminiscent of the Bezold-Brücke effect in vision occurs in audition. It will be recalled that increasing or decreasing the intensity of most spectral lights will produce shifts in hue. Only certain "invariant points" are exempt. Similarly, the auditory apparatus responds to changes in intensity by effecting shifts in pitch. Low tones, when increased in intensity, become lower, whereas high tones are raised in pitch when intensified. There is likewise an "invariant point"; it appears on the frequency scale in the region of maximal auditory sensitivity.

The experiment demonstrating pitch shifts with change of intensity is performed by presenting, in succession, two tones of slightly different frequency. The intensity of one of the tones is adjusted by the observer until the two tones appear to be of identical pitch. On the basis of results from such an experiment Stevens (547) has derived curves showing the correspondences which must obtain between frequency and intensity to preserve constant pitch. Figure 7–9 presents a family of "equal pitch contours" from his work.

This phenomenon of shifting pitch as an accompaniment of intensity changes is an important one for auditory theory. Accordingly, it has prompted a fair amount of experimental work and no little speculation (628, pp. 340–346). Even though the shift is a relatively small one, it is definite and measurable. One would like to know what characteristics of the auditory system permit its occurrence. The available evidence suggests that the explanation is to be found in the mechanics of neither the middle ear nor the cochlea. Some crucial experiments performed by Thurlow (573) demonstrate that the same pitch changes occur—lowering of low tones and raising of high ones—when the initial tone is presented to one ear and the "loudening" occurs exclusively through the introduction of a second tone to the other ear. While the effect is most prominent if the second tone is identical in frequency to the first, this is not a necessary condition. Any frequency, higher or lower, produces the effect.

One would suppose that pitch changes induced by intensitive variations would play havoc with music. After all, the pitch shifts are appreciable ones, amounting in some instances to a whole musical tone. However, it is found that pitch variations of the type under discussion occur noticeably only with relatively pure tones. Musical instruments, with their complex timbres, produce tones which are perceived as of very stable pitch, and this occurs whether the instrument is played loudly or softly—happily for music! The explanation of this difference between the behavior of pure tones and that of complex ones is at present far from complete. It may be that musical tones, which characteristically have many and prominent harmonics in the region of maximal sensitivity (2000 Hz to 4000 Hz), are "anchored" by overtones falling in the invar-

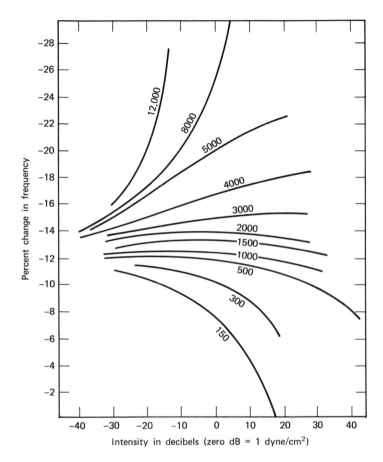

Fig. 7–9. Pitch as influenced by intensity. Contours of equal pitch from the experimental results obtained by Stevens (547). There is plotted the percentage change in frequency needed to keep the pitch of a tone constant as its intensity is changed. "The ordinate scale was arbitrarily chosen so that a contour with a positive slope shows that pitch increases with intensity" (553, p. 71). Courtesy of the editor, *Journal of the Acoustical Society of America.*

iant region. Or it may be that complex patterns of stimulation, once being set up in the central nervous system, are not easily altered by energy changes.

Makeup of the Auditory Area. Having seen something of the nature of Δ*f* and of Δ*I* it is now pertinent to ask what the results would be of integrating all the just noticeable differences of both frequency and intensity throughout the entire auditory area. How many separate tones are distinguishable in the region bounded by the intensitive threshold, the threshold of feeling, and the upper and lower frequency limits? The calculation has been performed by Stevens and Davis (*553*, p. 153) on the basis of the Riesz data for ΔI and those of Shower and Biddulph for Δf. The result shows that approximately 340,000 discriminable tones are contained in the auditory area. This figure may be a conservative one; it will be recalled that the Δf results doubtless err in the direction of containing too few steps.

Time and Auditory Sensitivity.   In vision we saw that time entered the picture at every turn—the relations determining sensitivity at brief durations (Bloch's Law and the critical duration), the conditions surrounding measurement of the various thresholds, afterimagery and contrast phenomena, light and dark adaptation, etc. Time is even more of the essence in audition. Hearing is predominantly a temporal sense, as we have already had occasion to note.

Time of stimulus exposure becomes a factor in the appreciation of both pitch and loudness. If a tone in the range of audible frequencies is shortened to a brief burst of sound, no longer than 200 msec, say, it will lose its rich, tonal character and become somewhat noisy. If it is reduced to about 100 msec or less it will be no more than a "click." How long must the exposure last for the click to become a tone, that is, how long is the *atonal interval*? The question is complicated by the consideration that clicks may possess a tonal quality! Indeed, the progression from click to tone is a three-stage affair. If duration of a click begins at a few milliseconds and is progressively lengthened until the stimulus lasts 400 to 500 msec, there will first be heard a toneless click, then one having some pitch but still constituting predominantly a click, and finally a stage in which pitch is both easily identifiable and unvarying with further lengthening. It seems convenient to distinguish the second and third phases as *click-pitch* and *tone-pitch*, respectively. Both kinds of pitch will be found to be dependent on both frequency and intensity of the stimulus, as well as on duration of exposure.

Figure 7–10 describes the results of one well-known experiment on thresholds of click and tone perception (*171*). Tonal intensity was held constant at the substantial value of 110 dB SPL, and liminal durations for click-pitch and tone-pitch were found for a wide range of frequencies. It is clear that time is not only related to the production of pitch but also to two separate varieties of it.

Loudness, as well as pitch, is partially determined by time. As with visual sensation, which we learned has an "action time"—the time

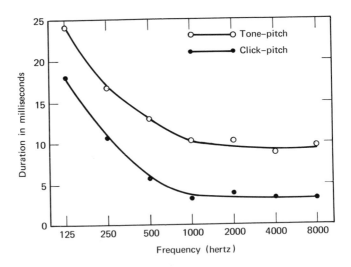

Fig. 7–10. Frequency and duration as determiners of click-pitch threshold (solid circles) and tone-pitch threshold (open circles). Stimulus intensity was uniformly 110 dB SPL. From Doughty and Garner *(171)*. Copyright 1947 by the American Psychological Association, and reproduced by permission.

between the onset of the stimulus and the reaching of the peak of excitability—auditory sensation has a time period following initial stimulation in which it shows a loudness development. A classic set of measures here is that of Békésy *(60*, p. 106) who matched to a constant 800-Hz tone of about 40-dB intensity and 0.2-sec duration a variable one at different times following the onset of the standard. The result is depicted in Figure 7–11. The ordinate states how much of an intensive change had

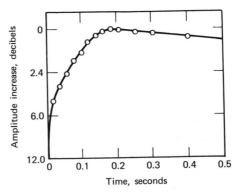

Fig. 7–11. Growth and decline of tonal loudness in time. From Békésy *(60*, p. 106).

to be introduced to produce a match. Apparently, loudness increases throughout a period of about 180 msec, then declines gradually with the intervention of the adaptation process. If another and quite different index of sensation growth is appealed to, the evidence is that loudness continues to make gains for a much longer time. Ekman and his colleagues (*185*) employed the magnitude estimation method and had observers judge 1000-Hz tones of varying durations and intensities. Estimates of loudness were still rising slightly when the test tone lasted as long as 600 msec. This is not the first time we have encountered different conclusions coming out of radically different methods, nor will it be the last.

Other Dimensions of Auditory Sensation.   Pitch and loudness we have already seen to be two separately discriminable aspects of auditory experience. Both are dependent on frequency and intensity, but they are quite different functions of the same two variables. Observation shows that there are two other dimensions of auditory sensation, *volume* and *density* (*84*, p. 375 ff.).

"Volume" is a word of several meanings. Because it has been used so freely in everyday speech as a synonym for "intensity" ("volume controls" on radios, e.g.) we do well to inquire carefully into its technical meaning when applied to auditory sensations. Tones appear to be big or little, massive or small; they vary with respect to volume. Typically, low-pitched tones are large tones; they seem to pervade space. High-pitched tones are tiny; they seem not to take up much room. If it is difficult to think of the shrill tones of a fife or piccolo as "massive" it is equally difficult to picture the pedal notes of a pipe organ as "pointed" or "minute." Perhaps it is entirely a matter of "picturing" it that way. Perhaps volume is a pseudo-dimension coming out of the common association of low tones with the large instruments that produce them and of high tones with the small ones from which they come. However, the case for volume as a sheer association is defeated by the experimental approach. Several researches have been directed at the measurement of "volumic limens." The variables of frequency and intensity may be manipulated to produce a just noticeable increase or decrease in observed volume. It is found that there is better than fair agreement among observers; in fact, it is possible to state with some accuracy the functional dependence of volume on intensity and frequency (*570*). Figure 7–12 shows the relation by way of presenting an "isophonic contour" of volume (as well as contours for other dimensions). The reduced volume consequent upon raising frequency may be compensated by an increase in intensity.

The same figure reveals the nature of the remaining dimension,

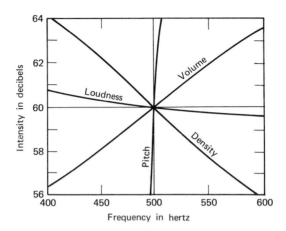

Fig. 7–12. Isophonic contours for loudness, volume, density, and pitch. Each line represents a set of coincidences between tonal intensity and frequency which will yield the same observed loudness, volume, etc. Thus a tone of 450 Hz and 58 dB and one of 550 Hz and nearly 62 dB are judged to be of equal volume. From Stevens (*546*). Courtesy of the National Academy of Sciences.

density. Tones vary with respect to their "compactness" or "thinness." High-pitched tones are typically "hard," "compact," "beady"; low tones are "loose," "rare," "thin." But, within limits, intensitive changes may make up for the densitive shifts brought about by frequency, as the iso-phonic contour for density demonstrates. The same compactness present in a high tone may be induced in a lower tone by raising its intensity.

The minor dependence of pitch on intensity and that of loudness on frequency, with which we are already familiar, are also shown in the remaining curves of Figure 7–12.

The contours of Figure 7–12 have not always gone unchallenged and, indeed, they have encountered some measure of disbelief. Such a limited range of intensities and frequencies is spanned in them as to provide no more than a suggestion of the broad generalities that might obtain for these dimensions. In particular, it has been thought that volume and density must be names for reciprocal aspects of auditory experience. As frequency increases, volume becomes smaller while density grows greater. At the same time, both volume and density are positively related to intensity, and this, of course, does not bespeak reciprocity.

Since the original contours were derived, there have been more thorough and more extensive studies of both dimensions. Terrace and Stevens (*568*) made use of the magnitude estimation technique and showed that tonal volume is a power function of sound pressure; as intensity is increased, volume grows at one rate or another, depending on tonal frequency. Figure 7–13 shows the log-log plots (power functions)

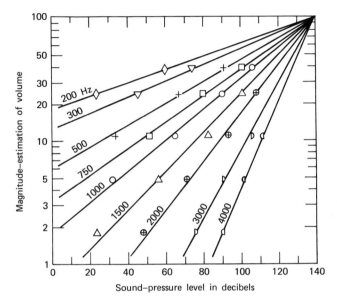

Fig. 7–13.   Power functions, for nine different frequencies, relating tonal volume to intensity. From Terrace and Stevens (*568*).

for nine different test frequencies ranging between 200 and 4000 Hz. All functions converge toward a single point in the neighborhood of 140 dB.

A volumic unit has been proposed, the *vol*. It is defined as the apparent volume of a 1000-Hz tone at 40 dB SPL. If volume, in vols, is graphed against frequency, in a double logarithmic plot, there results a considerably curvilinear function, not the nearly linear one implied by the volumic contour of Figure 7–12. See Figure 7–14.

Comparable experiments, with tones and ¼–octave bands of noise as stimuli, have been carried out for the dimension of density (*255*). Isophonic contours for a range of densities can be drawn relative to intensity and frequency axes (Figure 7–15), and they converge upon a point lying between 130 and 150 dB. Again, a unit has been proposed, the *dasy* (from the Greek word for "thickness"), defined as the auditory density of a 1000-Hz tone at 40 dB SPL. As with volume, a plot of density, as a function of frequency, yields a family of curvilinear relations, absolute density (in dasys) revealing its dependence on intensity. See Figure 7–16.

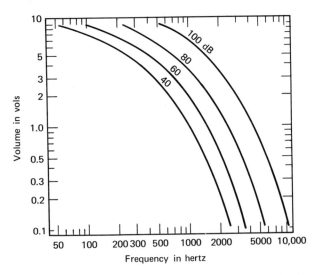

Fig. 7–14. Tonal volume as a function of frequency. From Terrace and Stevens (*568*).

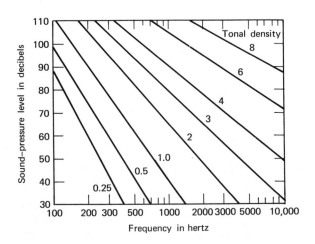

Fig. 7–15. Contours of equal density. Unit density (1 dasy) has been selected as that of a 1000-Hz tone of 40 dB SPL. From Guirao and Stevens (*255*).

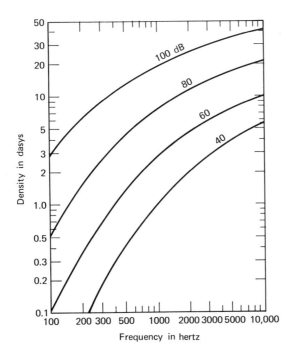

Fig. 7–16. Density as a function of frequency at four intensity levels. Narrow bands of noise were used in this experiment, though tones give much the same result. From Guirao and Stevens (255).

An amusing manipulation is that of plotting loudness estimates against the product of density and volume estimates (557). The data came from magnitude judgments of ¼–octave noise bands which, compared to pure tones, seem to yield estimates carrying a greater feeling of certainty with them. A wide range of intensities (42 to 100 dB) and center frequencies (200 to 6000 Hz) characterized the noise samples, which were independently judged for loudness, volume, and density. A log-log plot of loudness against the product of volume and density yielded a power function with an exponent of unity, a result which implies that loudness is strictly proportional to the multiplicative combination of the other two dimensions, that is, $L = V \times D$. A check on the accuracy of the relation involved a supplementary experiment in which the inverses of all three aspects, that is, softness, smallness, and diffuseness, were judged. Softness proved to be proportional to smallness times diffuseness, thus seemingly confirming the relation obtained earlier.

Other "dimensions" have been suggested from time to time, and certain of them have enjoyed brief careers of scientific acceptance. Thus *brightness, tonality,* and *vocality* have all had their day. We should have some familiarity with the concepts, for there is no doubt that the words refer to *something* discernible in auditory experience. The pitch scale may be thought of as a scale of "brightness." High tones are "bright," while low tones are "dull." However, two independently variable dimensions, pitch and brightness, are not found, nor are the differential thresholds for the two significantly different (*494*). Moreover, it is found that tones may be "brightened" by permitting high-frequency transients to enter into their production (*85*). "Tonality" refers to the intimacy of the octave relation. High c sounds more like low C than any tone between the two. In fact, we say in music that these are the *same* tone an octave apart. The confusion of octaves is the easiest error to make in identifying tones. But such confusions do not make tonality a dimension. The current judgment, influenced by the failure to discover experimentally the quantitative relations a dimension should yield, would seem to be that tonality is simply a name for the fact that octaves are confused more readily than are other tonal intervals. "Vocality" has made a more determined bid for recognition as a separate dimension of tonal sensation. By "vocality" is meant "vowel similarity." Tones are vowel-like or possess "vowel quality" in the sense that an observer, instructed to listen to simple tones and state which of the vowel sounds it most "resembles" will, after some preliminary training, make his reports with a fair degree of assurance and with surprisingly good consistency.

The classic experiment is that of Köhler (*366*), who, in 1910, used a series of tuning forks for low frequencies, and a variable-pitched whistle (the so-called Galton whistle) for high frequencies, and attempted to ascertain the frequencies that most nearly resembled selected vowel sounds. His results are of interest, quite apart from the question of their bearing on a separate vocalic dimension. The *u* sound (tr*u*e) was most intimately connected with a tone of 263 Hz; *o* (r*o*ll) gave 525 Hz; *a* (f*a*ther), 1053 Hz; *e* (t*e*n), 2100 Hz; *i* (mach*i*ne), 4200 Hz. The successive vowels: *u, o, a, e, i* were thus spaced approximately an octave apart. In addition to the vowel sounds the nasal *m* was linked with a frequency of 132 Hz and the sibilant *s* with 8400 Hz, thus adding an octave to either end of the vowel range. The current status of vocality as a dimension is not unlike that of tonality. Indeed, some have identified the two. On the other hand, Rich's repetition of Köhler's experiment (*494*) tended to equate vocality to volume, since the sizes of the differential thresholds for the two aspects of tonal sensation did not clearly warrant their separation.

Distortion in the Auditory Mechanism.   Strictly speaking, it is doubtful if anyone has ever heard a really loud "pure" tone, at least, heard it as pure. All systems responding to sound energy display distortion of one kind or another. The departure from fidelity takes several forms. Distortion of the driving force characteristics may be in amplitude, frequency, or phase. Of these, amplitude distortion is the most serious. The ear, in keeping with this general principle, distorts in a nonlinear fashion sounds falling on it. The main consequence is that it tends to introduce harmonics, overtones of the fundamental frequency being received. For human hearing the important questions are: How extensive is the distortion? How important to hearing is this introduction of *aural harmonics*? What elements of the hearing mechanism are responsible?

There was a time in the history of the study of auditory sensation when these questions were more readily answered than they are now. Helmholtz, for example, had a firm answer. It was the middle ear, in its failure to reproduce faithfully the gyrations imposed on it, that was responsible for aural distortion. Specifically, he singled out the tympanic membrane and the articulation of the malleus and incus. His general view of the mode of operation of the ear required that the chief complicating factors in hearing—overtones and combination tones—must all be present before the cochlea is reached, for the organ of Corti is capable of resolving the complexities by analyzing out the components.

The distorting action of the ear was brought under measurement for the first time in the 1920s, when the Bell Telephone Laboratories undertook a systematic investigation of it by an ingenious technique (*200*, p. 175 ff.). Noting, in experiments dealing with "masking" (later to be discussed), that frequencies corresponding to the higher harmonics of a pure tone behaved in a curious fashion, the Bell Laboratories investigators isolated the phenomenon and studied it. In the presence of a continuous pure tone of high intensity a second "exploring" tone, variable in frequency and intensity, was introduced. Whenever the variable tone came into a region corresponding to one of the overtones of the steady stimulus, audible beats were produced. On the reasonable assumption that the intensity of the exploring tone which gave the most prominent beats was a measure of the magnitude of the aural harmonics present (beats are most readily detectable when the tones producing them are equally strong) there were charted the frequencies and intensities of several of the aural harmonics. Their frequencies are, of course, exact multiples of the tones producing them. Their strengths depend both upon the fundamental frequency of the inducing tone and its intensity. Thus, for a pure tone of 60 Hz, all the first four overtones have made their entrance as detectable aural harmonics before a sensation level of 25 dB has been reached. For pure tones in the region of 1500 Hz no over-tones are noticed until a 50-dB sensation level is reached, where the first overtone is just detectable, and an intensity of 86 dB is necessary to render the fourth overtone audible.

But there is now considerable doubt about the efficacy of the "best beat" method. Extensive experiments by Békésy have led him to the conclusion that ". . . the method of best beats does not give a measure of the overload of the organ of Corti" (*628*, p. 588). What happens when a search tone is combined with the first harmonic (whose distortion products would comprise the large range of overtones being explored) is that, depending on the relative strengths of the two, their frequencies, and their phase relations, a new wave envelope is created. If the two components are slightly off-tuned, periodic surging of the maximal amplitude occurs and produces the waxing and waning characteristic of "beats." It does not follow that the beating complex has "isolated" any higher-order components. If there were no distortion at all, the same complex variations of amplitude would occur. Indeed, the known dynamic characteristics of the most obvious of the cochlear structures which might be expected to be nonlinear with respect to the driving force and thus initiate distortion products, that is, the basilar membrane, are such as to discourage the notion that an array of higher harmonics would be generated by a sinusoidal wave of a single frequency.

It may be, of course, that aural harmonics come on the scene a little later in the chain of events making up the overall response of the cochlear partition. Among theorists who take this position, Wever (*638*, p. 176) believes the distortion is introduced as part of the final stage of the cochlear action, at the point at which mechanical changes are being transmitted to the organ of Corti itself. Specifically, he has suggested that shearing motions in the *rods of Deiters*, which stand in most immediate relation to the hair cells, may generate the aural harmonics.

Wever's belief is prompted most obviously by the typical findings, his own and those of many other investigators, in recording from the cochleas of animals. Whenever the cochlea goes into operation there are generated within it electrical disturbances, the so-called "cochlear response" or *cochlear microphonic*. These waves are found to be exact counterparts of the sounds being led into the ear with, however, the important difference that they contain also the aural harmonics generated within the ear itself. Electrodes contacting the round window or some accessible inner ear structure may be attached to an amplifier and wave analyzer and the full structure of the sound spectrum present in the cochlea may be determined. Such an analysis should tell one quite exactly what is going on at the site of stimulation of the organ of Corti. By this means Wever and Bray *(633)* have measured the amount of distortion present in the ear of a cat when stimulated by a 1000-Hz tone. There were found, as well as the 1000-Hz fundamental, a large group of harmonics, as many as 16 being identifiable in some experiments. At high intensities of stimulation the aural harmonics were so prominent in the wave analysis as to make a total contribution over half that of the fundamental. At very low intensities no components other than the fundamental were present; the cochlear response was "pure." Figure 7–17 shows the elaborate pattern of harmonics generated in the cat's ear by 20 intensities extending over a wide range.

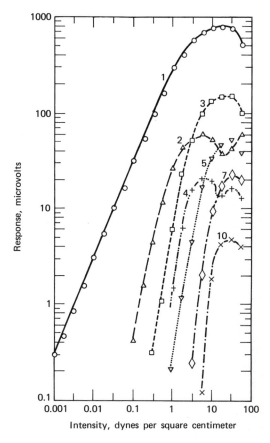

Fig. 7–17. Relative strengths of the harmonics created in the cat's ear by a pure tone (solid line, labelled 1) of 1000 Hz. Each of the other curves (2, 3, etc.) represents a multiple of the fundamental tone. From Wever and Lawrence *(638)* after Wever and Bray.

In general, when stimulation is of moderate intensity and distortion is not great, the harmonics appear in descending order of magnitude; for example, the first overtone is more prominent than the second, the second larger than the third, etc. However, at high intensities, when the transmission system of the ear is being "pushed," another phenomenon appears, that is, certain harmonics (3rd, 5th, 7th, etc.) become proportionately greater at the expense of the remainder (2nd, 4th, 6th, etc.). This fact goes far to identify the characteristics of the ear as a sound receiver. Sound-conducting systems may be broadly classified as linear or nonlinear, and as symmetrical or asymmetrical. Under forced vibration a nonlinear but symmetrical system will generate only odd-numbered harmonics. An asymmetrical system yields even-numbered harmonics. It is apparent, from the manner in which aural harmonics behave, that the ear's distortion is both nonlinear and asymmetrical when the system is forced into vibration by sinusoidal waves of moderate amplitude. At larger amplitudes the departure from linearity is the major feature of its response.

Why, even though the "best beats" method can no longer be regarded as demonstrating the existence of aural distortion, should there be any question about the reality of the phenomenon? The electrical response of the cochlea clearly seems to prove the presence of easily aroused and widespread distortion products. Part of the mystery is dispelled when it is found that not all observers agree on the sheer presence of aural harmonics in situations in which, one would suppose, they ought to occur. Plomp (474) has conducted an experiment on the audibility of aural harmonics in which he made available to a single receiver three tones, a fundamental and two higher frequencies (one of them pitched at a harmonic of the fundamental). By switching back and forth between frequencies and adjusting the intensities of the comparison tones it was possible to ascertain whether the overtones of the test frequency (the second to eighth harmonics) could be identified in the fundamental when sounding alone. The striking result was the large individual differences. Two of the ten observers never heard any aural harmonics at all, although intensities of the fundamental ran as high as 100 dB SL. Not more than half the observers ever reported hearing any particular harmonic and, on the average, only 17% of the trials led to positive identifications. Such uncertainties perhaps suggest why views as to the importance and origin of the phenomenon should not have been univocal.

Some of the anomalies connected with aural harmonics may ultimately be cleared up by the recognition that aural distortion is possibly more than a single-stage process. Experiments have been conducted which suggest that the two chief hypotheses concerning origin—nonlinearity in the vibration of the cochlear partition versus that in the final mechano-electrical transfer of energy at the organ of Corti—may both be correct. Dallos and his associates (*143*) have tested the effects of passing direct polarizing currents through the cochlear partition of guinea pigs and stimulating it with a variety of tones. Different things happen at different intensities. At high intensities changes in the distortion products are best interpreted as connected with the mechanical response of the cochlear partition. At low intensities changes are such as to be most readily identified with the final stages of cochlear action, triggering of the hair cells.

Lack of certainty is still with us here. What happens, in the final analysis, to the rich information about distortion revealed by the electrical response of the cochlea? Is it lost somewhere in the peripheral nervous system? Or is it that the loss is a positive gain—that the auditory message, having started out complexly, gets simplified, at least clarified, in transit to the brain?

Multiple Stimulation: Combination Tones and Beats. We have seen what happens through aural distortion when a single loud pure tone is led to the ear. What will be the result of stimulating with two such tones simultaneously? The nature of the response will depend upon the nature of the two tones. If they are of quite different frequencies there will be set up, in addition to the aural harmonics of each stimulus, some new products of interaction called *combination tones*. If the frequencies are quite close together there will result the phenomenon of *beats*.

Combination tones may be studied by either of the techniques used to identify aural harmonics. Certain of them are directly observable in the presence of the two interacting fundamentals, and additional ones may be located by the "exploring-tone" technique. Also, wave analysis of the electrical response of the cat's or guinea pig's cochlea yields a large number of combination tones.

There are two varieties of combination tones: *difference tones* and *summation tones*. The former have been known since the early eighteenth century and were noted by the celebrated Italian violinist, Tartini. He observed the presence of a third tone in double-stopping and came to use it as a check in tuning his strings. Difference tones are still sometimes called "Tartini's tones." The discovery of summation tones awaited the systematic researches of Helmholtz in 1856. As the name implies, a difference tone has a pitch determined by the difference between the frequencies of two other tones; a summation tone's pitch results from the addition of frequencies. Thus the first difference tone, D_1, which is easily detectable when two properly selected generating tones are used, has a pitch number coming from a simple subtraction of one frequency from the other; e.g., if the higher tone (h) has a frequency of 1000 Hz and the lower one (l) is 700 Hz, $D_1 = h - l = 300$ Hz. The first summation tone, S_1 would come from the summing of the fundamentals; $S_1 = h + l = 1700$ Hz. There are two "second-order" difference tones: $2h - l$ and $h - 2l$; three of the third order: $3h - l, 2h - 2l, 3l - h$; four of the fourth order: $4h - l, 3h - 2l, 2h - 3l, 4l - h$; etc. The general formula is: Order $= m + n - 1$, where m and n are all possible integers. A similar series exists, of course, for summation tones. The pitch number for any particular combination tone is therefore given by the expression: $N = mh \pm nl$.

Obviously a very large number of combination tones are obtainable, though from direct observation few appear. The reason is that combination tones lying at or near the location of either of the fundamentals or any of the prominent overtones of either fundamental may be masked to the point of inaudibility. Strong fundamentals are necessary to produce the distortion pattern to which the combination tones owe their existence; this situation also produces powerful masking. Analysis of the electrical potentials in the guinea pig's cochlea, under strong stimulation by tones of 700 Hz and 1200 Hz has, however, revealed the existence of 64 combination tones simultaneously present (446). Another similar experiment (634) found difference tones of the 20th order from fundamentals of 10,000 Hz and 100 Hz ($h - 20l$, a tone of 8000 Hz).

Now, what of the case where the two interacting fundamentals do not differ sufficiently in pitch number to generate combination tones? As has been stated, beats result when the two tones have frequencies quite near each other. If two tone generators are only very slightly mistuned, say 1 Hz apart, a very slow beat will result. Once each second there will be a regular loudening and softening of the heard tone. Similarly, two tones 30 Hz apart will produce 30 beats per second, etc. The rule is that the number of beats occurring each second tells one the frequency difference, in hertz, separating two tone generators. As has been seen, this fact may be put to use in the identification of unknown tones. Also, the fact that two perfectly tuned generators will not beat with each other is a convenient one; piano tuners make use of it constantly to bring two or more strings to the same pitch.

Beats may be detected when the mistuning of the primaries creating them is only very slight. The waxing and waning of loudness, which constitutes the "beat" under these conditions, may occur as infrequently as once in 2 minutes and still be noticeable. The exact lower limit for the detection of beats cannot be stated generally, since it is dependent upon the absolute as well as the relative intensities of the beating components. The problem is clearly that of determining how gradually ΔI may be introduced and still remain ΔI.

In the middle pitch range, when the frequencies are such that not more than four or five beats per second are created, the periodic surging is readily observed as a smooth rise and fall of loudness, commonly judged to be pleasant in character and effectively used in music. Beyond this point, with further separation of the generating frequencies, the smooth surging gives way to an intermittence which, if the tones are sufficiently intense, may be quite unpleasant. The intermittent effect consists of individual pulses separated by brief silences. With larger frequency differences, say 25 to 30 Hz, intermittence goes over into a roughness which continues so long as beats are observable. The point at which roughness appears and the further point at which it fades out, leaving only two clearly separate tones, are dependent upon the absolute frequencies involved. If the frequencies are high and of sufficient intensity tones may be heard to beat even though they are separated by as much as 250 Hz.

The apparent pitch of a beating complex is a matter of some interest. Beats are easily heard, but what is it that beats? Most investigators agree that, when the two primaries are close together, the heard pitch lies between them; the beat comes from an *intertone*. When the frequency difference is made larger the intertone remains and "carries" the beat, but the two fundamentals make their entrance on either side of it. Finally, the intertone drops out, only the roughness remaining along with the primaries to signal the presence of tonal interference.

The occurrence of beats is a testimonial to the fact that the ear is far from a perfect analyzer of sound. If analysis were complete, if Ohm's Acoustic Law held exactly, two tones differing by a few cycles would not beat with each other but each would be heard separately and distinctly, as they are when the tones are sufficiently separated to produce a resolution of the conflict.

Although both beats and combination tones arise from multiple tonal stimulation, care should be taken not to confuse them with respect to their probable physiological bases. Because the pitch number of the first difference tone is mathematically equivalent to the number of beats produced between the two fundamentals, many have been misled into regarding difference tones as "beat tones." Actually, beats and combination tones have nothing to do with each other. Combination tones, as we have seen, depend upon the ear's distorting action. If the response of the auditory mechanism were completely linear and symmetrical, which it is not, we should still hear beats, though combination tones would never occur.

Consonance and Dissonance. When two or more tones are sounded together, the various possible combinations differ very markedly with respect to their capacity to produce pleasing or displeasing effects. This is, of course, a matter of basic concern in music. Those tones that "fuse" well, when presented simultaneously, produce *consonant* intervals; those that have a "jarring" and generally unpleasant effect, which do not fuse intimately, are said to be *dissonant*. Although it has not always been a matter of universal agreement among musicians—musical styles, like others, change—those intervals, falling within the compass of an octave, generally regarded as consonant are: the octave itself (frequency ratio of 2:1), the major fifth (3:2), the fourth (4:3), the major sixth (5:3), the major third (5:4), the minor third (6:5), and the minor sixth (8:5). The last four have sometimes been called "imperfect" consonances, and, indeed, the various intervals differ, from person to person and in different ages of music, with respect to their relative "perfection" of consonance. One may, through repetitive hearing of a pair of tones, become so habituated to an interval as to change radically his judgment of its pleasantness or unpleasantness. The intervals commonly regarded as dissonant are: the minor second (16:15), the major second (9:8), the major seventh (15:8), the tritone (F–B, 32:45), and nearly all the intervals in which one term of the ratio is 7 (7:5, 7:6, 8:7, etc.), though some find the minor seventh (7:4) not unpleasant, especially as a transitional chord.

The language of music is an ancient one, and men in all ages have speculated about possible bases for consonance and dissonance. Galileo, in his *Dialogues* (1638?), addresses himself to the "splendid subject" of music and says, ". . . we may possibly explain why certain pair of notes, differing in pitch produce a pleasing sensation, others a less pleasant effect, and still others a disagreeable sensation. Such an explanation would be tantamount to an explanation of the more or less perfect consonances and dissonances. The unpleasant sensation produced by the latter arises, I think, from the discordant vibrations of two different tones which strike the ear out of time. . . . Agreeable consonances are pairs of tones which strike the ear with a certain regularity; this regularity consists in the fact that the pulses delivered by the two tones, in the same interval of time, shall be commensurable in number, so as not to keep the ear drum in perpetual torment, bending in two different directions in order to yield to the ever-discordant impulses. . . ." (*215*, pp. 99–100).

This perspicacious explanation does not sound too strange to the modern ear. In fact, the theory of consonance most favored at the present time, that of Helmholtz, is not very different in basic conception. It was Helmholtz' belief that relative consonance occurs when the upper partials of the tones producing the interval are coincident and that the 'roughness" accompanying dissonance results from the beating of partials separated by too small frequency differences to give unique impressions. Thus, the octave is the most consonant interval because all the even-numbered partials of the two coincide and reinforce each other. A dissonant interval such as the minor second not only produces beats between the fundamentals but also between a multitude of combinations of higher harmonics.

This view of Helmholtz' has not always met with ready acceptance. There have been many competing theories of tonal fusion (*451*, Chapter 6). However, the chief objection raised against Helmholtz, that consonances and dissonances remain when entirely pure tones are used in producing the intervals creating them, necessarily had to subside with the discovery of the aural harmonics. The ear provides the mechanism for beating upper partials if the stimuli do not.

A contemporary reworking of the consonance-dissonance relations has been undertaken by the Dutch workers (*475*), who have demonstrated with modern instrumentation and methods that harmonic interference is indeed the basis of the roughness of dissonance, thus supporting in essence Helmholtz's interpretation. The new note they add is to relate the whole matter to so-called *critical bandwidth*, a central concept in pitch and loudness discrimination and in the phenomenon of *masking*. We shall encounter it almost immediately in the latter context. For the present, let us simply note that tones whose frequency differences exceed critical bandwidth are always judged to be consonant, while the most dissonant intervals are those corresponding with frequency differences of approximately one-quarter of the critical bandwidth.

Masking.   Several effects of multiple tonal stimulation have now been considered: difference and summation tones, beats, and consonance-dissonance. There remains another, the phenomenon of *masking*.

If two tones of different frequency, one of high and the other of low intensity, are simultaneously led to the same ear it is likely that the weaker one will not be heard at all. It is said to be "masked" by the stronger. To reach audibility, to "cut through" the masking tone, the weaker one has to be intensified considerably. The amount by which the threshold of a tone (or noise) is raised by virtue of the presence of a second one may be taken as a direct measure of the masking strength of the latter.

This suppressive influence is nonspecific in the sense that it extends great distances throughout the frequency range, though the masking effect is greatest on closely adjacent frequencies. Loud, low-pitched tones, in particular, may extend their masking influence great distances throughout the sound spectrum. Finck (*196*) tried masking stimuli of 10, 15, 25, 30, and 50 Hz at relatively high intensities: 100, 115, and 130 db SPL. Whereas the lowest frequencies did not generate very spectacular effects, the loudest tones in the lower audible frequency range (25, 30, and 50 Hz) gave large threshold shifts. A 50-Hz masker operating at 130 dB SPL, for example, elevated the threshold of a 1600-Hz tone by 55 dB and even shifted upward by 23 dB the threshold of a 4800-Hz tone. Nor is there any reason to suppose that the spread of the masking effect stops there; higher frequencies were not tested in the experiment in question. There is every reason to suppose that maskers of the lowest frequencies ought to have very widespread influence throughout the audible spectrum; recall that Békésy's direct examination of the cochlear partition shows the basilar membrane's motions to be essentially in phase throughout its entire length when driven at low frequency, and it is presumably competition between the masker and the masked tone for peaking or "funneling" of the mechanism that is involved here.

Quantitative determinations of masking have been carried out systematically by Bell Telephone Laboratories, and the data obtained there by Wegel and Lane (*614*) are classic for this phenomenon. Figure 7–18 provides a picture of: (1) the degree of masking produced by a steady (primary) tone of 1200 Hz and 80 dB SL; (2) the complex phenomena occurring once the masking level is exceeded by the masked (secondary) tone; (3) the occurrence of beats in those regions where the secondary

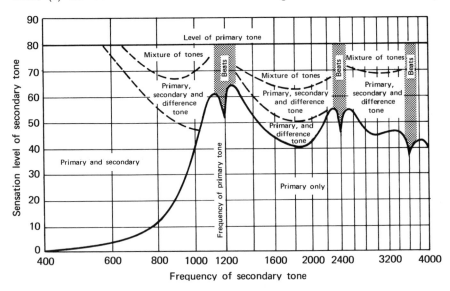

Fig. 7–18.   Tonal interrelations in masking. The data of Wegel and Lane (*614*), revealing the complex phenomena produced by a steady "masking" tone of 1200 Hz and 80 dB (sensation level) as a secondary tone of variable frequency and intensity, are introduced.

tone lies close to the fundamental or overtones of the primary. The continuous, irregular curve (the "masking audiogram") is the locus of thresholds of all frequencies of the secondary tone in the presence of the primary, masking one. Obviously, for all points under the curve the masking tone only will be heard. Above it, in those places where the intensity of the secondary tone is relatively low (roughly, less than 40 dB), both tones will be detected. In certain regions, for example, at 1800 Hz and 45 dB, the primary and the first difference tone are perceived; the secondary tone has emerged above threshold but makes its presence felt only through the generation of a difference tone. At higher levels the secondary tone enters the complex as a separately perceived component, and, at still higher intensities, the mixture of tones becomes elaborate as a result of the addition of prominent aural harmonics.

It would appear from the Wegel and Lane data that upward masking (toward the higher frequencies) is more effective than that in the downward direction. Such a conclusion would be hasty; there is an artifact here. If one consults curves derived from the same set of experiments but those in which lower masking intensities were employed, it is found that masking effects in the two directions are about the same. As is suggested by the locations of the irregularities of outline in the masking audiogram at high intensities, the primary tone receives an assist from its octaves. Of course, these are generated as aural harmonics by the powerful primary masker. If the primary tone is reduced below 40 dB SPL the masking audiogram no longer shows any appreciable skewness.

It is here that the concept of critical bandwidths, already alluded to in connection with our last topic, comes to perform a valuable service. The idea of critical bands goes back a certain distance in the history of auditory thinking. In some important experiments on masking, reported in 1937 by Fletcher and Munson (203), tones were masked by wideband noise rather than by other pure tones. Once there had been ascertained the distribution of energy throughout the sound spectrum that would mask all tones uniformly, it was found that the whole broad band of noise could be raised or lowered in intensity and the masking effect would still be uniform on all test tones. But something more important was discovered also—that the range of frequencies in the noise could be cut down considerably without altering in any way the masking capability of the noise. The width of the frequency band that would do this varied from one part of the spectrum to another. In general, low frequencies called for relatively narrow critical bands; high frequencies needed considerably wider bands.

Subsequently, it has become apparent that the concept of the critical band is indeed a basic one. Several different auditory phenomena can be united under its aegis. One of these concerns the reception of complex sounds. At threshold level, the acoustic energy needed to arouse a liminal sound is independent of the frequency composition of the sound so long as all components fall within the critical band. At higher levels, it appears that the loudness of a complex sound is independent of bandwidth until the critical band is transcended. At this point loudness begins to grow.

Similar considerations enter into the experimental manipulation called *two-tone masking*. Just as noise can mask tones, tones can mask noise. Two loud tones, separated on the frequency scale, are selected to "bracket" a band of noise, the threshold of which is to be measured. The noise threshold remains constant so long as both masking tones are within the critical band; when bandwidth is increased to fall outside the critical one the noise threshold promptly drops.

There are other effects that may be related to critical bandwidth, such as the ear's response to modulation of different kinds. These also are in harmony with the critical band concept. See Scharf's cogent review (*510*). Since the implication is that a short length of the basilar membrane behaves in a more or less unitary fashion, pitch discrimination ought to be a related phenomenon. It seems to be, the width of the critical band at any position along the cochlear partition being roughly 20 times the size of Δf. The human basilar membrane, about 31.5 mm long, on the average, may be thought of as divided into a succession of 24 small functional segments, perhaps averaging 1.3 mm in length and each supporting a critical band of frequencies. If the idea is valid, the distribution of sensitivities will have to check with the curve of Figure 7–19, which shows both the increasing size of the critical band (in terms of frequency range embraced) as the absolute frequency scale is ascended and the Δf curve, derived from the classic pitch discrimination experiment of Shower and Biddulph (*526*).

A question long asked about masking concerns its essential locus. Where in the auditory system is it initiated? It is easier to specify some regions where it presumably is not generated. The evidence is strong that it does not put in its appearance up to the point at which the hair cells of the organ of Corti go into action. At least, the chief electrical changes of the cochlea in response to stimulation—cochlear microphonics, later to be examined in some detail—fail to show masking effects in their repertory. If masking is peripheral in its origin it does not occur at the receptor cells themselves.

What about the auditory brain centers? One would suppose that a crucial experiment here would be to take advantage of the fact that we have two ears and two ascending pathways that must come together at

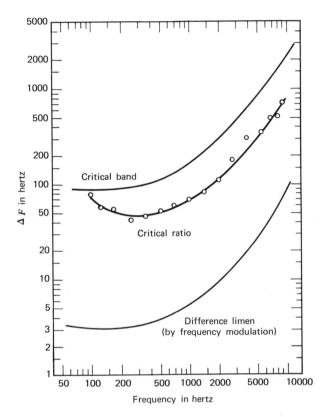

Fig. 7–19. Three measures of critical band width. The top ("critical band") curve shows how the band increases in width as the center frequency of the band is raised. The middle ("critical ratio") curve defines the width of the critical band in terms of "the ratio between the intensity per cycle of a noise and the intensity of a pure tone that is just masked by the noise." The lower ("difference limen") curve shows the width of the just noticeable "warble" or range of frequency modulation. From Zwicker, Flottorp, and Stevens (*666*).

the brain. A test signal can be led to one ear and a masker to the other. With suitable insert-type phones, relatively high energies can be delivered, well over 75 dB SPL, without inducing "cross talk" by way of transmission through the bones of the head. If this is done it is found that masking occurs, but not nearly to the same extent as when masker and test signal impinge upon the same ear. The size of the effect will depend upon the composition and mode of application of the two. The threshold of a test tone in one ear is raised only slightly by even a relatively strong pure tone in the other unless the two tones fall within the same critical band. Then the test tone may have to be increased very appreciably (by 10 to 15 dB) to be heard (*667*).

Pure tones are unnecessary to binaural masking. Noise also will mask contralateral test signals, whether they be tones or noises. It was found by Sherrick and Albernaz (*522*), who were the first to perform the experiment, that pulsing the masker and the test tone simultaneously, for short, relatively transientless bursts, brought about more binaural masking than when steady stimuli were employed. Figure 7–20 shows the amount of

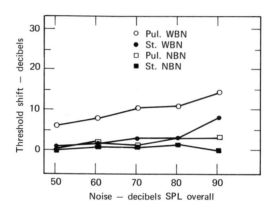

Fig. 7–20. Size of threshold shift, for a 1000-Hz tone, produced by steady (St.) or pulsed (Pul.) noise in the opposite ear. In some experiments wide-band noise (WBN) was employed; in others the noise was narrow-band (NBN). From Sherrick and Albernaz (*522*).

threshold shift produced for a 1000-Hz tone when both wide-band and narrow-band contralateral maskers were at work. Intensity of the masker is of some importance but not nearly so much so as keeping masker and test tone within neighboring frequency regions (*165*).

Where, then, does masking occur? It looks very much as though masking may occur anywhere in the system that neural interaction can take place. It is too early to guess about details of the process, but the best candidate for explanation would seem to be the intricate interplay of excitation, facilitation, and inhibition that must be occurring all along the ascending pathways. As we have seen, a minimum of four neurons comes into play—five, if we include the cortical cells themselves—and there are collaterals and alternate longer paths present at several points en route. A study of Ades' description of the central auditory mechanisms is revealing in this context (*4*).

Auditory Adaptation.   The ear, like the eye, adapts in response to steady stimulation, although the evidences that it does so are not too obvious in everyday experience. Listen to a prolonged tone and it is not apparent that it is undergoing a loudness reduction. There is nothing to reveal that the ear's sensitivity is being altered. But, then, in the absence of some comparative stimulus the brightness reduction occurring in vision during light adaptation is not ordinarily remarked, either. A more sensitive approach is obviously needed.

There are several experimental avenues to the measurement of auditory adaptation (or "fatigue"—the older term has not yet evaporated completely). Some of the techniques are direct analogs of those used in vision; some are peculiar to audition and derive from special properties of the auditory system. Let us consider the visual analogs first. In general, these are the more "solid" methods.

Just as one may determine the extent to which steady stimulation of the retina has produced a diminished sensitivity by ascertaining what elevation of threshold has been brought about, it is feasible to measure the

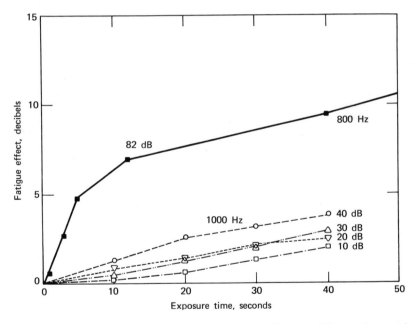

Fig. 7–21.   Elevation of thresholds through adaptation at different intensities. The curves for 1000 Hz show the raising of the threshold for tones of low and moderate intensity. The results for the high-intensity 800-Hz tone reveal more clearly the curvilinear nature of the function connecting fatigue effect and time. After Wever (*628*).

reduction of auditory sensitivity by making a rapid determination of absolute threshold immediately following a period of unvarying auditory stimulation. Figure 7–21 presents Wever's combining of the results of two different but comparable experiments (628, p. 320), both conducted by the threshold method. Low and moderate intensities of adapting stimulus (10 to 40 dB) lead to a simple exponential loss of sensitivity—(the "fatigue effect" is plotted in decibels)—while a strong tone (82 dB) produces an initial rapid drop in sensitivity which is followed by a more gentle threshold rise. More recent studies of auditory adaptation by the threshold method have prompted consideration of a most elaborate set of variables generally subsumed under the concept, "temporary threshold shift" (TTS). A valiant effort to untangle its considerably confused literature has been made by Ward (607). Knowing, as we do, about the complexities attending manipulation of the absolute visual threshold, it should not be surprising to find that alteration of the auditory threshold through adaptation should be a function of many variables, among them intensity, overall stimulus duration and energy distribution through time, wave composition of the adapting tone or noise, especially in relation to that of the test tone, prior state of adaptation, the psychophysical method used in threshold measurement, and certain well-recognized observer variables, for example, age and experience at the observer task.

The other chief method of measuring the course of auditory adaptation is also analogous to a visual technique. It involves the provision of a "comparison field" that may be matched, in apparent intensity, to the adapted one (Chapter 3). In audition the two "fields" are provided by the two ears, the adapting stimulus being allowed to work, for a preset time and intensity, on one ear and a comparison stimulus, presented immediately on concluding adaptation, in the other. Two early experiments were those of Békésy (55, p. 354 ff.) and Wood (649). Very similar conditions were imposed upon the subjects in the two experiments, which were performed quite independently of each other, and very similar results were obtained in the two. Figure 7–22 presents a typical adaptation curve from Wood's work. The stimulus was a 1000-Hz tone of moderate intensity. After steady stimulation of one ear for intervals ranging from 5 sec to 2 min the adapting tone was cut off and a 1-sec comparison tone was delivered without delay to the other, previously unstimulated ear. In successive trials the intensity of the comparison tone was changed systematically, and a match to the loudness last heard from the adapting tone was established.

The course of the curve of Figure 7–22 shows that there is a quite precipitous reduction of loudness (expressed as the remaining percentage of the original loudness) in the first few seconds, then a negative accelera-

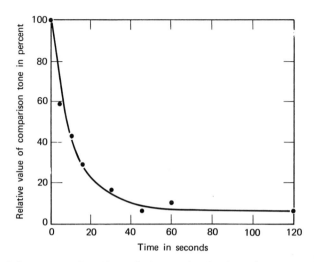

Fig. 7–22. The course of auditory fatigue. The decline of apparent loudness of a steadily exposed tone of 1000 Hz. Percentages of the initial intensity required to produce a loudness match in the unfatigued ear are plotted on the ordinate. From the unpublished work of Wood (*649*).

tion of the declining sensitivity to a new equilibrium level. Wood's results have been confirmed by several subsequent experiments. Figure 7–23 brings together a representative curve from Wood's work, one from that of Egan (*182*), and, by way of comparison with the analogous process in vision, one of Wallace's (cf. p. 57) light adaptation curves.

There are still other ways of investigating auditory adaptation, both its course and its extent. The differential threshold may be used, for example, rather than the absolute one. One method puts the continuous adaptation stimulus in one ear and an adjustable comparison tone in the other, the latter giving a 200-msec burst and alternating with equal periods of silence. In essence, the comparison of balancing stimulus "tracks" the intensity of that heard in the adapting ear. An obvious question concerns how much adaptation is taking place in the measuring ear, which must as a result be giving false indications. Palva and Kärjä (*457*), who tracked adaptation in 38 adults by such a method for 3-min periods, using 7 frequencies (250 to 6000 Hz) and 4 intensities (20 to 80 db SL), found huge individual differences. Half the subjects showed slow reductions in sensitivity, maximum adaptation being reached near the end of the 3-min test. Nearly all the remainder showed a rapid drop in sensi-

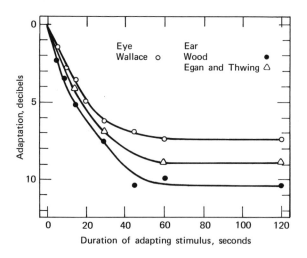

Fig. 7–23. The course of adaptation for eye and ear. Adaptation curves for vision (Wallace, *600*) and hearing (Wood, *649;* Egan and Thwing, *Journal of the Acoustical Society of America,* 1955, **27**, 1225–1226) are compared. Cf. Figs. 3–12 and 7–22. From Small *(535).* Courtesy of Academic Press, Inc.

tivity in the early stages (much as would be expected from the classical studies), while 5% gave no evidence whatever of any adaptation having taken place! One sees why observer variables must be listed among the parameters complicating the story of adaptation.

Another method takes advantage of the fact that unbalanced loudness in the two ears will produce a displacement of localization from the median plane of the head. One can thus give a prolonged period of adaptation in one ear, then either determine what intensity in the other will produce a median localization or present the initial adapting intensity to the unadapted ear and measure the time for the displaced "phantom" to move back to its original locus.

Clearly, any stimulus manipulation that will sensitively and reliably measure differences of sensitivity between the two ears can be put to work in the study of auditory adaptation, for reduction of sensitivity and recovery of it are the two sides of the shield, here as in vision.

"Persistence," "Flutter," and After-Effects of Stimulation. We have already noted that a short but appreciable time is required to bring auditory sensation up to peak (p. 200). The sensory system needs a little time to develop its product. It has an "action time." It should be no surprise, therefore, to learn that it also needs time to subside. Auditory sensation briefly outlasts its stimulus.

There are several ways of going about the measurement of the decay time of auditory sensation. One technique is to make comparisons between the sound created when a stimulus is cut off abruptly and when it is made to subside more slowly. If a decay rate can be found that just fails to sound different from a sudden termination, presumably the fading time at such a setting is the physiological decay time. Békésy found the subsidence of an 800-Hz tone to take about 140 msec, and Miller found white noise to decay in a somewhat shorter period. The two experiments are in agreement on the fact that intensity is not a factor. Both tones and noises fade to threshold in a uniform period, the slope of the decline necessarily being greater for the stronger stimuli.

Another method of measuring decay time is to present two brief tones or, better, two bursts of white noise, the two separated by a silent interval. The observer's task is to find the separation at which, 75% of the time, the gap can be detected. Presumably, when this limen is reached, the sensation of noise is just carrying over from the end of the first burst to the onset of the second. The time needed proves to be a function of the intensities of both pulses (473). By systematically varying the energies of both bursts, it is possible to derive functions which, extrapolated downward, will tell us how much time must elapse before the absolute intensitive threshold would have been reached. The linear functions plotted in Figure 7–24 show all decay lines converging at a point a little above 200 msec. This, then, is the total decay time.

It is only one step from a consideration of persistence of auditory sensation to the question of whether such a sensory lag provides the basis for the fusion of repeated discrete pulses. Does there occur in audition anything analogous to the flicker phenomenon in vision? Is there, for example, a point of fusion which, like the CFF in vision, might serve as a useful index of auditory sensitivity?

The question is not a new one. Before auditory research was revolutionized by electronics, an attempt was made by Weinberg and Allen (615) to establish the validity of the auditory "critical flutter frequency". In front of an orifice that conducted a tone to the ear, they rotated a disc having four symmetrically disposed holes cut in it. The disc, like the sector wheel of flicker experiments, was supposed to produce alternate "on" and "off" periods. What actually happened was that the disc only succeeded in yielding periodic fluctuations of intensity. It was amplitude-modulating the stimulus, as Wingfield's careful repetition and improvement on the original experiment clearly demonstrated (644). "Flutter" was produced, of course. This happened when modulation

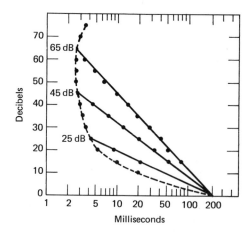

Fig. 7–24. Total auditory decay time. On the abscissa are plotted just detectable intervals (Δt) between two noise pulses. Intensity (SL) of the second pulse is given on the ordinate. Four experiments were performed: (1) intensity of the first pulse was uniformly 65 dB SL (top solid line); (2) first pulse intensity was 45 dB (middle line); (3) first pulse intensity was 25 dB; (4) the two pulses were equated in sensation level (dashed line). All four functions have been extrapolated to a common value of 225 msec. From Plomp (*473*).

changes exceeded ΔI. When they did not, there was apparent "fusion," that is, there was insufficient fluctuation of intensity to give flutter, and the tone naturally appeared steady.

It should be clear that such a manipulation in no way resembles the flicker-fusion-point situation of vision. The "flutter point" of the Weinberg-Allen experiment was sheer artifact. However, through other arrangements (electronic ones), it is quite possible to produce sharp onsets and cutoffs of tonal envelopes or of brief "packages" of noise. The latter is the preferable medium because with white noise, composed as it is of a wide spectrum of frequencies, there is introduced no differentiating cue at the instant of change. Transients, which contaminate sudden tonal presentations, are themselves noise, of course, though typically not "white," since they are likely to have peaks in their spectra.

In 1948, Miller and Taylor first proposed that a true auditory flutter, analogous to visual flicker, could be obtained by suitable "chopping" of white noise (*421*). Gating a noise signal with an electronic switch, they obtained a series of bursts that could be varied in interruption rate, duty cycle, and amplitude. As will be recalled, these are precisely the variables manipulated in flicker experiments. It was arranged that the chopped signal would alternate with a continuous noise at 1.5-sec intervals. Thus, when flutter gave way to fusion, as it would when intensity was lowered sufficiently to stay within the bounds of ΔI, there would simply be a steady "rushing" sound. This "critical flutter frequency" was found to be measurable over a wide range of interruption rates, from a few to well over 1000 per second (at a 0.5 duty cycle), but discrimination of flutter rate became quite poor in the upper frequencies, over about 250 pulses per second. Up to that point the flutter produced a recognizable pattern that could be matched for pitch with a pure tone.

The parallelism of auditory flutter and visual flicker seems considerably less intimate in some subsequent work. In one experiment that sought to isolate the important parameters of flutter (266), it was found that neither intensity nor sound-time fraction (duty cycle) seemed to matter. The only variable controlling flutter fusion point proved to be "off time," that is, the duration of the silence between pulses. Both rise and decay times were varied to given sloping onsets and offsets rather than a simple rectangular envelope. "On time" was of no consequence. When off time was such as to permit a 0.4-dB fall in intensity during decay, the flutter point was reached. It was even possible, with the more gradual onsets and offsets, to let the envelope contain pure tones rather than white noise, with substantially the same result for tones as for noise. Figure 7–25 shows the dependence of the critical flutter point on off time and the lack of it on signal intensity.

A curious aftereffect of relatively prolonged stimulation has been dis-

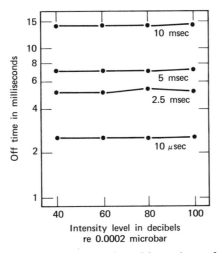

Fig. 7–25. Critical flutter fusion points for white noise at four different sets of rise and decay times and intensities. Duration of the silent period between pulses is completely controlling. From Harbert, Young, and Wenner (266).

covered in the Harvard Psychoacoustic Laboratory (*386*, p. 1013). After listening for a half-minute, say, to a continuous series of strong sharp pulses, which appear as a steady, intense buzz, new sounds presented to the ear take on a peculiar "metallic" or "rasping" quality temporarily. The noise of a typewriter in action, of two pieces of sandpaper being rubbed together, or of any other familiar sound pattern, especially if it is discontinuous and complex in harmonic content, takes on this ringing or jangling timbre immediately following the conditioning exposure. The aftereffect lasts only a short time, from 1 or 2 sec up to 10 or 12, depending on exposure time, stimulus strength, constitution of the pulse train, and probably the character of the test stimulus. Attempts to discover the optimal conditions for the effect (*506*) reveal that: (1) A certain kind of stimulating pattern is necessary. Random noise, whether continuous or interrupted, is ineffective. (2) A square-wave pattern produces the effect but not nearly as vividly as rectangular pulses of the same peak intensity; (3) prominent high-frequency components must be present in the acoustic pattern for the best aftereffect to result; (4) duration and intensity of exposure may be substituted for each other to a certain extent; that is, brief strong stimuli and long weak ones operate in an equivalent manner; and (5) a relatively narrow range of pulse frequencies (30 to 200 per second, with a maximum slightly above 100) may be used effectively. The aftereffect displays itself only in the presence of a test sound. It does not assert itself against a background of silence. For this reason it is best to characterize the phenomenon as an *aftereffect* of stimulation, not as an auditory "afterimage," as its codiscoverers have unhappily called it.

An effect more nearly meriting the designation, "auditory afterimage," has been described by Zwicker (*665*). He arranged that a white noise would have a half-octave band of frequencies suppressed and the remainder presented at a moderate intensity level of about 60 dB SPL. With an exposure of one minute there is heard, immediately following the stimulus cutoff, a tone that lasts for about 10 sec. The "afterimage" can be matched in pitch to a pure tone having a frequency within the suppressed band.

The effect apparently does not appear in response to either high- or low-intensity stimuli, only moderate ones. It does, however, occur with both long-lasting and brief noises; when stimulus duration was reduced to as little as 300 msec the tonal afterimage was there. If a wider band of frequencies is suppressed, for example, a whole octave, the afterimage is weakened and its tonal character degenerates. The phenomenon is apparently monaural. Two different band suppressions, one in each ear, leads to two afterimages forming a chord! With repeated brief bursts of band-suppressed noise, 100 msec on and 100 msec off, there is created a weak, continuous tone lying within the range of the missing frequencies.

8

Electrophysiology
and Auditory Theory

The Microphonic Action of the Cochlea.   Electrical potentials recorded from the region of the round window can serve as a revealing index of events transpiring within the cochlea. The story of the discovery of the cochlear potential is one of the most dramatic in the history of psychophysiology. In 1930 Wever and Bray, working in the Princeton Psychological Laboratory, attempted to study action potentials in the auditory nerve of a cat by hooking a pair of electrodes to the short extent of nerve leading into the medulla, amplifying, and reproducing the electrical changes in a loud speaker. They were successful in picking up electrical waves accompanying tonal and vocal stimulation of the cat's ear. The waves proved to be faithful reproductions of the stimuli, so faithful that an observer listening at the receiver could identify, by the quality of his voice, the person speaking into the cat's ear! It appeared that the cat's auditory nerve was serving as one part of a telephone system and was reproducing with considerable fidelity all the complex waves delivered to the ear, even those of relatively high frequency.

The phenomenon reported by Wever and Bray naturally aroused considerable scientific interest, and several repetitions of the experiment were undertaken almost immediately. Not only did the "Wever-Bray effect," as it came shortly to be called, seem to be crucial for auditory theory, but the finding that high frequencies of nerve impulses could apparently be conducted by the auditory nerve seemed in a fair way to revolutionize modern neurology. Hitherto it had been thought that the maximum frequency any nerve could conduct was of the order of 1000 per second, being limited to this value by the "absolutely refractory period," known to be about 1 msec in duration. The Princeton investigators had reproduced tones of 5000 Hz over their cat-telephone, and this would call for a refractory period lasting no longer than $\frac{1}{5}$ msec.

The work stimulated by the Wever-Bray experiment was extensive and valuable. More solid facts were added to auditory psychophysiology in the next ten years than in any other similar period of research in this field. It turned out that the first interpretation—that the counterpart of the stimulus was being carried over the auditory nerve—was incorrect. The Wever-Bray effect proved to be compounded of two phenomena: auditory nerve action potentials and aural microphonics, the latter generated not in the nerve but in the cochlea. Since the two may be picked up simultaneously from the auditory nerve close to the cochlea—and will be, unless special steps are taken to isolate one or the other—it is not greatly to be wondered at that they were intermingled in the initial Wever-Bray study.

The two effects have important points of difference, however, and it is possible to separate them analytically, even though their physical separation requires a considerably more intimate electrode arrangement than was obtained in the original study. Let us examine briefly some of the differentiating features. Whereas, in experimental animals, both the nerve response and the electrical response of the cochlea are adversely affected by cold, reduction of blood supply, anesthetics, or death of the animal, the cochlear response is considerably more resistant to such changes. The waveforms of the two are also different. The cochlear microphonic follows relatively faithfully the waveform of the stimulus (except for the addition of aural harmonics, as we have seen); the nerve response displays "spikes" characteristic of action potentials in other nerve preparations. The temporal characteristics of the two responses also differ. The time lag of the cochlear microphonic is inappreciable; its onset follows the introduction of the stimulus by only about 0.0001 sec or less. The nerve response always shows a considerably longer delay. The cochlear microphonic has no "threshold" in the same sense that the nerve has one. The lower limiting value for the former is that of the instruments used to record it; the nerve response requires considerably more energy to set it off. It does not display the adaptation or "fatigue" phenomenon. In one experiment (486), continuous exposure of a cat to a moderately loud, 1000-Hz tone produced an undiminished cochlear microphonic for 85 hours, the full period of physiological unimpairment. Perhaps the outstanding difference, however, has to do with the frequencies displayed by each. Action potentials never have the extremely high-frequency components found in aural microphonics. The latter presumably go at least as high as the upper-frequency limit of hearing (16,000-Hz waves have been recorded), while frequencies much above 4000 Hz yield nerve responses that are not well synchronized with the stimulus. The high frequencies in the Wever-Bray experiment were a part of the cochlear microphonic.

In sum, then, the cochlear microphonic has no refractory period or any of the other "all-or-nothing" features connected with nervous action. This indicates that the two phenomena, nerve response and cochlear microphonic, probably have quite different origins.

What can we say about the probable origin of the cochlear microphonic? There would seem to be only a few ways in which alternating electrical currents can get generated in biological tissues: (a) by movement of ions, (b) by displacement of electrical charges, and (c) by variations in electrical impedance between two stable charges. The movement of ions is perhaps too slow a process for the task at hand but either of the other principles can be and have been applied to the problem of accounting for the cochlear microphonic. It has been widely assumed that the hair cells of the organ of Corti are the generating elements, though Reissner's membrane was at one time suspect, as was the tectorial membrane.

Are there clear evidences that there exist the basic electrical potentials for such generation? There can be no doubt of it. Living cells are potent energy producers. In general, they tend to be electrically polarized, that is, there is a characteristic difference of potential between the two sides of the cell membrane. The cell is typically negative internally and positive externally. Since there are many different types and conditions of cells in the cochlea, it should not surprise us to learn that several d.c. potentials have been found to exist there. There is a relatively large potential, amounting to 50 to 80 millivolts, known as the "resting" or *endolymphatic potential* of the cochlear duct. This potential, discovered by Békésy in 1952, can be recorded with one electrode in the duct and the other in the perilymph of the scala tympani or, indeed, by "grounding" almost anywhere in the inactive tissues of the head. Other, lesser potentials can be found by entering Reissner's membrane (about -20 mv) and other structures of the cochlear partition. Just how these potentials are generated is still something of a mystery, as is the way in which their general level may be shifted. Davis at one point hypothesized a "summating potential" that influenced the baseline of the endolymphatic potential through neural summation but subsequently concluded that it was brought about by asymmetry of Békésy's traveling waves. Cf. Davis's (*148*) and Wever's (*630*) accounts.

Figure 8–1 shows one conception, that of Wever (*628*, p. 149), of the electrodynamic changes occurring when the hair cells are stimulated. The hair tufts, embedded as they are in the tectorial membrane, produce a strain on the cell membrane when the cochlear partition is forced into vibration. Corresponding changes in polarization result, as indicated in Figure 8–1. The motion imparted to the cells may be more of a shearing

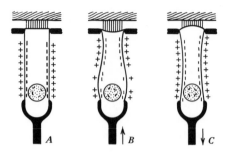

Fig. 8–1. Wever's hypothesis concerning the electrodynamic events in the hair cells. The hair tufts, embedded in the tectorial membrane (top) remain immobile as the basilar membrane (below, not shown) moves, forcing a distortion of the hair cell (bulging in *B*, the reverse in *C*). The change in shape affects the state of polarization of the cell's limiting membrane, as indicated by the distribution of positive and negative ions. From Wever (*628*).

movement than is indicated by *B* and *C* but the electrodynamic alterations could be expected to be essentially the same.

Why should attention have settled on the hair cells as the generators of the cochlear microphonic and, by extension, the crucial excitatory agent for hearing? There are other supporting facts, but the most telling evidence comes from work with animals. Albinotic cats and certain strains of dogs, mice, and guinea pigs ("waltzing") are born deaf. Examination of their cochleas shows hair cells to be absent, though the supporting tissues are intact. From such animals cochlear microphonics cannot be elicited at all. Another line of evidence comes from experiments in which animals have been subjected to prolonged tonal stimulation sufficiently intense to produce cochlear damage. There proves to be a close correlation between hair cell loss and extent of impairment. Especially significant are experiments in which damage is controlled by regulation of the sound exposure. It is possible to manage just a reduction of the cochlear microphonic—no other important functional change—and find hair cells to be the sole damaged elements. Finally, there is the critical evidence from tissue damage induced by drugs of the mycin family. Streptomycin and its relatives, originally introduced to combat tuberculosis, proved to have most unfortunate side effects. One of these is impairment of hearing, usually accompanied by vertigo and other symptoms of malfunctioning of the organs of equilibrium. In an effort to pinpoint the locus of damage, small animals were given one or another of the mycin compounds, either by subcutaneous injection or by perfusion of the ear. Guinea pigs, treated with large doses of streptomycin, kanamycin, or especially, neomycin, showed rapid deterioration of hearing and, significantly, total abolition of the cochlear microphonic as recorded from the round window. Subsequent sacrifice of the animals and examination of the cochleas revealed that the basilar membrane had frequently been denuded. Hair cells and cochlear microphonics had disappeared together.

Nowadays, it is so much taken for granted that the cochlear microphonic is the instigating agent in the triggering of the eighth nerve that widespread studies of animal auditory functions rely exclusively on this response to establish sensitivity curves. The degree of correspondence between such curves and various behavioral indices is sufficiently close as to provide a justification for doing so. Moreover, the magnitude of the response is linearly related to stimulus energy. That is, it is directly proportional to input up to the point where overloading of the system occurs. Then, the cochlear microphonic not only does not mirror stimulus intensity but also the lessened response serves as a warning that the elastic limits of the system are being exceeded.

Responses of the Auditory Nerve.   Certain characteristics of the nerve response, differentiating it from the cochlear microphonic, have already been considered. Other features are disclosed by studies of action potentials originating in the auditory nerve bundle.

The response of the nerve as a whole is necessarily somewhat elaborate. In general, while one finds the kind of complexity that would be predicted for a bundle containing perhaps as many as 35,000 fibers, there is also a characteristic sequence of responses whenever very brief stimuli are employed. Record with gross electrodes the electrical changes brought about by a strong, sharp click and there is found a chain of three impulses of descending size, spaced about a millisecond apart. Each consists of a well-synchronized volley of action potentials. The three have been labeled N_1, N_2, and N_3 and are salient landmarks in auditory nerve records. At moderate intensities N_3 is missing, while at low energy levels N_2 is likewise engulfed by asynchronous discharges. N_1, N_2, and N_3 are presumably the result of repetitive discharge of fibers and are spaced, not unexpectedly, in accordance with the schedule of absolute refractoriness that ensues upon such discharge. If, instead of a click, a pure tone under 4000 Hz is the stimulus, there will be a regular succession of bursts synchronized with the stimulus. Above this frequency level the nerve's response becomes somewhat irregular.

A more intimate picture is obtained when small electrodes, commensurate in size with the cells from which they are to record, are substituted. If a small hole is drilled in the base of the cat's or guinea pig's cochlea, a tiny pipette electrode may be inserted and there may be contacted the twisted bundle of the eighth nerve near the base of the modiolus. The tip of the microelectrode is forced into the bundle where, with favorable placement, it picks up electrical activity in individual fibers of the nerve. Only a little further in the central direction it will be immersed in a mass of cell bodies, in the area of the cochlear nucleus of the medulla, where the first synapse in the auditory tract occurs. See Figure 8–2.

Recordings of action potentials at both loci, nerve and cochlear nucleus, have proliferated to the point where much is known about the propagation of impulses, yet it cannot be said that the overall picture is either simple or clear. Contradictory findings there are in abundance, and this implies that the phenomena are correspondingly complex. For one thing, while there is considerable similarity to the human mechanism, and their use is therefore justified, experiments on guinea pigs, cats, and monkeys lead to results that are far from easy to interpret; no one supposes that there is anything simple about auditory organization in these or any other mammal. As yet there has been little inquiry, of a systematic and comprehensive kind, of primitive auditory systems. Doubtless such will be needed before it can be expected that fundamental principles will emerge.

However, many important facts are known. One of these came to light with the very first studies ever to be made on single units (*212, 147*). When Galambos and Davis, who performed the experiments, made their initial analysis they believed their electrodes to have been contacting axons of fibers whose dendrites originate at the base of the hair cells of the organ of Corti and whose cell bodies lie in the spiral ganglion. Subsequently, from detailed microscopic study of similar segments of the cat's eighth cranial nerve, it could be deduced that the original records must have come mainly from cell bodies of the cochlear nucleus (*213*). Second-order, rather than first-order, neurons had been involved. Nevertheless, the second nerve cell in the chain of four from the cochlea to the cortex presumably carries much the same information as does the first one; probably the two do not differ radically from each other in mode of operation. As Wever has said (*628*, p. 184), "The cochlear fibers must perform at least as well as the second-order neurons; they may do better in their representation of the stimulus, but they cannot do worse." Since the second-order nerve cells behave in a quite elaborate and revealing fashion, it is of interest to see what phenomena they displayed in response to external stimuli.

When tones of low intensity were delivered to the cat's ear it was found that individual elements responded in a quite specific fashion. At threshold intensity a particular element might show potentials only in response to tones of a very limited frequency range, for example, 690 Hz to

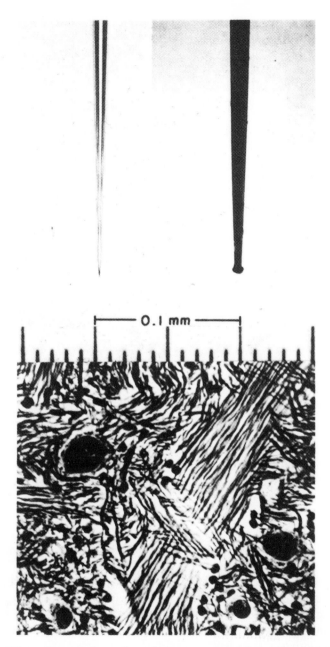

Fig. 8–2. Dimensions of electrodes relative to structural details within the cochlear nucleus. The electrode on the left is a pipette filled with KCl solution (3 M); that on the right is filled with indium and has a platinum ball plated at the tip. The diagonally disposed fibers belong to the eighth cranial nerve, while the globular structures are cells of the cochlear nucleus. From Kiang (*358*).

710 Hz. To all other tones it would be entirely unresponsive. Other units had, at threshold, similar specificities. If the stimulus intensity were increased, however, a wide band of frequencies became effective in bringing about discharge. The spread of response as the energy of the stimulus was raised was an asymmetrical one favoring the lower frequencies. Figure 8–3 shows the roughly triangular "response areas" for four dif-

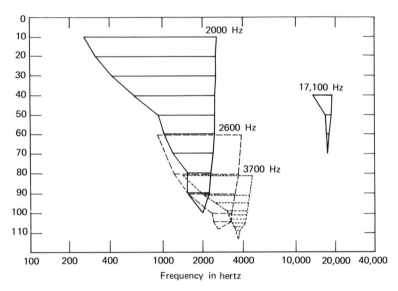

Fig. 8–3. The "response areas" of four neurones in the cat's cochlear nucleus. At threshold only a single narrow range of frequencies is effective. The higher the intensity, the less critically "tuned" is the responding element. After Davis (*147*). By permission of the publishers and the authors.

ferent units. The behavior of the "2000-Hz element" (the one responding at threshold only to tones in the immediate vicinity of 2000 Hz) may be taken as typical. When stimulated with high-intensity tones, at a level corresponding to about 90 dB human sensation level (10 dB below 2 volts, on the chart), this unit has become so nonspecific in its response that tones from 250 Hz to 2500 Hz will excite it. In other words, an element "tuned" to respond at threshold only to a very small range of frequencies will, if stimulated intensely, respond to tones three octaves below and one-half octave above its "characteristic" frequency. Cells having characteristic frequencies as low as 200 Hz and as high as 50,000 Hz were found in the cat. The "low-pitched" neurons were rare.

Subsequently, there have been many explorations of the two sites, cochlear nucleus and base of the spiral ganglion. Several studies have made direct comparisons of the two, very similar techniques having been applied to both. It turns out that there are similarities and differences to be considered. Response areas—"tuning curves," they have come to be called—are much the same in the two places, though there may be differences in sharpness of tuning and, also, a second kind of tuning curve has been found to characterize some nerve units. Whereas fibers having a high CF (characteristic frequency) also have a sharp upper-frequency cutoff, fibers tuned to lower frequencies may have broad tuning curves, sloping gently upwards in both directions. See Figure 8–4. Apparently, all fibers respond to low-frequency tones if stimulus

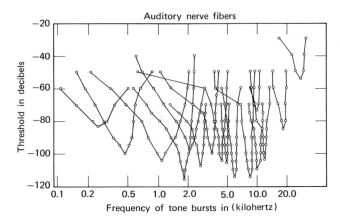

Fig. 8–4. "Tuning curves" of 16 auditory nerve fibers. The stimuli were transientless tone bursts of 50-msec duration presented at a rate of 10 per second, at the indicated frequencies. From Kiang (*358*).

intensity is high enough, whereas the presumption is that those originating near the apex of the cochlea are restricted to low frequencies in their responding (*567*).

There are many who picture tuning as getting progressively sharper from the periphery to the cortex, and this is an attractive hypothesis in attempting to account for frequency analysis in the system and for the extraordinary tonotopic localization we have seen operating in the brain. But the facts do not array themselves this conveniently. Kiang (*358*) finds somewhat broader tuning of elements in the cochlear nucleus than in the nerve, and Katsuki (*343*) finds progressive narrowing of response areas only up to the level of the medial geniculate body. At the cortex they are very broad. Units of the reticular pathways of the midbrain that connect with cells of the "classical" auditory afferent system seem to have no frequency specificity at all. There are obviously some things to be learned.

Except for the feature of specialized frequency reception the individual auditory nerve components behave very much as do fibers belonging to the other senses. They show characteristic random discharges ("spontaneous" activity) in the absence of external stimuli. Discharge rate in the "resting" state may vary from a few to about 100 spikes per second, and this seems not to be related in any way to the CF of the unit (*357*). However, it has been asserted that "the average time pattern of response for any auditory nerve fiber to simple acoustic stimuli is predictable from the 'tuning curve' and rate of spontaneous discharge" (*358*, p. 186). Nothing else, so far, does seem to be predictable. Thresholds of different auditory nerve fibers differ greatly among themselves, encompassing a range of as much as 60 dB, despite the fact that there is a relative uniformity of constitution in them. Auditory nerve fibers do not vary much in their physical dimensions; all appear to lie between 2.5 μ and 4.0 μ in diameter. Their conduction velocities, then, should not cover a wide range.

Other features of the auditory nerve fibers' response are not unexpected. Their refractory periods are not found to be unusually short (as was suspected in the days of the "Wever-Bray effect"). They also respond, individually, to intensity increases by discharging with greater rapidity, though there is a limit to which this occurs; most units show a maximum discharge rate with an actual rate decline with further increase of energy level. Frequency of discharge in the auditory nerve is thus determined by two variables, stimulus frequency and intensity.

The question may be raised, as it was for the cochlear response, as to how the nerve discharge is initiated. Once more we have to appeal to hypothesis to some extent, for the facts are far from being all at hand. One view is that the genesis is mechanical; vibratory distortion of the hair cells of the basilar membrane produces both the nerve impulse and the cochlear response, the latter as a by-product. Another hypothesis is that the auditory nerve, like other nerves in which such a mechanism has been pretty well demonstrated, has to be discharged by a chemical mediator. Recent researches on acetylcholine as the initiator of nervous impulses lend credence to this idea. In the transmission of impulses from nerve to muscle the role played by acetylcholine is beyond dispute. Perhaps the final step in the excitation of all nerves is the same. At any rate, the appreciable time delay in the arousal of auditory nerve action potentials demands some such explanation and the facts fit the chemical mediation theory well.

A third hypothesis has been that the cochlear potential, the aural microphonic, is itself the initiating agent, that the nerve is stimulated electrically by the currents generated in the cochlea. This view is an attractive one because nerve impulses can, of course, be set off by direct electrical excitation, and the cochlear potential is known to be a large one, appropriately located and possessed of some of the other requisite properties for service as a nerve excitant. However, it does not have all of them, and this fact has led to the search for some intermediary process, some set of events standing in more immediate relation to the discharge of the nerve twigs at the base of the hair cells.

The discovery that there is a local excitatory potential does not, of course, necessarily invalidate the mechanical and chemical hypotheses. All three could be right. The mechanical motion is certainly there, and it is still a mystery as to how mechanical distortion or changing tension can initiate a nervous discharge. Moreover, the chemical hypothesis is not incompatible with the mechanical and electrical ones. Biochemical processes may be triggered by mechanical deformations; they also usually have electrical manifestations. The mechanical, chemical, and electrical accounts may simply provide three different but related pictures of the same set of basic events. At any rate, until we have a more intimate knowledge of the ways in which receptor cells act as energy transducers we shall not be in a position to reject any of the current guesses concerning initiation of nerve impulses.

Responses of Higher Auditory Centers.   Somewhat parallel to what we have already encountered in vision (Chapter 3) are the electrical signs of nervous activity appearing at higher levels of the auditory tract. What is found there depends, in general, on two items of technique—electrodes and anesthetics. Electrodes may not be too gross and still record the activity in individual brain units; if too many cells are "within range," a summed effect, lacking specificity, will be obtained. If they are very small, the result obtained will depend on adventitious placement. In any case, microelectrodes plunged into the cortical mass cannot be expected to yield uniform records for more than a relatively short time at any one locus, and this is a hindrance to putting the whole, integrated picture together. The other limiting factor, anesthetics, is currently less of an obstacle than it was formerly. Moreover, the growing use of indwelling electrodes in totally unanesthetized animals is bringing to light many phenomena hitherto unavailable for study.

For many years after the first crude recording of neural changes to clicks and tonal stimuli had been made, there were severe restrictions on the "messages" that could be gotten through to the highest levels. It seemed to be true that nervous responses to tonal stimuli, faithfully present at the lower centers, were not capable of transmission to the cortex. The answer lay in the effects of anesthesia. A general anesthetic always influences the highest centers first and extends its effects downwards, neurologically speaking. When techniques were found for immobilizing an experimental animal without inducing general anesthesia—several curarelike drugs will do this—there was found the expected cortical activity in all its complexity.

"Complexity" is clearly the correct term, for cortical cells unquestionably have a most elaborate division of labor. If microelectrodes pick up impulses from individual cortical cells of the cat while the ear is being stimulated with clicks, tone bursts, noise bursts, and tones briefly swept through the audible frequency range, there are found units performing in one or another of the following ways: (a) response only to onset; (b) response only to termination; (c) response to both "on" and "off" but not to a sustained stimulus; (d) steady response with the stimulus present; (e) response consisting of suppression of previously ongoing "spontaneous" activity; (f) a change in response pattern to a shift of frequency; (g) a changed pattern from shifting intensity; (h) display of a best frequency (CF), evidenced either by showing a very low threshold to that frequency or responding with its strongest burst to it. In one thoroughgoing analysis of single-unit activity in the primary projection area (AI) of the cat (238), of 68 units successfully recorded, 39 were "broadly tuned," that is, they gave responses to frequencies extending over more than half an octave, 29 were narrowly tuned (less than $\frac{1}{2}$ octave), while 12 showed activity in two or more separated frequency ranges. In the same study, still other patterns of response were encountered, for example, cells that reacted only to sweeping of the frequency but that, presented the frequency band to which it had previously responded, gave no response whatsoever. And there were other seemingly anomalous patterns of response. The authors of this study were led to the conclusion that ". . . coding of acoustic stimuli by units of the primary acoustic cortex of the cat appears to be a highly individualistic and variegated matter, which almost defies quantification" (238, p. 454).

It is evident from the interesting work of Whitfield and Evans (639), on the responses of single cortical units to frequency-modulated (FM) tones, that the repertoire of cells functioning at the highest centers cannot be predicted from a knowledge of their responses to clicks, tone bursts, or steady tones. Many units were found that would give no response whatever to steady tones that would, nevertheless, react to an FM stimulus. Moreover, a fair proportion of the units for which steady tones were effective stimuli would respond more readily and over a wider frequency range when "moving" rather than "static" tones were used. This recalls the roughly analogous finding of Hubel and Wiesel (Chapter 3) in the visual cortex: cortical neurons that made no display to steady retinal illumination but that promptly reported movement in the same retinal area. The analogy is even closer, for the direction of "movement"—actual spatial direction in the visual case and in the direction of increasing or decreasing frequency in the auditory one— seems to have much to say about the capacity of the cortical cells to respond.

It does not necessarily require recording of the degree of intimacy found in the above studies to unearth important general relations between activities at different levels of the afferent tract. Glass electrodes giving only extracellular records are adequate for registering, at lower centers, neural responses to clicks, while even larger electrodes can be used to detect the passage of the click response at the white and gray cells of the cerebrum. Etholm (*191*) has recorded from four levels in the cat: inferior colliculus, medial geniculate body of the thalamus, white matter, and cortex. It is striking how closely the responses at these four places resemble each other, both qualitatively and quantitatively. Figure 8–5 shows the dependence of response strength on click intensity.

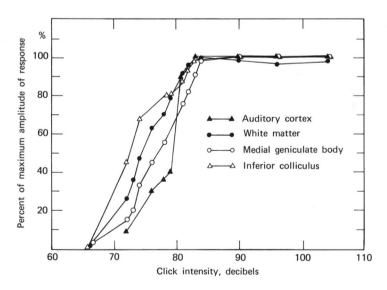

Fig. 8–5.   Responses at four neural levels in the cat. As click intensity is raised, response strength grows in much the same fashion at colliculus, medial geniculate body, white matter, and cortex. From Etholm (*191*).

Within a relatively narrow range of 15 dB, all four centers have swung into action and all reach peak at about the same energy level. There would appear to be some fidelity of transmission of the simple information contained in a click all the way from the ear to the cortical projection center.

Of possibly more importance is the finding, in the same experiment, that two successive clicks, separated by a silent interval, show the basic nature of inhibition in these centers. At the colliculus, if the double clicks were spaced within 50 msec of one another, the second one gave a diminished response. The inhibitory state created by the first one carried over that long. At the medial geniculate body, the interclick interval could be extended to 150 msec with the same effect. In the white matter and at the cortex the volley of impulses induced by the first click completely suppressed the appearance of the second one if it followed within 100 msec, and there was evidence of continuing inhibition up to intervals between 150 and 200 msec.

Just how sustained inhibitory states are mediated in the auditory tract is far from completely understood. However, as we have already had occasion to note when we were examining the neuroanatomical provisions for hearing (Chapter 6), there are efferent pathways that presumably play such a role (Rasmussen's tract). Also, Desmedt (156) has drawn attention to a "loop system" paralleling the classical auditory afferent pathways and terminating in the cochlear nucleus which may also exercise a measure of inhibitory control over ascending paths. The central nervous system obviously plays a management role that is far from being simply permissive or passive.

Theories of Hearing.   The chief facts of hearing are now before us. Into what sort of framework shall we put them? Are there available for our use any embracing conceptions which will permit us to arrange our facts in more meaningful patterns and, looking past them, enable us to foretell where new facts are to be found? This is the service good theories perform.

We should understand at the beginning that there exists no general theory of hearing any more than there exists a general theory of vision. There are theories of accommodation, theories of contrast, theories of color quality, etc. No one has attempted the almost superhauman task of bringing all the visual facts together and formulating a theoretical structure that will relate all of them to each other or, indeed, that will encompass the major portion of them. In the same way, auditory theories are part theories with their own restrictions and limitations. Generally, they are theories of cochlear operation that attempt to account for just one central phenomenon, pitch. There are some exceptions. At a crucial time in the development of auditory knowledge, Boring brought into relation with the frequency principle the phenomena of loudness, volume, and localization (*81*). There is the monumental work of Wever, who, in his *Theory of Hearing* (*628*), related his own volley theory to many different auditory phenomena: absolute and differential sensitivity, loudness perception, adaptation, auditory defects, tonal interaction phenomena, temporal variations of stimuli, binaural relations, as well as the acoustic, clinical, and neurological evidence. More recently, Licklider has attempted to explicate the overlap among three sets of auditory phenomena, those of pitch perception, speech intelligibility, and signal detection (*387*). And there are others, but, by and large, under the heading of auditory theory one expects to find discussed the mechanism of pitch production by the cochlea and auditory brain. We need to take a look at history here.

More than a score of pitch theories exist, but there are few which, over the years, have prompted research leading to significant discoveries. If this is made a criterion we are reduced to two major theories and three minor ones. The "resonance" theory of Helmholtz and the "telephone" theory of Rutherford and Wrightson fall into the category of major theories; the minor ones are Ewald's "sound-pattern" theory, Meyer's "hydraulic" theory, and a "frequency-resonance" theory due to Troland. We shall consider each in turn, though devoting more attention to the first than to the others, for Helmholtz' theory, now over a century old, has stood well the test of time and continues to prove its worth as a stimulator of new investigations.

The Helmholtz resonance theory is sometimes called the "harp" or "piano" theory, since the central idea is one which pictures the transverse fibers of the basilar membrane as acting very much like harp or piano strings. Everyone is familiar with the fact that, if the sustaining pedal of a piano is held down and a tone is sung near by, the strings corresponding to the vocal frequencies will vibrate sympathetically, that is, will resonate to the sounds striking them. The fibers of the basilar membrane, varying as they do with respect to length (long at the apex of the cochlea and short at the base) and perhaps variable also in tension and "loading," seem admirably suited for service as a series of graded resonators. Here is a mechanism which, because it can respond selectively to different frequencies, may be an adequate tone analyzer and thus meet the requirements of Ohm's Acoustic Law. A given "place" (a particular fiber or group of them) on the basilar membrane is responsible for a particular pitch; overtones stimulate a series of fibers spaced down the membrane. Tones so close together as to affect overlapping portions of the membrane produce local interference and hence the beat phenomenon. Consonance and dissonance yield no disturbing facts; as we have seen, the beating of upper partials may be responsible for creating dissonant intervals.

The theory, as left by Helmholtz, had little to say about loudness. Intense tones produced vigorous movements of the membrane and strong impulses in the nerve fibers attached to the hair cells. It was not until much later that anyone questioned this aspect of the theory. Meanwhile, some objections had been raised concerning the basic notion that the transverse fibers could vibrate independently of each other. They are, after all, closely connected with each other in the tough, fibrous tissue of the basilar membrane, and sharp tuning would not be expected of such a structure. The objection was formally met by A. A. Gray, in 1900, though the principle he employed was inherent in Helmholtz's own statement of the theory (628, Chapter 5). Gray pictured the basilar membrane's response to a pure tone as involving, as well as the "in-tune" fiber, other fibers adjacent to it. The extent to which neighboring fibers will be called in depends upon the intensity of the stimulus. However, the "in-tune" resonator reacts with the greatest vigor and gives its pitch to the complex response; those flanking it have progressively diminishing amplitudes the further situated they are from the center of the responding group. Gray called this the "principle of maximum stimulation," and this amendment to Helmholtz' original theory is commonly called "Gray's modification."

The first real difficulty encountered by the resonance theory came in 1912 with the discovery of the "all-or-nothing" principle of nerve discharge. It was clearly demonstrated by Lucas and Adrian that nerve fibers normally respond by discharging "at full strength." Either a nerve discharges completely or it does not discharge at all; except under special circumstances there are no graded responses within the individual nerve fiber. What of the correlate for loudness in the Helmholtz theory? Amplitude of sympathetic vibration was supposed to be translated into strength of nerve discharge to take care of the intensity-loudness correlation.

At first the discovery that there are no graded "strengths" of nerve discharge seemed to present an insuperable difficulty. Then, in 1915, there came a new theoretical formulation of sensory intensity. Forbes and Gregg (204) surmised that varying intensity of stimulus might be reflected in variable frequency of discharge within a single fiber. Whereas, in conformity with the all-or-nothing principle, a fiber must always discharge with its full capacity to do so, it may fire only a few times a second or may deliver very rapidly successive discharges, depending upon the amount of energy acting upon it. Immediately following discharge there occurs a brief period, of the order of a millisecond, in which the fiber is "absolutely refractory"; no amount of stimulation can affect it. Following this there occurs a "relatively refractory period," in which the original sensitive state is being rebuilt and in which the fiber can again respond. A weak stimulus must wait until quite late in the rebuilding period to effect discharge, and the fiber's response will thus be infrequent. A strong stimulus, by invading the relatively refractory period early, will produce more frequent responses. In this way stimulus intensity comes to be translated into discharge frequency. The demonstration that single nerve fibers actually behave in this manner did not come for another dozen years. The Forbes-Gregg hypothesis, meanwhile, rescued the Helmholtz theory from the temporary embarrassment into which the all-or-nothing discovery had plunged it.

There is another way in which intensity may be mediated. A strong stimulus may call into action a large number of fibers in a nerve bundle, while a weak one will involve only relatively few. This principle is commonly employed to account for graded muscular responses and may be used to explain variations in sensory intensity as well. However, as applied to the auditory nerve, it would seem to introduce complications for the Helmholtz theory. To bring into play any large number of fibers is to involve somewhat remotely situated nerve endings and these, being at other "places," would generate a conglomeration of pitches. Loud tones should be "muddy" tones. There is a question as to how far Gray's modification can be relied on to preserve tonal purity. The matter of aural harmonics is not concerned here. Harmonics have, of course, pitch numbers demanding wide spacing on the basilar membrane.

What were the evidences for the "pitch-place" correlation, the very heart of the Helmholtz theory? Unless it can be shown that tones have individual loci of reception in different portions of the basilar membrane, that low-frequency tones are analyzed out by fibers terminating near the apex of the cochlea, and that high-frequency tones are mediated by those in the basal turns, the whole theory falls to the ground. The chief relevant facts are those concerning (1) localization of the microphonic effect within the cochlea, (2) pathological findings in partial deafness, and (3) results of "stimulation-deafness" experiments.

That the aural microphonic arises in different portions of the cochlea, depending upon the stimulating frequency, seems certain. Electrodes situated at the base of the cochlea show high-frequency responses to be favored; records from the apex reveal low-frequency waves to have the greater magnitude. (264, 554). The most convincing early evidence of a fairly specific localization came from the work of Culler (134, 135) and a confirming experiment by Kemp and Johnson (349). Culler explored the external surface of the guinea pig's cochlea, determining at each of 23 points the frequency requiring the least intensity to produce a small, constant electrical response. The presumption was that the most effective frequency, at any given point, must be generated in the immediate vicinity. A schematic representation of the results is given by Figure 8–6. Even though an elaborate mathematics and set of corrections were required to establish the individual points, the results would seem to imply that low frequencies of the aural microphonic are generated in the apical turns; high frequencies have their origin near the base.

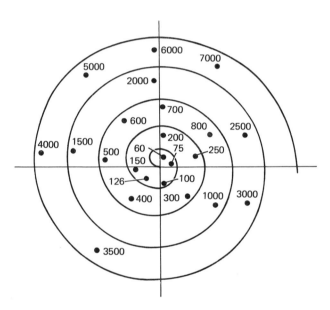

Fig. 8–6. Topographical variations in the size of the cochlear potential. The guinea pig's cochlea is represented schematically, apex at the center. There are shown optimal positions for obtaining the cochlear potential at each of the stimulus frequencies indicated, according to the reports of Culler and his associates (*134, 135*). By permission of the editor, *Annals of Otology, Rhinology, and Laryngology.*

The evidence from pathology, as is so often the case, is not without internal contradictions. However, the clearest results support a general "place" differentiation for pitch. In cases of high-tone deafness, whether characterized by gradual losses toward the higher frequencies or more abrupt ones, post-mortem examination of the cochlear structure most commonly shows partial atrophy of nerve fibers and other degenerative changes in the basal turn (*132*). These findings, while not crucial, are at least consistent with the "place" theory.

Considerable work has been devoted to "stimulation deafness," the production of lowered or abolished sensitivity in experimental animals by exposing them to intense tones for a matter of days or weeks. The early experiments connecting local degeneration with tonal gaps seemed decisive and were frequently cited in support of the Helmholtz theory. However, by now there have been many such experiments and the conclusions seem far less certain. There is little doubt that cochlear lesions can be produced in this way, providing the stimulating tones are sufficiently intense and prolonged, but the losses as well as the lesions are often quite general, and, in the better-controlled experiments, the zone of greatest loss (as determined by diminished electrical response) has not always coincided with the "place" one would expect the "deafening" tone to occupy. High-frequency tones quite typically produce degeneration in the basal turn of the cochlea, near the stapes, and damage to hair cells, nerve fibers, and ganglion cells, and supporting tissues may be confined to a stretch of basilar membrane no greater than 1 mm. Low-frequency tones, on the other hand, are likely to extend their damaging effects over a considerable distance at the apical end. Figure 8–7 depicts

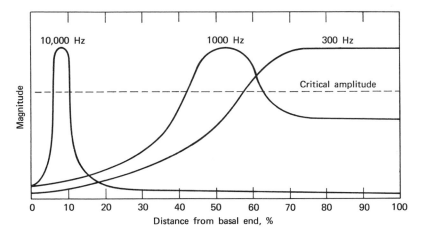

Fig. 8–7. The extent of damage found in stimulation deafness experiments suggests the above mode of action of the cochlear partition. "Critical amplitude" is the threshold of tissue breakdown. From Wever and Lawrence (*635*).

the general set of relations between stimulating frequency, vibration amplitude, and extent of tissue degeneration. The "critical amplitude" marks the threshold of tissue destruction as pictured by Wever and Lawrence (*635*).

In arriving at a tentative evaluation of the Helmholtz theory it must be said that its "place" feature is not the least of its virtues. In addition to the evidences just cited there are some other facts that are accommodated well by the assumption that there is a systematic pitch localization along the length of the basilar membrane. The way in which various frequencies contribute to total loudness and to speech intelligibility and the operation of critical frequency bands in the production of masking find most ready interpretation in the light of the pitch-place assumption.

On the other hand, the resonance feature of the original Helmholtz theory must be said to have appeared more and more improbable as the evidence on cochlear mechanics has accumulated. There is little doubt that a kind of "resonance" occurs. The relative amplitudes of vibration of different parts of the basilar membrane and its attachments change in a regular manner as stimulus frequency is changed, the point of greatest displacement moving towards the base of the cochlea as frequency is raised, but a large portion of the membrane is in operation for all frequencies. This is especially the case for low tones. Moreover, the phase differences existing between widely separated parts of the vibrating system clearly prove that we are dealing with a traveling wave rather than with a simple resonance of the "harp-string" variety. The basilar membrane, it turns out, is not a series of stretched transverse fibers. The membrane is not even under tension. This is demonstrated by making fine cuts in it, either longitudinally or transversely. The cut edges do not pull apart; they should, of course, in an elastic tissue under tension. As one estimate has it (*61*, p. 1094), "Had the theory of hearing not started with the notion of a vibrating piano string, the basilar membrane might never have been regarded as under lasting tension at all."

The place idea, then, we do well to preserve, while rejecting the crude notion of "resonance through sympathetic vibration." For it we must substitute Békésy's "traveling wave," even though it must still be regarded as a matter of theory. The traveling wave, of course, calls for a "place" correlation. The great question that remains is how the gentle peaking that goes along with realistic basilar membrane mechanics—relatively great stiffness of the cochlear partition and close coupling from point to point along its length—permits the degree of specificity of neural response that must obtain if the requirements of pitch recognition and discrimination, timbre, critical bands, beats, and a host of related phenomena are to be accounted for in theory. Békésy has appealed to the principle of sensory inhibition to produce the necessary "sharpening" of the stimulation pattern as it advances from the periphery to the nervous centers (*60*), and this exciting idea bids fair to explicate many a phenomenon lying, as yet, outside the pale of auditory (and general sensory) theory.

And it must not be assumed that traveling wave theory is complete in all details. Is it that energy is "passed along" from one segment of the basilar membrane to its neighbor as the wave "travels," or is it that successive portions of the membrane go into action in an orderly sequence because differential local tissue characteristics require it whenever vibratory forces are imparted practically simultaneously to all parts of the membrane by way of the cochlear fluids? Wever (*636, 637*), who does not question the accuracy of Békésy's observation that there is a progressive movement along the basilar membrane, speaks of the activating force in cochlear stimulation as a "pseudo-traveling wave," since, he contends, equally plausible with the interpretation that vibratory energy is flowing apically along the basilar membrane is the possibility that neighboring segments respond successively because their loading, stiffness, etc. demand that they do so. A crucial experiment that would decide between these opposing interpretations of a single set of facts is hard to devise, much less execute.

Before entering into the history of the Helmholtz theory's great rival, the telephone theory, there are some facts, neglected up to now, that must be placed in evidence. These concern what has come to be called *periodicity pitch*, in contrast with "place" or *spectral pitch*. Some of the considerations engendering the spectral pitch concept we have already examined—peaking of the traveling wave, loci of best reception of the cochlear microphonic, specificity of damage in stimulation deafness experiments and in partial deafness. Others might be cited, for example, the spacing of frequencies along the basilar membrane demanded by the psychophysical measurement of Δf and, especially, by the facts of masking of pure tones by white noise. Figure 8–8, taken from Fletcher's account of his and Munson's experiments at the Bell Laboratories, shows optimal frequency positions along the 2½ turns of the cochlea demanded by masking calculations.

The evidence for periodicity pitch is not nearly so imposing, though the idea it embraces is neither without merit nor is it very new. The notion that pitch might be generated quite simply by nerve impulses of the same frequency as the stimulating tone is encountered in the theorizing of some of the founding fathers of experimental psychology, Wundt (1880) and Ebbinghaus (1902), not to mention the much earlier hypothesis of the German histologist, Hensen (in 1863, the year of Helmholtz's formulation) and the influential theories of William Rutherford (1886) and Max Meyer (1896), to which we shall return later.

Perhaps the best demonstration of the operation of periodicity pitch

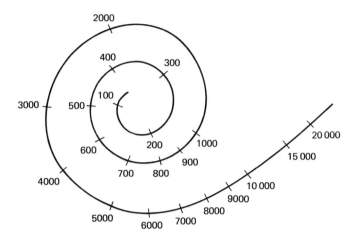

Fig. 8–8. Pitch localization along the basilar membrane. Loci were derived from measures of tonal masking by white noise. Courtesy of Dr. Harvey Fletcher and the National Academy of Sciences.

is the one connected with what, in the literature of audition, has come to be called "the case of the missing fundamental." If, in a tone of complex timbre, the kind that is typically produced by most musical instruments, there are progressively filtered off the fundamental and several of the lower overtones, leaving only the upper partials, it will be found that the tone gets increasingly "thinner" but does not seem to change pitch. Degree of tonal complexity is not entailed, for identical results may be obtained with speech sounds. Moreover, one could begin with a synthetic tone, for example, the sum of the frequencies 500, 600, 700, 800, 900, and 1000 Hz and get a pitch identified by a listener as 100 Hz. When this startling phenomenon was first discovered there seemed to be an easy explanation available. The fundamental was being reintroduced by way of aural harmonics; the cochlea's nonlinearity was responsible.

Nowadays, we think we know better. Not only is nonlinearity of response regarded to be a less potent factor in producing distortion than it was formerly thought to be, but there are also direct experiments, especially those of Schouten and those of Licklider (see *387*, pp. 108–119), which obviate such an explanation. Licklider set up a situation in which a band of low-frequency noise (below 1300 Hz) "flooded" the auditory system while spaced, high-frequency harmonics of low-frequency fundamentals were sounded in synchrony. The masking noise was sufficiently powerful to prevent any low-frequency fundamental from being heard when it was present as the sole stimulus. When the high harmonics were sounded, however, there was reconstituted a low-pitched fundamental in the presence of the masking noise! Obviously, the "fundamental" arrived at in this way cannot be occupying the proper "place" on the basilar membrane. It must be created by repetitive firing of nerve cells in the unmasked region. This, then, is pitch produced by periodicity.

It is apparent that a low frequency need not be physically present for a low pitch to be perceived. A group of narrowly spaced higher harmonics of a periodically pulsed signal join to form a pattern that generates the low pitch. This pattern is called the *residue* by Schouten (*512*). It is not essential that the pattern be complicated. Thus, in some of Schouten's early experiments only three harmonics of the (missing) fundamental, 200 Hz, were involved: 1200, 1400, and 1600 Hz. A low-pitched "residue" was heard, one that would not beat with an exploring tone in the neighborhood of 200 Hz, yet it sounded like 200 Hz. If the filter were adjusted to pass only the frequencies, 1800, 2000, and 2200 Hz, the residue again sounded like 200 Hz but was judged to be "sharper" than in the former instance. Pitch had not changed but timbre obviously had.

With this struggle between place and periodicity concepts of pitch before us—a theoretical issue as yet unresolved except in the minds of those for whom compromise of principles is an acceptable solution—let us return to auditory history.

The "telephone" or "frequency" theory of hearing, first devised by Rutherford in 1886 and given more elaborateness of detail by Wrightson in 1918, also deserves serious consideration. Its assumptions are quite different from those of the Helmholtz theory; in fact, in a sense, the two are diametrically opposed. This opposition has, more than once, served to provide the impetus and the setting for an experimental problem. Thus the frequency theory, like the resonance theory, has proved its value as a guide to research.

The basic tenet of the frequency theory is that the basilar membrane vibrates as a whole and thus behaves very much as does the diaphragm of a telephone or a microphone. Whatever complexities are present in the vibrations transmitted by the foot of the stapes are also present in the movements of the basilar membrane and hair cells. The latter discharge their nerve fibers, and the entire pattern of stimulation is reproduced in the response of the auditory nerve. Loudness is accounted for by the assumption that a vigorous response on the part of the basilar membrane, arising from energetic motions of the transmission system, will bring into play a large number of fibers, while a weak stimulus will involve relatively few. Thus the correlation between intensity and number of fibers, not readily accommodated by the Helmholtz theory, is the naturally acceptable one to adherents of the telephone theory.

It is to be noted that the whole matter of tonal analysis is shifted, under the frequency theory of hearing, to the brain. The central nervous system must perform the dissection of the complex wave demanded by the Fourier analysis and Ohm's Acoustic Law, for the pictured mechanism is one which makes of the cochlea simply a device for detecting and faithfully transmitting to higher nervous centers the complex waveforms falling on the ear.

An objection that may be fairly urged against the telephone theory in its unmodified form is that it calls for the transmission of impulses over the auditory nerve at rates of repetition which are probably impossible of realization. If the nerve is to report to higher centers precisely the frequencies present in the basilar membrane's movements, and the latter are in step with those of the eardrum, it follows that the highest audible frequencies must be represented by nerve discharges of 20,000 per second. This requires a refractory period as short as 0.05 msec, and the weight of experimental evidence places the shortest refractory period at about 1.0 msec, perhaps slightly less.

It was this circumstance that led Wever and Bray to propose a modification of the frequency theory which they called the "volley" theory. They supposed that, up to a point established by the absolutely refractory period, individual fibers will yield increasingly frequent responses as the stimulus intensity is raised. All responses are synchronized with the stimulus because it is only at a particular phase of the sound wave's action that the hair cells are stimulated. It is further assumed that not all fibers are identical in their response characteristics. Some have short refractory periods, others long. For a low-frequency tone it may be possible for all fibers to "keep up with" the stimulus and thus respond to every wave. Meanwhile other fibers, having other refractory periods, are responding to waves skipped by the first. At the highest frequencies it may not be possible for even the most sensitive of fibers to respond more frequently than to every tenth wave; however, its neighbors will be responding at their own pace to the missed waves. The "regiment" of fibers thus fires by "platoons," and the net result is a high frequency of response on the part of the bundle of nerves but only relatively infrequent discharge on the part of the individual components. Figure 8–9 illustrates the operation of the volley principle. For Intensity A, each of the fibers is discharging only to every third wave, but the refractory periods of a, b, c, and d are so chosen that no period of the sound wave is without its discharge. For the higher Intensity B, each of the

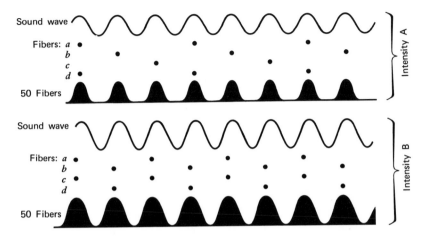

Fig. 8–9. The operation of the volley principle. At Intensity A (low) all fibers represented are responding to every third wave. At Intensity B (high) each fiber responds to every other wave. In both cases synchronism with the stimulus is preserved. The sum of responses of many fibers is represented by the black hillocks. These reproduce both the frequency and intensity of the stimulus. After Wever and Bray *(631)*. By permission of the *Psychological Review* and the American Psychological Association.

fibers is responding to every other wave (more frequently, in accordance with the Forbes-Gregg principle), and the integrated response for a large number of fibers shows a larger (louder) response. The frequency of the stimulus is also preserved, as demanded by the telephone theory, through synchronization of the impulses with the sound waves. Thus, by way of addition of the volley principle, the frequency theory again becomes plausible and acceptable as an explanatory framework for the chief factors that must be handled by auditory theory, pitch and loudness.

Perhaps the most spectacular validation of the volley theory is found in the ingenious work of Rose et al. *(504)* on single auditory nerve fibers of the squirrel monkey. Recording from units in the spiral ganglion with micropipettes less than 1μ in diameter, they were able to verify what Kiang and others had found, that responses to tones up to about 5000 Hz could be obtained in individual units. Their most important finding was that cochlear nerve fibers transmit their information at least up to this point on the scale (and perhaps still higher) by discharging at intervals closely grouped around the period of the stimulus or integral multiples of it. Figure 8–10 shows a typical set of results for a single neuron having a response area extending from about 100 Hz to slightly

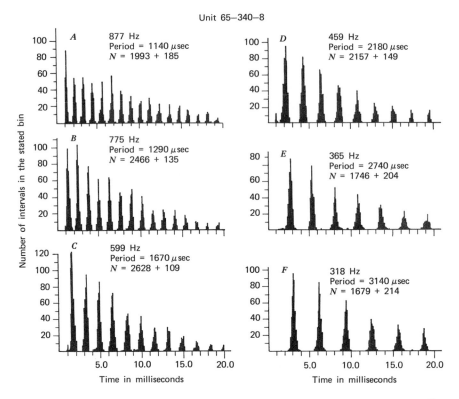

Fig. 8–10. Responses of a single neuron having a "response area" extending from 100 Hz to 1000 Hz, approximately. Pure tones ranging from 877 Hz (*A*) to 167 Hz (*K*) stimulated this cell. The fact that the vast majority of action potential spikes occurred in strict synchronism with the stimulus is evidenced by the location of the tiny dots (just below the abscissa). These mark off time intervals representing multiples of the stimulus frequency. From Jerzy E. Rose, John F. Brugge, David J. Anderson, and Joseph E. Hind. Phase-locked response to low-frequency tones in single auditory nerve fibers of the squirrel monkey. *J. Neurophysiol.*, **30**:769–793, 1967.

above 1000 Hz. The little histograms are distributions of interspike intervals, some extending up to 20 msec. The dots below the abscissa indicate multiples of the stimulus period. It is clear that, in all instances, the cadence of the response was set by the stimulus, not by an inherent discharge rate. The nerve was discharging in quite strict synchronism with

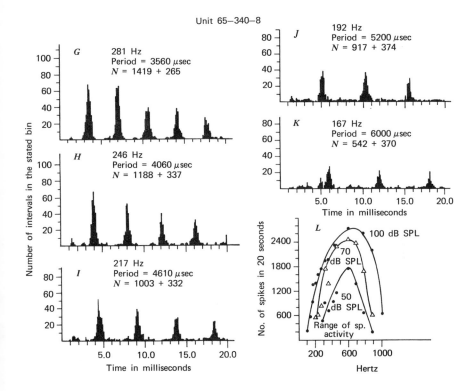

Unit 65–340–8

the stimulus cycles. This, of course, is precisely what is demanded by volley theory. The surprising thing is that the fiber's intrinsic properties have so little to say about when it will respond.

In the 40 or 50 years since the volley theory was devised, its basic correctness has been everywhere evidenced. Indeed, volley theory is in somewhat the same situation as in duplexity theory in vision. We should perhaps stop talking about volley *theory* and duplexity *theory* and, instead, refer to the *fact* of locked-to-the-cycle neural coding in hearing and the *fact*, in vision, that rods and cones are the instruments of two separate sense channels, not one.

The remaining theories need not detain us long. While containing some interesting ideas they do not offer the possibility of accommodating any large assortment of hearing facts, at least in a manner suggestive of crucial experiments.

The "sound-pattern" theory of Ewald gets its inspiration from the phenomena displayed by vibrating plates and diaphragms. If a metal plate on which sand has been sprinkled is set into vibration by striking or bowing the edge there are created elaborate patterns in the sand, these reflecting the complex motions of the plate. Each tone, indeed each variation in intensity, has its own pattern. Ewald, experimenting with diaphragms and photographing the patterns formed on them by standing waves, became convinced that the basilar membrane must behave in a similar manner. His theory of hearing therefore supposes that each combination of frequency and intensity must have its unique pattern, what Ewald called its "acoustic image." The sound pattern of a complex tone, replete with overtones, must be very elaborate indeed. Analysis of tones, recognition of voices and musical instruments, and discrimination of the nuances of musical passages must place a very heavy burden on the brain. The scientific judgment of the sound-pattern theory has been that there is no need to admit so much complexity for the reception of even a simple tone until forced to do so by the failure of more parsimonious principles.

The hydraulic or "displacement" theory of Max Meyer (*415, 416*) is essentially a "frequency" theory but one which denies resonance to the basilar membrane or any of its components. In fact, it holds that the basilar membrane is not an especially elastic tissue and that it behaves as one might expect a stiff piece of leather to act. When pushed into one position by the pressure of the cochlear fluids it remains there until pushed into another. Meyer's theory has been dubbed the "leather chair-seat" theory for this reason. The foot of the stapes, on its inward excursion, communicates pressure to the basilar membrane, which is depressed progressively along it length just so long as a positive pressure continues. As much of the membrane ("phragma," as Meyer persisted in calling it) is pushed out of position as is required to make room for the fluid displaced by the stirrup's motion. When the stapes comes to a stop and describes a return movement the basilar membrane bulges in the opposite direction, again beginning at the base. A length of the membrane will reproduce the motions of the stapes and thus preserve synchronism with the stimulus, even though the waveform be an intricate one. The extent of the membrane involved will determine loudness. A weak stimulus will jerk the membrane out of position for only a short distance before the disturbance dies out; a strong one may involve the entire membrane up to the apex. Unlike other adherents of frequency theories, who have left analysis to be cared for by the brain, Meyer has worked out a mechanical analysis within the cochlea. This involves differential action by successive sections of the membrane and accounts peripherally for Ohm's Law and combination tones. The analysis, rather than being based on the Fourier series, is essentially a geometrical one.

The displacement theory possesses all the virtues of any frequency theory and certainly provides a unique picture of cochlear mechanics. It does this, moreover, without bringing in the concept of resonance. It has not been a popular theory, however. Perhaps this is because it is inherently a difficult theory to understand, as Wever has pointed out (628, p. 88). Perhaps it is because, until only quite recently, no one has been able to demonstrate the plausibility of some of the mechanisms hypothesized by the hydraulic theory. At any rate, it can safely be said that over the years it has not provided a great impetus to research and discovery. Perhaps it may yet come to do so.

A theory which is essentially eclectic in spirit, in that it borrows both from the resonance theory and the frequency theory, is one devised by Troland in 1929. A not too dissimilar one was outlined by Fletcher in 1930 (201). As much of the Helmholtz theory as assigned different pitches to separate locations on the basilar membrane is preserved in order to make of analysis a peripheral event. However, pitch is determined by the frequency of impulses in the nerve, regardless of the point of origin of the discharging fibers. As in other frequency theories, synchronism between the stimulus and the neural pattern of discharge is assumed. This use of resonance for analysis and frequency for pitch demonstrates that the central conceptions of the two most successful of the auditory theories are not necessarily incompatible. Troland's theory and Fletcher's theory are notable in another respect—they anticipated (somewhat in advance of the "Wever-Bray effect") the volley theory by correlating loudness with "the total number of impulses passing a fixed cross-section, per second, in a group of cooperating fibers" (582). Thus, by a division of labor, there was avoided the refractory phase difficulty encountered by earlier frequency theories.

Other combinations of principles contributed by the classic theories are possible. There is no reason to assume, because history would seem to have it that way, that either the place theory or the frequency theory is generally applicable to all auditory phenomena. The current state of our knowledge would seem to prejudice us toward a place theory for high tones and a frequency theory for low ones. Somewhere in the middle range of tonal frequencies one principle may give way to the other, the two thus complementing each other. This is the view championed by Wever in his modern statement of the volley theory (628). Of course, there is always the possibility that there will eventually emerge an idea of a higher order, a "master principle," capable of subsuming under it all known auditory phenomena. Our current auditory theories have, after all, attained a riper age than most good scientific theories ever achieve.

9

The Skin and
Its Stimuli

The Classification of the Senses. Two avenues of sense, vision and audition, having already been dealt with in the foregoing chapters, it may seem odd that only now is there being raised the question of how, in general, the senses are to be classified. The reason becomes clear when it is learned that there are five senses, or more than a score of them, or some intermediate number, depending upon what decision is made concerning sensations originating in the skin and internal organs of the body. Classically, there are five special senses: vision, audition, smell, taste, and "touch" or "feeling." Aristotle had it that way (though even he expressed some doubt about "touch" as a single sense), and his five-fold classification of the senses has upon it the sanction of the centuries.

Current popular usage is, of course, completely in the Aristotelian tradition. At various times, however, and especially of relatively recent years, the list has been expanded. Always the "extra" senses have come out of the sense of feeling by a process of subdivision; whenever the number has shrunk back to five the additional senses have gone back into "feeling" again. Boring (*82*, p. 34), listing the "sense-qualities" of feeling for which some fair claim to independent status had been made by 1915, includes: pressure, contact, deep pressure, prick pain, quick pain, deep pain, warmth, cold, heat, muscular pressure, articular pressure, tendinous strain, ampullar sensation or dizziness, vestibular sensation or sense of translation, appetite, hunger, thirst, nausea, sex, cardiac sensation, and pulmonary sensation. Others, including itch, tickle, vibration, suffocation, satiety, and repletion, at one time or another have been raised to independent status.

In the intricate history of the classification of the senses there have been, in general, three logically distinct approaches. Sensations may be grouped together (1) *qualitatively*, on the basis of their observational similarity, (2) *stimuluswise*, with respect to the objects or forms of physical energy that typically set them off, or (3) *anatomically*, in accordance with the system of sense organs or tissues initiating them. The last of these seems to provide the best organizational principle, and, wherever knowledge about the bodily structures responsible for originating sensation has been sufficiently complete, the anatomical basis of classification has been preferred. We could talk about the "sense of green" and the "sense of gray," but since we know the production of these qualities to be the work of a single anatomical unit, the eye, we are accustomed to grouping the two classes ot sensation together as "visual." Similarly, we might appeal to stimuli and, in hearing, speak of the "sense of tone" and the "sense of noise," but both kinds of sensation are mediated by the ear and hence are classed as "auditory." In the cases of smell and taste the anatomical reference is natural. Olfactory sensations are "nostril sensations"; those of taste belong to the tongue and palate.

When we come to consider the sensations aroused in the skin and internal organs of the body there is some indefiniteness of classification, mainly because we do not have entirely certain knowledge of the anatomical mechanisms involved. Indeed, the question of what nerve endings in the skin and deeper-lying tissues respond to common touches and pressures is still far from settled. As to the detailed manner in which they operate to elicit sensations we can as yet only make shrewd guesses. Despite the fact that the skin is, from the evolutionary standpoint, the oldest of the sensitive tissues of the body, it has yielded up its secrets reluctantly. It houses a multitude of variously constituted and differently disposed structures, and the opportunities for variation in their performance are many. Perhaps it is not surprising, therefore, that its phenomena are complex and hard to master. Perhaps, too, it is not greatly to be wondered at that its sensations are difficult to bring under simple classificatory concepts. If, under one set of prejudices, the cutaneous and internally aroused sensations all seem to belong together and thus indicate the existence of a single sense of "feeling" and, under another bias, seem to bespeak a veritable plethora of separate and distinct "senses," this is but a reflection of our current ignorance of the basic facts and uncertainty as to the interpretation of those we have. Actually, the available criteria for separating out "modalities of sensation" probably have to yield, in the long run, to the almost universal contemporary conclusion that somesthetic receptors are specialized in their function through the operation of the principle of *patterned response*. We know that some cutaneous end organs will answer to more than one form of energy—for example, mechanical pressure and thermal change—and that a particular receptor may be quite selective with respect to the range of intensities within which it will respond. Moreover, it is likely to belong to a local organization of peripheral nerve endings of one size of receptive field or another and having one or another degree of overlap with its neighbors. It has its own range of adjustment through the operation of such neural mechanisms as accommodation, adaptation, recruitment, and afterdischarge. Its pathways to the central nervous system may converge greatly or little; they may give off many or few collateral fibers en route. Since it is highly improbable that a single end organ ever reports by itself—if it did, it would impart no "information"—the conclusion is inescapable that each aroused receptor must contribute to an elaborate spatiotemporal pattern of impulses which, presumably at the level of central projection, brings about "sensation." Considering the number of continuously varying factors that must enter and the practically infinite number of patterns that must be possible, the wonder is that we are ever able to classify into a relatively few somesthetic "senses."

For convenience in considering somesthetic phenomena we shall consider the skin as housing three more or less separate systems of sensitivity, one for pressure reception, one for pain, and one responsive to temperature changes. Mainly because there are anatomical similarities and analogies with the superficial skin senses but also because they frequently participate in responses to identical environmental events, the systems of sensitivity associated with deeper-lying tissues, muscles, visceral organs, and the nonauditory labyrinth of the inner ear will be thought of as constituting the "internal senses," also somesthetic.

The Skin and Its Sensitivities.   The first thing to be noted about the skin is that it is not uniformly sensitive. If a pencil point is moved gently across the back of the hand there are aroused at some places sensations of touch or pressure, at others cold sensations may flash out, and there may be felt tickling or even itching at others. Moreover, if the stimulus is changed to a sharper or duller object, or if the mode of attack is varied to involve direct pressure into the skin, or if warmed or cooled metal points are used, a considerable range of sensations may be brought forth. This suggests that the skin's potentiality for yielding a great diversity of sensations can be gauged only by exploring sample areas in a systematic manner, controlling the many variables that must enter to produce such widely differing phenomena.

To make systematic exploration possible it is obviously necessary to resort to some kind of mapping procedure so that the same local skin area may be readily found again, either to investigate its constancy of response when uniformly and repeatedly stimulated or to isolate it for systematic variation of the stimulus in successive trials. The common laboratory technique is to utilize a rubber stamp prepared in the form of a square grid, 20 mm on a side and thus containing 400 mm² squares. An ink impression of such a grid is stamped on the skin area to be explored, and the center of each tiny square becomes the locus of stimulation. Since there is nothing permanent about such marking (perspiration and accidental rubbing of clothing readily smear or even obliterate it), a technique making the grid lines reproducible has been devised by Dallenbach *(140)*. This consists of injecting into the skin with a finely drawn-out glass tube or a hypodermic needle, at the four corners of the grid marking, a small "dot" of India ink. The corners of the grid pattern, thus being permanently tattooed into the skin, make possible exact placement of the grid in successive stampings. With the aid of such "anchor points" the author has been able to stamp the skin and relocate spots especially sensitive to cold and pressure a dozen years after they were first found.

If a somewhat more intimate map of a skin area is desired, a freehand sketch of the surface as seen through a low-power ($10\times$ to $30\times$) binocular microscope may be made. Better still is a microphotograph of the area. With judicious lighting, furrows and ridges, hair stumps, and other distinguishing marks may be brought out and used as orientation signs to assist in stimulus placement. An ingenious method to provide a somewhat temporary but perfectly reproducible set of marks is to make use of the method of electro-osmotic staining *(233)*. A solution of methylene blue or other dye is used to saturate a piece of filter paper, which is then placed over the skin region to be marked. A positive electrode of appropriate shape and size is then pressed firmly on the filter paper, the negative electrode being attached to the body at some indifferent point. A direct current of 1–2 ma, at 20–40 v, is allowed to flow through the circuit for 5 min or more at the termination of which the dye has been carried into the skin by way of the sweat duct openings. A few days after such a dyeing operation the individual sweat duct openings are clearly marked and remain so for long periods of time, perspiration depositing particles of dye in tiny "craters" at the skin surface.

With the aid of any of these marking methods the skin's sensitivities may be explored. The system of sensitivity called into action will, of course, be a function of the type of stimulus used in the exploration. Here the possibilities are many, for the skin proves to be responsive to a wide range of stimuli: *mechanical, thermal, electrical,* and *chemical.* For the arousal of "touch," "contact," and "pressure" any thermally indifferent solid or liquid will, of course, suffice, and even air blasts have been used in some experiments. For these sensations the technique of exploration developed by von Frey, at the end of the last century, has become standard procedure. This involves the use of hairs, both human and animal, of various lengths and diameters, attached at right angles to the end of a match stick or other wooden holder. Following von Frey's lead, most investigators of touch and pressure sensations have made point-by-point serial explorations of skin samples with hairs varying from 0.05 mm to 0.2 mm in diameter. The end of the hair is placed over the spot to be stimulated, and the holder is then depressed in such a way as to make of the hair a long cylindrical column with its force exerted perpendicularly to the skin surface. Fair constancy of stimulation is assured by reason of the fact that the greatest force of which a given hair is capable must be expended in each stimulation; "loading" is maximal at the pressure at which the hair bends as the holder is moved downwards. Moreover, its force is exerted practically instantaneously. The intensity of the stimulus depends, of course, both on the stiffness and length of the hair. Because stiffness may be expected to alter with changes of humidity some investigators have substituted nylon threads and glass wool filaments. Calibration may be effected by determining, with a sensitive balance, the heaviest weight that can just barely be raised in one scale pan by the hair, pressed down to the point of bending, in the other.

To elicit warm and cold sensations any device which will conduct heat to or away from the skin will serve. Immersion of an area of skin in previously warmed or cooled water is one readily available procedure. For the rapid raising of skin temperature the delivery of radiant heat to an exposed skin area from an electrically heated coil or thermocautery is convenient. "Infrared" lamps of the type now generally available may be used effectively for this purpose. To produce cooling of the skin convection currents from evaporating "dry ice" may be directed against a general skin area.

Such "macroscopic" stimuli fail, of course, to reveal the great local variations in thermal sensitivity of the skin, and a point-by-point exploration is needed to bring them out, as in the case of pressure sensations. Several different devices have been designed to accomplish local thermal stimulation. The Dallenbach temperature stimulator (Figure 9–1) is well known. This instrument has its contacting point limited to an area 1 mm in diameter. In addition to the feature that circulating water keeps the stimulus point at a constant predetermined temperature, it possesses the advantage that concomitant pressure on the skin can be controlled. To explore cold sensitivity in a truly punctiform manner von Frey and his students have employed tiny copper and brass cylinders constructed of bits of wire, the stimulating ends of which have been fused into small knobs. In these heat conductivity is a function of the composition and

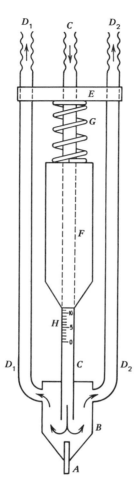

Fig. 9–1. The Dallenbach temperature stimulator. Either warm or cold water enters the instrument through C and is exhausted through D_1 and D_2. A sufficiently rapid flow keeps the chamber, B, and thus the 1-mm stimulus point, A, at constant temperature. The handle, F, is lowered to a given point on the scale, H, after A has contacted the skin, partially relieving the spring, G, and controlling mechanical pressure. After Dallenbach (*138*).

dimensions of the wires, and a graded series can be easily prepared by manipulation of these factors. The common laboratory instrument for the mapping of warm and cold sensitivity is the "temperature cylinder" (Figure 9–2). A series of such cylinders, preheated or precooled, may be used successively, each one serving until its temperature has changed significantly. The cylinders, being solid and thus having considerable

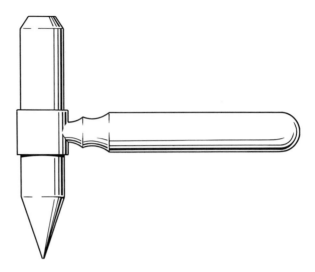

Fig. 9–2. A temperature cylinder. Adapted from Boring, Langfeld, and Weld, *A manual of psychological experiments*. New York: Wiley, 1937.

heat capacity, may be used continuously for several minutes at a time without returning them to their water bath. At least, this is the case for temperatures not greatly divergent from that of the surrounding air.

There is obviously added precision of control and some convenience in any thermal stimulator that will supply both warm and cold stimuli on demand. Circulating water will do this, of course, albeit a little clumsily, and there has been some elaboration of "thermode" systems. The thermode, a small plastic chamber with a metallic bottom resting on the skin, can have its temperature changed rapidly by two water jets directed into it. Interruption of one or the other permits quite accurate regulation of temperature, and this is continuously monitored by strategically located thermistors. Hensel et al. (*304*) and Kenshalo et al. (*355*) have realized high precision of threshold measurement with this technique, changes of as little as 0.05° C being reliably presented to the skin.

Somewhat less cumbersome stimulus control has been achieved (*352*) through the utilization of the Peltier effect, an old principle that could not be put to work practically until there were suitable developments in the area of semiconductors. The Peltier principle is essentially the reverse of that operating in the thermocouple. Where the latter generates a current across two dissimilar metals when heated or cooled, the Peltier refrigerator initiates a temperature change when a direct current is passed through its junction. By reversals of current flow, both warming and cooling effects can be created, and these can be obtained rapidly.

For "prick," "pain," and allied sensations any strong stimulation will suffice, though typically needles or other sharp-pointed devices which will actually penetrate the skin surface or produce a steep declivity in it have been used. Thistles, attached to the ends of von Frey hairs to permit pressure control, have been used commonly for punctiform exploration. For the pain associated with extreme thermal stimulation extensions of any of the procedures outlined for temperature sensations may, of course, be used. Chemical stimuli have been worked with in the arousal of pain, though not entirely in a systematic fashion. Chemicals and drugs have been, in general, of more interest for their possibilities in allaying pain and have been studied chiefly for their anesthetic properties. However, some facts of stimulation are known.

Water-soluble materials have little effect upon the horny surface of the skin and, to stimulate receptors, must be injected hypodermically, driven into the tissues electro-osmotically, or introduced into injured surface areas. Whereas generalities concerning the differential effects of the various classes of chemical stimuli are difficult to arrive at, it appears that the hydrogen ion is particularly effective in the arousal of pain. Solutions varying in hydrogen-ion concentration (pH values of 5.8 to 8.0), when injected into the skin, have been shown to produce pain at pH values below 7.2, the intensity of pain increasing progressively with degree of acidity. At pH 5.8 the pain may be unbearable. The introduction of alkalis of pH values above 7.2 produces an immediate quelling of pain. However, figures such as these are valid only for certain prescribed stimulating conditions. If, instead of an ordinary hypodermic needle the "jet injection" technique is used, the accompanying mechanical pressure may radically change the threshold value. One investigator (389) employed such a procedure while controlling pH with an acetate buffer. He found liminal pain at a pH of 6.2 and the most intense pain at 3.2. Another (346), jet-injecting HCl into the skin, had to go below pH 3 to get any pain at all, then it was rapidly dissipated because the tissues themselves serve as a buffer for this acid. With organic acids it appears impossible to separate out the effects of the dissociated hydrogen ion and the remaining undissociated acid, so pH, at the site of stimulation, is indeterminate.

Of the inorganic salts only those yielding excess potassium ions seems capable of arousing pain. Indeed, one of the theories of the origin of the painful sensation (63) states that the release of potassium by body cells is a necessary precursor to pain. Direct action of intracellular potassium, it says, causes pain; analgesics are agents that inhibit potassium release. However, at the level of the chemical stimulus, as it is applied directly to tissues, several different classes of organic compounds are effective. The most persistent pains come from amines and peptides derived from venoms, but severe pain can also be generated by materials "natural" to the skin, for example, histamine and acetylcholine, when present in sufficiently high concentrations. It is interesting that the latter two compounds, as well as potassium, when applied directly to the raw, abraded skin, produces a pressury sensation which is not unpleasantly painful but which changes to unmistakable pain when concentration is raised sufficiently. The "zone" below outright pain Keele and Smith (See 527, p. 113) have proposed calling the *metaesthetic range of pain*. The analogy with mesopia, the dimly defined region between twilight vision (scotopia) and daylight vision (photopia), is obvious.

It is not only "painless pain" that can be created by chemical stimuli. By bringing about rapid heat interchanges between the skin and surrounding air, by altering blood circulation and thus distributing the heat equilibrium of the skin tissues, and by direct action on nerve endings, many chemical agents are capable of arousing warm or cold sensations.

It should be obvious that chemicals introduced to the skin, circulatory system, or muscles by injection—all procedures that have been used both experimentally and clinically—constitute a method that leaves much to be desired in the matter of precision of control. In an effort to improve reliability of method and to bring the locus of action as close as possible to the receptor structures, Keele and his associates (*346*) have introduced a technique of blistering the skin in a standard fashion and imposing chemicals directly on the blister base. The vesicant, cantharidin ("Spanish fly"), is applied overnight in a plaster to the skin of the forearm. In the morning the 1-cm-diam blister is opened, the fluid is drained, and the superficial epidermis is cut away. A 15-min period of bathing the blister base in Locke's solution (physiological saline) allays any pain from the "operation." Periodically, the bathing solution is removed and the chemical under test is substituted. The observer makes a judgment on a prearranged scale as to the degree of pain elicited.

Many pain-arousing materials have been investigated in this way. Figure 9–3 shows the results obtained with one of special interest, KCl. As potassium ion concentration ($\log_{10}[K^+]$) increases somewhat over tenfold, there is a clearly linear increase in the severity of pain experienced, on the average, by the 15 observers. The method obviously has close limits of error.

The remaining form of energy to which the skin responds is electricity.

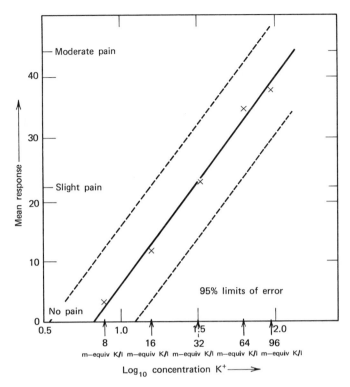

Fig. 9–3. Severity of pain as a function of potassium concentration. Sixty applications of KCl were made at intervals of 10–15 min. There were 15 observers. From Keele (*346*) after Smith, *UFAW symposium on assessment of pain in man and animals,* Edinburgh, 1962.

This is the great "inadequate" stimulus, inadequate in the sense that it has no specialized receptor of its own on which to operate. Electricity may be counted on to discharge nerves wherever they are contacted by electrodes, if the current is of sufficient strength. The presumption is that, led to the intact skin, electric currents do not require the intermediation of receptor organs and that they stimulate nerves directly by altering their membrane potentials. All kinds of currents, galvanic and faradic, continuous and interrupted, are effective. The curious thing is that steady, direct current does not feel "steady." The sensation is a quite lively one, describable as "whirring" or "tingling." Pulsed d.c. and a.c., at least at low frequencies, have an additional periodic surging quality. At high frequencies they may be indistinguishable from d.c.

The direct stimulation of the skin by electricity is not as simple a matter as the operations performed in bringing it about would imply. The skin, down to some indeterminate depth, must complete a circuit that has sufficient voltage to drive a liminal or supraliminal amperage through an impedance, chiefly that of the superficial layers of the skin, which is rarely stable in value for any appreciable length of time because it acts like a leaky capacitor. With direct currents, pulsed or continuous, the system polarizes and changes the skin's apparent resistance. There are problems associated with electrodes, whether wet or dry. Also, it must never be forgotten that electrodes come in pairs and, accordingly, the body fluids beneath the skin participate, as a volume conductor, to an incalculable depth from the neighborhood of one electrode to that of the other. Indeed, it is the current density at the site or sites of nerve stimulation that constitutes the true electrical stimulus, and there are obviously great difficulties in the way of getting the stimulus specified at this point.

It should not surprise us if all cutaneous qualities can be aroused through electrical stimulation, just as through chemical stimulation. Application of currents to the optic nerve produces visual sensations (phosphenes), to the auditory nerve clicks, buzzes, and tones (electrophonic phenomena), and to the chemical senses characteristic odors and tastes. Pass a suitable d.c. current through the head, with electrodes contacting the temples, and there will be felt, at the moment of make or break of the circuit, a stinging, pricking sensation under the cathode, a light flash will be seen, a click will be heard, a slightly acrid odor and a "metallic" taste will arise and, additionally, there is likely to be a hint of dizziness, for the current also stimulates the nonauditory branch of the eighth cranial nerve, and the head reflexly tilts to the side in response to it.

Of all forms of human sensitivity the most confined "dynamic range" belongs to the skin's response to direct application of electric current. This means that the distance, on the scale of stimulus intensity, between absolute threshold and the point at which sensation strength becomes too uncomfortable to tolerate is a short one, embracing a range of about 10 dB only. However, not all bodily loci are identical in this respect. Indeed, the same electrode placements yield somewhat variable ranges, depending especially on current duration, but also on the history of immediately prior stimulation, the bodily area involved, and a host of lesser variables. The horny portions of the hand and foot, for example, are relatively resistant to electrically aroused pain, the sensation in these areas having a somewhat "dull" quality that is readily tolerated, while the hairy portions of the arms and legs are characterized by an unpleasant "stinging," even at quite low stimulus values.

One of the best of the methods of electrical exploration is that devised by Bishop (70). It involves the creation of high-voltage potentials which are allowed to spark across from the exploring electrode to the skin, the discharge taking place at very low amperage. Single or multiple shocks may be delivered to any desired point. One of the chief advantages of this technique is that it provides uniform stimulation devoid of any accompanying mechanical distortion of the skin surface. With its aid it is possible to arouse, at different points, the full range of basic cutaneous sensations: touch, pressure, pain, warmth, and cold in all their intensitive variations.

Structure of the Skin. Some of the conditions for the experimental investigation of cutaneous sensations now having been set forth, it will be well for us to inquire into the makeup of the tissues concerned.

Considered from its external and superficial aspect, the skin presents a highly variegated structure. Of relatively smooth appearance in some parts of the body, it is deeply creased and furrowed in others; in some parts hairless and in others richly endowed with hairy appendages; in some places, especially over bony protuberances, stretched to the point of tautness and in others highly mobile and even flabby; in some regions thickened, horny, and tough but in others thin, pliable, and vulnerable to injury; in some portions dry and scaly but moist and flexible in others. If widely differing reactions to uniform stimulation are found to accompany these differences of composition it should not be surprising. Owing largely to the manner in which underlying structures are disposed, areas in different parts of the body display radically different properties. The larger part of the skin surface presents many small furrows which intersect in such a manner as to enclose rectangular, triangular, and polygonal spaces. On the palms of the hands and soles of the feet the furrows run in close parallel rows separated by slender ridges, and the eminences contain the openings of sweat ducts with which these regions are liberally supplied. Contrasted with this high degree of structural organization are the smooth and relatively undifferentiated surfaces of the calf of the leg and the area of the upper arm over the biceps. Something of the variations in surface consistency may be judged from the photographs of Figure 9–4. Were it not for some fundamental similarities of subsurface structure one might even suppose that different parts of the skin surface ought to be regarded as a collection of quite separate organs. However, there are uniformities, and we should see of what they consist.

Though classification of the successive layers of the skin is somewhat arbitrary, it is conventional to mark off three major groupings: the *epidermis* or cuticle, the *corium* or true dermis, and *subcutaneous tissue.*

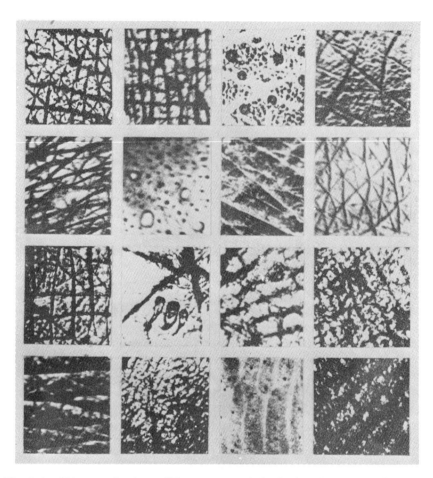

Fig. 9–4. Skin samples from different parts of the body. Photographs from von Skramlik (*532*).

The epidermis (see Figure 9–5) consists of two chief layers: the horny, most superficial tissue, called the *corneum*; and a deeper *germinative* layer (stratum germinativum or Malpighian layer) from which the cells of the corneum arise. The transition from the germinative layer to the corneum is, in some parts of the body, quite abrupt. In the process of growth and replacement the cells of the lower layer move up toward the surface of the epidermis, become closely packed and flattened, lose their nuclei, and acquire a horny consistency. The surface structure, only a few cells thick in most areas, is constantly being sloughed off and renewed

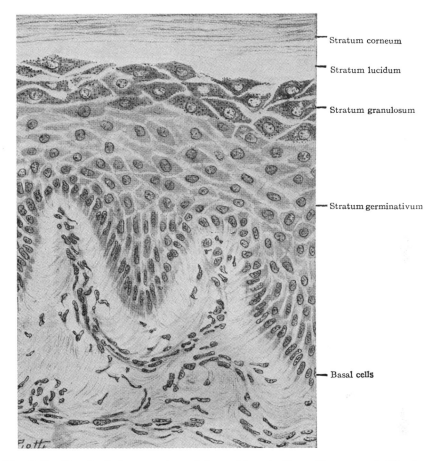

Fig. 9–5.   Detail of the structure of the epidermis. From Bremer and Weatherford (*89*). By permission of the Blakiston Company, Philadelphia.

from beneath. Two additional states of transition may be marked off in
some regions. In the process of cornification there may be distinguished
a layer just above the germinative layer. This, because of the appearance
in it of coarse granules in the cell material, is called the *stratum granu-
losum.* The cells here are in process of losing their nuclei and are becoming flattened and angular. The granule cells quite abruptly acquire a
shiny, translucent appearance and thus give rise to the differentiation of
a fourth epidermal layer, the *stratum lucidum.* In some tissue preparations the latter, usually only two cells thick, is indistinguishable from

other parts of the cornified surface tissue but, because it is deeply colored by several stains commonly used by the histologist, may serve as a distinct ribbonlike lower boundary of the corneum.

As is seen in Figure 9–5, the separation between the epidermis and corium is a highly irregular one, the uppermost layer of the corium (papillary layer) consisting of conical mounds of connective tissue, *papillae*, projecting into the floor of the epidermis and almost completely surrounded by the basal cylindrical cells of the Malpighian layer. The papillae are made up of finely interwoven fibers and house the greater portion of the smallest blood vessels and nerves of the skin. Some of the papillae contain capillary loops and are hence classed as vascular; in others are found specialized nerve endings, the *corpuscles of Meissner*, and are thus of the nervous or tactile type. The papillae vary greatly in length, some of those found in the sole of the foot projecting into the germinative layer as much as 0.2 mm, those in the facial region being but 0.035 to 0.040 mm long. It is the regular and fixed lineal disposition of the papillae that gives to the fingers and toes the orderly arrangements that make fingerprint and toeprint classification possible. Below the papillary layer of the corium is the *reticulated dermis*. This has a looser texture and consists of interlacing bundles of connective tissue. It is almost devoid of capillaries and nerve endings but contains many larger blood vessels, small nerve trunks, the tortuously coiled ducts of the sweat glands, the smaller hair follicles, and a considerable amount of elastic tissue that forms a bond with the lowermost layers of the skin.

The subcutaneous tissue consists chiefly of fibrous bundles which extend down to the muscles and bones. In some parts they are loosely meshed, and the spaces between them are occupied by fatty lobules; in others they are more tightly interlaced and give a firmer texture to the whole skin mass. In general, the more nearly parallel to the skin surface the connective tissue bundles are disposed, the greater is the skin's mobility. In the subcutaneous tissue are also to be found most of the larger blood vessels, nerve trunks, sweat glands, and hair follicles of the skin. The sebaceous (oily) glands have their secreting tissues here. Several types of encapsulated nerve endings, with which we shall later become acquainted, are found in subcutaneous tissue. Figure 9–6, which is a composite diagram with emphasis placed on the nervous connections and terminations of the skin, will serve to provide an overall view of the skin's structure, the relative depths of the various layers, and the disposition of many of the tissues that have been described. It should be apparent, from what has been said of local variations in skin structure, that no single section of skin will reveal all the features of importance to us, nor can any such single representative be thought of as "typical."

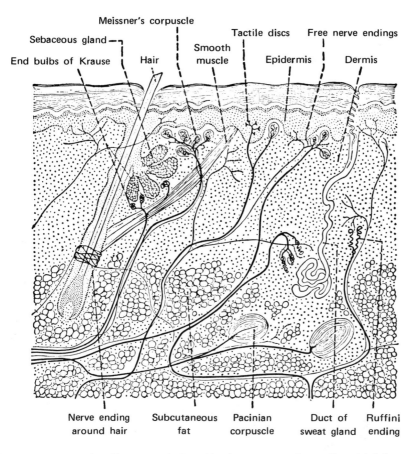

Meissner's corpuscle

Sebaceous gland

End bulbs of Krause

Hair

Smooth muscle

Tactile discs

Epidermis

Free nerve endings

Dermis

Nerve ending around hair

Subcutaneous fat

Pacinian corpuscle

Duct of sweat gland

Ruffini ending

Fig. 9–6. Composite diagram of the skin in cross section. The chief layers, epidermis, dermis, and subcutaneous tissue, are shown, as are also a hair follicle, the smooth muscle which erects the hair, and several kinds of nerve endings. In the epidermis are to be found tactile discs and free nerve endings; in the dermis are Meissner corpuscles, Krause end bulbs, Ruffini endings, and (around the base of the hair) free terminations. The subcutaneous tissue is chiefly fatty and vascular but contains Pacinian corpuscles, the largest of the specialized endings. From Gardner (*216*) after Woollard, Weddell, and Harpman (*652*). By permission of W. B. Saunders Company, Philadelphia.

Nerve Endings in the Skin. A considerable variety of nerve terminations is to be found in the skin layers. They range in size from that of the deep-lying Pacinian corpuscles, large enough to be seen with the unaided eye, to that of the finest naked fibrils in the epidermis. The latter terminations, so-called *free nerve endings,* are the most numerous. In histological skin sections they are found to terminate at all levels, in the epidermis, corium, and subcutaneous tissue. A great many endings may derive from a single nerve fiber, so that an appreciable area may contribute to the discharge of a particular nerve cell. Free nerve endings are best studied in the cornea of the eye, where no other type of termination can be discovered. It has been shown (*580*) that free terminations covering as much as an entire quadrant of the cornea belong to a single sensory fiber. Moreover, other fibers supplying the same general area have endings which maximally overlap and ramify into each other's fields, though functional independence of each network seems to be preserved despite the close anatomical proximity of endings. The supposition is that in the skin generally a single fiber may, through successive branchings, have a great number of separate terminations, covering in some instances areas of several square millimeters or even centimeters, but that a single fiber does not alone "possess" the region. Interlocking and proliferating endings, forming an intricate network and arising from other fibers, also lay claim to the region and participate in its response.

Free endings are derived from both myelinated and unmyelinated fibers but they are most commonly traced to small fibers of the former class. As they proceed from subcutaneous levels toward the skin surface they appear to have two chief destinations, one in *glabrous* (smooth) skin and one in hairy skin. In glabrous tissue, some terminate below the papillary level while others pass up into the papillae. Where there is a thick epidermis they may even pierce the top of the papilla and extend some distance into the epidermis. The other area of termination is in the vicinity of hairs. There they form an elaborate network around the middle portion of the hair follicle, encircling it (*circular* fibers) and extending along its length (*palisade* fibers). Because they so completely enclose the hair follicle for a distance they are often called *basket endings,* and there are some histologists who regard these endings, together with the connective tissue into which they have ramified, as constituting an encapsulated corpuscle (*422*).

If one regards the free nerve ending as the prototype of all cutaneous nerve terminations the remaining "types" of endings found in the skin may be regarded simply as elaborations of or developments from this fundamental form. Indeed, many histologists believe that if a completely systematic examination of all representative tissues were made there would be found an unbroken continuum of nerve endings in which the free terminations, at one end of the series, would be found to have been transformed, at the other, into the most elaborately formed of corpuscular endings. There is by now a long history of investigation of the skin's nerve terminations. In the earlier days of such study there was a strong tendency to look for differences and to proliferate distinctions into elaborate classifications. As many as 34 end organs had been catalogued at one time. However, many of the "discoveries" were traceable to the introduction of methods of tissue preparation and staining which themselves created artifacts, easier to come by than to avoid in this difficult field. Nowadays, the similarities are being stressed and, while there is far from complete agreement in the matter of classification, it is currently more a question of whether all terminations are to be regarded as variations on a single theme, or whether two or three categories will embrace all forms of ending. The answer is likely to be some time in coming, since, typically, silver and gold stains yield one result, methylene blue another, perfusion and immersion techniques provide different pictures, and the light microscope is giving away to the electron microscope for study of fine detail. Moreover, biochemical differences between terminals are beginning to be investigated, and the descriptions coming from this effort are not likely to simplify end organ classification.

The first step toward anatomical complication would seem to have been taken by certain of the skin endings on the tips of which appear tiny knoblike swellings. These are variously known as expanded-tip receptors, hederiform ("ivylike") endings, and Merkel discs. In glabrous skin they are very common and appear in great numbers high in the corium, just under the germinative layer of the epidermis. They are also found on the highly branched fibers making up the complex that surrounds hair follicles.

All other forms of endings have acquired sufficient structural complication to be classed as *encapsulated endings*. Several varieties have been described and named (See Figure 9–7). *Meissner corpuscles*, found in the papillae of hairless skin regions, vary from 40 to 150 μ in length and 20 to 60 μ in width. There may be as many as 20 or 30 of them packed into a square millimeter. One to five sensory fibers enter the lower end of each, lose their protective sheaths, and coil into the corpuscular ending. *Krause end bulbs*, somewhat smaller on the average than Meissner corpuscles, are also found in the dermal layers. They have been observed in the eye, near the margin of the cornea, and also in the tissues of the external genitals and of the tongue. Some authorities view the Krause end bulb not as an encapsulated ending but simply as an elaborate intertwining of fine fibrils having somewhat the "organization" of a ball of yarn. Because the Krause end bulb appears most characteristically in transitional tissue between glabrous skin and mucous membrane, Winkelmann (*646*) has given it the name, "mucocutaneous end organ"; he regards it to be the analog in nonhairy skin of the nerve network

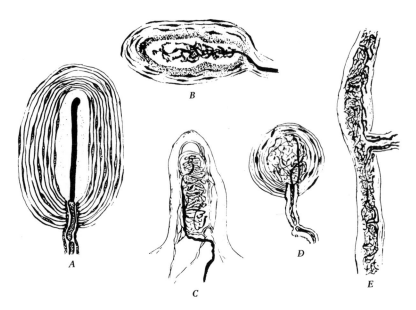

Fig. 9–7. Encapsulated nerve endings of the skin. *A,* a Vater-Pacini corpuscle; *B,* a Golgi-Mazzoni corpuscle; *C,* a Meissner corpuscle; *D,* a Krause end bulb; *E,* a Ruffini cylinder. Drawn from descriptions and photomicrographs of Boeke (*76*), Ramon y Cajal (*487*), and Ruffini (*385*).

surrounding hair follicles. The basket ending is a tangled mass of fibers that has attached itself to the follicle sheath; the Krause end bulb is one that had no hair to invade. *Cylinders of Ruffini,* also known as terminal cylinders and arboriform terminations, occur in the dermis near the junction of the subcutaneous layers and have also been found in deeper tissues. Most of them have their nerve entrances at the side, as shown in Figure 9–7, though some have been observed with connections at the end. A single dividing nerve fiber is occasionally found to connect with several Ruffini cylinders. Current opinion is running in the direction of regarding the Ruffini termination as merely a particular pattern of expanded-tip (Merkel) endings that have "rolled" or otherwise acquired constraints that give the collection of fibers its characteristic cylindrical form. Like the Krause end bulb, it may not really be an encapsulated receptor.

   The largest and in some respects the most elaborate of the encapsulated endings are the *Pacinian corpuscles* (Vater-Pacini) or lamellar corpuscles. These are 0.5 to 4.5 mm long and 1.0 to 2.0 mm wide. They occur deep in the corium and subcutaneous tissue and are abundant in the hand and foot regions. They are found also in the tissues of the joints, ligaments of the leg and forearm, in the external genitals, in the coverings of bones, in the connective tissue of the abdominal cavity, and near the walls of large blood vessels. Pacinian corpuscles have a thick coat composed of 10 to 50 successive layers of connective tissue arranged concentrically around a central granular core in which the nerve fibrils terminate. Minute blood vessels enter the basal pole, and the capillary network may be found between the onionlike layers. Apparently closely related to the Pacinian corpuscles are the similarly complex *Golgi-Mazzoni corpuscles.* These also have a somewhat general distribution, and very probably should be viewed simply as smaller Pacinian corpuscles, judging from their encapsulation, or perhaps as very deeply situated end bulbs of the Krause variety, considering their elaborate cores.

The Pacinian ending is of special interest on more than one account. It has been known as a skin receptor for a long time, since the middle of the eighteenth century, and has been studied assiduously, both structurally and functionally, more than any other cutaneous nerve ending. Moreover, along with the nervous network formed by free endings, it is invariably found as a sensory component in every organized nervous system beyond a certain degree of complexity (*485*). It is the first end organ to have yielded to experimental methods aimed at determining how receptor cells are able to transduce energy impinging upon them and initiate impulses in their attached nerves. Loewenstein and his associates (*391*) accomplished this with the lamellar corpuscle and thus provided a prototypical account with important implications for all of sensory psychophysiology.

A warning has already been given that we should not be too complacent with our current knowledge of the receptor population. Anatomy abounds in descriptions of nerve terminations that are "Meissner-like," "Ruffini-like," etc. At different stages of development and in different body loci end organ shapes and sizes vary. Some have been led to the belief that free nerve endings, tapering off into the upper reaches of the dermis and epidermis, are the only receptors to have properly reached their destination. All others are rejects, so to speak. Having encountered an obstacle, they spend their growth force in adjusting to local conditions. One kind of evidence favoring such a hypothesis is that adduced by FitzGerald (*199*) who has demonstrated an expansion of the number of terminations in growing skin, whether this occurs in the fetus and neonate during normal growth or during recovery from wounds and damaging skin diseases, such as psoriasis. But there appears to be a "ceiling" beyond which the mature epithelium will not go in accepting available fibers. Similar considerations come out of the interesting and provocative work of Speidel (*538*), who has followed, with time-lapse photography, the growing tips of nerves in the transparent tail of the tadpole. Indeed, until an analogous attack becomes possible for human skin, we are unlikely to be able to supplant our somewhat static picture of neural organization with a more dynamic one.

Central Pathways for the Cutaneous Senses.   There exists such a multiplicity of end organs and sensory fibers in the skin and underlying tissues as to lead one to suppose that their attached nerve trunks in the spinal cord must be hopelessly confused. Fortunately, however, it is possible to see some order in the constitution of the central pathways. In fact, far from being haphazardly and chaotically combined, nerves from the periphery become organized progressively in the direction of functional simplicity once they enter the central nervous system.

If any of the sensory nerves traveling through subcutaneous tissue were to be traced out to individual fiber terminations it would be found that the bundle contains components serving all types of endings. Some of the fibers constituting the nerve would be relatively large (15μ or more in diameter) and a great many would average about 8μ, while perhaps three-quarters of them would be quite small (1.3μ or less) and would lack myelin sheaths. The picture, then, of a cutaneous sensory nerve is one of anatomical complexity. Apparently the bundle is a conduit carrying fibers from a fairly definite skin area but serving several different kinds of sensation. It follows that injury to such a nerve will result indiscriminately in loss of sensations of touch, warmth, cold, and pain in the area supplied by the nerve. There is no way in which the various modalities can be sorted out at the peripheral level. This is also the case just before entrance to the spinal cord. All cutaneous impulses are carried to the cord by way of 30 of the 31 pairs of spinal nerves—the first cervical pair has no sensory roots—and 4 of the cranial nerves (V, VII, IX, X). Up to the point of entrance to the central nervous system these nerves are still serving as functionally undifferentiated conductors, and it therefore follows that interruption of a spinal nerve will abolish all systems of sensitivity in the area housing its terminations.

The region of skin supplied by a particular spinal nerve is called the *dermatome* of that nerve. Since there is considerable overlapping, with branches of two or more spinal nerves typically invading a given skin area, it follows that peripheral exploration will not establish the extent of the dermatomes. However, there are ways of mapping them. One of the best is to make use of Sherrington's method of "remaining sensibility," a procedure involving the sectioning, in animals, of three dorsal

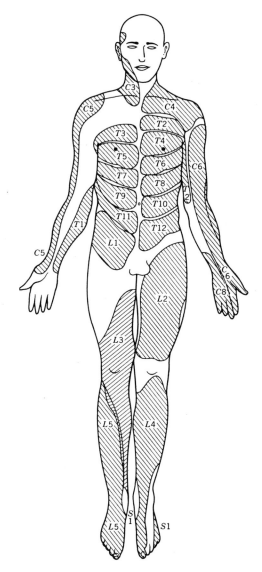

Fig. 9–8. The dermatomes. Each area is supplied by a single posterior root of the spinal cord. Half the dermatomes are shown on one side of the figure, half on the other side. Extensive overlap is the rule; a single local region of the skin may be innervated by two or even three roots. From Lewis (*384*). By permission of The Macmillan Company.

spinal roots above and three below the one to be studied. This eliminates overlapping nerve supplies in the skin region belonging to the now isolated spinal root, and there is left at the skin "an island of sensitivity in a sea of anesthesia." By systematic sectioning there have been mapped the dermatomes corresponding to spinal nerves at all levels. They are depicted in Figure 9–8. Another way to explore the dermatomes is to inject strychnine into a dorsal root zone. This elicits sensations localized in the corresponding peripheral region, and the licking, biting, and scratching of an animal so injected reveal the extent of the skin area affected. In humans comparable data may be obtained by noting the distribution of skin eruptions in "shingles" (herpes zoster), a virus infection of posterior root ganglia. The pattern of eruptions coincides with the dermatomes. Still another technique with human subjects is to inject hypotonic saline solution into the dorsal roots and induce pain of the angina variety in the corresponding skin area. This is the method by which Figure 9–8 was derived. Information supplementary to the data obtained by any of these methods is to be had from surgery for prolapsed spinal discs when direct electrical stimulation of dorsal roots reveals the peripheral projection. It would be most surprising if all these procedures yielded univocal results, and they do not, of course. Although wounds near the peripheral site may result in a highly delimited area of anesthesia,

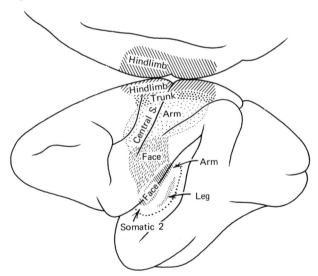

Fig. 9–9. Somatic sensory projection areas in the monkey. From Terzuolo, C. A., and W. R. Adey. Sensorimotor cortical activities. In: *Handbook of Physiology. Neurophysiology.* Washington, D.C.: Am. Physiol. Soc., 1960, Sec. 1, Vol. II, 797–835.

damage to the dorsal root inevitably brings less well-defined boundaries because of the relatively extensive overlap of dermatomes.

There are two main pathways to the brain: (a) the *lemniscal system* and (b) the *spinothalamic system*. Fibers, chiefly larger ones of the "A" group, which are faster-conducting and which subserve touch, pressure, and kinethesis (at least) proceed from the dorsal horn directly upwards, by way of the posterior white columns of the cord. Then, without crossing, they terminate in the lower medulla. Those from the lower trunk and legs have their synapse in the *gracile nucleus* of the medulla, nearest the body midline, while fibers from the upper trunk and arms end in the neighboring *cuneate nucleus*. From these two medullary centers new connecting neurons cross to the other side of the body and ascend in the medial lemniscus, terminating, for the most part, in the ventrobasal nucleus of the thalamus. Third-order neurons now synapse and radiate upward to the cortex, arriving in one of two somatic sensory projection areas, S1 or S2. The two areas are diffusely outlined in Figure 9–9. S1 is situated in the postcentral gyrus, S2 in the upper bank of the Sylvian fissure. The presumption is that most lemniscal fibers go to S1; this route has shorter latencies and sharper localizations. Comparable fibers from the face region join the medial lemniscus by way of secondary neurons from the trigeminal nuclei which, in turn, receive their input from the fifth cranial nerve (the trigeminal).

A second main component of the lemniscal system, sometimes called the *neospinothalamic pathway*, runs a different course in its lower reaches. Collaterals from A-fibers, at the level of entrance to the dorsal horn, cross over fairly abruptly to the contralateral side and ascend in the *ventral spinothalamic tract*. In the medulla these join (crossed) fibers of the medial lemniscus. There is some evidence that this tract projects chiefly to S2 in the cortex.

There is a third constituent of the lemniscal system, the *spinocervical tract* (also known as Morin's pathway), which consists of large, rapidly conducting fibers that conduct impulses from the dorsal horn to the *lateral cervical nucleus*, a gray patch immediately below the medulla, thence to the medial lemniscus. This is important to many lower forms, such as the cat, but need not detain us long. Humans have presumably phylogenetically "outgrown" it. It is represented by the dotted line of Figure 9–10A.

The other main somatic system, the *spinothalamic*, differs in many ways from the lemniscal system, both structurally and functionally. Peripheral fibers contributing to it are primarily those of the "C" group, but small myelinated fibers participate also. This means, in the first instance, that the spinothalamic system is a relatively slowly conducting

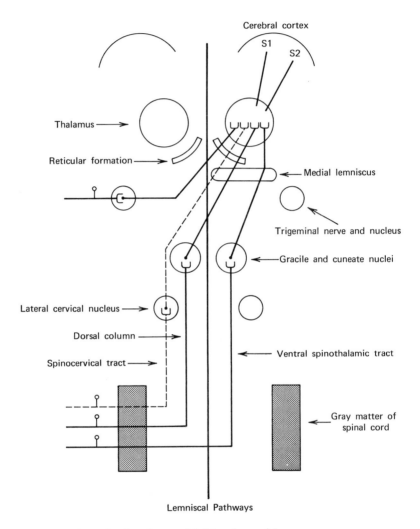

Cerebral cortex

S1

S2

Thalamus

Reticular formation

Medial lemniscus

Trigeminal nerve and nucleus

Gracile and cuneate nuclei

Lateral cervical nucleus

Dorsal column

Spinocervical tract

Ventral spinothalamic tract

Gray matter of spinal cord

Lemniscal Pathways

Fig. 9–10A. Lemniscal pathways (highly schematic).

one. Moreover, the synaptic provisions are such, in the ascent to the cortex, that there may be several delays en route. First-order neurons, entering the cord through *Lissauer's tract* (see Figure 9–11), terminate abruptly on large dorsal horn cells at which point they are freely interconnected. Second-order fibers having short axons end one or two segments above or below the level of entrance. Many cross to the opposite

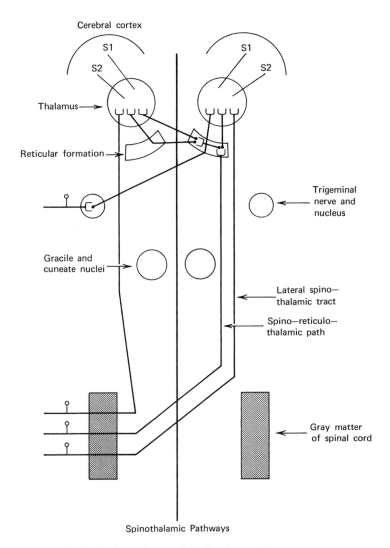

Fig. 9–10B. Spinothalamic pathways (highly schematic).

side of the cord and ascend in the *lateral spinothalamic tract*. But the fact that many components of the spinothalamic tract are found to be bilaterally represented in the thalamus indicates that both crossed and uncrossed fibers participate in the system's responses. It is also clear that some ascending fibers enter the reticular formation of the brainstem and there connect, sometimes polysynaptically, with fiber groups ascending to the thalamus. Although lemniscal pathways project mainly on the ventro-basal complex of the thalamus, those from the spinothalamic system go chiefly to the posterior group of thalamic nuclei and project bilaterally on it.

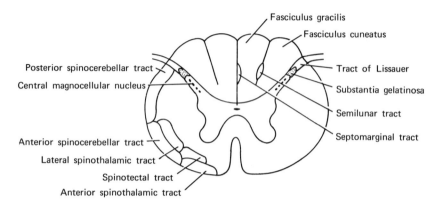

Fasciculus gracilis

Fasciculus cuneatus

Posterior spinocerebellar tract

Central magnocellular nucleus

Tract of Lissauer

Substantia gelatinosa

Semilunar tract

Anterior spinocerebellar tract

Lateral spinothalamic tract

Septomarginal tract

Spinotectal tract

Anterior spinothalamic tract

Fig. 9–11. Cross section of the cord showing the location of several ascending pathways. Lissauer's tract is of special interest. From Sinclair (*527*).

Impulses passing over the spinothalamic system are undoubtedly responsible for the reporting of pain, temperature, and touch, though not exclusively so in the case of touch and perhaps not exclusively so in the case of temperature. There is widespread belief that pain is the system's specialty, but here again there is enough doubt about pain pathways to make one hesitate to indulge in sweeping generalizations. Small C-fibers, which make up the bulk of the contributors to this system, have been shown, by the technique of producing a "collision" between impulses passing centripetally (*orthodromic*) and those generated centrifugally (*antidromic*), to carry messages reporting light touch (*172*). Figure 9–12 diagrams this ingenious experiment, made necessary because ordinary methods of microelectrode recording are extremely difficult with such fine strands of nerve.

As a practical matter, it is often possible surgically to block out pain by transection of the anterolateral spinothalamic tracts, though by no stretch of the imagination could such operations be regarded as "surefire". Most often temperature insensitivity accompanies whatever degree of analgesia is attained, and frequently the elevation of pain threshold is so small as to be clinically unimportant. There is probably not just one pain pathway, nor does it seem likely that there is only a single variety of pain. We shall confront this important question later.

If peripheral excitation is to be effective at the highest levels of the central nervous system the receptor activity must, of course, be "rep-

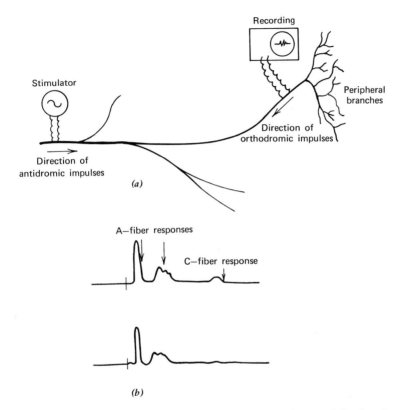

Fig. 9-12. The Douglas-Ritchie experiment. *(a)* Electrical activity in the peripheral branch of a small sensory nerve is induced by antidromic stimulation and is recorded on an oscilloscope. *(b)* In the absence of peripheral stimulation, the full reaction of the nerve (both A- and C-fiber responses) occurs. See upper trace. However, as is shown in the lower trace, suitable stimulation of the peripheral twigs sets up an orthodromic impulse that "collides" with the C-component and greatly attenuates it. From *Physiological Psychology,* by Peter M. Milner. Copyright 1970 by Holt, Rinehart, and Winston, Inc. Reproduced by permission of Holt, Rinehart, and Winston, Inc.

resented" in some adequate way at every neural level. One way of tracing the progress of the message—and hopefully of finding out how the nervous system "codes" it—is to plot the *receptive field* for each accessible recording site. The size of a skin area contributing to activity in a particular afferent fiber varies tremendously from one skin sample to another. In the cat, receptive fields as small as 1 mm^2 and as large as several square centimeters have been found when recording was at the primary neuron, the nerve leading directly to the skin. In general, the larger diameter fibers have small, restricted fields, while small, slowly conducting fibers are associated with large receptive fields (*321*).

Nerve potentials may be picked up at almost any available site, all the way to the cortex, though interpretation of what is happening en route is not equally easy at all levels nor are all forms of peripheral stimulation equally efficacious. Potentials can be evoked at the cortex from peripheral stimulation in the forms of joint rotation, light touch, heavy pressure, and hair movement. Thermal stimuli are less certain in their action, though cold on the tongue is known to arouse cortical units (*373*), and noxious stimuli designed to initiate pain are generally not successful in evoking cortical potentials.

At the level of the first synapse in the cord, at the dorsal horn, receptive fields are larger than in the peripheral nerve, and this is to be expected in view of the impingement of a single peripheral axon on several central cells and the convergence on a single cell of several axons. This arrangement suggests that receptive fields must not be homogeneous, the overlap favoring a central, higher-sensitivity region. In general, this proves to be true, with the center of the field yielding highest-frequency discharges, shortest latencies, and longest adaptation times. Still larger receptive fields may be found at higher levels. At the gracile nucleus and at the cortex there are single cells that have the whole body as a receptive field! In addition to convergence and divergence of neurons, there is also the principle of *surround inhibition* to be reckoned with—this we have encountered before, in vision—and, at the cortex, so-called *complementary inhibition*, whereby excitation of corresponding limbs with like stimuli may reduce the effect of the primary stimulus.

In tracing out the progress of impulses from receptor to cortex, two stations come to be of special interest for the vital roles they play, the thalamus and the cortex itself. We have seen that the lemniscal and spinothalamic systems project to the thalamus in a somewhat different way, the former unilaterally to the ventrobasal nuclear complex, the latter bilaterally to the posterior group of nuclei. Considering their origins—rapid A-fiber transmission over somewhat discrete pathways, in one instance, and predominantly slow, diffuse C-fiber transmission, in the other—it would be surprising if the two nuclear regions in the thalamus showed identical properties. And they do not, whether one judges in terms of receptive fields or modality specificity. Figure 9–13 contrasts the two areas along both dimensions. It is clear that the ventrobasal centers have relatively confined receptive fields; contributing to the posterior centers are broad skin areas, in many instances encompassing half the body.

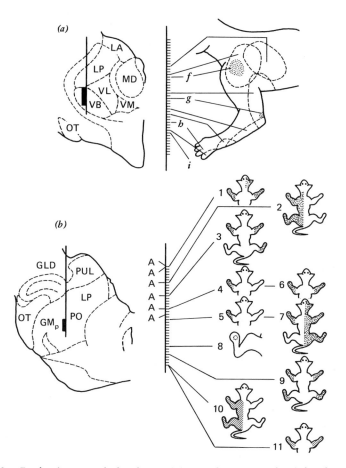

Fig. 9–13. Projections to thalamic nuclei. *(a)* shows: on the left, the path of an electrode penetration to the cat's ventrobasal nuclear complex (VB); on the right, the location of contralateral skin areas, stimulation of which produced records from this electrode. *(b)* shows a similar penetration of the posterior nuclear group (PO), on the left. The figurines on the right side of *(b)* show the location of receptive fields served by paths contacted by this electrode: 1–9, light mechanical pressure; 10–11, strong and destructive stimuli; A, levels at which cells were found that responded exclusively to auditory stimuli. There is no regular lineup of topographic fields as there is in *(a)*. From Thompson *(572)* after Poggio and Mountcastle *(476)*. Copyright, The Johns Hopkins Press.

Individual cortical units can be found that are even more diffuse, their fields covering the entire skin surface. But, this is only to say that receptive fields of individual cortical cells are more variable than are those

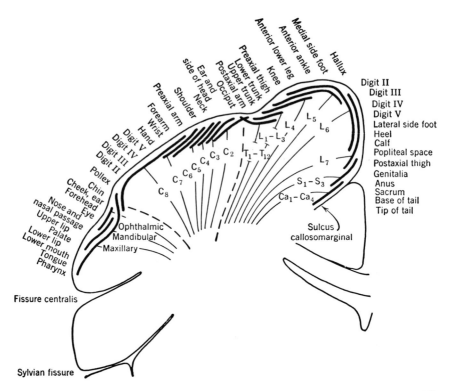

Fig. 9–14. Projection of the body surface on the central gyrus of the cortex. The left cerebral hemisphere of the monkey is shown in cross section. Correspondences between cortical loci and specific body areas were established by the evoked potential method. After Woolsey, Marshall, and Bard *(654)*. By permission of the Johns Hopkins Press and the authors.

anywhere else in the nervous system. There are also units that receive from relatively confined fields and, altogether, the receptive-field size and specificity seem to be pretty much the same in the cortex as they are in the thalamus.

In view of all the complexities—the varying densities of peripheral innervation, the devious routes and connections, the several kinds of facilitatory and inhibitory interactions—it seems surprising that any kind of topographic arrangement representing the body surface can be retained once the cortex is reached. Yet, a meaningful map can be constructed; indeed, several different maps are possible. The exact form it will take will depend upon what degree of anesthesia is present when the data are taken, whether, in the case of the evoked potential, the

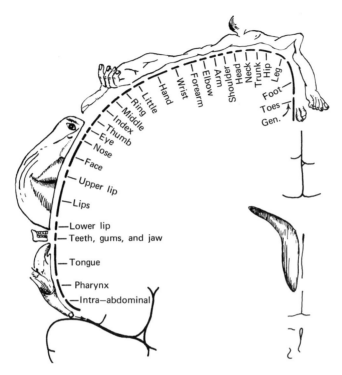

Fig. 9–15. A sensory homunculus. Projection of the human somatic system on the brain's post-central gyrus. Obviously, the face region, the mouth and tongue in particular, claim disproportionate amounts of cortical tissue. From Rasmussen and Penfield, *The cerebral cortex of man.* New York: Macmillan, 1950.

significant variable plotted is the response magnitude or its latency, or whether the essential information entering into the construction comes from the reverse procedure, that is, direct electrical stimulation of the cortex in humans undergoing exploratory brain operations. Also, it must be remembered that a point at the skin surface is inevitably represented by an area, large or small, at the cortex, and this means that the map will necessarily lack precision in any case. Such constructions are thus not to be taken too seriously. They merely serve to demonstrate that some topographic order is preserved. Not all is chaos.

Two of the "classics" in this effort are reproduced in Figures 9–14 and 9–15. One comes from projection of the body surface on the post-central gyrus of the monkey (S1); the other incorporates results, with human patients, of direct cortical stimulation and the ensuing feelings of tingling and numbness in the corresponding body area.

10
Pressure Sensitivity

A variety of names has been applied to the sensations falling under the general rubric, "pressure." Not all pressures have the same "feel." "Contact" designates a bright, lively sensation as contrasted with the dull and heavy feeling of "deep pressure." Some pressures are "dense" and "pointed," some feel "granular," while others are "diffuse." Some have a superficial localization; others seem to have originated in deeper tissues. It has been contended that pressure sensations vary along a continuous scale of "brightness-dullness." Differences in the characteristic manner of arousal are also observable. Some pressures rise to peak in an abrupt fashion, while others develop slowly; others are discontinuous or vacillating. Careful observation leads to the conclusion that no cutaneous sensation is entirely simple in its composition. All have temporal, intensive, and spatial aspects. Each pressure feeling constitutes a "pattern" having these and perhaps other separately variable dimensions. Certain patterns, occurring frequently and familiarly, we come to endow with names: "touch," "contact," "tickle," "vibration," "dull pressure," etc.; others, their particular combinations of attributes coming only occasionally to observation, go unnamed or are indefinitely dubbed simply "pressure."

The usual stimulus for the arousal of pressure is, of course, mechanical deformation of the skin tissue. It can be shown that an essential feature of the deformation, in order to be effective, is the production of a "gradient" of sufficient magnitude. The mere application of mechanical pressure to a skin region does not guarantee that pressure sensations will result. Thus, if a finger is dipped into a jar of mercury only the "ring" at the surface of the liquid is felt. Considerable pressure is being exerted on the immersed part of the finger, but the pressure is evenly distributed, and one local area of tissue is not deformed with respect to its neighbor except at the region of transition from mercury to air. Whenever a sufficiently steep gradient is formed the necessary mechanical condition for the arousal of pressure sensations is present. The intensity of stimulation is also to be related to the steepness of the gradient, sharp gradients arousing more intense sensations. It is of no consequence whether the gradient is formed inwardly or outwardly with respect to the skin surface. Traction applied to a thread glued to the skin provides an effective pressure stimulus and demonstrates that the only necessary condition is tissue distortion.

In the final analysis it is, of course, tension within the cutaneous tissues that constitutes the physical stimulus for pressure sensations. Deformation is effective only because it invariably creates such tensions. Using a series of small stimulus hairs von Frey and Kiesow (*209*) were able to demonstrate that pressure thresholds were reached at an approximately constant level of tension (about 0.85 gm/mm). Thus a force of 17 mgm operating through a stimulus hair of 0.02 mm radius and one of 85 mgm imposed on a hair of 0.1 mm radius are both just capable of eliciting pressure. It is neither force per se (grams) nor hydrostatic pressure (grams per square millimeter) but tension, expressed in terms of force per linear extent of skin surface contacted, that constitutes the significant variable. The relationship, obtaining uniformly for tiny skin areas, breaks down for larger stimuli and forces.

If, with a von Frey hair or a needle, a gradient of constant moderate

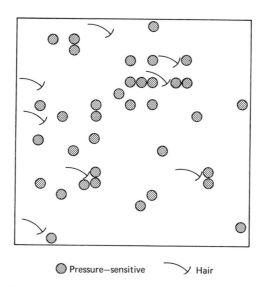

◉ Pressure—sensitive   ⌇ Hair

Fig. 10–1. Distribution of pressure-sensitive "spots" on a sample skin area located on the underside of the forearm. Each dot represents the locus of stimulation evoking a report of "pressure" when a constant, moderate gradient was applied systematically 400 times in the area. From unpublished data of the author.

magnitude is maintained while exploring, point by point in a systematic manner, a sample area of skin on the underside of the forearm, a map of pressure-sensitive "spots," such as that illustrated in Figure 10–1, will be obtained. Some points stimulated will respond with clear sensations of touch, contact, or pressure. Others will yield these qualities but with diminished intensity. Many points stimulated with the same gradient will produce no sensation whatever. Obviously there are great sensitivity differences even within a relatively circumscribed area. It is notable that a close correlation exists between the location of sensitive spots and that of hairs, in the great majority of instances the point of high sensitivity being located on the "windward" side of the hair (the side from which the wind appears to be "blowing" the hair). This peculiar distribution is very suggestive and points either to an intimacy of anatomical relation between pressure receptors and hair follicles or to participation of the hair in the process of effecting tissue distortion. Of course, both could be the case. The former possibility should be considered seriously in view of the profuse network of nerve fibers surrounding hair follicles. That the portion of the hair embedded in the skin serves to facilitate transmission of distorting forces applied to the skin surface can hardly be doubted. Obliquely disposed relative to the skin surface, the hair provides a relatively massive, solid, and unyielding column which could account for tissue displacements at all points along its length. Whereas "pressure points" are found, even with moderately weak stimuli, at other spots than over hair follicles, it is these areas that display the greatest constancy of response as measured by reproducibility of results in successive tests of the same sample skin area.

Something more of the skin's provision for pressure reception may be learned by using a graded series of stimulus hairs and making a number of successive explorations. As the intensity of the stimulus is increased there are found more and more sensitive "spots," and eventually, if a sufficiently stiff hair is used, it will evoke a positive response wherever it is applied. Guilford and Lovewell (254) have performed an experiment demonstrating this, with results as shown in Figure 10–2. The stimuli ranged from 0.01 to 1.60 gm, in nine steps, and each was set down on 200 equally spaced loci in a 1 cm² patch on the shaved back of the hand. As is shown by the curve connecting stimulus intensity with proportion of points responding, the weakest intensity evoked sensations in less than 1% of the trials, while the strongest did so 100% of the time. The shape of the function is interesting, being of sigmoid form, and suggests that any given "unit area" of the skin's surface has a statistical probability of responding to a stimulus of a given intensity.

Further evidence that there is indeed a statistical distribution of

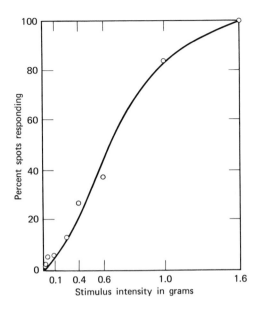

Fig. 10–2. Pressure sensitivity as determined by intensity of stimulation. Proportion of spots responding in a 1 cm² area as hair stimuli of graduated strength are used. From the data of Guilford and Lovewell (*254*). By permission of the Journal Press.

response from pressure points comes from some interesting records obtained on nerve discharges in macaque monkeys (*624*). Successive papillary ridges on the animal's finger were stimulated with brief pressure pulses by means of an electromagnetically driven lucite probe. Intensity, measured in terms of extent of skin indentation, was held constant for any given set of stimulating conditions but was systematically varied in different experiments from weak to strong. Figure 10–3 shows what happens when a series of eight papillary ridges is traversed. The average number of impulses generated is a function both of stimulus intensity and position within the receptive field.

Absolute and Differential Pressure Sensitivity. The intensive threshold for pressure sensation has been seen to depend primarily upon the locus of stimulation. Assuming, however, that the most sensitive local region is selected for measurement, an important question remains. We have raised it before for visual and auditory sensations. What is the order of magnitude of the absolute threshold for pressure? How much physical energy must be expended to arouse a just detectable pressure sensation? Several

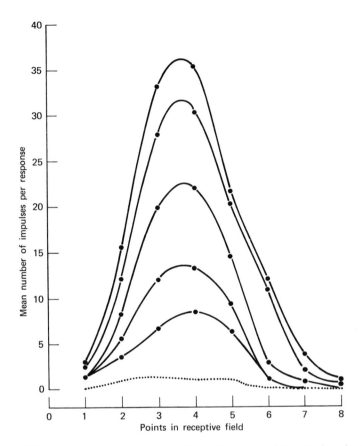

Fig. 10–3. Nerve responses and pressure intensity. Each of the "points in receptive field," on the graph's abscissa, is a papillary ridge lying within a single receptor field of the monkey's finger. Stimulus intensity was varied in six steps, the highest curve coming from the heaviest skin gradient. From Werner, Gerhard and Mountcastle, Vernon B. In: D. R. Kenshalo (Ed.), *The Skin Senses,* 1968. Courtesy of Charles C. Thomas, Publisher, Springfield, Illinois.

investigations have been directed at this point. If a von Frey hair is used one answer will be forthcoming. If a gentler gradient is created by the use of a larger mechanical contactor the threshold value will be found to be higher. In the hairy portions of the skin one can take advantage of the fact that a hair itself serves as a lever of the second class (i.e., with its follicle more or less firmly anchored below the skin surface) to create disturbances in the superficial skin layers. Moving the distal end of the hair ever so slightly is likely to arouse lively sensations of touch. It has been found by von Frey (207) that a minimal energy of 0.04 erg, applied to the end of a hair 1.0 cm long, was sufficient to exceed the threshold of sensation. Other determinations by Wolf (647; 532, pp. 134–138), with the aid of an ingenious apparatus making possible the delivery of carefully measured tiny impacts to the skin, yielded the following representative values: 0.026 erg, on the ball of the thumb; 0.037 to 1.090 ergs, on the tips and balls of other fingers; 0.032 to 0.113 erg, at various positions on the underside of the forearm. These values seem small indeed but, compared with the energies needed to excite the retina or the cochlea, they are of tremendous magnitude. Direct comparisons of absolute intensitive thresholds in the visual, auditory, and tactual realms show that the skin absorbs from 100 million to 10 billion times the energy required by the eye or ear in getting into minimal action.

The figures just cited come, of course, from psychophysical experiments on intact human skin. If it were possible to measure threshold at the receptor cell itself, what might we expect the order of magnitude of the effective mechanical displacement to be? In its purest form that experiment, on humans, would seem to be a long distance away in time, but there are several very close approximations to it in animal preparations. Tactile receptors in frog and toad skin and with Pacinian corpuscles of the cat's mesentery and footpad have been the "subjects", action potentials being taken off the attached nerve fiber. In the mesenteric Pacinian corpuscle (245) there is required movement of a mechanical stylus contacting it of no more than 0.5μ (the motion being completed in 100 μsec) to reach threshold. The delay in discharging the nerve is trivial, 1.5 msec; at larger, suprathreshold displacements latency gets down to 0.5 msec.

One might suppose that the Pacinian corpuscle, with its onionlike construction and its volume 10,000 times as great as the nerve ending it surrounds, would behave somewhat exceptionally, certainly differently from a free nerve ending. Many have thought that the capsular arrangement in the Pacinian and Meissner corpuscles give these end organs a mechanical advantage over other receptor forms, perhaps concentrating energy on the nerve tips where the impulse is generated. An instructive experiment germane to this point was performed by Loewenstein and Rathcamp (391). They undertook to dissect away the successive lamellar coats of the Pacinian corpuscle in an attempt to localize the seat of impulse generation. To everyone's surprise they found that all the layers could be removed, leaving only the bare core with its enclosed fibril, without altering in any way the action potential of the corpuscle's attached nerve. Even small pieces of the core material could be removed without changing the nerve response. Clearly, the generation of the afferent signal does not depend on the large superstructure surrounding the nerve tip. By systematically compressing various portions of the stripped-down receptor it was possible to demonstrate that two major electrical events occur within it: (a) there is set up in the unmyelinated fibril at the core of the corpuscle a graded response (the *generator potential*) which reflects the intensity of the mechanical stimulus and which, in the normal condition, is brought about through the summated action of many independent sites scattered throughout the capsule; (b) the all-or-nothing discharge of the attached myelinated fiber comes about through a flow of current between the active generating area of the terminal fibril and the nearest node of Ranvier, still within the capsule, a relatively uninsulated portion of the afferent nerve.

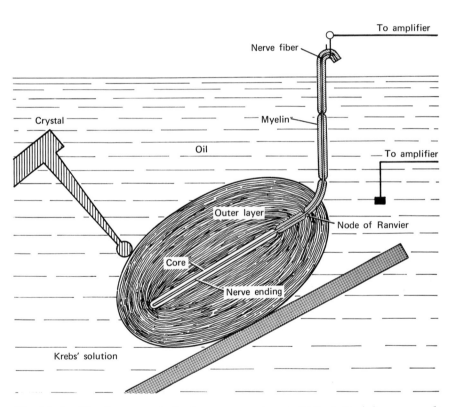

Fig. 10–4. The Loewenstein-Rathcamp experiment (*391*). A Pacinian corpuscle is stimulated by a rod actuated by a vibrating crystal, the nerve impulse being picked up a short distance away. Reprinted by permission of the Rockefeller University Press, *J. gen. Physiol.*

Of course, there remains some considerable mystery about the intimate steps between mechanical distortion of tissue and generation of an electrical potential (see *111*), but this remarkable experiment—imaginative if not entirely decisive—goes some distance toward our ultimate understanding of the process. The experimental arrangements are shown in Figure 10–4.

The question of the differential threshold exists for pressure sensitivity, as for vision and hearing. If we begin with a threshold sensation and add energy until a just perceptibly stronger pressure is felt, what will be the size of the needed increment? What is the magnitude of ΔI for pressure sensitivity, and what of the relation between ΔI and I, that is, what is the size of the Weber fraction, $\Delta I/I$? Is it constant, as Weber's Law requires, or does it vary in some systematic fashion?

The available answers are not as clear-cut as we might wish, despite a considerable amount of experimentation over the years. The major variable is, of course, locus of stimulation. In general, those parts of the body surface displaying high absolute sensitivity show small values of ΔI, while the reverse is true for relatively insensitive regions. Thus ΔI has a large value on the abdomen and thighs; it is small at the lips, finger tips, and on the soles of the feet (*532*, p. 142). Other variables have been shown to affect the measured size of ΔI. The period for which the initial intensity has been effective, before the addition of the increment, is important, as is the rapidity with which the additional pressure is applied. Moreover, if ΔI is computed as a decrement, i.e., from unloading rather than loading experiments, its value appears to be approximately doubled (*249, 250*). If both stimuli (I and $I + \Delta I$) are kept brief the time interval between the two makes a difference, short intervals yielding larger values of ΔI (*367*). The size of the skin area contacted is important in both absolute and relative measures of sensitivity.

The question of the constancy of the Weber fraction, $\Delta I/I$, can be answered in much the same fashion as it was for vision and hearing. It is not constant throughout the entire intensity scale, $\Delta I/I$ showing relatively large values at low intensities and smaller (and roughly constant) ones throughout the middle range of intensities. Perhaps the clearest data are those of Gatti and Dodge (*218*) and those of Schriever (*532*, pp. 138–144). Figure 10–5 reproduces the former set. The Weber fraction, at least for a single pressure-sensitive "spot," appears to pass through a definite minimum in the middle reaches of the scale of effective stimuli.

Comparative data on differential sensitivity come from animal experiments. Recording from individual fibers in the medial nerve of the monkey's arm, the distal terminations of which were in the glabrous skin of the palm, Werner and Mountcastle (*623*) obtained a series of records

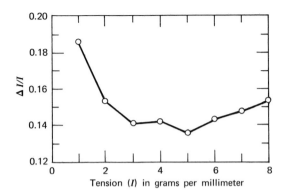

Fig. 10–5. Differential pressure sensitivity as a function of intensity level. The Weber fraction, $\Delta I/I$, varies with the absolute intensity (tension in grams per millimeter) of the base stimulus. The data were obtained by Gatti and Dodge (*218*) on an isolated pressure spot. After Boring (*84*). By permission of the copyright owners, Appleton-Century-Crofts, New York.

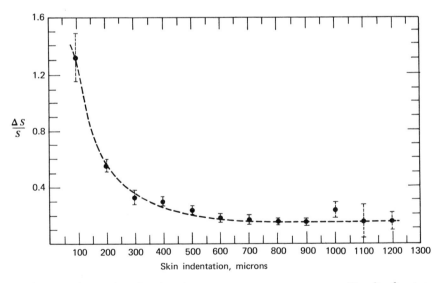

Fig. 10–6. The Weber fraction in cutaneous nerve response. Results for ten different fibers, averaged, in the palm of the monkey's hand. An increment of five impulses is taken to be just discriminable. Vertical bars at each data point lay off confidence intervals of three standard errors. From Werner, Gerhard and Mountcastle, Vernon B. In: D. R. Kenshalo (Ed.), *The Skin Senses*, 1968. Courtesy of Charles C. Thomas, Publisher, Springfield, Illinois.

permitting nerve responses (number of impulses discharged) to be plotted against stimulus intensity (amount of skin indentation) for a fixed observation interval. The relation proved to be a strictly linear one, although the slope of the function varied from one fiber to another. If, now, it is assumed that a just discriminable response increment is associated with the addition of a definite number of impulses to the preexisting response —a reasonable assumption in view of the linear relation just alluded to— it becomes possible to plot a kind of "Weber fraction." Figure 10–6 combines the data for ten fibers. The rule adopted for this purpose is that the addition of five impulses will produce a just discriminable increment. The resemblance of the overall function to other $\Delta I/I$ curves is obvious.

Pressure Adaptation.   A decline in sensitivity with continuing action of a stimulus is a very general phenomenon in sensory psychophysiology and one which intervenes significantly in nearly all experimental situations. Pressure is no exception. Let a pressure stimulus, whether areal or punctiform, be applied steadily to the skin, and the sensation will fade, eventually to the point of disappearance. The rate of decline and the total time required for complete obliteration ("adaptation time") depend on several variables. Bodily locus is doubtless one, though it has never been investigated systematically. Intensity of stimulus and area over which it operates are known variables. Adaptation time is longer in the case of intense stimuli and briefer with large cutaneous areas (661).

In considering the light and dark adaptation processes in vision we commonly think of them as mediated by reversible photochemical reactions, that is, as resulting from altered states of sensitivity of the receptors. The temptation is great to extend such thinking to the cutaneous realm and to picture altered chemical equilibrium states in or near end organs as responsible for adaptation. The fact that the essential process may be of quite a different nature is indicated by some interesting results of Nafe and Wagoner (442). They arranged a carefully controlled apparatus to permit weights varying between 8.75 and 70.0 gm to be placed gently on the leg just above the knee. The progress of the weight as it "sank" into the skin and compressed underlying tissue was followed with a sensitive recording system. Their results show that a weight, once placed on the skin surface, does not rest there but continues to move downward for a surprisingly long time. Pressure is felt just so long as a supraliminal rate of movement is maintained. When tissue resistance reduces motion to an undetectable level the sensation fades out. The end point of "adaptation" has been reached. The conclusion is obvious: "complete adaptation" represents stimulus failure. The fact that the answer is not to be found in "fatigue" or depletion of the resources of the end organ is easily proved by increasing the load on the tissue once adaptation has apparently run its course. In such a situation there is a fresh response, a new sensation accompanying the further compression, until the stimulus once again "fails." The stimulus for felt pressure is tension set up within the pliable cutaneous tissues, and the intensity of the sensation presumably is correlated with the degree of tension produced. Another interesting consequence of this view is that removal of a weight from the skin, once adaptation is complete, should result in the rearousal of pressure sensations, since tissue elasticity will cause new tensions to be created in the return to the original equilibrium state. The evidence is in line with expectations. So-called "after-sensations" of pressure are of regular occurrence under such circumstances. "Stimulation" is produced in the absence of any external stimulus.

The psychophysical experiment pointing to stimulus failure as the explanation of pressure adaptation was subsequently supplemented and its conclusions fortified through a neurophysiological study of the dorsal cutaneous preparation of the frog and of the rat's femoral and lingual nerves (440). The receptor responding in the frog, a single-fiber preparation, is of the rapidly adapting variety, what Adrian (5), following an earlier distinction made by Sherrington for motor mechanisms that are

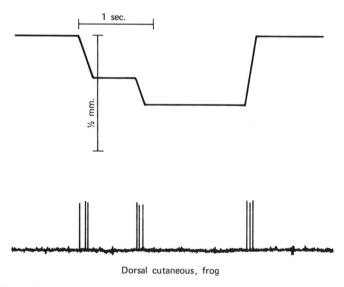

Dorsal cutaneous, frog

Fig. 10–7. The nerve's response to pressure. Impulses from the frog's dorsal cutaneous preparation accompanying two steps of forced pressure, followed by abrupt release of pressure. From Nafe and Kenshalo (440).

prompt in their action, termed "phasic" receptors. Figure 10–7 shows the neural response in the frog during the process of adaptation to do just what pressure sensations had done in the Nafe-Wagoner experiment, that is, adapt out completely as the mechanical force is steadily applied, show a second burst of action when the force is increased, and produce a third response when the force is released and the frog's skin regains its original posture. Tissue movement does indeed seem to be the necessary condition for the eliciting of impulses reporting pressure.

To get a more intimate picture of what is happening at the receptor, it becomes necessary once more to ask what the relevant findings are in the functioning of the only specialized skin receptor cell thus far intensively studied, the Pacinian corpuscle. It is possible to take advantage of the "stripping down" technique developed in the Loewenstein-Rathcamp experiment, already described (p. 295), to ascertain what role, if any, the laminar features of the corpuscle may play in the adaptation process. Mendelson and Loewenstein (413) first recorded the generator potential at the nerve tip with the lamellae in place. In response to deformations having rapid onsets and offsets and lasting about 30 msec there was set up a single transient current, lasting but 6 msec, at the beginning and again at the end of the pulse. When the corpuscle was pared down to leave little more than the core intact, the generator potential behaved quite differently. It showed a sustained response that lasted, though not entirely undiminished, about as long as the mechanical deformation did. In the optimal preparation, the most thoroughly denuded one, the generator potential lasted 12 times as long as in the intact corpuscle.

Evidently, the lamellar superstructure of the end organ, while being quite unnecessary for stimulation, serves another function, that of mechanical filter of nontransients, a so-called high-pass filter. The fact that following of the mechanical changes is not quite perfect, that in the stripped-down preparation there is some slippage, may only mean that the small amount of tissue still protecting the terminal fibril is functioning as a minor buffer in the system. Loewenstein believed that the mechanical filter is not the only one present. Because prolongation of the generator potential seems not to lead to increased nerve discharges in the attached axon it has to be assumed that a second filtering process intervenes between the generator potential and the nerve discharge. Perhaps this one is electrochemical and has the effect of limiting nerve excitation so as to keep the system "phasic."

Temporal Pressure Patterns: Vibration. It has been seen that each feeling of pressure, far from being simple, is organized in a pattern having intensitive, spatial, and temporal aspects. Certain of them are mainly notable for their temporal features. Chief among these are the feeling patterns commonly called "tickle" and "vibration."

That tickle falls in the family of pressure patterns is fairly obvious from direct observation. To and fro movement of a hair brings it out, as does light brushing of the lips or other sensitive hairless regions. It is less clear that the vibratory pattern is based on the operation of pressure receptors. Indeed, until relatively recently, when full proof became available, much doubt existed concerning the essential connection between vibration and pressure. A very considerable controversy, elsewhere reviewed by the author (222), continued for a half century between those who viewed vibratory sensations as "pressure in movement" and those who held that there existed a separate "vibratory sense" with its own special receptors and nerve supply. We cannot go into all the arguments. Suffice it to say that the controversy may now be said to have been resolved in favor of the conclusion that the vibratory pattern is in fact "pressure in movement." It is only necessary to know something of the skin mechanics involved in vibration to come to an understanding of the phenomena that led to the mistaken postulation of a special "vibratory sense."

Let the base of a tuning fork or other vibration generator be placed on the skin, and there is felt an intermittent "whirring," somewhat indefinite in localization especially if bony tissue lies directly under the point of application of the fork. Vagueness of localization, a misleading cue in that it seems not to suggest mediation by the somewhat precise pressure sense, can be shown to arise from the fact that vibratory motions impressed on the skin travel great distances, with very little loss, through cutaneous and subcutaneous tissues. Bones are especially good conductors. Widespread transmission of the vibratory disturbances, in all directions from the generator, prohibits the possibility of confining the stimulus to a local region. A very extensive feeling pattern, poorly localized, is set up as a result. From such gross experiments one gets little hint that the mechanism responsible for pressure reception is actually involved.

However, it is possible to design an experiment in such a way as to show the basic identity of the two sensitivities. If, instead of a broad contacting surface, one uses a small, very weakly vibrating needle or hair and makes a systematic exploration of a given skin area, one finds the kind of local variations in sensitivity so characteristic of pressure. Vibration, like pressure, is distributed in a punctiform manner. If, now, within such an area there are isolated for study two populations of "spots," one highly sensitive to pressure and the other having very low sensitivity (requiring gentle and steep gradients, respectively, to elicit pressure sensations from them), one can ascertain with some precision their responsiveness to vibration. It is necessary only to set the exploring needle in motion, at some preselected frequency, and determine the minimal amplitude that will bring out a just detectable "whirring" sensation. If this is done one finds pressure-sensitive spots to have very low and consistent vibratory thresholds, while those showing poor pressure reception require large amplitudes, varying greatly from spot to spot, to produce feelings of vibration (*223, 225, 617*). The results of one such experiment, involving extensive measurements on ten pressure-sensitive and ten pressure-insensitive spots lying within an area of 2 cm² on the volar side of the forearm, are presented in Figure 10–8. Five test frequencies, from 64 Hz to 1024 Hz in octaves, were used. On the average, pressure-sensitive spots in this region require about 0.025 mm excursions of the needle point, apparently irrespective of the rate of repetition, to call forth the discontinuous, vibratory sensation. Insensitive spots need many times this amount, some of them requiring amplitudes of the order of half a millimeter. Moreover, there is a distinctly different feel at the two kinds of loci. Pressure-insensitive spots yield dull, vaguely localized sensations.

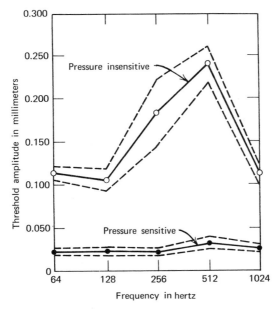

Fig. 10–8. Vibratory thresholds for two populations of cutaneous "spots," one highly sensitive to pressure, the other highly insensitive. The loci previously determined to be pressure-sensitive have low thresholds to vibratory motion at all frequencies. Pressure-insensitive spots are relatively insensitive to vibration. The dotted lines show variability of measurement. From Geldard (*224*).

One can "tune in" pressure-sensitive spots by dragging a gently vibrating needle across them; tuning being optimal, the sensation is "bright," highly discrete, sharply localized. The presumption is strong, from such experiments, that pressure sensitivity and vibratory sensitivity go hand in hand, the activity of identical receptors being involved in both.

Whereas, in the lower curve of Figure 10–8, frequency of stimulation seems not to be a determining variable, this conclusion cannot be generalized for all skin areas under all conditions. On the contrary, vibratory sensitivity has been shown under certain circumstances to be a function of frequency. If, instead of delivering the vibrating stimulus to a highly sensitive pressure point situated in a region having a somewhat sparse distribution of receptors, one applies a relatively large contactor to the fingertip, say, it will be found that the vibration frequency selected is a matter of some importance. Several well-controlled experiments are in virtual agreement as to the shape of the frequency function. Figure 10–9

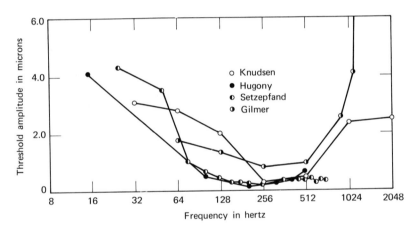

Fig. 10–9. The frequency-intensity function for vibration at the fingertip. The results of four investigators have been combined in a single plot. All used relatively large contactors applied to the tip of the index finger. Compare Fig. 10–8 for needle-point stimulation at the wrist. From Geldard (*224*).

combines the results of four such experiments, all using the fingertip as the stimulated area, and shows that there is an optimal frequency in the neighborhood of 250 Hz. There can be little doubt that, for areal stimulation in a highly sensitive region, thresholds will in part be a function of the frequency with which impacts are repeated. The difference between the shapes of the curves in Figures 10–8 and 10–9 has never been satisfactorily accounted for, and further research along these lines is certainly indicated. Both Sherrick (*521*) and Verrillo (*587*) have subsequently verified the essential nondependence of absolute threshold on vibration frequency for "spots," at least small contactors, the former sampling the frequency range at 20, 150, and 1000 Hz, the latter at seven frequencies between 25 and 640 Hz. Several recent investigators (*588, 235, 566,* to single out only a few highly reliable sets of measurements) have reconfirmed the U-shaped function for broader contactors.

Another question poorly answered as yet concerns the upper and lower frequency limits for vibratory sensation. What, in cutaneous vibration, corresponds to the 20 to 20,000 Hz range in hearing? The problem of the vibratory upper limit is complicated, as it is to a lesser degree in hearing, by the necessity of producing very high-frequency oscillations of a mechanical contactor at relatively large amplitudes of movement. Driving a phonograph "cutting head" at frequencies of the order of 10,000 Hz and with a 50-watt amplifier, the author has succeeded in getting, at the fingertip, fleeting but definite "bursts" of vibratory sensation. That the tissue is actually conducting forced vibrations of this frequency and that the phenomenon is thus not artifactual is attested by the fact that the stimulus frequency, and no other, may be detected by a crystal "pickup" several millimeters distant on the skin surface from the stimulus needle. The upper limit may be even higher than this; thus far instrumentation has not been entirely adequate to a correct solution.

The lower limit is also in doubt, though the failure to provide a definite answer here is not the result of inadequate apparatus. The observational difficulties are similar, in most respects, to those confronted in establishing the lower limit of tonal perception. As frequency is raised, at what point does the appreciation of discrete impacts pass over into "vibration"? Some experiments have placed it as low as 10 per second; others would have it as high as 80. Knudsen (*365*), taking as a criterion the entrance of a "tingling" sensation, as opposed to the feeling of separate shocks, got an average lower limit of 15.3 Hz.

We have considered only two kinds of loci of stimulation, the somewhat sparsely populated volar forearm and the densely innervated finger pad. Does this represent the sensitivity range? Not at all. Although the fingertip is perhaps the most sensitive region, there are also others that require little energy to excite them (palm, sole of foot, skin over the sternum). As for the forearm, there are many areas of the body having poorer sensitivity. With regard to low-threshold regions, Sherrick (*520*) has carefully measured the minimal vibrator sensitivity of the tongue. In its range of best response, around 200 Hz, it is only a little less sensitive than the fingertip. Concerning the high-threshold regions, it will be observed in Figure 10–10 that there are few body areas having better

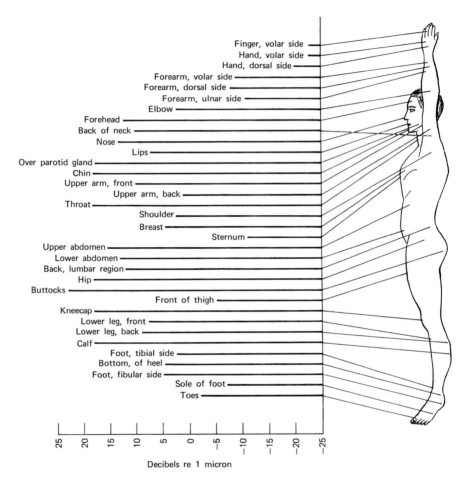

Fig. 10–10. Bodily distribution of vibratory sensitivity. Thresholds, in decibels, of 34 skin areas to 200-Hz sinusoidal vibration. Absolute threshold varies from −23 dB (re 1 micron of amplitude) at the fingers to +23 dB, at the buttocks. From the data of Wilska *(641)*.

sensitivity than the volar forearm. To be sure, the data are confined to those derived from an exploring probe of appreciable size (1-cm² contact), vibrating at 200 Hz, and a frequency change upward alters things a little but, in general, the forearm is a relatively sensitive region when tested in such an experiment. These data were gathered by Wilska *(641)* who will be remembered for his classic measurement of the tympanic membrane excursions at auditory threshold (p. 184).

A variable that was mentioned as possibly influencing absolute vibratory threshold is skin temperature. Precise measures of the effect of warming and cooling the skin on thresholds of vibration have been obtained by Weitz (*617*). Figure 10–11 reproduces the threshold-temperature func-

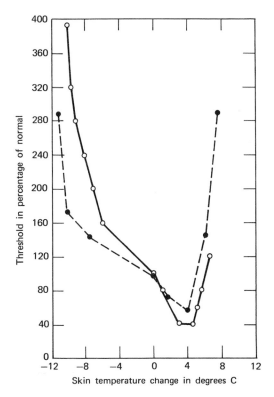

Fig. 10–11. Vibratory sensitivity as a function of skin temperature. There is an optimal point, about 4° C above normal skin temperature, for the arousal of vibratory feelings. The two curves are for different regions of the skin. From Weitz (*617*). By permission of the *Journal of Experimental Psychology* and the American Psychological Association.

tion for two separate loci at the wrist. Threshold amplitude at normal skin temperature is taken as unity, and percentage changes in amplitude of excursion necessary just to elicit the vibratory feeling are plotted against decreases and increases in surface temperature of the skin region in which the stimulated point lay. The complexity of the function— marked reduction in sensitivity (raised thresholds) with initial cooling, enhancement of sensitivity with mild warming, and subsequent sharp decline with continued heating—seems to call for interpretation in other than mechanical terms. Some form of chemical hypothesis, perhaps one which entails the operation of a catalyst and its destruction at high temperatures, seems more congenial to the facts. Incidentally, if further proof were needed, the correspondence between vibratory and pressure sensitivities is made even more certain by the fact that pressure receptors show a similar dependence on temperature, pressure thresholds being related to skin temperature by a concave function with maximal sensitivity between 36° and 38° C (*15*), just as with vibration.

Vibratory Dimensions.   In hearing we found it necessary to make clear distinctions between the psychological dimensions of loudness, pitch, volume, and density and the physical dimensions of the stimulus, intensity and frequency, that give rise to them. We also found some interesting correspondences between the durative features of auditory sensation and the temporal properties of tones and noises. It should not surprise us, then, that vibration imparted to the skin rather than to the ear generates some analogous phenomena. Indeed, in somesthesis we also talk of vibratory "loudness" and "pitch," there being available in the lexicon of feeling no really suitable words to describe these aspects of experience.

Vibratory *loudness*, the apparent intensity of vibratory sensation, like auditory loudness, is a joint function of physical intensity and frequency. Figure 10–12 presents a family of loudness contours, each of which reveals the intensity-frequency dependence for one stimulus intensity (Sensation Levels—decibels above absolute threshold, it will be recalled from audition—of 5 to 55 dB). All loudnesses falling on a particular contour are of equal subjective magnitude. They were derived by an estimating technique and are for a 2.9-cm² contactor on the fleshy portion of the hand at the base of the thumb. The familiar U-shaped threshold function for large contactors becomes a natural reference; it is the lowermost of the collection of curves. The essential similarity between these contours and those with which we are familiar in audition expresses the kinship between feeling and hearing. The two sets are very much alike; the cutaneous one is simply transposed downward on the frequency scale.

Vibratory *pitch* on the skin is the analog of musical pitch in hearing. In general, as frequency is increased, felt pitch goes up. However, although auditory pitch depends mainly on frequency, it has a minor dependency on intensity. Louden low tones and they drop in pitch; louden high ones and they are raised. A somewhat simpler but more dramatic thing occurs in somesthesis. Any increase in vibratory amplitude will be felt both as a loudening and slowing of rate, a fall in pitch; any decrease of amplitude will be interpreted both as a reduction of loudness

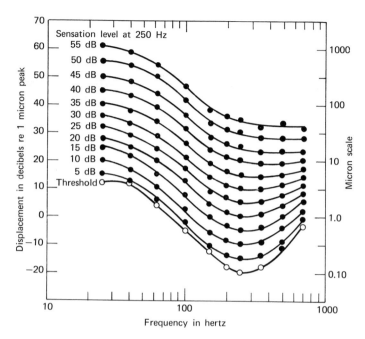

Fig. 10–12. Vibratory "loudness" contours. Estimated loudness as a function of frequency of vibration. Intensity (in decibels SL) is referred to threshold for 250 Hz. From Verrillo, Fraioli, and Smith *(590)*. Courtesy of *Perception and Psychophysics.*

and a raising of pitch. The effect is a vivid one. Békésy *(54)* has shown that the apparent pitch of a vibratory stimulus applied to the skin may be changed by as much as three octaves by altering amplitude only, frequency being held strictly constant meanwhile.

Another revealing comparison between feeling and hearing comes out if we raise the question for touch, as we did for audition, of the discriminative capacity for frequency, Δf. The fundamental experiment here is that of Goff *(235)*. Most earlier work suffers from one or another of two major defects, either failure to control for differences in subjective intensity when different frequencies were to be compared or the presence of contaminating transients at the onset and offset of the stimulus envelope. Goff avoided these faults, first assembling a group of equal-loudness stimuli of differing frequencies within the available range, then measuring Δf in a systematic manner throughout that range. This was done at two intensity levels, 20 and 35 db SL. At both, differential frequency discrimination proves to be good at very low frequencies—up to about 50 Hz,

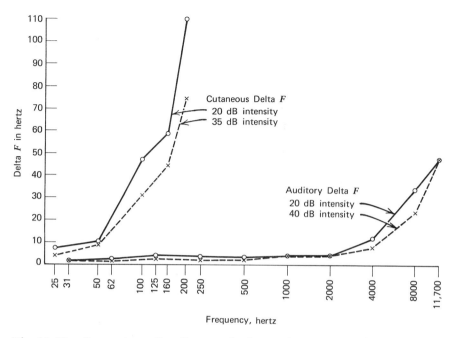

Fig. 10–13. Comparison of auditory and vibrotactile frequency discrimination. The auditory data are those of Shower and Biddulph (*526*); the vibrotactile measures are from Goff (*235*).

say—but it deteriorates rapidly as the frequency scale is ascended. At 20 dB and 200 Hz, for example, Δf has climbed to a value of 110 Hz. The Weber fraction is 55%! Figure 10–13 makes the startling comparison between skin and ear by juxtaposing the Goff data and the classical Bell Laboratories measures of auditory Δf.

The phenomenon of "action time," the duration of the interval between stimulus onset and peak sensation, has been encountered in both vision and audition. It can be measured in cutaneous vibration as well. Indeed, the two investigators whose results we considered in connection with auditory action time (p. 200) have performed a similar service in the vibrotactile realm. Here they are in closer agreement, however, despite their divergent methods. The approach by way of comparing sensory intensity of a brief vibratory burst with that of a longer one that has attained full loudness was adopted by Békésy in a classical experiment (*55*, p. 536). Whereas it took about 180 msec for tones to reach peak, it will be recalled, a 100-Hz vibratory pulse of moderate intensity required about 1.2 sec to attain full loudness. The skin obviously responds somewhat sluggishly as compared with the ear.

The approach by way of magnitude estimation, interestingly, yields a similar value. Berglund et al. (67) measured sensory intensity, for a 250-Hz vibratory burst at eight durations (30 to 1200 msec) and five intensities (32 to 54 dB SL), and found it growing as a log function of stimulus duration up to about one second. Variations of intensity were unimportant.

Another way in which time comes to be a major parameter in vibratory sensitivity is through the working of adaptation, a thoroughly familiar phenomenon by now. In the field of vibration, vision, rather than audition, provides the prototypical experiments. Of the several possible approaches to the measurement of adaptation, two of them, the altered threshold method (perhaps the commonest of all in other sense channels) and the comparison stimulus ("matching") method have been used most effectively. One excellent study, that of Hahn (261) employed them both in a comparative fashion. Uniformly applied 60-Hz vibration at an amplitude of 200μ was delivered to the pad of the index finger for varying durations. At planned intervals, either the absolute threshold at the stimulation site was determined (threshold method) or a comparison burst of

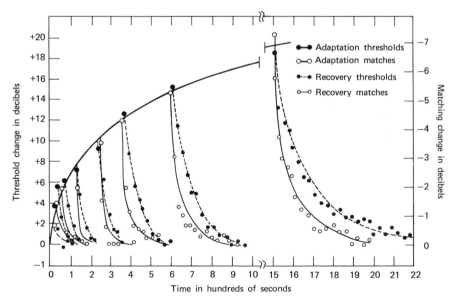

Fig. 10–14. Adaptation and recovery of vibratory sensitivity. Threshold data are referred to the left ordinate, those for magnitude matching to the right. From Hahn (261). Copyright, 1966, by the American Psychological Association, and reproduced by permission.

vibration was given to the contralateral index finger (matching method). Recovery curves were also obtained, both methods being used for various lengths of adaptation period. The results of all these operations can be read from Figure 10–14. Although the threshold technique indicates that adaptation reduces sensitivity nearly three times as far—compare right and left ordinates of the figure—it is clear that the course of adaptation is very much the same, regardless of method of measurement. Sensitivity is still declining at the end of 25 min of vibratory stimulation.

It seems natural to relate this experiment to the Nafe-Wagoner experiment with which we became familiar earlier. Can the sensitivity loss from a continuous vibratory "pounding" of the skin be interpreted, as that from a static weight was, to be "stimulus failure"? Here the adapting stimulus is acting like a small but powerful trip-hammer which must be producing some complex effects under it. Before we can have an assured answer we shall need to make a more intimate analysis of the relative roles of static and dynamic pressure changes in the skin and learn much more about viscosity and elasticity of the tissues housing the receptors.

Other Pressure Patterns: "Touch Blends." If we forsake, for the moment, the approach to the study of cutaneous sensitivity by way of carefully controlled experiments and pay some attention to the role of the skin in its daily task of gathering information about external objects and situations, we are led to view it as a remarkably discriminative organ of sense. We commonly make entirely correct judgments, on the basis of "feel" alone, concerning hardness or softness, roughness or smoothness, wetness or dryness, stickiness, oiliness, and a host of other object qualities. Even with auditory cues excluded, tapping with a finger nail is often sufficient to determine whether an object is made of wood, metal, or plastic. In nearly all such discriminations movement of the skin relative to the object is a necessary condition; a spatial-temporal pattern of cutaneous excitation is involved. Let the fingertip rest gently on an unfamiliar surface, and, whereas something of its hardness or softness may be estimated, nothing will be learned of its roughness or smoothness. Movement of some degree is essential to the latter judgment. The amount of relative motion can be very slight and still yield a correct impression. A brief tap, lasting no more than $\frac{1}{300}$ sec, has been found in some experiments to be enough for complete identification of the material touched (*344*). The "threshold for roughness," if sufficient movement of the exploring fingertips is allowed, is also surprisingly small. A lightly etched piece of glass having eminences no higher than 0.001 mm can be successfully discriminated from an entirely smooth one. Assuming a little familarity with the characteristic "feel" of materials one can make very nice discriminations of roughness and smoothness; "cloth feelers" are able to make their living at it. Since movement is the cue, there is little mystery about the essential mechanism responsible. Slight disturbances imparted to a sensitive skin area send vibratory "shock waves" relatively unimpeded, to large numbers of pressure receptors. Coating the fingers with a thin layer of collodion or interposing an unyielding stick between the material to be "felt" and the fingers makes very little difference in accuracy, as might be expected. The important thing is that the shocks be transmitted to the sensitive receptors, there to set up the complex spatial-temporal excitation pattern characteristic of "roughness."

Since the advent of magnitude estimation methods, roughness-smoothness has been a dimension of some interest, perhaps mainly because it is a convenient one for the methodological study of perceptual opposites— others are lightness-darkness, loudness-softness, denseness-diffuseness (of tones or noises)—but also because it is relatively easily manipulated in cross-modality experiments. One may take a series of emery grits, graded either by the sieve sizes used in preparing them or, more precisely, their relative coefficients of friction, and get their roughness or smoothness beautifully ordered on a power function. Stevens and Harris (558) have done the experiment and obtained an exponent of the log-log plot of grit number against estimated roughness of -1.5 ($+1.5$ for smoothness).

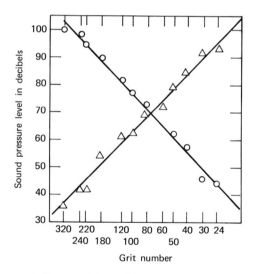

Fig. 10–15. Cross-modality matching of loudness of noise and cutaneous roughness-smoothness. Triangles give roughness points; circles are those for smoothness estimates. From Stevens and Harris (558). Copyright, 1962, by the American Psychological Association, and reproduced by permission.

Figure 10–15 shows what happened when tactual roughness and smoothness were matched to loudness of a noise. Although seemingly unrelated dimensions of sensation, they can obviously be predicted one from the other with considerable accuracy. These authors have suggested the amusing term, *ruk*, as suitable for the unit of roughness, and have provided a formula that predicts subjective roughness, in ruks, from emery grit numbers ($R = 5724 \ G^{-1.5}$).

Pressure sensations enter into a number of other complex cutaneous patterns or "touch blends." The pressure component can be analyzed out by painstaking observation and, once identified, can sometimes be artificially recombined with the other constituents of the blend to produce, synthetically, the original complex. As in chemistry, the test of analysis is synthesis. Thus "wetness" seems always to have a pressure component and one of cold. Is moisture also necessary in the stimulus? The analysis and subsequent synthesis were originally performed about a half-century ago by Bentley (*65*). He demonstrated that a cold pressure, uniformly distributed over the stimulated area, would produce the feeling of "wetness." Moisture is quite unnecessary. Dip into cold water a finger kept dry with lycopodium powder or with a thin rubber membrane, and the feeling will be quite as "wet" as without such protection.

Other synthetic experiments have been performed with more or less success (*84*, p. 509 ff.). Thus "oiliness" reduces to weak pressure accompanied by warmth, with movement enhancing its reality. "Hardness" is an even, cold pressure with a good boundary, while "softness" requires an uneven, warm pressure of poor boundary. "Stickiness" takes a variable and moving pressure, while "clamminess" is essentially "a cold softness perceived with movement and supplemented by unpleasant imagery." Complications of a still higher order are possible, of course. Indeed, it is held by one school of theorists that felt emotions are made up in just this way and that a thoroughgoing analysis of anxiety, love, or disgust would reveal them to be compounded of simple qualities belonging to the cutaneous and internal senses.

The Search for Pressure Receptors. Since we shall encounter similar questions in conjunction with forms of sensitivity other than pressure, perhaps we should first think a bit generally about the problem as a whole. The history of speculation about receptors and nerves in relation to their modal responsibilities is replete with claims and counterclaims, guesses and half-formed beliefs, and temporary enthusiasms coming out of histological discoveries. To link up any form of sensitivity with the operation of a particular receptor organ or kind of nerve fiber it would obviously be necessary to demonstrate that there exists an invariable relation between the two, sensitivity and mechanism. The type of sensation in question should never occur in the absence of the mechanism and, wherever the appropriate afferent system is present and functioning normally, it should be possible to arouse the sensation. Sinclair has indicated what would constitute acceptable proof (527, p. 101): "A definite relationship between a given kind of ending and a given kind of sensation could only be established by stimulation of an isolated ending of a known type in a conscious human subject who could record his sensations, and this experiment has not yet been done." Moreover, it is almost a certainty that it never will be done, at least in a way permitting generalizations about entire modalities. If individual endings were to have their messages carried intact to the highest levels of the central nervous system, it should be true that dorsal horn cells and nerve cells at progressively higher centers all the way to the cortex would display modality specificity. But we know of no such principle at work in the afferent pathways. The rule is convergence, inhibition and facilitation, integration. The relations are far from chaotic—an orderly psychophysics is the hope of all of us—but they surely do not reduce to a simple one-to-one arrangement between periphery and cortex with respect to the qualitative "tag" a sensation bears.

Obviously, in view of the above, the question of what constitutes a pressure receptor comes down to the question of which of the nerve endings in the skin seems probable as a transducer of mechanical change.

The widely accepted belief is that pressure sensations and their variants are mediated by two sets of cutaneous receptors, (1) free endings of nerves proliferating around hair follicles, in hairy regions of the skin, and (2) Meissner corpuscles, in hairless parts of the body. It should be said straightway that this is a matter of belief; it is far from being one of incontrovertible fact. The argument for these two structures as *the* pressure receptors rests almost exclusively on the known facts of distribution. The common occurrence of high points of pressure sensitivity "to the windward of hairs" is, of course, very suggestive. As has been seen, histological examination of skin sections reveals hair bulbs to be well supplied with sensory terminations, the masses of bare nerve endings proliferating so freely around the bases of hairs as to have earned for them the name "basket endings." These, then, are probable pressure receptors. What about the hairless regions of the skin? Pressure receptivity and discriminability are very high in the lips and parts of the hands and feet where there are no hairs. The guess has been that Meissner corpuscles, conveniently situated in the papillae of the corium in these regions, have the proper location and distribution to serve as pressure receptors. Indeed, histologists have designated the papillae housing Meissner corpuscles as "tactile" papillae out of deference to this belief in their function. Yet, competent histological authority (*645*) is nowadays denying the existence of any Meissners at all in lips, tongue, or other areas verging on mucous tissue. Instead, there are found *muco-cutaneous organs* (Krause end bulbs) and these are present in neither hairy nor glabrous skin.

Vital staining with methylene blue of a finger about to be amputated has successfully revealed, in subsequent sectioning of the skin, the distribution of Meissner corpuscles and their innervation (*610*). It appears that Meissner corpuscles occur in groups of two or three, rarely singly, and that ten such groups may be found in an area as small as 1 mm². The nerve fibers leading to corpuscles approach the cluster from various directions, suggesting that considerable overlap from disparate sensory fibers may be the rule of innervation.

Over against this conventional view are several strong bits of evidence which can only be interpreted as indicating that still other structures participate in the pressure response. Slicing down the epidermis at the fingertip with a sharp scalpel arouses only sensations of pressure and, so long as any of the epidermal layers are left, pressure sensations can be elicited. Cutting further, into the corium, produces pain. Since the only known structures to penetrate the epidermis are free nerve endings, these are naturally suspect as pressure receptors. Moreover, microscopical analysis of the parings reveals endings of fine nerve fibers terminating in "loops and figures" (*609*). There is also presumptive evidence, from their high frequency of occurrence and their general distribution, that hederiform endings (Merkel cells) participate in responses to pressure changes in glabrous skin.

It seems highly probable that the Pacinian corpuscle is a pressure transducer, but one responding only to relatively rapid pressure changes. We have seen it to be clearly a phasic type of receptor, answering to transient changes of pressure and adapting quickly. It obviously could not signal steady deformations of tissue. The belief is firmly held by some (*566, 589*) that the Pacinian corpuscle is the vibratory receptor par excellence, mediating that pressure pattern at frequencies above about 80 Hz.

11
Pain

Cutaneous Pain.   Pain may be brought forth by a great range of stimuli, in fact by agents belonging to all classes of stimuli capable of arousing the skin to sensory activity: mechanical, thermal, electrical, and chemical. As a consequence, pain has a great many modes of appearance. The following terms descriptive of pain, demonstrating the richness of our language in this respect, have been catalogued by Dallenbach (*142,* p. 614): achy, beating, biting, boring, bright, burning, clear, cutting, dark, digging, dragging, drawing, dull, fluttering, gnawing, hard, heavy, itchy, nipping, palpitating, penetrating, piercing, pinching, pressing, pricking, quick, quivering, radiating, raking, savage, sharp, smarting, squeezing, stabbing, sticking, stinging, tearing, thrilling, throbbing, thrusting, tugging, twitching, ugly, vicious. It is clear that some of these terms characterize the temporal aspect of the feeling pattern, others its spatial dimension, others the blend with pressure or temperature, while some appear to have reference to associated forms of emotional response. Pains are patterned so variously, in fact, that it is difficult to find a common principle holding them all together.

The independent status of pain as a separate cutaneous sense remained in doubt for a long time. Indeed, some scientists currently defend the position that pain is not a distinct unitary form of sensibility but that it always results from overstimulation of one or another of the other senses. Throughout the ages pain has been considered, in various philosophical systems, as very general and pervading in its nature and has, in consequence, been juxtaposed to pleasure as a form of emotion. For both Plato and Aristotle pain was a "passion of the soul," and this traditional view was a long time with us. Only comparatively recently, on the basis of compelling experimental findings, has pain come to be thought of as an independent member of the family of cutaneous senses.

Pain then, like other cutaneous sensations, comes patterned. It seems possible to distinguish two radically different sorts of pains on the basis of typical "feel" and localization and, since the histological discoveries of Weddell and his associates (*611, 613, 194*), on the presumed anatomical bases for them. In general, pain from the superficial layers of the skin is "bright" in quality, ordinarily is relatively sharply localized, and tends quite uniformly to elicit prompt withdrawal reactions. It does not matter which of several methods of stimulation are used. Pain resulting from a light, quick touch with a heated wire, a brief pulse of electric current, a quick tug of a hair, or a jab with a fine needle all feel exactly alike to a subject if care is taken to keep away from him supplementary information concerning the stimuli employed or if their nature is masked by a neutral accompanying stimulus. All pains induced by these means are brief ones; they are all uniformly reported by the subject as "pricking" pain. Similarly, if any of these stimuli is allowed to function in a more prolonged manner the uniform report will be that of "burning" pain. Sir Thomas Lewis (*384*, p. 39) has said, "The difference between 'pricking' and 'burning' pain is not one of quality or tone, it is purely one of duration." There is some doubt that the difference is "purely" one of duration. When later we come to consider the debated question of the "double pain response," we shall see that there are other possible differentia of pricking and burning pain.

Pain sensations originating in deeply disposed tissues are quite unlike skin pains. Deep pains have a dull, aching, much more unpleasant character, and lead more commonly to immobilization of the affected part. They are ordinarily far more difficult of exact localization; in fact, gross errors of localization are the rule. If intense, they have widespread reflex accompaniments—slowing of the heartbeat, a fall in blood pressure, nausea, and sweating. These organic complications are never accompaniments of superficial cutaneous pain.

Intensitive and Differential Thresholds for Pain.   Whereas pain can be aroused in a great variety of ways, it is not easy to find a stimulating device which will permit quantification of painful effects. Mechanical stimulators must either impair tissue or produce radical deformations in it if they are to arouse pain. Chemical stimuli are practically impossible to control in that they cannot be spatially confined. Electrical stimuli pose problems that we shall confront later. Thermal arousal of pain is somewhat more controllable, but the physical and physiological events intervening between the application or withdrawal of heat and the discharge of sensory impulses must be a very complicated affair in a system having as a prominent feature a self-regulatory temperature mechanism. However, the production of pain by thermal stimuli currently offers the best possibility of experimental control for measurement purposes, as we shall see.

Classic techniques employed in attempts to measure pain thresholds have involved a considerable variety of "algesimeters," for the most part weighted needles, stiff hairs or hairs to which thistle spines have been attached, glass fibers, and similar graded mechanical contrivances. In the hands of von Frey remarkable consistency of measurement was achieved with calibrated hairs. He was able to demonstrate that the pain threshold for a given skin area is constant and is proportional to the hydrostatic pressure (grams per square millimeter) exerted on the tissue. A nice confirmation of these old experiments has resulted from the work of Bishop (71). He prepared stimulators consisting of tiny balls of solder impaled on and cemented to needle tips and arranged a graded series of them. With such stimuli and over the range 0.2 mm to 1.5 mm diameter, the threshold of pain is reached, irrespective of stimulus diameter, when the lower hemispherical surface of the ball tip has just been pressed into complete contact with the skin surface. The formula covering all cases is, as it was for von Frey's 1896 experiments, $gm/r^2 = K$. It may be inferred from this general relation that the constant factor in pain arousal is lateral stretch of cutaneous tissue. Bishop goes further and believes that "lengthwise stretch of nerve terminals appears to be the effective stimulus for pain endings in mechanical distortion of the skin." There are several known facts of pain sensitivity that make this supposition credible. Unless inflammation has intervened to complicate the situation, any sharp cut through the epithelium will prove painful when the skin encompassing it is stretched. However, under the same general circumstances relative immobilization of the tissue with collodion will prevent the appearance of pain. It is a well-known surgical phenomenon that pain may be produced by the stretching of unanesthetized internal organs, whereas cutting of the same tissue may not be an effective precipitant of pain. A normal appendix may be pinched without hurting the patient; an inflamed one may not.

Pain as a by-product of intense thermal stimulation is a familiar phenomenon. Experiments with the "burning glass" extend back into the last century. A radiant-heat method of measuring pain thresholds which has come into clinical prominence recently is that devised by Hardy and his associates (271). The schematic arrangement of their apparatus is shown in Figure 11–1. Light (and heat) from the 1000-watt lamp, L, is focused by a lens, C, through an aperture onto the forehead of the subject, H. S is a secondary shutter, operated manually and opened just before the stimulus is to be given. The primary shutter, P,

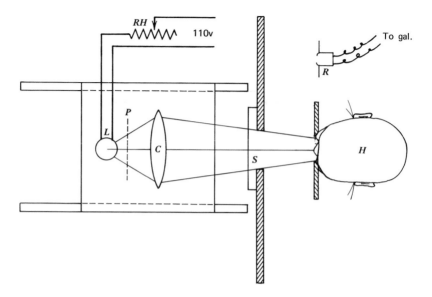

Fig. 11–1. The radiant-heat technique for measuring pain thresholds. Radiation from lamp, *L*, is directed by the condensing lens, *C*, through a shutter, S, to the forehead of the subject. An automatic shutter, *P*, allows an exposure of exactly 3 sec. In successive trials the level of operation of the lamp is increased, by variation of the rheostat, *RH*, until the subject feels a sharp stab of pain just before the closing of the shutter. Substitution of the radiometer, *R*, for the forehead permits calibration in energy units. From Wolff and Wolf *(648)* after Hardy, Wolff, and Goodell *(271)*. By permission of Charles C. Thomas, publisher, and the authors.

is regulated by a pendulum and provides a stimulus duration of exactly 3 sec. Heat intensity is regulated by the rheostat, *RH*. *R* is a radiometer, substituted for the subject's forehead at the time of stimulus calibration. If the radiometer itself has been calibrated against a standard, threshold may then be stated in gram-calories per second per square centimeter. The method of measuring the pain threshold is to step up the intensity, in successive trials, until the subject feels a sharp stab of pain, the culmination of an intense sensation of warmth, just before the termination of the 3-sec exposure. The subject's forehead is usually blackened with India ink to provide a highly absorptive and uniform skin surface. Care must also be taken to permit dissipation of heat between trials; a 30- to 60-sec intertrial rest period is therefore allowed.

Measurement of the pain thresholds of a large number of normal, healthy people by this technique revealed remarkably little variation from person to person, or from day to day in the same person (*513*). A group of 150 subjects gave a mean threshold of 0.206 gm-cal/sec/cm².

The same method has permitted measurement of the differential pain threshold, a practical impossibility with mechanical techniques. Hardy, Wolff, and Goodell (*272*) determined first the approximate limits of painful stimulation with their radiant-heat apparatus. For the standard 3-sec exposure the absolute threshold for pricking pain lay at 0.220 gm-cal/sec/cm² (220 millicalories, for short). The practical upper limit was found to be at about 480 mcal; above this value inconvenient burns were induced. Between the limits of 220 and 480 mcal there were found 21 j.n.d.'s of intensity. Between the threshold and about 320 mcal, ΔI increases in such a way as to render the Weber fraction, $\Delta I/I$, roughly constant at 0.03. Above this point the ratio grows larger. Hardy, Wolff, and Goodell have suggested that the intensive series in pain is capable of scaling, and they have accordingly proposed the "dol" as a unit of pain intensity. The dol is equal to 2 j.n.d.'s. This roughly provides a decimal scale between pain threshold and "ceiling" pain. Figure 11–2 is

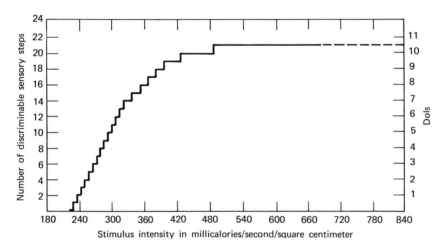

Fig. 11–2. The "dol" scale of pain intensity. The dol is equal to two successive "just noticeable differences" in pain intensity. From Hardy, Wolff, and Goodell (*272*). By permission of the editors, *Journal of Clinical Investigation,* and the authors.

a graphic representation of their pain scale (considerably idealized, because the ΔI measurements are really very crude ones statistically). The energy range between lower and upper thresholds is, of course, a narrow one. The 21 discriminable steps are embraced within an energy ratio of little more than 2:1. It is interesting to compare the lower pain threshold and the point farther down the scale at which warmth is first detected. There are some 90 steps in this range, and the two energy values involved stand in the ratio of 2000:1.

The essential correctness of the dol scale, at least in its lower reaches, has been verified by the use of the direct magnitude estimation method (3). The relation between estimated pain and thermal irradiation to the forearm and forehead, over the range of the first six dols, was found to be a power function with an exponent of 1.0.

The radiant heat technique has not been without its critics. In clinical use, especially, it has proved to possess some basic faults. Whereas there is little difficulty in measuring the temperature of the stimulus at the delivery aperture—radiometers are currently fast-acting, sensitive, and highly reliable—determination of the temperature of the affected skin is another matter. The skin's temperature is not solely a function of the energy impinging on it; in part, it is determined by local blood circulation and sweating. Moreover, radiation of the skin, especially if it occurs repeatedly, leads to release of histamine by the tissues. This, in turn, makes the skin more sensitive. It is not safe to assume that moving the test spot about will obviate local heating effects; different patches of skin are unlikely to be equivalent in this respect.

Much attention has been given to the various subjective factors that may radically alter pain threshold, attitudinal matters in general, and the effects of suggestion in particular. One team of investigators (46) could find no effect whatever on pain threshold, as measured by the Hardy-Wolff-Goodell method, of sizable doses of morphine and codeine, though there was a reliable threshold rise to aspirin! They used the "double blind" procedure in which neither the subject nor the experimenter knows whether a drug or placebo is being administered on a particular trial. Since others had claimed large reductions in sensitivity with "single blind" methods, the conclusion seems inescapable that suggestibility may play a decisive role in forcing the typical result. This and other attitudinal determinants has been thoroughly discussed by Beecher (45).

It is obvious that electricity can be used to arouse pain; indeed, the problem with electrical stimulation is to find ways of avoiding pain. It is in the context of cutaneous communication systems that the question arises as to how pain can be prevented when electrical signals are delivered to the skin. One would like to use them since they possess the clear advantage over mechanical stimuli that with them elaborate energy transducers are not needed and power requirements are extremely modest. Thus far, in their application to the communication problem,

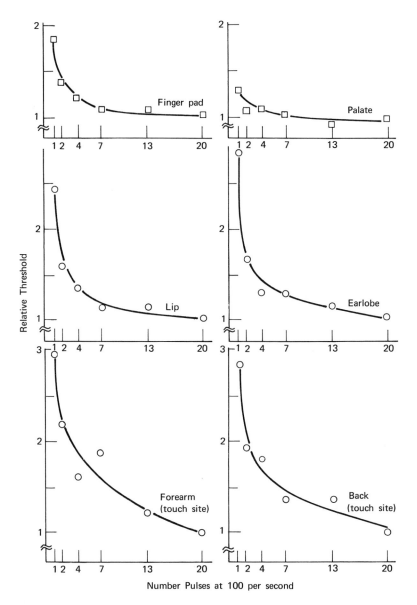

Fig. 11–3. Relative pain thresholds, plotted as multiples of peak current (with current at 20 pps as unity), as a function of the total number of successive pulses, delivered at a constant repetition rate. From Gibson, R. H. *(232).* Figure reproduced from D. R. Kenshalo (Ed.), *The Skin Senses,* 1968. Courtesy of Charles C. Thomas, Publisher, Springfield, Illinois.

the best compromise with pain has come from using very brief pulses of direct current (0.5 msec) in trains of not more than three or four in a burst lasting no more than 40 to 50 msec. Figure 11–3 shows the rapid lowering of threshold, for six different body sites, as the pulse train is increased beyond a few (232).

The chief difficulty connected with the electric current as a tool to investigate pain phenomena is that its specification, within the skin tissues where it operates, is an exceedingly dubious matter. Electricity, being the great "nonadequate" stimulus—it will arouse every sensory and motor system—affects every conductor in its path and does so differentially, depending upon what impedance (resistance and capacitance) it encounters locally. Electric currents do not uniformly produce the same pain under any and all conditions. High-frequency currents (1000 Hz and higher) are considerably less unpleasant to "take" than those of low frequency (100 Hz and below) for the same amount of power expenditure. The most commonly used electrical stimulus, 60 Hz a.c., delivers a peculiarly "ugly," "digging" pain at even moderate intensities. In measuring pain thresholds to either d.c. pulses or a.c. currents it is important that a uniform criterion of pain be adopted. By general agreement, since it seems to be the only available indicator, the point at which a pressury "tap" becomes a pricking "stab" is taken as the sought-for end point. But the evidence is good that the pricking sensation can only be elicited where skin impedance is high (436); then the sudden stab comes about when the impedance is suddenly surmounted by an increasing voltage driving sufficient current through the tissue. The pricking sensation is a signal that the skin's dielectric properties have been precipitously altered. It follows that all the carefully taken readings of stimulus intensity—amperage (ideally), voltage, power, or whatever—become simply a measure of the skin's dielectric strength and not a measure of threshold stimulation.

It might be supposed that the selection of the proper electrodes would go some distance toward guaranteeing that constancy of stimulation would be maintained. Electrodes are not inconsequential; selection of inappropriate ones can lead to faulty results. However, within limits, electrode size and constitution are not really important beyond certain limits. What happens is that, as voltage builds up at various points within the "active" electrode's compass, there proves to be a single point (perhaps more—electrical equivalents) having the poorest dielectric properties. This is the one that "breaks over" first and causes the "stab." All available current is funneled through this channel. The true stimulus thus becomes the density of current impinging directly on receptor or nerve. If we could measure current density at the site of stimulation, we should have the important proximal stimulus under control. As it is, we have to be satisfied with remote measures of total current flow in the circuit, an approximate and perhaps misleading indication.

Distribution of Pain Sensitivity. Pain has an interesting distribution throughout the body. For most areas of skin and with appropriate stimuli pain "points" or "spots" appear in great profusion. (We can be sophisticated about "spots" now, after having seen in connection with pressure sensitivity that the "spots" are artifacts of experimental procedure!) Table 11–1, derived from the work of von Frey's laboratory,

Table 11–1. Distribution of Pain Sensitivity

Skin Region	Pain "Points"/cm^2
Back of knee (popliteal fossa)	232
Neck region (jugular fossa)	228
Bend of elbow (cubital fossa)	224
Shoulder blade (interscapular region)	212
Volar side of forearm	203
Back of hand	188
Forehead	184
Buttocks	180
Eyelid	172
Scalp	144
Radial surface, middle finger	95
Ball of thumb	60
Sole of foot	48
Tip of nose	44

After H. Strughold (562).

gives some representative results of systematically exploring various regions of the body with a spine-tipped hair. Whereas the absolute number of "points" found in a unit area may not be too significant, since alteration of the sharpness of the stimulus point or of the force exerted by the hair attached to it would certainly change the number of pain "spots" reported, identical procedures were used for all skin samples, and the results for the several regions are therefore presumably comparable with each other.

It is interesting to note that the "hollows" of the body conformation, the fossae, are among the most readily responsive areas. In passing from the base to the extremity of a limb provisions for pain reception tend to decrease; the reverse is the case for pressure sensitivity.

Two highly sensitive tissues, not included in Table 4, are the cornea of the eye and the tympanic membrane of the ear. The most exquisite pains in the body can originate from these sources. The cornea is of special interest, since it is widely held that this tissue is devoid of all sensitivities except pain. In fact, the cornea may be said to be a veritable battleground on which has been waged for at least half a century a crucial theoretical struggle concerning the neural basis of pain. We shall have to take a good look at the evidence for unique properties of the cornea when we come to the question of the receptor system for pain.

Certain areas of the body are relatively analgesic, and a few are apparently totally so. Among the former may be counted the mucous lining of the cheeks and back parts of the mouth, including the rear portion of the tongue. The lower half of the uvula is completely insensitive to pain, as is also a small region of the inner cheek opposite the second lower molar, sometimes called Kiesow's area. Evidence coming chiefly from surgical experience points to the generality that the "solid" organs of the abdominal cavity are insensitive to direct stimulation, assuming no inflamed or diseased condition to be present. The same may be said for the alimentary canal from the stomach to the rectum and for the gall bladder. The "hollow" viscera, especially those lying in the upper part of the abdominal cavity, may produce pain, sometimes quite severe, when under traction. Probes inserted into skeletal muscle, tendons, fascia, and periosteum reveal these tissues to be supplied with pain endings, though not too liberally in the case of large muscle bundles. Hypodermic injection of irritant solutions into these organs demonstrates the same thing. The bone coverings are especially sensitive, pain from them partaking more of the quality of superficial cutaneous pain and being capable of somewhat accurate localization.

One would hope to learn something useful about pain from study of people who are bereft of it. Many alleged instances of total congenital pain insensitivity are to be found in the literature. Sternbach, who has carefully reviewed the problem's history *(541, 541a)* and who has described cases of his own, has concluded that, if a rigid criterion of congenital pain insensitivity is adopted—defect present from birth and no instance of pain having been felt, general insensitivity to pain over the entire body with no significant involvement of other senses, no mental or physical retardation, achievement of some maturity (children being suggestible and difficult to test)—"there is no case which appears to be a genuine instance of congenital insensitivity to pain" *(541,* p. 254). However, there are a score or so that come close to meeting the requirements. Certainly one would have to so categorize the "human pincushion" case described by Dearborn *(155)*. Studied at the age of 54, this man had experienced pain only three times in his life: "headache" at age seven after having had "an axe buried in his skull," pain from a finger, at 14, from the probing by a surgeon for an imbedded bullet, and the setting, at 16, of a broken fibula, which "hurt a little." His analgesia obviously did not prevent his "living dangerously"!

There are many other vivid reports of pain insensitivity attending self-mutilation, especially by children: bone and flesh injuries from banging the head against a wall, chewing off tips of fingers or tongue, serious burns from leaning against a stove or sitting in scalding water. Perhaps the Canadian case reported by McMurray in 1950 (402) more nearly meets the severe criteria laid down by Sternbach. The subject's only pain experience came at age 29, shortly before her death from complications following a hip operation. Autopsy revealed no hint of structural change in the pathways presumed to conduct pain, including the positive finding that the free nerve endings of the skin were normal in appearance.

Pain Adaptation.   Pain has been widely held to be incapable of adaptation. Its apparent failure to fade out on continued stimulation has led to this belief, and certain biological views concerning the survival value of pain have tended to perpetuate it. Dallenbach (141) has summed up the classic argument (preparatory, it should be added hastily, to showing its falsity): "Pain is deleterious; adaptation would be of anti-survival value, as organisms that become adapted to pain would, in the long run, not survive; hence pain is non-adaptable."

The failure to recognize the adaptability of pain arose from the same sources that prevented for so long a time any sort of quantification of results where pain is concerned—difficulties inherent in control of the conditions of stimulation. Headaches, toothaches, and pains from injuries inevitably involve constantly changing conditions at the site of stimulation, chiefly rhythmic ones based on circulatory events. It is the case in all the other sense fields that the course of adaptation is revealed only when steady stimulation is maintained. Pain should be no exception.

The simple fact is that pain is not an exception in the sensory realm, and it is revealed when care is taken to provide an unvarying stimulus. Many experiments, some of them performed more than 50 years ago, have demonstrated the reality of pain adaptation. A particularly helpful series of studies has been made by Dallenbach and his students (141, pp. 345–346). They aroused pain by mechanical means (sharp needles, the applied pressure being carefully regulated), by intense warmth (radiant heat, without pressure accompaniment), and by cold (a dry-ice stimulator, likewise pressureless). With the needles the typical course of adaptation was a gradual reduction of pain intensity to the point of disappearance, residual pressure sensations replacing the pain. When heat was used the first sensation reported was naturally warmth; this developed into weak pain which became progressively intensified. From the peak intensity it gradually subsided, returning eventually to warmth. Likewise, cold stimulation produced feelings of "cool," then "cold," and eventually pain. After remaining at a high degree of intensity for a time it declined gradually to "cold" and, finally, to "cool." These events are precisely what would be expected if pain adapts independently of the other cutaneous modalities. All three experiments reveal, as residual effects, the types of sensation inherent in their appropriate stimuli. Strong pressure elicits pain but leaves as a residue, when pain has adapted out, a pressure sensation. Heat leaves warmth, and cold, cold.

A temporarily puzzling set of facts concerning adaptation came out of a series of experiments performed by the Hardy group with radiant heat. An observer was set the task of continuously adjusting heat intensity to maintain threshold pain (247). This he did by keeping skin temperature within a narrow range (about 44 to 46° C) for prolonged periods, sometimes close to an hour. The presumption is that, had pain adaptation been going on steadily all this time, a gradual increase of skin temperature would have been needed to keep the sensation supraliminal. The conclusion seems indicated that pain from radiant heat does not adapt. Yet this is contrary to the older, well-established findings and also to those of some more recent investigation (379, 443) that have found pain thresholds at considerably lower temperatures.

Accordingly, fresh experiments were undertaken in which warm water immersion was substituted for radiant heat. Two kinds of procedure were instituted: (1) exposure of the lower back, the subject sitting in a shallow tub of rapidly circulating warm water until it felt neutral, then quickly bending back to subject relatively large skin areas to temperatures of 36 to 41° C (269); (2) immersion of the hand, first in hot water of 40 to 48°C for 30 sec, then to water in the neutral range of 32 to 35°C (270). In both instances both pain and adaptation occurred, but there were variations in felt pain intensity and in latency of onset and obliteration of pain, depending mainly on the temperature to which the skin was exposed. There also were significant individual differences. Figure 11–4 shows estimated intensity of the pain sensation on an 11-point scale (because of the range of dols) as a function of time of immersion of the hand. Five observers are represented. It seems clear that both of the earlier conclusions are correct, that is, low and moderate intensities do adapt out, while those close to the injury point on the temperature scale do so only transiently. Apparently, pain receptors have both a

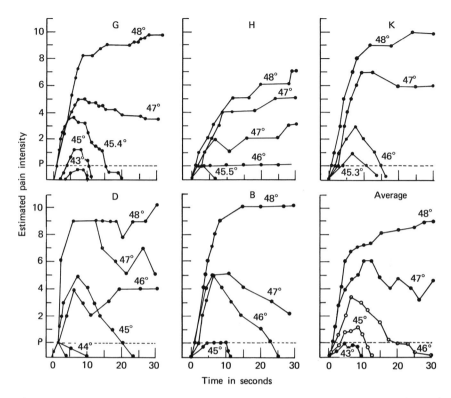

Fig. 11–4. Pain from hot-water immersion. The intensity of pain was estimated, on an 11-point scale, by five observers, over a 30-sec period of stimulation. From Hardy, J. D., Stolwijk, J. A. J., and Hoffman, A. D. *(270)*. Figure reproduced from D. R. Kenshalo (Ed.), *The Skin Senses,* 1968. Courtesy of Charles C. Thomas, Publisher, Springfield, Illinois.

"phasic" function to perform (weak stimulation) and a "static" one (strong stimulation). This does not solve the mystery of the pain mechanism, of course, but it does add an important dimension to the problem.

These adaptation experiments have a significant bearing on an old controversy. Earlier in this chapter it was pointed out that the view still persists that pain is not a separate and distinct form of sensibility but that it invariably results from overstimulation of some other sense mechanism. This theory is an old one and was chiefly espoused by Goldscheider. His controversy with von Frey on the subject is classic. It still resounds in the literature.

That pain is a separate and distinct sense is a belief of great antiquity.

The crude beginnings of a theory incorporating this supposition have been traced to Avicenna in the eleventh century (*141*). On the basis of a considerable body of accumulated evidence—and not a little speculation—von Frey made the theory quite specific. For him not only was pain a system of sensitivity apart from pressure, warmth, and cold but it was mediated by receptor organs of its own, free nerve endings. The "factual" evidence, in 1894–1897 when von Frey was stating his theory, was concerned largely with: (1) the distribution of pain points; (2) the differential action of anesthetics on pain and other tactual sensitivities; (3) threshold determinations; (4) the apparent pathological separation of pain from other tactual systems in diseases of the cord and brain; (5) the relatively long latency of pain sensations following stimulation; and (6) the uniqueness of certain areas, such as the cornea of the eye, in yielding only pain sensations.

Goldscheider, on the other hand, believed that the body possessed no separate system of nerves for the mediation of pain. He did not fall into the error, made by so many earlier theorists, of supposing that pain was a very general consequence of overstimulating just any sensory nerve. Dazzling lights, loud noises and shrill tones, intense heat and cold, and pungent odors can all be "painful," but this is to be explained satisfactorily on the basis that pain has an entirely ubiquitous distribution in the body. There is no mystery about this. Pain endings are found associated with all organs of sense as with many other organs, and, given the appropriate muscular tensions and other reactions of associated tissue, pain is likely to result. Goldscheider's view was that pain is relatively specific in the sense that only one cutaneous system was responsible for it; the system was that responsible also for pressure. Pressure and pain differ from each other intensively. What is pressure on weak stimulation is pain on more intense application of the stimulus. Summation of pressure impulses in the gray matter of the cord produces painful sensations.

One of the consequences of this view is that pain, upon being sufficiently weakened, should change into pressure. The adaptation experiment becomes critical for deciding between von Frey and Goldscheider, and, as we have seen, it fails to support the latter's contention. Pain, in the course of adapting, becomes progressively less intense and finally disappears without passing over into pressure. That is, it fails to leave a residue of pressure unless the adaptation stimulus is a pressure stimulus as well. Mechanical stimuli cannot answer the question, but thermal stimuli do so quite decisively.

Identification of the Pain Receptor.   As we have seen, the widespread distribution of free nerve endings throughout the body very early formed the basis for the belief that these organs are the receptors for pain. The view has not often been challenged. That the free nerve ending is the pain end organ is a common textbook statement. We need not accept it entirely on faith, however; there is imposing evidence to be considered.

The best support for the correlation of pain sensitivity with activity of free endings is perhaps the incontrovertible fact, which impressed von Frey and others long ago, that unencapsulated terminals of sensory nerves exist generally throughout the body. Plexiform arrangements of fibers ending in minute skeins, loops and whorls, brushes, knobs, and fine twigs abound within and beneath the epidermis and are present in mucous membrane and in a great variety of somatic and visceral organs. These elaborate neural designs seem anatomically to be but variations on a main theme. Their distribution is sufficiently widespread to coincide with that of pain sensibility, so far as can be judged from the available evidence. At least, there is no encapsulated ending having a similarly broad and rich distribution.

If an area could be found which possessed only pain sensitivity and which, at the same time, revealed only a single neural mechanism to be present, this would be strong evidence indeed for a firm correlation between mode of sensation and neural structure. Logically, of course, the possibility would remain that, in other areas, different mechanisms might also mediate pain, but at least one certain correlation would exist. The cornea of the eye has been held to provide exactly the instance sought. It has been repeatedly claimed that the cornea contains only free nerve endings and that pain is the only sensation of which the cornea is capable. It does indeed seem to be the case that the central portion of the cornea has but one type of sensory innervation. Its neural arrangements, a somewhat elaborate network of interdigitating free terminals, have been described in careful detail by Tower (580). So much for one side of the correlation. However, in completing the other side, pain as a unique product of corneal stimulation proves to be a factual disappointment. The cornea, to be sure, has tremendous capacity for generating pain. Ask anyone who has suffered from a corneal ulcer! Indeed, very special conditions have to be imposed to arouse anything other than pain in the cornea. However, it can be and has been done. Nafe and Wagoner (441) carefully lowered onto the cornea brass cylinders of the type used in thermal exploration of the skin. Stimulation was controlled mechanically by a pulley and counterweight arrangement in such a way that a pressure not exceeding 1.5 gm was exerted on the tissue. A large series of stimulations of six subjects resulted in almost uniform reports of simple contact or pressure. One report was of "sharp contact." No stimulations were painful. Apparently, direct observation under carefully controlled conditions reveals the central cornea to be capable of pressure sensations as well as painful ones.

The Nafe-Wagoner experiment does not stand alone; there has since been ample verification by others. If there is applied a wide range of different stimuli, intensity being scaled down to suit the special circumstances present in the cornea, "almost as many qualities of sensation can be evoked as can adequately be expressed linguistically," according to one outstanding authority (612, p. 114). This is a strong claim, and we shall have to examine it again in the next chapter when we raise the question of temperature sensitivity in different parts of the body. Meanwhile, it obviously makes more than adequate room for corneal pressure in addition to pain.

Another line of evidence points to the multiple sensitivity of the cornea. In 1938 there was introduced to neurosurgery Sjöquist's operation for the relief of intractable facial pain. This operation involves cutting the bulbospinal tract of the fifth (trigeminal) cranial nerve and leaves the face completely analgesic. In cases so operated the cornea is found to have a remnant of sensitivity; appreciation of touch is retained, although pain is missing. The cornea, then, fails to provide the unique relationship sought. Perhaps there are other tissues with which we could do better. The inner reaches of the external ear, the tympanic membrane in particular, have been similarly considered capable only of pain. Careful study of this region has not been attempted, mainly because of its relative inaccessibility, and an answer is not yet forthcoming.

Meanwhile, there are other lines of attack on the problem. One revolves around the much-discussed question of "double pain" and some interesting experimental findings connected with it. If pain is elicited by pinprick or intense heat applied to a finger or toe there may be noted two phases in the temporal course of the sensation. There is first a sharp, sudden pain, followed by a longer-lasting second pain. These two phases have been called "fast pain" and "slow pain" or "first" and "second" pain. There is not uniform agreement about the qualities possessed by the two. Some observers have called fast pain "pricking pain" and slow pain "burning pain." Other, equally well-qualified investigators have come to the conclusion that the two are qualitatively identical. See Sinclair's excellent summary (527, pp. 197–202). Of the temporal separation there seems to be little doubt. Figure 11–5 gives a schematic representation of the courses of the two pains and shows, in addition, the prolongation of "second" pain in cases of peripheral neuritis. The significance of the double pain response is that, since both slow and fast pain must be set off at the receptor practically simultaneously, differences in nervous conduction rates must be responsible for their temporal

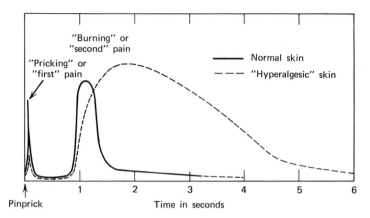

Fig. 11–5. The course of "double pain." The solid line suggests the normal temporal course of "first" (pricking) pain and "second" (burning) pain resulting from a pinprick. The dotted line shows the heightening and prolongation of "second" pain in cases of hyperalgesia. From Bigelow, Harrison, Goodell, and Wolff (*69*). By permission of the editors, *Journal of Clinical Investigation,* and the authors.

separation in experience. This was Zotterman's hypothesis in 1933; by now it is so widely believed as almost to have the status of fact.

Not all who have looked for double pain have found it. Some have denied its reality altogether (*565, 335*). Much depends upon how one goes about investigating it. Electric shocks, under ordinary circumstances, will not yield two pains. The reason seems to be that slowly conducting, unmyelinated fibers have very high thresholds to electric currents as compared with fast, myelinated ones. If the shock is sufficiently strong to arouse C fibers it produces an overwhelming response in A fibers, and this "swamps" second pain. Brindley (*93*) cleverly let the two sets of fibers compete on more even terms by partially anesthetizing the nerve trunk carrying the messages. He had his observers sit on a narrow rail for about 30 to 40 min, thus partially blocking the sciatic nerve, then delivered brief electric impulses to the foot. The two separate pains occurred regularly with an interval of 1.5 to 2.4 sec between them (individual differences). Suitable control experiments ruled out both delay at the block itself and differential receptor latencies as possible causes. The most reasonable explanation is that first pain is carried over fast A fibers— from their latencies, probably of the delta group—while the second pain message was transmitted over slow C fibers. The "sting" or "prick" of first pain is associated with a mechanism that responds phasically to the stimulus; the long lasting "burning" pain is the product of nerves that typically display a persistent afterdischarge, and this seems to be the substrate for the characteristic radiating and slowly subsiding pattern of second pain.

Double pain is not the esoteric phenomenon some have thought it. Sinclair and Stokes (528) tested its appearance in 40 medical students who were without benefit of prior indoctrination as to what to expect. A standard stimulating situation was created in which a finger was slipped into a water bath heated to 57°C, and it remained there for one second. Two-thirds of the subjects felt the two pains. Elapsed time to the onset of second pain was 2.13 ± 0.42 sec. First pain arrived in less than a second. Repeated trials with the same finger led to a buildup of sensation that felt like more or less continuous second pain. The finger tingled and felt hot for more than an hour.

A smaller number of highly reliable observers subsequently were subjected to asphyxial block of the arm with a pressure cuff, reaction times to first and second pain being taken at 6-min intervals. The experiment was carried as far as safety would permit—very prolonged cessation of blood flow in a limb can result in gangrene—and some individuals continued on for 36 min. Second pain was present on every trial and showed an unchanging latency of a little over two seconds. First pain, however, started out with a delay of about 0.8 sec, became slower to arouse as asphyxia progressed, and ended up at a value of 1.58 sec, on the average. Some observers dropped out after about 20 min, the temporal distinction between first and second pain having already disappeared.

The explanation of double pain in terms of two sets of pathways, fast A fibers and slow C fibers, is not the only one ever to have been proposed. Indeed, any mechanism demanding a delay of the message en route would take care of the differential latencies. Thus, it has been held that second pain is to be accounted for by double processing in the central nervous system, either a significant portion of the excitation flooding the gray matter of the cord or being shunted through the reticular formation of the brainstem. As early as 1922, von Frey (208), revising his earlier opinion that the dual sensations were really an initial pressure followed by pain, suggested that first pain comes from direct stimulation of the nerve but that an ancillary reaction is the liberating of a chemical, and the subsequent action of this on the nerve ending accounts for second pain. As the role of histamine has been pursued in skin physiology this hypothesis has seemed not at all improbable (507). It would be easier to choose among the various possibilities if so much did not depend on latency measures. Overall reaction time to a painful stimulus is an extremely complex indicator, comprising as it does action time of receptors, delays at a somewhat indeterminate number of synapses, possible though less probable variations in conduction times along efferent paths, and all these dependent for their absolute values on intensity of excitation.

"Protopathic" Pain.   Often, when cuts and other injuries to the skin produce a local anesthesia, there will be found an 'intermediate zone" bordering the insensitive region and separating it from surrounding normal areas. This "zone" has special sensory characteristics. In other instances, where the extent of injury is relatively slight, only a superficial branch of a sensory nerve being involved, there will be no absolute anesthesia but there will result a somewhat circumscribed area having the same special properties as the intermediate zone in more extensive injuries. The outstanding characteristic is the greatly altered quality of pain sensation evoked from the abnormal region. Though its threshold may be higher, the pain is exceptionally strong and unpleasant. Moreover, once aroused, it tends to persist and to radiate. Localization is diffuse and grossly inexact. Such a pain pattern is difficult to describe, and it has received a variety of names in the literature: protopathic pain, hyperpathia, paradoxic pain, hyperalgesia, "overreaction," dysesthesia.

The British neurologist, Henry Head, performed an experiment over a half-century ago that was destined not only to draw attention to this phenomenon but from which he was to derive a whole theory of cutaneous sensitivity (276). Several repetitions of Head's experiment, with modifications, have been performed over the intervening years. They have been as much directed at testing Head's ingenious and provocative theory as at the final establishment of the facts of cutaneous innervation (605).

Head, in cooperation with the psychologist, Rivers, and the surgeon, Sherren, cut two nerves in his forearm and studied the sensory losses resulting. Carefully following the course of the return of sensation as the nerves regenerated (see Figure 11–6) he believed he had discovered a basic separation between two types of cutaneous sensitivity. The immediate consequence of knocking out the sensory supply to the forearm was that there appeared a region of total anesthesia. Surrounding this during recovery was an "intermediate zone" having some remnants of sensitivity but behaving in most respects unlike the normal skin lying beyond. In the intermediate zone pain could be aroused, and it was a peculiarly disagreeable pain. High and low temperatures could be appreciated (above 45°C and below 20°C), but not moderate ones. Moreover, there was no discernible adaptation to these extremes of temperature. Pressures could be felt if heavy, but only coarse gradations of pressure

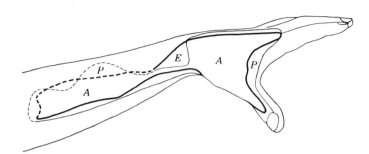

Fig. 11–6. Epicritic and protopathic sensitivity. Map of Henry Head's hand and arm 1 month after the radial and external cutaneous nerves had been cut. The area marked *A* is still entirely anesthetic, while "protopathic" sensitivity is found in area *P* and "epicritic" sensitivity, rarely occurring by itself, is in area *E*. From Boring (*84*). By permission of the copyright owners, Appleton-Century-Crofts, New York.

strength could be appreciated. Head believed these symptoms to be those of a primitive nervous structure, now artifically dissociated from another, more highly developed one which was also present in normal skin. The primitive system he dubbed the "protopathic." The later-regenerating system, the "epicritic," he considered to be a finely discriminative one and one which was probably phylogenetically a later development. The epicritic system was superposed on the protopathic system of nerves and was responsible for partially inhibiting the latter's action. Epicritic functions included the mediation of light touch, fine intensive gradations, temperatures between 25°C and 40°C (and their adaptation), and the spatial features of touch such as localization and two-point discrimination. Pain was never mediated by epicritic nerves.

The protopathic-epicritic distinction was appealing to many, and the concept has been used not only to interpret cutaneous sensory phenomena but, coupled with the further hypothesis that the protopathic system makes its appeal to the thalamus while the epicritic system has its central terminations in the cortex of the brain, the theory has been used quite generally as a basis for a broad neurological interpretation of behavior. Thus Rivers (*501*) has utilized the notions of protopathic and epicritic forms of *behavior* (essentially, instinctive and emotional responses as opposed to intelligent and manipulatory ones) as devices for explaining various forms of psychoneurosis, "substitution hysteria" in particular. But it is as a theory of cutaneous sensation that we are presently interested in the protopathic-epicritic distinction. As such, it stands in opposition to the classical theory of four cutaneous modalities: pressure, pain, warmth, and cold. To be sure, Carr (*110*) analyzed in detail the results reported in the Head nerve division experiment and came to the conclusion that, on the basis of his own results, Head should have logically found for no less than seven systems of sensitivity, not two. However, scientific theories never got established or abolished by merely arguing about them. What are the current facts and what shall we conclude about the usefulness of Head's theory?

The most recent and the best-controlled of the nerve division experiments is that of Lanier (*374*). In three subjects the two main nerves (the lateral and median cutaneous antebrachials) supplying the volar surface of the left forearm were destroyed by injecting their tracts with 95% alcohol. A considerable region corresponding to the peripheral projection areas of the nerves was thus left anesthetic. These areas, carefully located in advance, were explored systematically for several months before denervation. The same care in mapping was used throughout the 2-year period following the operation. Instrumentation and procedure were such as to guarantee comparability between successive tests, a matter too frequently overlooked in some of the earlier work. Moreover, quantitative measures of threshold were secured by means of a calibrated mechanical algesiometer (pain), a "limen gauge" (pressure), and a thermoesthesiometer (warmth and cold). All four modalities were found to recover continuously and gradually throughout the process of nerve regeneration, though the area of initial loss for the temperature senses was markedly greater than for pain and pressure. Pain, pressure, and cold recovered, by circumferential shrinkage of the area unresponsive to a stimulus of constant magnitude, at about the same rate. Warmth was considerably delayed; Lanier found Head's peculiarly unpleasant "protopathic" pain both in the intermediate zone shortly after denervation and in the central anesthetic zone once the regenerating nerve fibers began to grow back into it. But sensations best described as "protopathic pressure" also appeared, and pressure is, of course, not supposed to be a protopathic quality. While there was a return to near normality after 2 years or so, Lanier reported to the author that, more than 15 years after the operation, he still had occasional "protopathic" reactions from the region originally made anesthetic by denervation.

Boring, who undertook one of the several repetitions of the Head experiment (*80*), also found himself left with a memento. In a personal letter to the author, in 1953, he said: "I had the nerve in my forearm cut in 1913. When sensation began to return to the anesthetic area, I found that stroking the originally anesthetic area gave referred fluttering sensations in the proximal part of the palm of the hand. These are still there forty years later for this kind of stimulation of the affected region. In that sense the area never recovered." Head, by the way, was somewhat contemptuous of Boring's experiment, which concluded against the necessity for the protopathic-epicritic distinction. He felt that because only a superficial branch of the nerve had been severed, it was only a "miniature experiment." Boring quite properly retorted that "there is nothing in Head's theory that ought not to be demonstrable within a single square centimeter" (*84*, p. 474).

There was general qualitative agreement among Head's, Boring's and Lanier's studies. Nonconcurrence came in connection with details and, in particular, with the question of what constituted the simplest explanation of the phenomena. After weighing the evidence carefully Lanier concluded (*374*, p. 454): "The results of the study do not substantiate Head's theory of protopathic and epicritic systems of fibers in cutaneous nerves. Neither the patterns of sensory dissociations nor the sensitivity alterations in affected areas can be accounted for by his theory. The sensory dissociations observed point conclusively to the existence of four types of anatomical mechanisms underlying cutaneous sensibility."

A convincing histological study (*613*) added further to our understanding of the protopathic pain mechanism. Skin samples were taken from 59 patients who had scars or partially denervated skin. These were stained and subjected to microscopical analysis. In all instances in which pain of protopathic quality had resulted from pinprick in the affected area, the findings were consistently that the underlying nerve nets and terminals were isolated from their neighbors. There was no overlap or interdigitation of terminals in the region; only a single nerve fiber had supplied all the endings. Conversely, in no single case in which such isolation of terminals could not be found microscopically could "unpleasant" pain be produced. It would appear that protopathic pain owes its existence to simplification of the sensory nerve supply. Where normally intricate networks exist pain takes on a more subdued character.

Although the empirical facts seem pretty clearly to point to a renunciation of the protopathic-epicritic distinction, this has not proved to have been its fate. As neurophysiological investigations have mounted in number and avidity there has been both a preservation of the descriptive terms connected with the concept and, more importantly, the central idea of opposed dual mechanisms. The first may be only a matter of scientific usage but the second is vital to theory. We have just been considering double pain and its probable neural basis in fast and slowly conducting fibers. There could also be put in evidence the opposition between the highly discriminative lemniscal and the more rudimentary spinothalamic pathways; indeed, the whole recurring idea of excitatory-inhibitory relations at all levels of the nervous system calls for a balanced dual mechanism. As Rose and Mountcastle have insisted (505, p. 391): "The conclusion that Head did not prove his point is . . . irrelevant for an inquiry as to whether or not his central idea has merit . . . an unqualified rejection of these concepts may be premature. . . ." Bishop's view (72) is compatible with Head's, also. He pictures the phylogenetically earlier, more primitive sensory system as being constituted of small myelinated and unmyelinated fibers that mediate the full range of somesthetic sensation—pain, pressure, and temperature. A greater nicety of function, however, characterizes the phylogenetically later system mediated by the larger myelinated fibers. To the "bare" sensations have been added, through the operations of this latecomer, postural information, localization, and form recognition, the more discriminative of the somesthetic functions generally. Even though it was arrived at over a different pathway of reasoning, Bishop's conception is not inimical to Head's idea.

Pain Interactions and Itching.   We saw that pain comes patterned in a great variety of ways. One pattern of special interest is itch. Itching seems to bear about the same relation to pain as tickle does to pressure. It is a durative pattern, usually highly attention-demanding and, like tickle, leads ordinarily to reaction. One usually "does something about it," rubs or scratches the affected region. What are the conditions for the arousal of itch?

It is not possible to provide a complete answer as yet. A number of pathological skin conditions commonly accompanied by itching are known clinically. These presumably involve fairly low-level irritations of free nerve endings in the affected tissue. But itching can occur also in entirely normal skin. In mapping experiments with hairs and needles delays are often occasioned by the unwanted appearance of itching. One well-defined experimental situation for the production of itching has been discovered by Bishop (70) with the use of his electrical "sparking" method. Repetitive shocks, each so weak that by itself it will produce no sensation whatever, may induce a persistent itch not unlike that generated by an insect bite. Here is direct evidence of temporal summation in the pain receptors; in fact, summation occurs when the shocks succeed each other at a rate as slow as 5 per second. Itching may also be brought about as an aftereffect of the sharp pricking sensation produced by single shocks of greater strength. Weak but supraliminal single shocks induce pricking pain without itch, and, if the intensity is generally increased in slowly repetitive stimulations, the pattern passes over into sharp stabbing pain, eventually becoming intolerable.

It is not only electricity that will generate itching; mechanical, thermal, and chemical stimuli are effective under some conditions. Spicules of the plant, cowage (*Mucana pruriens*) are the active agent in "itching powder." The action of cowage on the skin proves to be both mechanical and chemical. Its sharp spines do injury by piercing the epidermis—and this part of the process has been successfully simulated with fine, springy wire of 0.001 in. diameter (*28*)—but the additional chemical effect comes from a proteolytic enzyme which is released from the plant and which has a histaminelike influence on the skin. Histamine itself is a powerful producer of itching, and any agent that will release the skin's own histamine (ammonia, morphine, the peptones, and others) will naturally generate itchy skin. Histamine injections and applications of cowage are the two most commonly employed experimental procedures for setting up itch sensations. With histamine there are always ancillary reactions; a wheal is raised and a prominent skin flare may be created at concentrations too low to cause itching, and this guarantees nicety of control and high sensitivity for the method.

It would be interesting to know the full details of the relation between itching and rubbing or scratching. Just how does the additional stimulation inhibit itchy feelings? Many studies have sought the answer. It has been shown, for example, that itch can be quelled, sometimes for long periods, by repeated pinpricks in an area previously made itchy by the application of cowage or histamine, by insect bites, or by injecting foreign proteins into the skin. This apparently works best if the same dermatome is involved in the two forms of stimulation. Thus, itching in a cowaged area of the back over a shoulder blade can be assuaged by painful pinpricks on the anterior wall of the chest. Similarly, if a skin fold on the forearm is made "touchy" by pinching it with forceps, developing a so-called secondary hyperalgesia, itch powder applied to the area may yield pricking pain from the spicules but not itching (*115*).

Itching can be reduced by other means; it is not necessary to "fight pain with pain." Melzack and Schecter first set up a moderate itching on the inner wrists of some 50 subjects by applications of cowage (*411*). Then, in various subgroups, mechanical vibration was applied (a) to the itchy wrist, (b) to the arm halfway to the elbow, (c) to the opposite wrist, or (d) to the opposite arm. There was also a control group that got contact at the wrist with a quiescent vibrator. Itching was significantly reduced in (a) and (c). Presumably, there was an interaction between the pressure and pain systems at the spinal roots common to the two.

Since itch is only one pattern in which low-grade pain appears, it is natural to ask whether interactions of the kind found in connection with itch can also be found at higher pain levels. The evidence is overwhelming that it can. One of the agents that has frequently been experimented with is electrical stimulation. Wall and Sweet (599) applied trains of electrical pulses (square waves lasting 0.1 msec each and repeated 100 times per second) at a current strength that would just bring about "tingling" or "buzzing" in the area supplied by the nerve. Eight patients having intense chronic pains were stimulated electrically either at the sensory roots in the cord or along the path of the sensory nerve leading to the affected area. While the current was on, prodding the skin with a finger did not evoke pain as it ordinarily would have. More importantly, by this treatment some of the patients were relieved of their pain for relatively long periods; analgesia lasted for a half-hour or more from 2-min "doses" of the electrical pulses.

Similar suppression of pain has been realized in cases of chronic trigeminal neuralgia. People who suffer from this affliction have intense paroxysms of facial pain. Typically, accompanying the pain, the facial muscles innervated by efferents of the fifth cranial nerve undergo prolonged spasms; the common name for the condition, *tic douloureux*, is derived from this symptom. There have been many approaches to its treatment: medication, alcohol injections, neural surgery of various degrees of severity, compression and decompression. Most measures are radical in that they are likely to leave some facial anesthesia, paralysis, or both. Ideally, relief of pain should have no permanent side effects, and one of the attacks made on this disorder has been to supply electrical shocks to the trigeminal nucleus with a view to breaking down any "polarization" of that center. At least, this is the thinking that induced Shelden (519) to implant a tiny radio receiver, imbedded in plastic and anchored to the temporal cranium, and supplied with platinum wires contacting the nerve close to the ganglion. A small radio transmitter (14 kc and 150 mW of power) was housed in a flashlight case which the patient carried about with him. When pain attacked, the transmitter was held against the scalp and a "shot" of high-frequency waves was delivered to the receiver. At the time the report of this vivid experiment was made, three participating patients who had many symptoms in common had been able to get instant and long-lasting relief for a period of 31 months.

It may be that some of the claims for obliteration or partial alleviation of pain from accessory stimulation will prove to be based on attentional distraction, attitudinal changes, or other central mechanisms of a cognitive kind. There is some sound thinking, however, that provides explanations at a more peripheral and neurophysiological level. One of the more successful attempts to concoct a theory that will recognize interplay of sensory impulses is that of Melzack and Wall (412). They call it the *gate control* theory. Figure 11–7 displays their model.

This is a theory of impulse competition at spinal cord locus. To under-

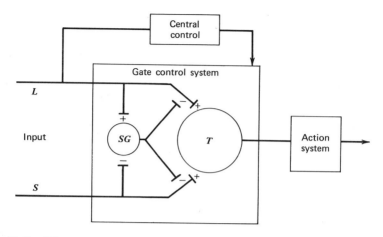

Fig. 11–7. The gate control theory of pain. *L*, large-diameter fibers; *S*, small fibers; *SG*, substantia gelatinosa; *T*, first central transmission cell; + = excitation; − = inhibition. From Melzack and Wall *(412).* Copyright 1965 by the American Association for the Advancement of Science.

stand the theory, three central features must be considered: (1) the role of the *substantia gelatinosa* of the dorsal horn of the cord (*SG* in the diagram); (2) the relative influences of large and small primary peripheral fibers (*L* and *S*); and (3) the transmission operation by so-called "*T* cells." The area bounded by the square constitutes the "gate control." It is supposed that this system modulates whatever input comes from peripheral fibers and thus determines what transmission there will be over *T* cells of the dorsal horn. Presumably the latter mainly involves anterolateral cord tracts. The input of large peripheral (mainly A) fibers, nearly up to the point where they synapse with *T* cells, is relatively straightforward. They either send their messages directly to the brain over the dorsal column system or impinge upon *T* cells. Small (mainly C) fibers discharge *T* cells directly. But both large and small fibers are known to enter the *substantia gelatinosa* of the cord where, by connecting with a multitude of short-axon cells and some long ones in Lissauer's tract, they have opportunity for free interplay with other units. It is this mechanism that supplies the "gate," for, as the diagram indicates, it imposes an inhibitory control, presynaptically, on both large- and small-fiber inputs. What will happen in the *T* cells, then, mainly depends upon the balance of activity in large and small fibers. A superfluity of activation from the small fibers opens the gate, and excess of large-fiber discharges closes the gate. Presumably, pain is the result of an open gate or a partially opened one.

It is to be noted that provision is made for feedback from the higher levels of the central nervous system. There are many evidences here, as in the auditory and visual systems, that efferent influences regulate operation in ascending pathways. Whatever is going on in T cells must be under continuous monitoring by central mechanisms. It is even possible that experiential and motivational concerns—perceptual, memorial, and attitudinal processes—effect the prime control of the gate. Melzack and Casey (409) think so, and they have, accordingly, put forward a major modification of the gate control theory. If it serves as well as its predecessor to suggest specific hypotheses for experimental test it will have been worthwhile indeed.

12

Temperature Sensitivity

The Thermal "Senses." One of the most persistently recurring questions in the whole realm of sensory psychophysiology is that concerning the basic nature of sensitivity to temperature changes. Are we dealing with a single "temperature sense," or are there two systems of sensitivity, a "warm sense" and a "cold sense"? If solely physical considerations were consulted, if stimuli alone could provide the answer, the problem should not detain us long. The absorption of heat by the skin is a simple, straightforward event, describable in the terms of calorimetry. Objects of higher temperature than the skin, upon coming into contact with it, transmit heat to it. The loss of heat by the skin to surrounding air or to objects contacted is the obverse process. There are not two sets of stimuli, warm and cold; there are only positive and negative transfers of a single form of physical energy, heat.

But, as we have seen, appeal to stimuli has never provided the best solution to the problem of classification of the senses. If it could be conclusively demonstrated that there existed in the skin a single anatomical mechanism capable of responding one way to heat gains and another way to heat losses we should doubtless decide in favor of a single "temperature sense." As the facts now stand the weight of evidence is against such a conclusion. Instead there are compelling reasons for believing that we are dealing with two systems of sensitivity, one for warmth and one for cold.

The chief argument for the separation of the two rests on the demonstration that cold and warm sensitivities are not distributed alike. If a sample area on the arm is explored, point by point, with a metal contactor cooled well below skin temperature a pattern of responsive "spots" will be found. Some points will "flash out" strongly with cold sensations, while others will yield moderate, cool feelings. In a 1-cm² area perhaps a

344

half dozen such spots will be found. If the experiment is now repeated with a warmed contactor the same area will yield perhaps one or two reports of warmth, perhaps none. The probability is that careful mapping of the region will show widely disparate patterns for the two qualities, cold spots nearly always being far more numerous than warm. Table 12–1, a composite of results from Rein (493) and from Strughold and Porz (563a) gives comparisons for several body regions.

Table 12–1.   Comparison of Warm- and Cold-spot Concentrations

	"Spots" per Square Centimeter	
	Cold	Warm
Forehead	8.0	0.6
Nose	8.0 (side) –13.0 (tip)	1.0
Upper lip	19.0	. . .
Chin	9.0	. . .
Chest	9.0	0.3
Upper arm, volar side	5.7	0.3
Upper arm, dorsal side	5.0	0.2
Bend of elbow	6.5	0.7
Forearm, volar side	6.0	0.4
Forearm, dorsal side	7.5	0.3
Back of hand	7.0	0.5
Palm	4.0	0.5
Fingers	2.0–9.0	1.6–2.0
Thigh	5.0	0.4
Lower leg	4.0–6.0	. . .
Sole of foot	3.0	. . .

After Rein (493) and Strughold and Porz (563a).

There is, of course, the same necessity here, as in our earlier considerations of pressure and pain "spots," to avoid the naive conclusion that the mapping of temperature spots implies the location of individual temperature receptors. "Spots" are products of certain experimental operations. The number found in a given area reflects, to be sure, the sensitivity in that area, but it also reflects the operation of a number of other variables. The number of warm or cold spots found in a given exploration is a function of at least the following factors, in addition to depending on receptor availability in the particular skin area being tested: (1) stimulus temperature, (2) size of stimulator, (3) concomitant mechanical pressure, (4) state of thermal adaptation, (5) duration of stimulus at each exposure, (6) interval between stimulations, and (7) the attentive "set" taken by the observer. Some of these are not as important as one might expect. Thus Heiser (*289*) systematically varied stimulus duration between 0.5 and 4.0 sec, in an experiment on warm sensitivity of the forehead, without finding any significant change in the number of reports of warmth. This is not only true of temperature sensitivity as measured by responses in small skin areas. With whole-body irradiation by heat it has been found, at levels ranging from weak to quite strong, that feelings of warmth change little over a 12-sec exposure, despite the fact that skin temperature is steadily increasing throughout that period (*403*). It is reasonably certain, though, that time could be shortened to the point where it would make a difference. Similarly, increase in stimulus pressure from 1.0 to 6.0 gm brought about an increase in number of warm spots which, however, was so small as to require treatment by probability statistics to make certain that the increase was a real one (*290*). The small increase accompanying a change from 1.0 to 2.0 gm was not statistically reliable.

The effects of stimulus size and stimulus temperature are difficult to separate. Both affect the warm and cold spot counts; increased size improves the probability that warm or cold will be reported in a given application, and increased deviation of stimulus temperature from that of the skin brings the same result. The two variables can, of course, be separately investigated in a systematic manner, but one hardly knows whether increase in frequency of temperature reports, in the case of an enlarged stimulus point, is the result of more end organs being stimulated or a more adequate delivery of heat to a fixed number of them. Increasing the contacting area of the stimulus may be tantamount to intensifying the stimulus. Conversely, increasing the effective temperature may be physiologically equivalent to spreading the stimulus over a larger amount of receptive tissue. Simple mathematical relations between either stimulus area or stimulus temperature and numbers of responsive "spots" have never been established with certainty. Everyone who attempts mapping

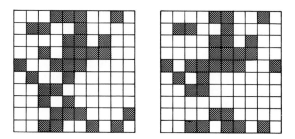

Fig. 12–1. Two successive mappings of cold spots in the same area. From the author's research records.

of cold or warm spots is impressed with the apparent fickleness of their behavior. Test-retest reliabilities are disappointingly low despite careful control of the obvious experimental variables. This is not to say that mapping and remapping of temperature spots inevitably leads to utter lack of consistency. The results are far from chaotic. One is likely to be able to see, in the charts of several successive mappings, strong pattern resemblances. See Figure 12-1. However, if exact correspondences are looked for square by square, agreement between any two maps is likely to run no higher than 70 to 80%. Indeed, far lower degrees of consistency are commonly found.

If, instead of mapping cold responses coming out of square-by-square exploration of a small area with the conventional 1-mm² cylinder point and doing so in an "all-or-none" fashion—"cold" or "not cold"—one varies the procedure by (a) covering a much larger skin area, (b) requiring graded reports of sensation intensity—"0" = no cold; "3" = "strong cold"—and (c) using a considerably larger stimulus point, one of 2.5-mm diam, both the patterning and the fluctuations from one testing to another show up strongly. Figure 12-2 displays an interesting set of maps obtained by this procedure, the first three and the last three separated by an interval of four hours (410).

In any extensive exploration of the skin with a cooled temperature cylinder there are likely to be found a few points at which cold comes out promptly and vividly. One can return to such spots time after time and get the same result. In fact, tests separated by relatively long periods of time, even years, will show unfailing responsiveness at the loci of of such peaks of sensitivity. There are, then, points of peculiarly ready reaction, and this may mean either that certain receptor aggregates possess abnormally high sensitivity or that they are extraordinarily favorably situated with respect to channels of heat transfer. There is some suggestion that the latter may be true in Gilmer's finding that about twice as many cold-sensitive spots are found on sweat duct openings as are found on loci of stimulation not involving mouths of sweat ducts (233).

The number of responsive spots in an area is not, of course, the only possible index of temperature sensitivity. One can report quite directly on feelings of warmth or cold in an attentively viewed region of the body. Hardy has done experiments of this kind, asking the observer to report on the thermal state of his forehead under various conditions (268). If, at intervals of 10 sec, the observer is required to give one of five indications—neutral, slightly cool, slightly warm, warm—even though he is surrounded by a strictly neutral thermal environment, his report will take the fluctuating form shown in Figure 12-3. Autonomous bodily changes

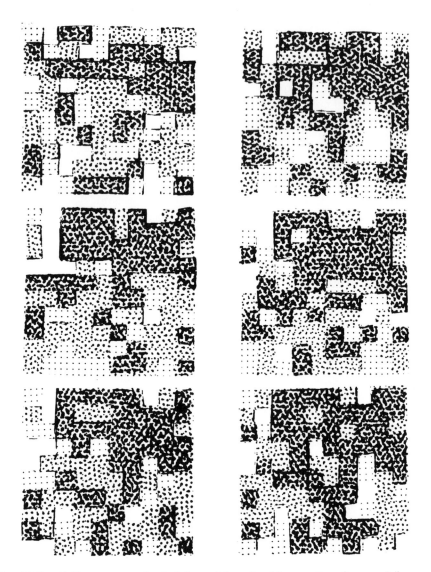

Fig. 12–2. Cold patterns. Graded intensities of cold sensation from a 2.5-mm stimulator. Open squares represent "no cold"; three grades of stippling show progressively greater cold intensity. The three maps on the left were made in quick succession; those on the right, also successive, were made four hours later. From Melzack, Rose, and McGinty *(410)*. Courtesy of Academic Press, Inc.

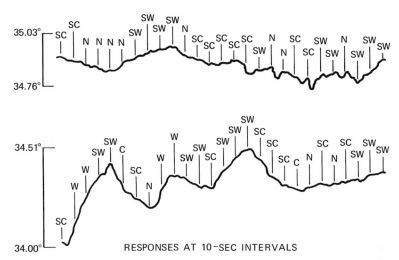

Fig. 12–3. Fluctuations of skin temperature. The upper record shows how forehead temperature moves up and down spontaneously in a constant-temperature (neutral) room. The lower record shows the course of temperature changes following gentle warming (a 30-sec exposure to 0.0002 cal/sec/cm² radiant heat). Every 10 sec, in each record, the observer gave sensory reports: SC, slightly cool; N, neutral; SW, slightly warm; W, warm; C, cool. From Hardy (*268*).

produce minor disturbances of skin temperature which, in turn, induce slight sensory effects. Sensitivity is best appraised by introducing small warming and cooling trends by radiant stimuli. In these experiments, of well over a thousand reports taken when the slight temperature decrement of 0.001°C/sec was in force, cool reports considerably exceeded warm ones (though the modal sensation was "neutral") and, when an increment of the same size was employed, warm reports were far more frequent than cool and neutral reports combined. Skin temperature by itself is hardly a trustworthy predictor of thermal sensations.

Thermal Changes in the Skin. One way we shall get a better picture of the probable stimulation process is to pay some attention to investigations of heat transfer by the cutaneous tissues. If the epidermis, with its relatively simple composition, may be regarded as a somewhat homogeneous conductor of heat, the same cannot be said of the more elaborate tissues beneath it. The dermal layers are, of course, considerably complicated thermally by reason of the fact that they house blood vessels—capillaries, venules, arterioles, and (at deeper levels) veins and arteries.

The vascular system has much to do with supplying heat to the skin and with regulating that supply. It obviously cannot be ignored in the thermal stimulation process.

Direct evidence concerning heat interchanges in the cutaneous tissues came first from the ingenious experiments of Bazett and his co-workers (36, 37, 38, 38a). Using tiny thermocouples inserted into the skin of the forearm under previously located warm and cold spots, they were able to measure accurately the extent of heat conduction through the tissue from a thermal stimulator applied to the surface. At a depth of about 1.0 mm below the surface (subsequently measured on X-ray photographs) there proved to be remarkably little heat gained or lost in arousing warmth or cold. With an applicator of 1.5 mm diameter a stimulus 10°C above the initial skin surface temperature, held on the spot for 6 sec, produced a maximum temperature rise of only 1.05°C 1.0 mm below the surface. A cold stimulus more than 15°C below initial surface temperature brought about a drop, 1.0 mm down, of only 0.4°C during a 5.6-sec period. Results with a much larger applicator (11.0 mm) produced more extensive shifts of subsurface temperature, though none was as large as might be expected. Moreover, the skin surface directly under the stimulator never attained the temperature of the physical stimulus, discrepancies between them of 8° to 10°C being common even at the moderate temperatures used.

The rate of heat penetration through the cutaneous tissues was found to vary from 0.5 to 1.0 mm/sec, depending somewhat on the vascular conditions at the time. If the blood vessels were in a dilated condition the velocity of heat transfer was reduced. Apparently the circulatory flow serves as a kind of cooling system, picking up heat and carrying it off, thus retarding direct heat penetration into the tissues lying beyond. Local inflammation is a particularly powerful inhibitor of cold sensations, reducing their intensity and exaggerating their latency of arousal. Conversely, hyperemic skin renders warmth easier to evoke.

The presence of blood vessels in the skin, more or less constantly varying in diameter as they do with consequent transient changes in warming and cooling effects, brings about an unstable thermal situation. It is little wonder that it has been impossible to establish experimentally the invariant relationships between stimulus temperature and sensitivity. Blood flowing past a given receptor must effectively contribute to the state of adaptation of that cell and must be regarded as constituting part of the thermal stimulation system. This means that a relatively large area of tissue may affect a given end organ. The situation is not unlike that obtaining in the radiation thermopile of the physicist. The thermocouple junction has soldered to it a metal disc or "radiation receiver" which collects over its relatively large surface enough heat to activate the thermocouple junction and thus greatly improve the sensitivity of the instrument. In like manner the blood supply of the skin imparts its heating and cooling effects to the relatively tiny nerve endings responsible for temperature sensations. In view of this condition it is remarkable that warm and cold sensitivities have anything like punctate distributions.

Out of the studies of heat transfers in the skin have come some interesting ideas concerning a possible mechanism of thermal stimulation. Bazett, McGlone, Williams, and Lufkin (38) performed the somewhat Spartan experiment of suspending with dulled fishhooks the skin of the prepuce, applied a thermal stimulus to one side of the fold, and picked up the transmitted heat with a thermocouple cemented to the other side. Since the stretched tissue of the foreskin is only about 2.0 mm thick, it was possible to stimulate or record from either side, thus permitting calculations of the probable depth of the receptor. Time relations for both sensation (reaction time) and heat conduction were carefully measured. The latency of the cold sensation is short (0.3–0.5 sec), and estimates from these experiments place the receptor at a depth below the skin surface of about 0.1 mm. Warm sensations are aroused more slowly (0.5–0.9 sec latency). Similar calculations place the receptor depth near 0.3 mm. These estimates would mean that the end organ for cold lies just above the most superficial venules; those for warmth are at depths where complex patterns of arterial and venous networks exist.

From his measurements Bazett was inclined to favor a "temperature gradient" theory of the stimulation process. This conception was apparently originated by Ebbecke in 1917 (180), and it has reappeared in the literature from time to time in different guises. It is supposed that, because there is a difference in temperature between the skin surface and the vascular structures underneath, this gradient represents the normal state of affairs (thermal indifference). A cold stimulus applied to the skin withdraws heat and steepens the existing thermal gradient. The situation for warm is somewhat different, though similar in principle. The application of heat to the skin surface will also disturb the gentle gradient existing in the (deeper) region of the skin where the receptors are and steepen it sufficiently to bring about stimulation. Both warm and cold, then, depend for their arousal on spatial gradients in the skin.

The idea is an attractive one, but the outcomes of several crucial experiments speak against it. Bazett himself eventually expressed doubt about its validity when he found that immersion of the hand in water at 42°C for an hour or more did not result in cessation of warm feelings. Temperature gradients should have flattened out completely by this time. Moreover, ancillary experiments with a tourniquet to control blood flow did nothing to enhance the gradient notion. Subsequently, there have been several other quite telling experiments. Hensel and Zotterman (307) recorded from temperature-sensitive fibers in the cat's tongue, and showed that a steady discharge is maintained over a long period despite the fact that the thermal situation in the tissue rapidly comes to an equilibrium. They could also stimulate the receptors, which lie close to the upper surface of the tongue, equally well from above or below. Spatial gradients must have been pretty thoroughly dissipated in both instances.

Since that demonstration, what is essentially a restatement of the gradient hypothesis was revived in a form that has been called the "ionic thermocouple theory" (379, 584). The proponents of this idea viewed the Hensel-Zotterman findings as being irrelevant because the initial temperature of the cat's tongue had been 37°C, which, being neutral, does not give a steady discharge. They believed that if a lower temperature, one that would steadily activate cold receptors, were present from the beginning, further cooling would accelerate the discharge frequency and demonstrate the thermocouple effect. The experiment was repeated by Hensel and Witt (305) with the upper tongue surface initially held at 32.3°C. In single cold fibers there was maintained a steady discharge until cold applied to the lower surface penetrated up as far as the receptors. Then there was an accelerated frequency of nerve discharge; the fibers were responding to increased intensity of stimulation. At no point was there any interruption of the cold discharge, not even when temperature changes within the tongue passed the turning point and reversed the gradient. All results were in harmony with the conclusion that the entire stimulation process was simply that of cooling and not the action of a spatial gradient.

The implications of quite a different kind of experiment are the same. Irradiation of the skin can be of two kinds: (a) infrared, which affects cutaneous tissue only to a depth of about 0.1 mm, since it is entirely absorbed within that distance; (b) microwave, which increases temperature of the skin more or less uniformly down as far as the subcutaneous fatty layer. This means that heat intensity will be substantially the same over the first 2.0 mm of transmission into the skin. Obviously, microwaves cannot set up gradients in the region containing nerve endings, whereas infrared radiation can. A direct comparison of the two would perhaps tell us something of the mechanism at work. Vendrik and Vos (585) performed the experiment, irradiating a 13-cm^2 area on the volar forearm both with 10-cm waves from a magnetron and with heat from the far infrared (a hotplate at 1000°C). Although there were individual differences in thresholds, all calculations point to there being no essential difference between the two forms of radiation so far as sensitivity of the skin is concerned. Thresholds obtained with the microwaves were comparable with those yielded by infrared at a depth in the skin of 0.3–0.5 mm, the presumed site of the receptors. The authors concluded that "a threshold sensation is obtained when the temperature of the warmth receptors is increased by a certain amount."

Adaptation, Thresholds, and Physiological Zero.   The phenomenon of adaptation, a very general one occurring in all the sense modalities, has always to be reckoned with in determining thresholds. Prior stimulation, if it is not too far removed in time, is likely to have reduced sensitivity and raised threshold values. This is the case in pressure and pain. When we come to consider adaptation in the thermal senses the situation is a bit more complicated. Adaptation is readily demonstrated for both warmth and cold. Prolonged stimulation with heat reduces warmth sensitivity (raises thresholds to heat), and prolonged cold stimulation reduces cold sensitivity (raises thresholds to cold). What complicates the situation, however, is that stimulation with heat also sensitizes the skin to cold. Adaptation to a hot stimulus brings with it an actual lowering of the cold threshold, in that temperatures which would normally result in thermal indifference or even produce mild warmth now feel cool. In like manner cold stimulation reduces the threshold for warmth; lower temperatures than are normally required arouse warmth.

The simultaneous moving of cold and warm sensitivities in response to a single condition of thermal stimulation is a fact of considerable importance. As might be anticipated, much is made of it by those who support the view that warmth and cold are simply different qualities belonging to a single "temperature sense." The analogy is drawn with color sensitivity in vision. Blue and yellow (or any other complementary pair) likewise move together; adaptation to blue builds up yellow sensitivity and vice versa. If there is this complementary relation between warmth and cold, as manifested in adaptation, there should also be an analogue of neutral gray in vision. There is. For a given area of the skin there is always some temperature representing thermal indifference. The temperature to which a response of neither warmth nor cold can be aroused is known as *physiological zero*. Assuming a normal heat equilibrium with the surrounding air and no immediate history of unusual thermal stimulation, physiological zero corresponds to the skin temperature. Thus, under these conditions, the skin over much of the exposed body surface has a temperature in the neighborhood of 32° C. This is physiological zero until warm stimulation raises it, or cold stimulation lowers it. Then it migrates temporarily to a new level. Some protected areas have normal temperatures much higher than this (36°–37° C);

some, such as the earlobe, where circulation is sluggish, normally stand at about 28° C. Gently grasp the earlobe between thumb and index finger. Ordinarily, the ear will feel cold to the fingers, the normal temperature differential being several degrees.

The concept of physiological zero is a little more complicated than has been indicated thus far. If physiological zero is to be defined as the temperature at which neither warmth nor cold will be felt, it is obviously not a point but a distance, since there exists a *neutral zone* on either side of it. Just how wide is the zone? It is not possible to answer this query in the absolute. The zone may be of the order of a few hundredths of a degree or it may be many degrees wide. The distance that must be traversed on the temperature scale is dependent on several factors. We are here raising, of course, the question of what the chief determinants of thermal thresholds are. There appear to be three: (1) the temperature at which one starts (physiological zero), for this establishes the state of adaptation; (2) the rate at which thermal change ($d\theta/dt$) is introduced in measuring thresholds; and (3) the size of the skin area involved.

Figure 12–4 shows how the first two factors interact. The data are from

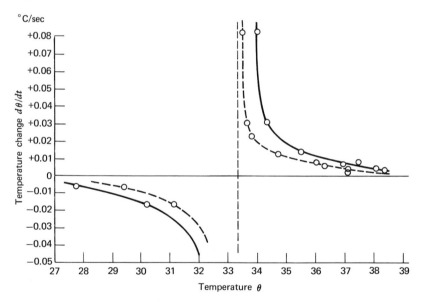

Fig. 12–4. Temperature sensitivity as related to skin temperature (θ) and rate of change of skin temperature ($d\theta/dt$). When skin temperature is far from physiological zero, threshold rate of change can be small. The dotted lines denote the first incipient change, solid lines the more conventional threshold where quality of sensation is identified. From Hensel *(298).* Courtesy of Springer-Verlag, New York.

an experiment by Hensel (*298*) in which a thermode contacted a 20-cm²
area of the forearm. Skin temperature was recorded intracutaneously by a
tiny thermocouple embedded a fraction of a millimeter below the skin
surface. Two thresholds were taken, one coming at the first detectable
change, the other at the point of clear identification of warm or cold.
Relatively precipitous changes of temperature are necessary to arouse
thermal sensation when the stimulus is close to physiological zero. At
extreme temperatures the rate can be very small. A more recent partial
repetition of this experiment (*354*) shows much the same outcome. If the
rate of addition or withdrawal of heat is small, larger deviations from skin
temperature are needed to reach threshold than if the temperature change
occurs rapidly. Something like constancy of temperature increment or
decrement is realized at rates of 0.1° C/sec and above; that is, neutral zone
width remains constant above that value, other things being equal.

The third factor affecting the width of the zone, stimulus size, raises
once more the subject of spatial summation. We encountered it first in
vision (Ricco's and Piper's Laws) but little has been said about it in
somesthesis. Pressures summate spatially; contactor size is an important
variable affecting sensitivity. The question is more moot in connection
with pain; it is only quite recently that slight areal summation of pain
has been demonstrated (*247*). However, there is no question about the
occurrence of temperature summation. An expanse of skin always feels
warmer or colder than does a small area, temperature remaining constant.
The wise mother tests the baby's bath with her elbow rather than her
finger. The facts of summation come out strongly in experiments with
both conducted and radiant heat (*353*). Figure 12–5 shows the extreme
reduction in the size of thresholds for warmth as the amount of skin
exposed is increased. Indeed, calculation shows that the formula uniting
area and intensity at thermal threshold is identical with Ricco's ancient
law: $A \times I = K$; that is, summation is perfect.

It is clear that, however sensitive the temperature receptors to thermal
stimuli impinging upon them, the sheer fact of adaptation prevents the
system from serving as a good thermometer. Where accurate temperature
judgments are required one does well to rely on the expansion and contraction of alcohol, mercury, or other substances rather than trust the
evidence of his cutaneous senses. At the same time the temperature system
of the skin is designed to preserve comfort and permit quite rapid accom-
modations to a constantly and sometimes quite rapidly changing thermal
environment. The phenomena associated with thermal adaptation will
bear looking into more intimately.

Numerous studies have been directed at adaptation rates and adaptation limits for large skin areas. A few have been concerned with puncti-

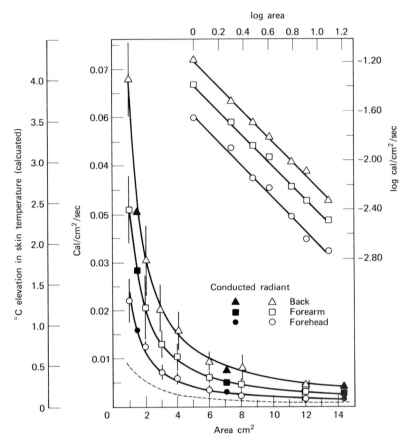

Fig. 12–5. Temperature sensation and skin area. Warm thresholds for both conducted and radiant energy on three bodily areas. In the curvilinear plot, radiant-energy values are referred to the ordinate to the immediate left (calories/ square centimeter/second); conducted-energy thresholds are referred to the "cal-culated" ordinate. The log-log plot in the upper right demonstrates the opera-tion of spatial summation for warmth. From Kenshalo, Decker, and Hamilton *(353)*. Copyright, 1967, by the American Psychological Association, and repro-duced by permission.

form stimulation. As early as 1846 Ernst Weber did the "three-bowl" experiment, perhaps inspired by John Locke's observation of a century and a half earlier *(390)* that water "... may produce the idea of cold by one hand, and of heat by the other. ..." Three containers of water at 20°,

30°, and 40° C were used. One hand was placed in the 40° water and allowed to adapt. At the same time the other hand was adapted to the 20° water. Then both hands were removed simultaneously to the 30° water where, of course, it was demonstrated that the same physical temperature can feel cold to one hand and warm to the other. Similar crude experiments can tell us a good deal about adaptation rates. The results of Hahn (257), shown in Figure 12–6, demonstrate that the course of thermal adap-

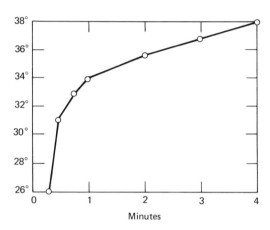

Minutes

Fig. 12–6. The course of temperature adaptation. The ordinate shows the temperatures (in degrees Centigrade) that yield the same thermal impression, to one hand kept in water at 38° C. until the time of testing, as that received by the other hand, kept in 26° C. water for the times shown on the abscissa. At the beginning of the experiment both hands were adapted to 38° C. From Woodworth (650) after Hahn (257).

tation, like all similar processes, proceeds in accordance with a negatively accelerated curve. These experiments were performed by simple immersion of the two hands in baths of varying temperatures and for various adapting periods, judgments of equality of cold sensations being required of the subject. At the end of 4 min (following an initial adaptation period of 5 min at 38° C for both hands) adaptation appears to be complete in that 38° feels the same to the right hand as 26° does to the left. Both are thermally indifferent.

Will all temperatures, however high or low, similarly induce complete adaptation, that is, will they all appear to fade out totally if stimulation is continued long enough? The uniform finding is that, for areal stimulation, extremes of temperature never proceed to complete adaptation. There is considerable blunting or dulling of the sensation but never total cessation. Hold the hand in chilled water at 10° C and, so long as the temperature of the medium remains constant, cold sensations will persist indefinitely. The same lack of complete adaptation is found for temperatures of the order of 45° C. Warmth never quite completely disappears. The zone within which total obliteration of thermal sensation can be produced through adaptation is usually put at 16° to 42° C. Within this range moderate temperatures reach physiological zero relatively rapidly, while higher and lower temperatures require longer to disappear.

Not all investigators have been in agreement about the upper and lower bounds of complete adaptation. The history of the problem, in general, is that there has been a progressive shrinkage of the range within which thermal sensation will fade out as techniques for the measurement of adaptation have been improved. The earliest studies found cold sensation to adapt out completely as far down as 5° C and warm sensation to do so as far up as 45° C. Subsequent experiments, conducted by the apparently straightforward procedure of keeping the warmth or cold under continuous observation for long periods of time while the adapting

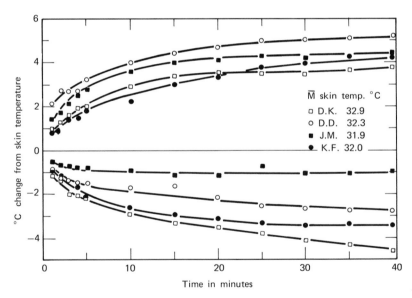

Fig. 12–7. The course of temperature adaptation. Each plotted point, the mean of four observations, indicates the amount by which the observer found it necessary to change the temperature stimulator from the initial skin temperature to maintain a just-detectable warm or cool sensation. Initial skin temperatures for the four observers are shown at the right. From Kenshalo and Scott (356). Copyright 1966 by the American Association for the Advancement of Science.

temperature was being held constant, tended to bring the lower limit up to 15–18° C and the upper limit down to 40–42° C. But there are difficulties with this technique, especially those of sustaining attention for observational periods of a half hour or more and picking a clear-cut endpoint of the fading-out process. An improvement would seem to be to "track" threshold throughout the adapting period, much as is done in testing hearing with the Békésy audiometer, that is, taking periodic measurements by the psychophysical method of average error, the experimenter occasionally upsetting the stimulus control in the interest of keeping the observer alert.

The negatively accelerated curves of Figure 12–7 depict the results of such an experiment. Threshold was tracked for 40 min, settings being obtained every minute during the early part of the course and every five minutes as the adaptation rate slowed. Two features are notable in the results: (a) the relatively narrow temperature range over which adaptation goes to completion, and (b) the large individual differences accompanied, however, by high precision of measurement. Each observer quite consistently remained on his trajectory. Apparently, complete adaptation can produce a zone of thermal indifference no larger than 8° wide, roughly from 29° to 37° C.

If there is some failure of adaptation to go to completion in the case of extreme temperatures and areal stimulation, there appears to be none where punctiform stimuli are concerned. Warm and cold spots have been subjected to continuous exposure to a wide range of temperatures (27, 381, 332) and, in all instances, complete adaptation has resulted. At extreme temperatures that would fail to extinguish sensation, were they applied to a large areal surface, local stimulation (1.00–1.25 mm diameter) produces total disappearance in a matter of seconds. The course of the fading-out process is generally observed to be an undulating or discontinuous one, especially in the case of warm spots. Adaptation times seem to be less related to the temperature of the stimulus than to the absolute sensitivity of the spot, the initially more responsive spots requiring longer to adapt. Moreover, the aftereffects are relatively prolonged and apparently cumulative. A recovery period at least equal to the adaptation time is required to bring the spots back to normal threshold. This factor is, of course, a complicating one in experiments involving serial exploration of spots with temperature stimulators.

Paradoxical Cold and "Heat."   In 1895 von Frey made a singular discovery with respect to the behavior of cold spots. He noted that spots previously identified as sensitive to cold would, on occasion, respond with cold sensations if touched with a very warm (45°–50° C) stimulus. Since it seemed paradoxical that a hot stimulus would yield impressions of cold, the phenomenon was named "paradoxical cold." The range of temperatures adequate for the arousal of paradoxical cold is, of course, well above that necessary to arouse warm spots and only a little below that needed to produce thermal pain. The latter normally has a threshold in the neighborhood of 52° C.

Paradoxical sensations of cold are encountered commonly enough in the mapping of warm spots. Cold sensations in response to other types of stimuli are occasionally found also. Thus the movement of a hair may elicit "flashes of cold." Alternating currents of low frequency applied to the skin by relatively confined electrodes may produce "cold vibration" (233). The fact that cold feelings result from the stimulation of a cold spot, whatever the nature of the effective stimulus, was regarded by von Frey and, indeed, by the vast majority of current theorists as the best possible evidence in support of Johannes Müller's doctrine of "specific nerve energies" and of the clear separation of warmth and cold as qualities belonging to two distinct cutaneous senses.

An analogous phenomenon to paradoxical cold, "paradoxical warmth," is alleged to occur, though even its co-discoverers (Rubin and Goldscheider, in 1912) specified radically different conditions for its arousal. Rubin believed faint warmth could be called forth by stimuli just below (0.1°–1.5° C) skin temperature. Goldscheider gave 6°–10° C below physiological zero as the temperature range necessary to paradoxical warmth. The fact seems to be that, if it is a genuine effect at all, the necessary and sufficient conditions have yet to be established. Many have sought it; few have ever reported finding it. In his long series of experiments Bazett reports with conviction on paradoxical warmth only once (37). Gilmer states (233, p. 324), "Out of a total of approximately 13,000 cold stimulations in this experiment only one report of paradoxical warmth was made. Repeated stimulation of this one spot on several different days failed to bring about another report of the experience." Since warmth, like cold, may occasionally be evoked by mechanical means the suspicion is strong that it is the mechanical rather than the thermal component of the stimulus that is responsible.

An effect presumably dependent on paradoxical cold for its occurrence is that known as psychological "heat." Although the designation is perhaps an unfortunate one, the word "heat" having a common physical meaning, there is no doubt that the phenomenon it refers to is a very real one in experience. The simplest condition for the perception of "heat" is provided by an areal stimulus between 45° and 50° C applied to a region, such as the forehead or arm, having good warm and cold sensitivity. Under these circumstances there should be aroused warmth (the normal response of warm spots) and in addition cold (paradoxical cold from cold spots). The two sensations fuse to produce an overall impression of intense "heat." To most observers the salient feature of the experience is a stinging quality added to the thermal background.

If psychological heat is indeed a fusion or mixture of warmth and cold sensations it should be possible to produce the effect synthetically, for all that is needed is simultaneous stimulation of warmth and cold (without depending on the latter's paradoxical arousal) in the same general cutaneous area. The experiment is made with the "heat grill" (see Figure 12–8), which provides the specified conditions. One alternate set of tubes gives

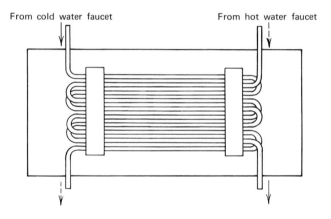

From cold water faucet   From hot water faucet

Fig. 12–8.   The "heat" grill. Warm water and cold water flow through alternate tubes. If a broad skin area, such as the underside of the forearm, is placed firmly on the grill "psychological heat" may be synthesized from mild warmth and cold. From Munn's *Laboratory manual in general experimental psychology*. Boston: Houghton Mifflin, 1948. With the publisher's permission.

a cold stimulus (12°–15° C), while the other is warm (42°–44° C). Although there is nothing really physically "hot" about the grill, the first impression on placing the arm on it is that it actually is dangerously so, and the uninitiated will quickly withdraw to avoid being burned.

This synthesis of psychological heat seems to bear out the analysis. "Heat" is compounded of warmth and cold. Whether it is a stable compound, so to speak, has been debated in what is by now a somewhat involved literature. To some, heat has seemed to be a complete fusion, a new quality which resembles neither warmth nor cold, just as gray is a fusion resembling neither the blue nor yellow of which it may be compounded. Others have viewed it as an imperfect fusion, in which warmth and cold are intermingled with heat. The visual analogy for this would be orange which, while neither red nor yellow, resembles both. Perhaps the most interesting result of experiments on synthetic heat has been the demonstration by Alston (*17*) that the stinging heat quality can be produced by simultaneous stimulation of a single cold spot (with cold) and a single warm spot (with warmth). The synthetic perception of heat occurs even though the two spots are separated by as much as 15 cm. This fact, as we shall see, is not easy to accommodate in theory.

The Classical Theory of Temperature Sensitivity.   As with pressure and pain, there exists no absolute certainty as to the identity of the end organs responsible for warm and cold sensations. There is no dearth of hypotheses, however, and we are led at once to the realm of theory to build up a picture of how the temperature senses operate. The classic theory is von Frey's. It is that warmth and cold are separately mediated, each having its own set of nerve fibers specific to the quality in question and each system having its own specialized receptor organs. The Krause end bulb is the receptor for cold; the deeper-lying Ruffini cylinder is the end organ for warmth.

The correlations hypothesized by von Frey have never been established as incontrovertible fact. As Dallenbach has pointed out (*139*), "Von Frey was duly cautious and conservative in stating his theory. He said, 'the end-bulbs are probably for that reason the organs of cold sensation'; 'there appears to me a probable correlation between Ruffini's end-organs and the sense of warmth.' He was, moreover, straightforward in pointing out the defects and weaknesses of his theory. . . . The further we get away from von Frey the more dogmatic in general become the statements regarding his correlation. The writers of textbooks during the first decade following the formulation of the theory were reserved in their statements concerning it, in the next decade they were less so, and during the past decade [1920–1930] the writers have very frequently given the correlation as established fact." In general, Dallenbach's remarks could be extrapolated into the following four decades. Meanwhile, there have been both strengthening and weakening experimental evidences and the appearance on the scene of a rival theory.

This virtue must be attributed to von Frey's theory (or the more dogmatic restatements of his theory): it is specific enough to have served as a powerful stimulus to experimental investigation. In the light of it several important studies were directed at testing the assumed correlations. Perhaps the most spectacular were those of Strughold and Karbe (*563*). They first amassed considerable presumptive evidence that the Krause end bulb was indeed the receptor organ for cold, finding that: (a) areas of the surface of the eye most sensitive to cold also showed, in anatomical studies, the greatest concentration of Krause end bulbs; (b) cold thresholds were low where end bulbs characteristically lay near the surface, and vice versa; and (c) the count of cold spots was in good agreement with the end-bulb counts made histologically. Their next step was to embark on an experiment in which they undertook, in three subjects, to produce vital staining of the eye. They used an aqueous solution of methylene blue, which has a strong affinity for nervous tissue, and continued to apply it to the surface of the eye at intervals until 1.5 to 2.0 mg had been used. Observation of the sclera with a corneal microscope and slit lamp revealed the successful staining, after several hours, of two end bulbs in one experiment and a group of four in another, while only nerve fibrils responded to the stain in the third. No cold responses could be aroused at the time of staining and, whereas the coloring faded out fairly rapidly, a generally anesthetic condition remained for some time. With a view to future exploration detailed maps were made to serve as guides. Three days after the application of the dye, cold stimuli (tiny wire cylinders, with a round bead at one end) produced weak responses. However, "after 8–10 days there were aroused in the previously marked places clear sensations of cold, while their nearest neighbors proved to be anesthetic or numb." Naturally, Strughold and Karbe concluded that the Krause end bulb was the cold receptor.

Another set of experiments upholding the von Frey correlations is that of Bazett, McGlone, Williams, and Lufkin (*38a*), previously described as the "prepuce experiments." Here the conclusions have to be less direct, since they depend solely on determinations of the population density of cold and warm spots, the calculated depths of the receptors, and histological studies of comparable tissue samples. For cold, the number of spots was found to be 6 to 12 per square centimeter and the depth to be 0.1 mm. About 15 end bulbs of the Krause type per square centimeter were found to be distributed at a depth of about 0.1 mm, just below the arteriovenous region immediately under the papillae. For warmth, the concentration of spots was found to be about 1 per square centimeter, with the receptor lying at a calculated depth of 0.3 mm or a little more. The histological results placed Ruffini cylinders at a depth of about 0.28 mm. Their distribution in the prepuce agreed fairly well with the warm spot count. Bazett's conclusion is constrained, despite the close agreements found. He states (*36*): "The special receptors for cold and warmth have received provisional, though not absolute, identification."

Other attempts to correlate structure and function have been, in the main, entirely disappointing. Excision experiments extend back to 1885, when Donaldson charted warm and cold spots, extirpated the tissue, and made a histological examination of it. "There were numerous nerves beneath these spots, but these were almost as numerous in neighboring parts. The result . . . is completely negative" (170). Häggqvist, in 1913 (256), similarly found no special end bodies. He did report bundles of smooth muscle tissue under cold spots, a finding which has never been confirmed by anyone since. Pendleton, in 1926 (461), excised tissue at carefully located cold spots; he found nothing of note in the tissue examinations. Dallenbach, in 1927 (138), plotted and replotted warm and cold spots, meticulously controlling for a number of the usually disturbing variables and getting in consequence good test-retest reliabilities. The mapped tissue was then extirpated, incisions being made to a depth of 3 mm, and prepared for histological study. Methylene blue was used as the staining agent. Not a single specialized end organ of any kind was found, though there were numerous nerve fibers and undifferentiated nerve terminations.

Somewhat more encouraging results, from the viewpoint of adherents of the classical theory, came out of the experiments of Belonoschkin in 1933 (62). He charted the cold sensitivity of female breast tissue about to be removed for carcinoma and postoperatively searched for nerve endings. Bielschowsky's silver stain was used. In the region of the nipple, where cold sensitivity is such as to present a practically continuous surface of high responsiveness, individual "spots" not being discriminable, nerve terminations were discovered in great profusion. In an area of 160 mm^2 more than 100 end bodies were present. The commonest had a form resembling the Krause end bulb. However, a diversity of other structures existed also. Simple terminal networks were of frequent occurrence. Other types of specialized endings were identifiable. So many variations appeared, in fact, that Belonoschkin found it useful "not to distinguish between them according to their customary designations but simply to speak of them as encapsulated and non-encapsulated nerve end-bodies." We saw earlier, in our general consideration of the nervous apparatus of the skin, that this view is gaining currency with histologists.

Now, with the major evidences before us, what shall we say of the adequacy of the classical theory of temperature sensitivity? It is clear that it leaves much to be desired. Resting as it does chiefly upon an assumed correlation between distribution of sensitivity and distribution of end organs, it cannot be said to be in a firm position so long as equally well-performed experiments point to diametrically opposed conclusions with respect to that correlation. As matters now stand we shall have to suspend judgment. Krause end bulbs and Ruffini cylinders may eventually prove to be specialized receptors for cold and warmth. That they are *the* receptors is far from having been established. On the basis of certain of the findings one might as readily conclude for free nerve endings as temperature organs, and yet, as has been seen, both pressure and pain can make some legitimate claims to these also. There is obviously much more to be learned before any of the systems of cutaneous sensitivity can be unequivocally assigned to a particular type of receptor organ.

If much uncertainty exists about the receptor organs responsible for warmth and cold there is somewhat less concerning the nerve fibers that carry the messages. Since the advent of refined neurophysiological techniques there has been a veritable plethora of studies directed at the identification of temperature fibers. The effort is, of course, part of a larger attack on the functional architecture of the nervous system begun with the classical experiments of Gasser and Erlanger. This work, for which they were awarded the Nobel prize in 1944, established the dependence of nerve fiber conduction velocity and spike amplitude on fiber size and permitted a certain amount of analysis of the behavior of individual fibers in complex nerve bundles. We cannot go into the intricate history of designations of fiber groups, often puzzling and somewhat arbi-

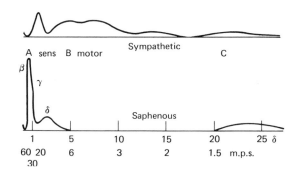

Fig. 12–9. Action potentials of two kinds of nerve. The sympathetic (top) is a mixed sensorimotor nerve and, while it lacks some of the components found in the saphenous (below), it has B (motor) fibers. The saphenous is a sensory nerve (no B fibers) and shows several elevations of the A wave. Both nerves contain large, rapidly-conducting A fibers, and both have slowly-conducting, nonmyelinated C fibers. From Bishop *(72)*. Courtesy of the Williams and Wilkins Co.

trary in any case, beyond indicating the general character of the compound action potential and its anatomical substrate. Figure 12–9 shows the electrical changes in two kinds of fibers of the cat, one the sympathetic nerve, a mixed sensorimotor bundle, the other the saphenous nerve, often regarded as a kind of standard afferent preparation because of the wide spectrum of fiber sizes, ranging from 17μ A fibers down to 1μ C fibers. The diagram is taken from Bishop's highly significant paper (72), which should also be consulted for an interesting view of the relation between somesthetic modality and fiber size.

As we have seen in other contexts, the larger the nerve fiber the more rapid the conduction rate ($v = kD$, for myelinated fibers; $v = \sqrt{D}$, for unmyelinated ones); also, the larger the fiber the lower its threshold to electrical stimulation. Cutaneous nerve bundles, which do not have fibers of the B class—these are always motor—typically have several groupings of discharges in their spectra: the prominent spike comprising the beta wave, which is ordinarily blended with a relatively inconspicuous alpha, and several "afterdischarges," minor modes of the action potential curve, each attributable to the more slowly conducting, smaller-diameter fibers. The prominent peaks are the delta elevation of A and the very much delayed C wave. The latter, of course, brings up the rear of the procession because it has the slowest rate of propagation, well under 5 m/sec as compared with 100 m/sec for the largest A fibers.

The evidence now seems relatively clear that both the delta group of the A fibers and C fibers mediate temperature sensations. They apparently also conduct messages in the touch-pressure category. And we saw, in the last chapter, that they are presumably responsible for first and second pain! Many have raised the question, quite naturally, about the possibility that "first" and "second" pressure and temperature also exist. Although the observational data do not directly encourage this kind of thinking, there are many evidences from studies of experimental nerve block and pathological states of feeling that do. Viewed in the large, the fact that all major somesthetic sensations: pressure, pain, cold, and warm, break up into two neural groupings, all four modalities being mediated by the smaller of the A fibers and all represented in the firing of C fibers, is probably best interpreted as the work of two systems, an old one and a new one, phylogenetically speaking, as indeed Bishop has urged (72).

The evidence favoring classical specificity theory would seem to have been considerably bolstered by much of the work done from 1951 to 1970 on single-fiber responses to cold and warm stimuli, though not all experimental findings during this period unequivocally point in this direction. To deal with the apparent exceptions first, several investigators have found fibers that respond both to mechanical pressure and to temperature changes, thus seeming to imply a lack of specificity. Douglas and Ritchie (172) conclude that the majority of C fibers are sensitive to both mechanical and thermal influences. Wall (598) found such double sensitivity to be not unusual in the smaller fibers entering the cord. Indeed, the very first investigation that concerned itself exclusively with afferent activity in C fibers (405) found some units responding only to mechanical stimulation, others to thermal stimuli, and still others to both. Iggo (326) isolated single C-fiber preparations in mammalian cutaneous nerves and, while he found many fibers that would answer only to mechanical stimulation, there were also others that would give discharges both to mechanical displacement and to thermal changes, if the latter were sufficiently extreme ($\pm$ 10° C). However, Iggo thought, and others have subsequently concurred in the conclusion, that it was probably pain, not temperature, that was being aroused by such large temperature shifts. But the common property of C fibers that renders them sensitive to two classes of stimuli, mechanical and thermal, is the feature that all biological tissues possess; that is, they are subject to functional changes when the thermal medium in which they operate is altered. Nerve discharge, like other physiological phenomena, has a temperature coefficient.

However, not all testimony is this indirect. It was demonstrated by Hensel, Zotterman, Dodt, and others, in an important series of experiments (307, 167, 303, 327) that there are fibers that will respond with a steady discharge to a fixed temperature. To classify a receptor as selective for cold stimuli, for example, Hensel has proposed (299, p. 287) that it meet the following specifications: (a) show a steady discharge that is clearly related to temperature; (b) display a frequency rise on cooling; (c) give no response to warming, if initially silent, or diminish its response, if active at the time; and (d) fail to respond to mechanical stimulation. Beyond this, "the electrophysiological findings should be in agreement with behavioural responses, thermoregulatory reflexes, and with temperature sense in man." Comparable requirements are placed on fibers for warmth.

Both warm and cold units meeting these specifications were found quite early among the A fibers supplying the tongues of dogs and cats. Then, as techniques for their quantitative investigation were developed, some C fibers began to meet the requirements. Now, it seems quite clear that there are both warm and cold fibers in both A and C groups. Figure 12–10 shows profiles for three individual C fibers, one responsive to warming, two to cooling. There are obviously individual differences among fibers and one will hardly know what impulse frequencies are to be regarded as typical until many species and nerve preparations within them have been charted. In single warm units from the cat's muzzle a steady discharge can be gotten to stationary temperatures in the wide range of 30° to 48° C, with a maximum between 45° and 47° (302). Raising temperature still higher brings about a sudden cessation of nerve response. A grad-

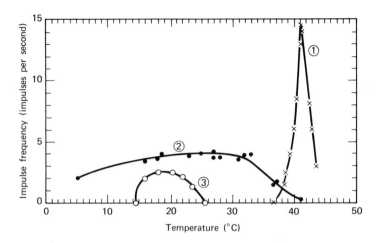

Fig. 12–10. Steady discharge frequencies of three selected fibers. No. 1 is excited by warming, Nos. 2 and 3 by cooling. Note the temperature range in which each operates. From Hensel, Iggo, and Witt (*303*).

ual reduction of temperature simply reduces discharge frequency, but sudden cooling, of course, brings with it prompt inhibition of response. In the rhesus monkey's saphenous and radial nerves, fibers were found that responded with frequencies up to 20 impulses/sec in the 40° to 44° C range. Higher temperature not only reduced frequency but caused impulses to be delivered irregularly or in short bursts (*300*).

As Sinclair has correctly urged (*527*, pp. 101–113), it is one thing to search for and find *stimulus* specificity of the kind we have been discussing, and quite another to find *sensation* specificity. Experiments on dogs, cats, and monkeys can serve the first purpose, not the second. Presumably, suitable experiments on humans could. For obvious reasons, there have not been many. Three widely differing studies, each vivid in its own way, bear especially on the question of fiber size and human pain (*288, 460, 124*); only one, the Hensel-Boman experiment (*301*), tells us anything about temperature sensitivity, and it can give no correlation with sensation quality or intensity, for the pathway to the central nervous system was cut and only the nerve record could speak for the subject. Seven volunteers in the Physiological Institute at Marburg, Germany, agreed to have the superficial branch of the radial nerve in the arm cut. This was done under general anesthesia, a 3-cm slit being made in the lower forearm to expose the nerve. A small bundle of fibers having been selected on the basis of its receptive field, which was revealed by weak electric shocks referred to the hand, the nerve was severed at a point proximal to the recording site. Except for a burning pain of a few seconds' duration at the moment of cutting, there was no discomfort to the subject, and he remained conscious throughout the period of several hours necessary to complete the experiment.

Altogether, 11 single-fiber preparations were found that would respond only to mechanical pressure at the hand. These were unaffected by warming or cooling. An interesting feature of the stimulation process was that the amount of pressure needed to arouse a single impulse in the nerve was precisely that required to reach touch threshold on a nearby "normal" skin area. Four fibers were found that yielded positive responses to both pressure and cold. In the absence of either they gave a steady spontaneous discharge; either pressure or cold would raise the discharge frequency.

Only a single fiber was encountered that met the specifications for a temperature unit; this was an A fiber that responded to cooling and only to cooling. Dropping temperature in the stimulating thermode increased discharge frequency; increasing temperature brought about a prompt inhibition of the discharge. Figure 12–11 shows a sequence of cooling

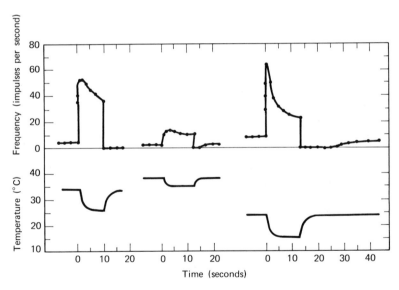

Fig. 12–11. Variations in impulse frequency in a single A fiber that responded to cooling and only to cooling. Discharge frequencies are shown above, temperature changes that produced them below. From Herbert Hensel and Kurt K. A. Boman. Afferent impulses in cutaneous sensory nerves in human subjects. *J. Neurophysiol.* 23: 564–578, 1960.

and rewarming from different initial temperatures and the nerve impulse frequency that accompanied each phase. By any definition, this appears to be a cold fiber.

The Neurovascular Theory.   The chief rival to von Frey's formulation is Nafe's neurovascular theory, first elaborated in the early 1930s and the subject of much discussion and no little controversy since then. Taking as a primary consideration the essential intimacy of relation between warmth and cold, forming as they do a single continuum passing through physiological zero, Nafe looked for one mechanism that might be responsible for both kinds of sensitivity. The only adequately distributed tissue which, moreover, might contain sensory nerve endings capable of generating impulses for temperature sensations he believed to be the smooth muscle walls of the blood vessels of the skin. As we know, the smallest of these extend to the upper reaches of the corium, vascular loops being common inhabitants of the papillae. Capillaries would seem not to be candidates; they are nonmuscular and are not supplied with sensory nerves. Venules are possibilities but appear not to have a sufficiently rich innervation to serve the purpose. The arterioles, then, are likely prospects. These and the smaller arteries house in their smooth muscle walls (at least in the outermost layers, the *adventitia* and *tunica media*) both afferent and efferent nerve terminations. Sensory termini in the forms of free nerve endings, button like endings, and terminal loops are found. They can be traced chiefly to relatively large myelinated fibers, though some have small myelinated and unmyelinated parent fibers. It should be noted that Millen, who has made a detailed anatomical study of the innervation of blood vessels both in the rabbit's ear and the richly vascularized stomach wall, states: "In none of the materials examined were fibers observed to end *directly* on the smooth muscle fibers of the arterioles" (*418*, p. 74). This does not necessarily mean that such nerve fibers are not stimulable. Contraction and relaxation of arteriolar walls could set up trains of impulses which, at the brain, could say "warm" or "cold." Temperature sensations are then, under this theory, kinesthetic sensations; they are proprioceptions of arteriolar movements.

The direct responses of smooth muscle tissue to thermal changes are such as to suggest that the correlations of movement and sensation necessary to a neurovascular theory of temperature sensitivity are possible. Nafe cited Sir Thomas Lewis as having shown (*383*) that denervated smooth muscle tissue responds directly to warmth by relaxation, to cold by contraction. These are then the assumed correlations. In response to a warm stimulus the arterioles dilate because their smooth muscle walls relax. Cold produces contraction of the arteriolar walls and constriction of the vessels. The pattern of nerve impulses created by relaxation (providing it is rapid enough) is interpreted as warmth; that produced by contraction is interpreted as cold (again, assuming the contraction to be vigorous enough).

Nafe also saw in the reactions of smooth muscle to relatively extreme temperatures the possible bases for "heat" and for thermally aroused pain. Table 12–2 reproduces his assumptions with respect to the action of

Table 12–2.   The Correlations Assumed by Nafe's Neurovascular Theory

Experience	Temperature (°C)	Action of Smooth Muscle
Pain		Spastic contraction
	52	
Heat	45	Constricting elements in dilating muscle
Warm		Relaxation
Zero	33	Physiological zero
Cold		Contraction
	12	
"Cold heat"		Muscle elements showing severe constriction in general contraction
	3	
Pain		Spastic contraction

After J. P. Nafe (439), p. 1055.

smooth muscle at different temperatures and the accompanying sensory events.

It is to be noted that "heat," with its pricking quality, is assumed to result from the complete constriction of scattered muscle elements in a general background of relaxation. Presumably those elements having the highest contractibility introduce the painful note. This happens normally just above 45° C. At about 52° C all or nearly all elements have constricted maximally, and pain alone is felt. "Cold heat" and the pain associated with extremely low temperatures are analogous occurrences at the other end of the scale. Here, however, the constricting elements superpose their effects on a general background of contraction. The essential continuity of the warm-cold series and the further continuity with heat-pain and cold-pain must be counted as strong supporting considerations for the neurovascular theory.

Several other temperature phenomena find ready interpretation within the framework of the theory. The shift of physiological zero with temperature adaptation and the resulting changes in warm and cold thresholds speak most strongly for a theory based on a single underlying mechanism. The occurrence of warm and cold sensations, reflexly aroused through vasomotor action as in the case of chills during fever, finds ready interpretation and may well constitute one of the best lines of evidence favoring the neurovascular theory. This would be true, of course, of any temperature theory that recognized the importance of blood vessels in the general temperature economy of the skin. The failure of high test-retest reliabilities to appear in the mapping of temperature spots—what we have spoken of as the "fickleness" of warm and cold spots—finds some accountability in the neurovascular theory. The shifting of responsive points may result from changes in state of tonus of the blood vessels. They are known to have their contractile state altered by blood pressure changes, variations in blood content, and other autonomous and reflex effects, including emotional reactions. The observational properties of warmth and cold also "make sense" in terms of the theory. Cold ordinarily puts in its appearance in an abrupt, clear, and well-defined manner, whereas warmth is more gentle in its mode of occurrence, "welling up" rather than "flashing out." Arteriolar contractions are more prompt and definite responses than dilatations. Even paradoxical cold produces no embarrassment for the theory. Smooth muscle is known to respond to intense stimuli with contraction, especially if the stimulus has a mechanical component, and it has been chiefly in connection with very warm thermal-mechanical stimulation that paradoxical cold is most commonly reported.

Not all is clear sailing for the neurovascular theory, however. Some serious objections may be urged against it. One wonders first about the obvious facts of relative distribution of warmth and cold. If the same underlying mechanism is responsible for both, why should the two have such radically different distributions? Why are there so many more cold spots than warm spots? Why do maps of the former yield so many discrete points as compared with the latter, and why do not warm spot maps fit exactly over those for cold? Moreover, if they are generated by impulses passing over the same fibers and constitute products of one and the same mechanism, why do not cold and warmth have similarities in observation? Why do not cold and warmth feel alike? If they are both basically kinesthetic in origin there should be some resemblances in their felt patterns, and yet they seem to be characterized more by a sharp qualitative difference than by similarity. Why are the intensities of warm and cold sensations differently related to stimulus temperature? In magnitude estimation experiments quite different exponents of the power function have been found: 1.0 for cold; 1.6 for warmth (545). Whereas the full meaning of the power function slope is not as yet clear, such a result would seem to imply two different mechanisms underlying the appreciation of warmth and cold.

A number of other established facts find no ready explanation in the neurovascular theory. Why should an increase in concomitant pressure bring with it an increase in number of warmth responses, as found by Heiser and McNair (290)? One would suppose that either heat or paradoxical cold would result, since the direct action of mechanical stimuli on relaxed smooth muscle tissue is to produce contraction. Why is the two-point limen, the separation of two punctiform stimuli that can just be discriminated as two, larger for warmth than for cold, and why is the normal error of localization for warmth greater than for cold? A mechanism common to warmth and cold should not produce differences of this sort. Why are the facts of intermittent stimulation with radiant heat as they are? It has been shown that a "critical fusion point" for radiant heat can be established; discrete and temporally equally spaced warm stimuli yield a continuous feeling of warmth when repeated every half-second or thereabouts. Picturing the direct responses of arterioles to such a mode of stimulation, one would suppose that a typical summation of smooth muscle responses might ensue and that the effect of such repeated stimuli might be tetanus (heat, then heat-pain?) or, at least, alternation of relaxation and contraction (alternate warmth and cold). How account for the findings of Alston (17) with respect to the generation of the heat experience from single warm and cold spots separated by as much as 10 or 15 cm? There is hardly provided a "general body of relaxation" within which constricting elements can operate, as demanded by the theory.

Many of the foregoing objections to the neurovascular theory deal with minutiae, of course, and it should be hastily added that the classical theory of temperature does no better with them. However, a completely satisfactory theory must deal with them. The basic difficulty with the neurovascular theory seems to be that, invoking as it does a complex and as yet only poorly understood mechanism, it both predicts too little and too much. One can find in the physiological literature of smooth muscle responses instances of nearly every kind of reaction. Thus, for example, although a strong mechanical stimulus produces sudden contraction of relaxed smooth muscle, such a stimulus, applied to partially contracted muscle, may produce a sudden relaxation. Why should not paradoxical warmth occur commonly and predictably, then? These are the necessary conditions for it. Other instances of unrealized predictions could be cited.

It is yet too early to attempt a final evaluation of the neurovascular theory. That it possesses both virtues and defects is apparent from the foregoing. In general, it meets the requirements of a good theory in that it comes into harmony with a fair share of the established facts in the temperature realm and it is, moreover, eminently testable. What is needed is serious investigation conducted in the light of it. Until much more is known about the reactions of arterioles in situ and of the correlations between their responses and sensitivity changes we shall not be in a position to decide whether blood vessels play a primary role or only a supporting one in temperature reception.

Temperature Sensitivity and the Cornea.   When, in the last chapter, we were asking what role the cornea of the eye might play to help identify the nerve endings responsible for pain sensitivity, we observed that there is good evidence for concluding that the bare endings of the cornea can mediate pressure sensations as well as pain. Indeed, we saw that some authorities (e.g., *612*) believe that the full range of somesthetic qualities may be called forth from the cornea if only stimuli appropriate to them are applied. Cold and warm are included, of course. Now, in connection with the evaluation of temperature theories, the question of the thermal sensitivity of corneal tissue becomes important, if not crucial.

What are the facts? It would be satisfying to be in a position to conclude that they stand out clearly for all the world to see. Actually, there is much disagreement among investigators and there are many pseudofacts to confound the unwary. Lele and Weddell (*378*), reviewing the literature of corneal sensibility in 1956, found 37 papers between 1878 and 1952 touching on the subject and three others, spanning a half century, that attempted to provide critical reviews. There was no disagreement whatever about pain; all evidences agree that it is the cornea's primary modality. If von Frey and his students are exempted—they invariably reiterated their belief that only pain could be aroused in the cornea proper—there was nearly complete agreement that touch or pressure could also be mediated by the cornea. What of cold and warm? Well over half the studies failed to investigate one or both. Of the remainder, about half had found for one or another form of temperature sensitivity, the other half had found against it.

But issues of this kind are rarely settled by the democratic procedure of taking a vote, and they shouldn't be, of course. The simple fact is that no investigator had ever replicated exactly the apparatus and procedure of another. There was thus no basis for comparison of results. Lele and Weddell, recognizing this, made an effort to account for past failures to find corneal thermal sensitivity, which they themselves found in abundance, by side experiments that left something to be desired.

Since then, there have been several new experiments but little progress toward univocality. Kenshalo (*351*), taking a leaf out of the Lele-Weddell book and using the bulb of a thermometer as a thermal stimulator, found the cornea responsive to both heating and cooling but interpreted his observers' reports as having no bearing on temperature sensations; instead, the patterns created were better characterized as "irritation" and generically related to pressure. Thermal sensitivity was also found to be higher in the forehead, lips, and conjunctiva of the eye than in the cornea. Dawson (154), in a meticulously conducted study of afferent impulses in the long ciliary nerve leading from the cornea and iris of the cat, demonstrated beyond any doubt that both increments and decrements of heat can be transduced by corneal nerve endings (though never both from the same fiber). Dawson (154, p. 208) performed the interesting service of juxtaposing the various studies in disagreement about corneal sensibility and concluding, as perhaps one must, that the major difference has to do with stimulator size. Small contactors (3 mm or less; von Frey, Nafe and Wagoner, Kenshalo), having low heat capacity and representing a minimum of spatial summation in the nerve network, give only pressure or pain. Large contactors (6 mm or more; Lele and Weddell, Sergeev [517]), capitalize on the deficiencies of smaller ones and evoke temperature sensations. This seems almost too simple a conclusion; it could easily be wrong. What is evidently needed is a more precise analysis of heat interchanges in and around the cornea during thermal stimulation. Some ground rules also need to be established concerning descriptive terms for thermal sensations when aroused at extraordinary sites, and this may easily be the more difficult of the two tasks.

13
Kinesthetic and
Organic Sensibilities

"Deep" Sensibility and Kinesthesis. All receptor systems thus far considered—those for vision, hearing, and the cutaneous senses—may be classed, according to the scheme introduced by Sherrington (*523*) long ago, as *exteroceptors*. All sense organs belonging to this class are stimulated from without the body and provide knowledge of events external to it. The chemical senses, smell and taste, likewise belong in the exteroceptive category. Many internal bodily changes also have their effects on receptor organs and result in sensation. These organs are the *interoceptors* and have as their receptive field the gastrointestinal tract. We shall encounter them later as the mediators of the so-called "organic" sensations.

Between the outer and inner bodily surfaces there exist other sense organs—in subcutaneous tissues, in the walls of deep-lying blood vessels, in muscles and tendons, in the coverings of bones (periosteum), and at the articulations of bones. Because these receptors are stimulated mainly by actions of the body itself they are called *proprioceptors*. This class of sense organs also includes, according to the original classification of Sherrington, the very special receptor system which is located in the nonauditory labyrinth of the inner ear and which, through the generation of an elaborate set of postural reflexes, is responsible for the maintenance of general bodily equilibrium.

Separate study of the receptors lying between the outer and inner walls of the body is not easy to arrange, and there is consequently something of a dearth of reliable information concerning them. If they are stimulated in their normal surroundings other tissues containing responsive nerve terminations are necessarily involved, thus producing confusion in experience. If they are investigated in physiological preparations the data are then restricted to electrophysiological indications, and the picture of the sensory process is only indirectly obtained and quite incom-

376

plete. Of course, it is possible to approach certain of the deep-lying receptor systems by way of the body surface, eliminating either by anesthetization or surgery the contributions of the purely cutaneous nervous components. This was what was done by Goldscheider in a series of experiments in which he investigated deep pressures and pains after dulling the overlying skin with cocaine. This was also what was done by Henry Head and a succession of researchers who repeated his experiment of dividing the median cutaneous nerve and rendering anesthetic a substantial area of the forearm and hand (see pp. 335–336).

It was, in fact, in connection with Head's original work that the designation "deep sensibility" first came into being. Upon severing the nerve and testing in the center of the affected skin area he found that, whereas light pressure, needle prick, and temperature stimuli aroused no response, heavy pressure evoked a deeply localized feeling of dull pressure which, if increased in intensity, passed over into dull pain. Presumably subcutaneous nerve endings were being stimulated. Just how deeply situated they were it would be important to know. Head believed them to be terminations of sensory nerves running their courses with motor nerves and thus unaffected by destruction of superficially disposed sensory nerves like the median cutaneous. The endings involved could, of course, be free terminations extending no further toward the surface than into the connective and adipose tissues of the subcutaneous regions. There are known to be many such. The endings could have been Pacinian corpuscles; in some parts of the body deep-lying tissues are somewhat freely supplied with these large, encapsulated end organs. Were sensory nerve terminations in muscles, tendons, and joints brought into play? They could conceivably have been. We know little of the distorting forces necessary to arouse these receptors. Possibly heavy pressures exerted on the skin are conducted to underlying muscles and bones with sufficiently small loss to be effective there.

Such "passive" appreciation of pressure properly comes within the meaning of "deep sensibility," as conceived by Head. A far more important set of sensations—important for its consequences in behavior—is that comprising the mass of feeling generated by movements of the body itself. This kind of sensitivity has been known, since the origination of the term by Bastian in 1880 (*84*, p. 525), as kinesthesis (literally, "feeling of motion"). Here belong the more or less continuous—and little-attended—sensations originating in muscles, tendons, and joints. Bastian included the labyrinthine receptors as part of the "kinesthetic" system. Current usage tends, in most contexts, to restrict the term "kinesthesis" to feelings aroused by movements of muscles, tendons, and joints or, in Goldscheider's terminology, the muscular, tendinous, and articular senses. Had they any peculiar qualities to contribute to experience these sensations would perhaps be better known and would receive distinctive names. As it is, they seem only to yield pressures and, very occasionally, pains. Their patterns are generally massive ones, deeply and diffusely localized and, moreover, combined in a multitude of ways with sensations arising from the superficial cutaneous senses. All of this makes observation of kinesthetic patterns difficult and uncertain. However, some facts are established.

Relative Roles of the Kinesthetic Receptors.   It was originally discovered by Goldscheider, in a notable series of experiments (*236, 237*), that the appreciation of passive movement imparted to the limbs comes chiefly from the joints rather than from the muscles. By cocainizing the overlying skin and muscles he was able to show that the "articular sense," joint sensibility, was mainly responsible for providing the sense data upon which discrimination of limb movement depends. Contrariwise, passing strong faradic currents through the joints rendered them much less sensitive, greatly elevating thresholds for the detection of movement. Historically, Goldscheider's discovery represented an interesting turn of events, for, since the days of Charles Bell (1826), the "muscle sense" had been pretty generally looked on as a sixth sense (to be added to Aristotle's original five), and it was believed that receptors embedded in muscle were chiefly responsible for originating the feelings underlying appreciation of posture, weight, resistance, and bodily movement.

Other proofs of the importance of the role of joint sensibility come from abnormalities. Cases are known in which anesthesia has invaded the muscles and overlying skin with, however, full retention of articular sensitivity. In such instances there is little, if any, disturbance of the ability to perceive passive movement in the affected limb. The converse type of pathological separation of function is also known. Bone disease may abolish the joint receptors and yet leave the muscles and skin unaffected. Here the result is also the predicted one; capacity to appreciate posture and movement is destroyed.

Discrimination of motion at joints proves, on measurement, to be remarkably good. Goldscheider (op. cit.) devoted a lengthy and thoroughly systematic set of experiments to threshold determinations, over 4000 observations being entailed. Whether measured in terms of the minimum angular displacement that could be detected (rate of movement being held constant) or in terms of the minimum velocity of motion that was discriminable, it was found that, of the nine joints tested, the shoulder was the most sensitive and the ankle was the least. Displacements of 0.22 to 0.42 degree (at a speed of 0.3 degree/sec) could be discerned at the shoulder. The wrist and knuckle of the index finger were nearly as sensitive (0.26–0.42 degree and 0.34–0.43 degree, respectively), while the ankle required relatively larger displacements (1.15–1.30 degrees). More recent measurements by Laidlaw and Hamilton (372) on 60 normal subjects yielded results generally in agreement with Goldscheider's figures, thresholds at different joints varying on the average between roughly 0.2 and 0.7 degree, though in these experiments the speed of movement was much less (10 degrees/min). The hip proved to be somewhat more sensitive than the shoulder, and the main joint of the big toe (the metatarso-phalangeal, not measured by Goldscheider) gave the highest values of the 12 joints investigated. In both sets of results it is clear that movement at the larger and more important joints, such as the hip and shoulder, is apprehended somewhat more readily than at the finger and toe articulations.

The chief value of subsequent repetitions and extensions of these experiments on passive movement is their discovery of some of the complicating factors. In one experiment (122) the elbow was moved in a vertical plane at rates of 6 to 15 degrees/min, and it was found that accuracy of judgments of motion was, in general, greater when the arm was being extended than when flexed. It was also greater with larger physical displacements than with smaller ones. The total duration of the trial was important; with brief exposures, kinesthesis was less accurate. The inclusion of occasional "dummy" trials (*Vexierversuche*, they are called in psychophysics), in which no motion whatever was imparted to the arm, resulted in reports of movement in nearly half of such instances. Some observers were regularly influenced in their judgments of direction by what had happened on the immediately preceding trial. In any case, one-third of the direction judgments were incorrect. Many reported reversals of direction during the progress of a smooth unidirectional motion. It is obvious that detection of motion itself has a much lower threshold than that for specification of direction. In this experiment, the former was of the order of 0.8 degree, the latter 1.8 degrees (for 80% correct identifications). Much of the uncertainty seems to be based on a characteristic waxing and waning of intensity of the kinesthetic sensation.

If active (voluntary) rather than passive postural adjustments are considered, a great many possibilities of testing present themselves. Almost any change of position of a limb, suitably quantified, might serve to provide information on the scope and precision of proprioception. Actually, there has been devised a great array of tests of muscle and joint sensibility, ranging from the clinical neurologist's simple procedure of touching the nose with the index finger, eyes closed, to very elaborate sequences of manipulative movements in certain aptitude tests.

The experimental literature is both vast and diversified; it is well beyond our purposes to attempt to deal with it systematically. (Consult *312*, Chapter 4, for a thoroughgoing review.) Suffice it to say that the following kinds of performances have all been used in attempts to assess precision of motor adjustment: duplication of posture in the contralateral limb, replication of a sequence of movements previously made or of a single position held earlier, initiation of a movement of a given magnitude, direction, or velocity, production of a prescribed pressure or tension, the prolonged holding of a fixed posture (steadiness tests), and the rapid repetition of a prescribed movement (tapping tests). Not all of these have contributed to our knowledge of underlying sensory mechanisms, to be sure, but they have tended to concur in stressing the prime role of articular sensibility, and many of them have made important additions to methodology by way of revealing the multiplicity of background conditions that make a difference in experimental outcomes.

For the appreciation of movement of a limb, whether the motion is passively imparted to it or actively initiated by the organism, the best evidence seems to indicate, then, that receptors in the neighborhood of joints are primarily responsible for providing the raw data on which the perception of such motion depends. Appeal to the neurophysiological facts confirms this. Figure 13–1 is an illustration in point. It charts the frequency of impulses coming from a single afferent neuron that terminated in the capsule of the knee joint of the cat (*87*). In the absence of stimulation there is a steady discharge that presumably provides information about position of the limb. Then, when the knee is bent through a 10-degree angle, there is a relatively high-frequency burst of impulses which, however, rapidly adapts to a lower, steady level. Removal of muscular tension by returning the limb to its starting position drops the nerve discharge to zero. Following a brief, silent period the nerve regains its initial "spontaneous" discharge level. Repetition reproduces the entire series of events with great fidelity. The joint receptors have obviously reported with some precision on positional changes. What of the role of receptor organs situated in muscle and tendon?

Their importance seems to lie chiefly in the feelings of strain added to the total kinesthetic picture when resistance to limb movement is encountered. Let something more than the normal demand of moving bones be placed upon their attached muscles, and evidence for feelings originating in muscular and tendinous tissue becomes evident by direct observation. Either require a heavy weight to be lifted or, more vividly still, continuously exercise a muscle group under conditions of diminished blood supply (by applying a tourniquet above it), and the feeling of

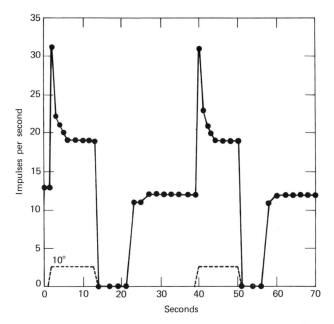

Fig. 13–1. Response of a single fiber terminating in the knee-joint capsule of the cat during a 10-degree flexion (dotted lines). The joint was moved at a rate of 16 degrees/sec. From Boyd and Roberts *(87).* By kind permission of Dr. Boyd and *The Journal of Physiology.*

strain—and, eventually, ache or even sharp pain—will assert itself. Most muscles and tendons are, indeed, well supplied with sensory endings. In the case of muscles the innervation is a somewhat complex one.

Kinesthetic Receptor Organs. Since the extensive and painstaking work of the British physiologist, B. H. C. Matthews *(406, 407),* the end organs responsible for initiating proprioceptive messages have been quite well understood. Four sets of receptors are involved, two in muscle proper, one in tendon, and one in the fascia associated with muscle. Matthews has designated them, respectively: A_1, A_2, B, and C endings. The anatomical arrangement of all but the last type is illustrated in Figure 13–2.

The form of termination picturesquely called "flower-spray ending" is the A_1 type and is found, in the diagram, at the end of the small-diameter fiber, *d.* A_1 fibers are found to be stimulated by passive stretch

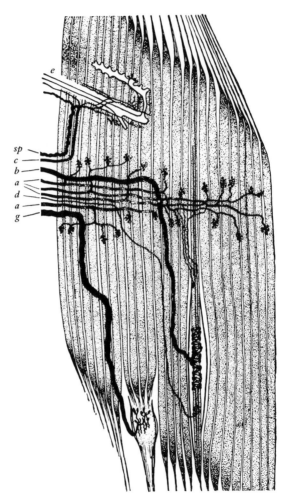

Fig. 13–2. Nerve endings in muscle. Innervation, both motor and sensory, of a group of muscle fibers. Motor neurones are those marked *a*. Three kinds of sensory fibers subserving kinesthesis are shown: Matthews' Type A_1 ("flower-spray" endings) at the termination of fiber *d*; Type A_2 (annulospiral endings) at the end of *b*; and Type B (Golgi tendon organs) terminating *g*. The structure labeled *e* is a small blood vessel innervated by sensory fiber *c* (pain?) and a sympathetic plexus, *sp*. From Fulton *(210)*. By permission of Oxford University Press.

of the muscle. Active contraction brings about an abrupt cessation of A_1 activity. A slight tension exerted on the muscle invariably brings the flower-spray endings back into play, and a strong, sudden stretch may excite a sufficiently high level of activity to produce sensory impulses from A_1 at frequencies up to 500 per second. A_1, then, signals muscle stretch and makes no report during active contraction. About 50% of the fibers in muscle are of the A_1 type.

A_2 fibers (*b* in the diagram) are of larger diameter, indeed, the largest class of afferents (so-called A-alpha or Group Ia fibers, 12 to 20μ in diameter, as compared with A-beta and gamma or Group II fibers, 5 to 12 μ, for the flower-spray endings), hence A_2 are more prompt to report. However, situated as their endings are, they provide much the same data as do the A_1 type. They likewise normally respond to stretch by initiating impulses and cease firing upon active contraction of the muscle. However, the terminations of A_2 (called "annulospiral" endings) do show heightened activity during a very strong contraction. This is presumably because they are wound around so-called "intrafusal" fibers, modified red muscle cells which also contract when the main body of the muscle contracts vigorously. Then the annulospiral endings are stimulated mechanically. Both A_1 and A_2 fibers will continue to fire with great regularity when the muscle is slightly stretched. Collectively, A_1 and A_2 have come to be called the *stretch receptor* or *spindle organ*. It is relatively slow to adapt, an important characteristic in a mechanism reporting postural adjustments.

Receptors of the B type are presumably the tendon organs of Golgi (see Figure 13–2*g* and Figure 13–3). These have been known since 1880,

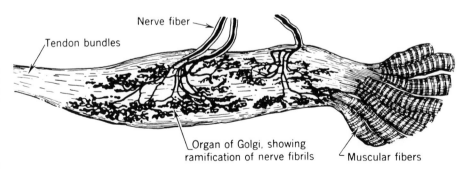

Fig. 13–3. Kinesthetic receptors in tendon. The B-type receptors of Matthews (*406, 407*) or Golgi tendon organs. From Lickley (*385*). By permission of Longmans, Green and Company, New York.

though no clear records of the responses of their attached fibers became available until the experiments of Matthews. B receptors have higher thresholds than do either A_1 or A_2. However, they respond with some regularity to tension, however it is imposed. Thus they signal both stretch and active contraction. Measurements of action potentials in their attached fibers show that their response (impulse frequency) is roughly proportional to the common logarithm of the tension. B receptors are, then, general tension recorders, and their function is somewhat less specialized than those of the A_1 and A_2 types. Figure 13–4 shows the

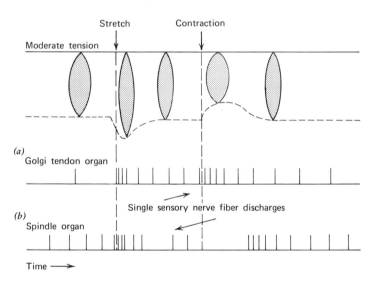

Fig. 13–4. Distribution of discharges of sensory fibers from a Golgi tendon organ (*a*) and a spindle organ (*b*) under conditions of stretch and contraction. From Thompson (*572*) after Granit. By kind permission of Dr. Granit and the publishers.

difference in performance between an afferent nerve fiber attached to a Golgi tendon organ and one coming from a spindle organ.

The receptor designated "C" by Matthews is perhaps the Pacinian corpuscle. Unlike the other forms of proprioceptors, this encapsulated ending is found to adapt very quickly. If the fascial sheaths of muscles are cut away the C-type endings disappear. In any case they are few in number and cannot be very important in the total picture of muscular response. They do, however, go into action during muscle movements, as do endings of the B type. The suspicion is strong that their contribution is to report mechanical deformations whether imposed from without ("deep pressure") or from within (muscle movement).

A word must be added about the motor nerves leading to muscle fibers, for there is an interesting feedback system in operation here. We have seen that the spindle organ quite abruptly ceases to send messages when the strong contractile elements of the muscle (extrafusal fibers) are activated, leaving the Golgi terminations to report on muscle tension. The overall contraction of the muscle bundle is brought about by large, rapidly conducting motoneurons of the alpha class. There is another efferent supply to the muscle, however. This is by way of the much more slowly conducting *gamma motoneurons*; these accompany the alpha fibers as they issue from the ventral root of the cord. But, whereas alpha motoneurons terminate in motor end plates on the contractile elements, gamma fibers go to the intrafusals, which do not contract vigorously. These, it will be recalled, also constitute the terminal sites of the annulospiral and flower-spray endings. The net result of this arrangement is that the gamma efferents are excitatory to the spindle organ. They, in turn, send afferent messages that reflexly excite the motor fibers returning to the muscle. This loop system must have much to do with regulation of reflex responses, especially in permitting the fibers from the spindles to have a full range of discharge rates, and per-haps—and this is strongly suspected—it plays a role in the initiation and control of so-called voluntary responses.

The foregoing analysis of the receptor systems in and around muscle is complete except for the omnipresent free nerve ending. Muscles are, of course, highly vascularized tissues, and blood vessels are sensitive structures. At least, they are well supplied with sensory nerves of the freely terminating variety. Whereas many of these doubtless have the primary duty of initiating reflex reactions concerned in the maintenance of thermal equilibrium, it is perhaps also the case that they can arouse sensation. Small, unmyelinated endings are found distributed widely throughout muscle, tendon, fascia, ligaments, and joints. The exquisite pains associated with muscle cramps and sprains, the severe aches connected with muscles exercised under conditions of diminished blood supply, and the breathtaking sharp pains consequent upon puncturing the fascia with a needle all bespeak a wealth of sensory innervation, and the free nerve ending is, of course, suspect as the originating agent. The details are as yet obscure, but the weight of evidence favors the interpretation that, in all these subdermal organs as in the skin, the free nerve ending is a pain receptor. As in the skin, whether it is *the* pain receptor future research will have to decide.

Proprioception and Psychophysics. One of the "founding" trends in experimental psychology, it will be remembered from Chapter 1, was the whole set of influences introduced by Weber and Fechner that brought measurement into the service of the new science. It will also be recalled that it was kinesthetic sensations, on which Ernst Weber did his first experiments, that led to the formulation of Weber's Law. Scientific history, like histories of other human activities, at times has a way of behaving much like a musical rondo; themes tend to come 'round and 'round again. The topic of proprioception is such a theme. Some of the fundamental changes that are currently taking place in psychophysics have as a common vehicle the study of sensations generated in the motor mechanisms of the body. The most basic change of all, substitution for Fechner's Law, in a wide range of situations, of the power law of Stevens—$\Psi = k(\Phi - \Phi_0)^\beta$, *equal stimulus ratios tend to produce equal sensation ratios*—has frequently been encountered in our discussions, especially those of audition and the cutaneous senses. We shall find the power function insinuating itself into still other contexts yet to come.

The classical proprioceptive problem is, of course, that of lifted weights. As Boring has said (*84*, pp. 529–30), "Fechner . . . made the discrimination of lifted weights the representative psychophysical experiment. There must have been lifted within the next sixty years hundreds of thousands of pairs of weights, all for the purpose of studying sensitivity and judgment, for the lifted weights contributed much more to the development of the psychophysical methods than to a knowledge of kinesthesis." Proprioceptive cues have naturally entered conspicuously into several of the experiments designed to test the power law. Lifted weights were, of course, a medium attacked early, since results with them would provide a ready comparison with all manner of experimental findings over the years.

Figure 13–5 brings together in a single graph lines expressing the relation between physical weight and judged weight (in units called *vegs*). The lines, all power functions, are derived from the results of eight different experiments, two of which used the fractionation procedure, two the constant sum technique, one ratio estimation, and three magnitude estimation. There are not unexpected variations in slope (1.13–2.07) and one hardly knows which exponent to single out as most representative. If the question were to get settled purely democratically, the average exponent would be 1.45, and that is customarily taken to be the slope constant for lifted weights (*555*).

In Chapter 1, when we were considering the development of modern psychophysics, we noted that power function exponents were likely to be quite constant for a given modality, but that there are other variables

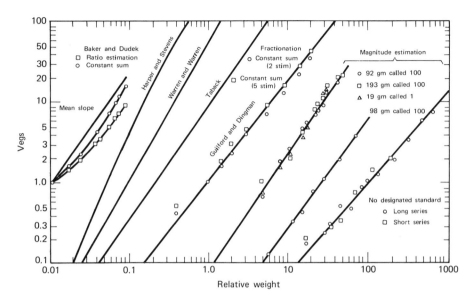

Fig. 13–5. Power functions, from eight different experiments on lifted weights, relating judged weight to physical weight. From Stevens and Galanter *(555)*. Copyright 1957 by the American Psychological Association, and reproduced by permission.

entering into sensory experiments that can influence them. In lifted weight experiments we may encounter one such variable, depending on how the experiment is performed. There is a well-known phenomenon connected with the lifting of weights; it is called the Charpentier or size-weight illusion. In accordance with the working of this illusion, a weight of large volume will almost inevitably be judged lighter than one of the same mass but smaller size. It follows that, if vision is permitted in a lifted-weight experiment, the illusion will operate. It is therefore common practice to blindfold the observer.

In an experiment designed to ascertain how apparent heaviness is influenced by observed size of the weight being lifted *(544)*, it was found that volumic changes not only altered the weight judgment but also the slope of the power function on which the judgments fell. The exponent, β, in the standard equation increased about 30% as volume moved from 58 up to 2375 ml in six steps.

If one searches for variables likely to influence lifted-weight judgments, a factor that is naturally suspect is adaptation. Knowing, as we do, how a motor performance can deteriorate in the presence of fatigue or other debilitating condition, it is of interest to find out whether the decrement is exclusively muscular or whether long-continued exposure of proprioceptive receptors to stimulation is likely to alter efficiency. Gregory and Ross (248), raising a question that was, indeed, discussed by Fechner, asked whether the addition of a superfluous weight to the forearm would impair discrimination in the conventional lifted-weight experiment.

A series of seven identical containers arranged in 3-gm steps was compared wth a standard of 111 gm at midseries. Each stimulus was compared 10 times with the standard, judgments only of "heavier" and "lighter" being allowed (Method of Constant Stimuli). At some point in each experiment, either before or during the taking of data, a heavy cuff (500 gm) was laid on the arm that did the weight lifting. The difference limen (DL) was computed from results obtained under four different conditions, two of which involved a 30-min wearing of the cuff prior to the weight judgments, and two not. In half the data-gathering series, judgments were given with the cuff in place, half not. Also, the cuff judgments came first half the time and last half the time.

Considering first the effect of having an additional weight on the arm during the weight comparisons, it was found that the observer did significantly better without the cuff in place: without the cuff the DL was 9.02 gm; with the cuff it was 12.65 gm. Such a result is not unexpected, of course; the increment in one case is being applied to the weight of the arm itself, in the other to the arm plus 500 gm. Now, however, consider the results when the observer wore the 500-gm cuff for a half hour before the weight lifting began. The DLs now were: without cuff, 10.65; with cuff, 11.00 gm. It appears that any change in loading, relatively, is deleterious. Discrimination becomes impaired to some extent whether arm weight is suddenly raised or lowered. The sensorimotor system works best at the level to which it is adapted. This principle of "adaptation level," first worked out with colors, lifted weights, memory phenomena, and reaction time effects, has come to be recognized as a very general one, entering into a great range of human judgments and adjustments (293).

Despite its classical importance, the lifted weight experiment is not the sole type of situation calling for proprioceptive triggering of movement. Cues mainly generated in muscles, their attachments, and bone articulations are responsible for guiding action in such diverse performances as handgrip, knob and lever manipulations, estimating the hardness or viscosity of compliant materials, spanning an object with the fingers, exerting pressure on pedals, not to mention such obvious motor adjustments as those involved in acrobatics, indeed the even more obvious gross motor functions of walking, running, swimming, and guiding food to the mouth! Not all these are exclusively kinesthetic and articular, of course. Indeed, the situation in which there is not cutaneous or other sensory involvement, with pure proprioception in control, is scarcely imaginable. And there is often a differential substrate of sensations from beneath the skin, playing an unassessed role, in discriminations seeming to be exclusively cutaneous. When, in Chapter 10, we considered the perception of roughness as a variant of pressure patterns we might reasonably have asked how much contribution is made by feelings of strain in muscles and joints as the rough surface is being actively explored with the fingers.

We cannot do more than sample the research output. Some motor adjustments, such as finger span, have had relatively little experimental attention over the years; others, such as handgrip, have been especially assiduously studied recently because of the strategic role they play in cross-modality experiments. There is better than fair agreement about the manner in which several quite different muscle groups yield stimulus-sensation relations that fall into a power function and, more than that, the way in which the exponents occupy the same relatively narrow range of values. Thus, handgrip, under a variety of conditions (542, 543) yields magnitude estimates that give a power function when related to force in a log-log plot. The exponents are found between 1.3 and 1.7. Foot pressure against a pedal that moved horizontally through a small excursion gave 1.65 (184). Feelings of strain coming from one minute of pedaling a bicycle ergometer that offered varying resistance yielded an exponent of 1.6 (77). Squeezing blocks between thumb and middle finger to judge apparent thickness gave one of 1.33 (559).

An interesting finding in the handgrip experiments was that, whereas longer durations of maintaining tension resulted in higher estimates of the amount of exertion at the end of the trial, as anyone who has taken a hand-dynamometer test can readily appreciate, the slopes within the family of power functions did not differ significantly among themselves (542). See Figure 13–6.

The fact that the power exponent may be quite stable despite considerable variation in experimental conditions is nicely illustrated by an experiment on perceived viscosity (556). Seven blends of clear silicone fluid ranging widely in viscosity (10.3–95,000 centipoises, a measure of internal friction) were judged by observers under three sets of instructions. The fluids were contained in screw-top jars that were half filled. In one series of trials, the observers shook and turned the jar while looking at it, and assigned a numerical estimate to its apparent viscosity. In another series, blindfolded observers were instructed to stir the liquid

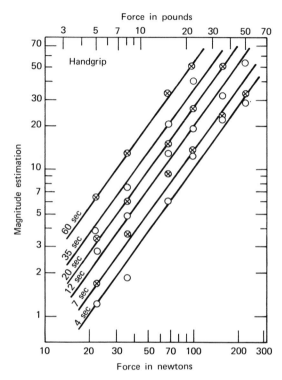

Fig. 13–6. Estimates of terminal force applied in a handgrip. Brief (4-sec) squeezes of a given magnitude are judged to be far less forceful than a prolonged one (60 sec). From Stevens and Cain *(542)*. Courtesy of *Perception and Psychophysics.*

with a rod. In a third series, they again stirred but with the fluid in full view as they did so. The judgments of viscosity in all instances fell into a power function, but slopes hardly differed from one experimental condition to another: 0.42, 0.43, and 0.46. These are low values in the family of power exponents; what meaning this has, if any of significance, the future will have to decide.

Organic Sensibility: Visceral Sensation. It has long been a commonplace in surgical experience that organs of the abdominal viscera may be freely manipulated, even squeezed, torn, or cauterized without benefit of anesthetic, provided only that traction on the mesentery and direct mechanical or thermal stimulation of the body wall be avoided. Visceral organs are, in general, peculiarly undemonstrative. Anatomically, it is the case that there are far more motor fibers supplying the viscera than there are sensory fibers reporting on their action. Moreover, the vast majority of afferents from the viscera have nothing to do with sensation. They are exclusively concerned with the mediation of reflexes, themselves controlled at relatively low levels of the central nervous system, which are necessary to the maintenance of the vast and intricate economy involved in circulation, respiration, digestion, excretion, and related vegetative functions.

However, it is not the case, as has frequently been stated, that "the viscera are insensitive." They are only relatively so. On occasions, when large distending forces are present (e.g., "gas pains"), or when their smooth muscle tissues go into a state of strong contraction (spasm, "cramps"), or when subjected to the action of unusual chemical irritants, certain of the viscera are demonstrative enough. It is no solace to the angina sufferer or the victim of a kidney stone to be told that "the viscera are insensitive"; he knows better, at least about some of them. But the large and sudden distentions responsible for such pains are not of usual or normal occurrence, and, fortunately, enough is known about their neural bases to permit a certain amount of management of them. A generality which is useful here is that pains originating in organs of the viscera are reported almost exclusively over fibers belonging to the sympathetic division of the autonomic nervous system. Contrariwise, afferent impulses concerned in visceral regulatory reflexes and in reporting non-painful visceral sensations are conducted over parasympathetic fibers. There are known exceptions to this rule in the case of some of the pelvic organs, for example, the bladder. This clear separation of function makes possible a variety of neurosurgical attacks on persistent and unbearable pain arising from visceral sources. By stripping the artery supplying the organ (since sympathetic axons usually follow the artery closely), removing the appropriate sympathetic ganglia, cutting several posterior roots at the proper cord level, or sectioning the anterolateral tract of the cord it becomes possible to interrupt the pain pathway without seriously disturbing the normal functioning of the organ so denervated.

By any practical criterion the problem of pain is, of course, the most urgent one to raise in connection with the visceral organs. But, as has been intimated, some of the viscera are capable of yielding other sensory patterns, several of them such as hunger, thirst, and nausea quite elaborate in their modes of appearance. Organs of the alimentary tract can, up to a point, be explored for their sensitivity to mechanical pressure, electric currents, and thermal changes. With somewhat less accuracy their reactions to chemical stimuli can be ascertained also. In the majority of the few studies directed at revealing normal sensitivity of the gastro-intestinal tract the technique has been that of the stomach balloon. Varying pressures, with slow or rapid onset, can be produced by inflation of the balloon, and the pneumatic system can itself be used as a recording device for muscular contractions of the stomach wall. Thermal sensitivity can be investigated by means of a simple stomach tube through which is conducted hot or cold water, a smaller rubber tube running through the larger one carrying the wires of a thermocouple to record temperature of the stomach contents. Similar techniques may be used for studying responses to pressure and thermal stimulation of the colon. Electrical sensitivity of the esophagus has been demonstrated with the use of a stomach tube bearing on its external surface a series of metal rings, each capable of serving as an "active" electrode in the stimulation process.

The classic study here is that of Boring (78, 79), who, repeating many of the earlier experiments that had yielded conflicting results and at the same time avoiding many of the previous errors of control, was able to show that parts of the gastrointestinal tract are sensitive to pressure, warmth, cold, and chemical stimuli. The pressures effective for the alimentary canal are not those of contact or simple deformation but relatively large distending ones. Slow inflation of a rubber balloon against the walls of the esophagus (or the colon) results in the eventual arousal of a broad pattern of muscular pressure. Rapid inflation may produce deeply localized pain or ache. Release of air pressure from the balloon promptly brings the painful or pressural feelings to an end. Similar pressure variations introduced in the stomach proper are without effect. However, the stomach does prove to be thermally sensitive, as is also the esophagus. An increase in stomach temperature of 5° F, brought about within 6 sec by pouring 25 cc water at 60° C through a stomach tube, is felt as warm. A similar amount of icewater will reduce stomach temperature by 5° C in the same period of time and will be felt as cold. That these changes are appreciated by way of deep-lying receptors in the stomach tissue is attested by the fact that skin temperatures, recorded simultaneously from the adjacent body wall, remain virtually constant throughout such experiments. Thermal conduction to cutaneous receptors thus cannot be responsible. Chemical stimuli such as alcohol, oil of peppermint, and mustard in suspension introduced directly to the stomach by way of a rubber tube can be appreciated.

Localization of visceral sensations is not infrequently faulty. So constant and reproducible is the error of localization in the case of certain pains that the phenomenon constitutes a commonplace of clinical practice, so-called *referred pain*. The classical example of referred visceral pain is that associated with angina pectoris. An acute pain arising in the heart is localized in the chest wall and is felt to radiate outward to the underside of the arm. Another clearly recognizable instance of referred visceral pain is that occurring in renal colic. A stone passing down the ureter produces a sharp pain which, however, appears not to move but to be referred constantly to the groin. This happens despite the anatomical fact that the upper end of the ureter is situated under the last rib! Not all referred pains involve such large errors of localization, nor are all referred pains of visceral origin. Certain somatic pains, for example, those originating in the margins of the diaphragm, may be referred considerable distances away from the site of stimulation. In general it seems that those sensations which have a fairly superficial and easily identifiable mode of initiation tend to be localized with some accuracy; those having a deeper origin are subject to larger localization errors. The full explanation of this is not obvious. It may be that the relative infrequency with which deeply disposed tissues are ever restimulated in identical fashion militates against the building up of a localization schema for these organs. Localization, so far as present evidence attests, is a product of learning, and, hidden from sight as the viscera are, the chances are remote of learning directly much about one's own viscera and particularly of verifying the sources of their stimulation.

Much of the apparent mystery surrounding the faulty localizations of "referred" sensations disappears when attention is paid to the underlying neurological facts. Spread of excitation within a dermatome (see p. 278) is a natural consequence of the intimacy of neurological relationship existing within a given spinal segment. Especially in the case of the strong stimuli necessary to the production of visceral pain, "flooding over" at the spinal level is to be expected. It is not surprising, therefore, that a common reference for pain is to the opposite side of the body to that affected, localization being in the area of the corresponding dermatomal segment. Nor is it surprising, once the dermatomal projections of the spinal segments have been studied, that certain unilateral anomalies of localization should occur. In the instance of the seemingly odd radiation of anginal pain into the left arm, for instance, it is actually the case that the same thoracic segment that sends fibers into the chest area over the heart also innervates the inner side of the upper arm. "Synthetic" angina has been produced by Lewis and Kellgren (*384*) by injecting the appropriate interspinous ligament with 5% saline solution, which produces a strong irritation of the spinal center and pain projected to its dermatome. The pain in this case was indistinguishable in localization from that of true angina pectoris.

One interesting anomaly of localization is that occurring in the esophagus. It may be noted that very cold or hot food seems to disappear, on being swallowed, only to reappear in the stomach region. The supposition would be that the esophagus is thermally anesthetic. Actually, if the esophagus is explored carefully it is found to be sensitive throughout its length to both warmth and cold. Why, then, the apparent contradiction between everyday experience and experimental result? This question was answered by Boring, who performed the instructive experiment (78) of electrically stimulating five levels of the esophagus, separated evenly by 5-cm spaces. The subjects were required to localize each internal stimulation by pointing to the appropriate place on the chest or neck. Whereas all five loci were effective, it turned out that there is not a one-to-one correspondence between position within the esophagus and that of the overlying thoracic wall. Stimulations near the upper and lower ends of the esophagus were fairly accurately localized; there was a tendency for higher stimulations to be referred upward to a point above the clavicle, while the lowest tended to be shifted still further down, below the end of the sternum. Stimulations in the middle reaches of the esophagus were rarely accurately localized, being commonly referred either up or down. Sometimes they had a double reference, both up and down.

Organic Sensory Patterns: Hunger.   It was suspected more than a hundred years ago that hunger pangs have their origin in contractions of the stomach walls. Ernst Weber, writing in 1846, said that "strong contraction of the muscle fibers of the wholly empty stomach, whereby its cavity disappears, makes a part of the sensation which we call hunger." Weber's conclusion was based on surmise; it remained for Cannon and Washburn (109), in 1912, to furnish what passed for many years as incontrovertible experimental proof. Their technique was that of the stomach balloon. (See Figure 13–7.)

Over a period of several weeks Washburn, the observer, introduced daily to his stomach a tube terminating in a small balloon. For several hours each day the tube was carried about, balloon in the stomach, until Washburn was thoroughly habituated to it. Then, when records were to be taken, the balloon was gently inflated to conform with the stomach walls. The stomach tube was joined to a manometer, and a float on its mercury column recorded on a kymograph variations in gastric size. A pneumograph was also attached about the waist to record any movements of the abdominal muscles. Washburn, out of sight of the kymograph, pressed a key whenever he felt hunger pangs. As the record in Figure 13–7 reveals, hunger indications were found to coincide exactly with the occurrence of powerful stomach contractions. The contractions were fairly rhythmic ones, each developing to a peak and subsiding again within a span of about 30 sec. They recurred at a frequency of 30 to 40

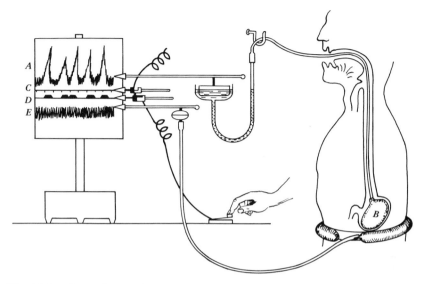

Fig. 13–7. Recording of hunger contractions. The Cannon-Washburn technique *(109)*, devised in 1911 and widely used since, for revealing motions of the stomach wall in hunger. Note the correspondences between record *D,* which registers hunger pangs, and record *A,* which is of stomach contractions. *C* is a time line, *E* a record of abdominal breathing. From Cannon *(108).*

per hour, though this was somewhat variable from one hunger episode to another. In any given "attack" of hunger the contractions are likely to begin somewhat feebly, long periods of relative quiescence separating them. As time goes on the contractions become more powerful and recur with greater frequency. Assuming that nothing is done to assuage the hunger, the series of contractions may be prolonged for an hour or more or, somewhat more typically, may run its course in one-half to three-quarters of an hour. The peaks of contraction may be as few as 20 or as many as 70.

The coincidence of stomach contractions and hunger pangs is certainly not accidental. Since the original Cannon and Washburn experiment gastric contractions in relation to hunger have been studied by many, notably by the Chicago physiologist, Carlson, and his students. Always the one-to-one correspondence between the sensory and the gastric events has been demonstrated. The simple conclusion would seem to be indicated that feelings of hunger are caused by stomach contractions and thus are kinesthetic sensations of a certain pattern. However, the mere fact that gastric contractions can be shown to be taking place when hunger is reported does not prove that vigorous motion of the stomach wall is either sufficient or necessary to arouse hunger feelings. Both events may be traceable to another, more deeply seated mechanism. That strong contractions are not of themselves *sufficient* to produce hunger pangs is demonstrated time and again in gastric records. Violent contractions may occur in the absence of any experienced hunger. There is, of course, nothing surprising about this; stimulation, however strong, does not necessarily result in either sensation or response. Inattention, fatigue, or some other inhibitory influence may prevent it. That stomach movements may not be necessary to hunger is a conclusion forced by clinical experience. In a case in which the stomach was totally removed and the esophagus joined directly to the intestines (*606*) desire for food continued to be felt, and the patient ate normally. Similar implications are involved in the finding that rats surgically deprived of their stomachs will perform normally in maze learning even though the "hunger drive" is used as a motivating force. The same animals show as much activity in hunting food as normal rats do, and they yield normal scores on an obstruction apparatus designed to measure the strength of the "hunger drive."

It is at this point in the search for an explanation of hunger that ambiguity of meaning begins to perform a disservice. "Hunger" is at once the name for an organic sensory pattern, the "pangs" or "aching pain" experienced when the stomach is empty, and also for the desire for food or urge to eat—in short, appetite. If eating were entirely a matter of satisfying hunger pangs, meals would become very brief affairs, for the first few mouthfuls of food are sufficient to reduce the strong gastric contractions to a level subliminal for sensation. Food is not the only agent having this effect. Even nonnutritive and indigestible substances—bits of leather, moss, or clay—will temporarily allay hunger pangs. Swallowing hard, tightening the belt, or smoking will do the same. It is well known that strong emotions will promptly produce a thoroughgoing cessation of all digestive activities. The prolongation of eating, then, is not in the interest of satisfying hunger pangs but must be accounted for somewhat more elaborately in terms of deep-seated desire or motivation—what it would be better always to call appetite. It is appetite, not hunger, that gets us as far along in a meal as dessert.

The origin of hunger contractions themselves is still veiled in mystery, though some facts concerning the relation between them and the organism's need for food have been unearthed. Blood transfused from a starved dog into a satiated one will set up vigorous gastric contractions in the latter. Conversely, blood from a recently fed dog will inhibit stomach contractions in a starving one. Clearly there is a chemical principle at work here. What is it? At one time the answer seemed entirely obvious and simple. Blood sugar level was thought to control the hunger mechanism. A deficiency of blood sugar, brought about either by abstention from food or by the use of insulin, has been shown to augment gastric contractions. Also, glucose injected into the blood stream will, under some circumstances, abolish hunger contractions. However, the close correlation between the onset of hunger and fluctuation of blood sugar concentration that would be predicted on the basis of these relationships did not materialize as further experiments were performed. Other ideas were substituted, including the views that overall stored fat (lipostatic theory) and bodily heat (thermostatic theory) provide the cues to eating and satiety. Yet, neither of these can be considered to have established itself. The amount of scientific work in this area is prodigious, well beyond the scope of our inquiry to consider in detail. (See 251, Chapter 6 for a thoroughgoing review.)

But what of the role of sensations of hunger? Two developments have come about in recent years that tend to minimize their importance in the general treatment of hunger viewed as a motivating force. The first is the questioning by Davis and others (152) of the initiatory role of stomach contractions as cues to hunger sensations and, indeed, of the universal reality of hunger "pangs" and "gnawing" sensations. Many observers were questioned about their feelings of hunger; the vast majority were innocent of "pangs" when hungry. In the absence of food in the stomach there appears to be much less activity on the part of the stomach walls than when food or other objects have been put into it. Indeed, it is the "other objects" that produce misleading indications. Davis recorded muscular activity of the stomach by using high amplifications and electrodes positioned on the body wall, externally. His conclusion was that strong stomach contractions occur only when there is something to digest, and the "pangs" of the Cannon-Washburn experiment represent nothing more or less than the effort of the stomach to digest the rubber recording balloon!

The other development concerns the strong emphasis placed on central mechanisms by the discovery, first, of a "satiety center" in the brain and, later, of a "feeding center." Hetherington and Ranson, in 1940 (308), found through selective destruction of the hypothalamus of the rat's brain that a highly localized area, containing the ventromedial nuclei, was the seat of the "turning-off" mechanism for eating. With this center impaired rats will eat food ravenously, become quite inert generally, and get progressively more obese. The second discovery, by Anand and Brobeck in 1951 (20), came from destruction of a small area of the lateral hypothalamus. Damage here, if bilateral, abolishes eating. An animal so operated will starve to death though surrounded by palatable food. So, there are two juxtaposed hypothalamic centers, one inhibitory, the other excitatory for eating; both must be intact for normal feeding behavior to be preserved. Both centers are found in higher mammals and the clinical evidence is that the human is similarly equipped.

This dramatic series of findings has, quite naturally, tended to deemphasize peripheral or "local" theories of hunger. What, then, are the relations among hunger sensations, hunger drive, and food intake regulation? How do centers in the hypothalamus "learn" of the depletion of energy stores and take appropriate action? There obviously has to be some avenue of communication between the midbrain and the gastrointestinal tract. In the general economy of the alimentary canal, the stomach does not have to be involved as a unique message center. Distentions and contractions, peristalsis, occur throughout its length. Perhaps the crucial information is created in the duodenum, intestines, or colon, where osmotic processes occur that bring about nutritive absorption. Perhaps the circulatory system provides the essential nexus through chemical balances of food elements and hormones. Perhaps the reporting machinery is basically neural, even though extensive denervations can occur without impairment of feeding behavior. A host of possibilities exist, so many as to suggest that the combination that effects the intricate linkage between tissue depletion, felt hunger, hypothalamic activation, and the taking on of nourishment is, in fact, under the sway of many different but cooperating principles.

Organic Sensory Patterns: Thirst. Just as hunger seems to be most immediately connected with strong contractions of the stomach walls, sensations of thirst can be shown to be set off by dryness of the mouth and throat. That local conditions in the throat region are directly related to thirst sensations is not only the conclusion from experience; it can be demonstrated by experiment as well. Any set of conditions which will produce drying of the tissues of the mouth and throat will induce thirst in some degree. Thus the breathing of hot dry air, the chewing of desiccated foods such as crackers, or prolonged speaking or singing are familiar thirst-provoking situations. In all these the normally moist surfaces of the buccal cavity become partially dehydrated, and distressful feelings of dryness and stickiness result. But the belief that dryness of the mouth and throat constitutes *the* stimulus to thirst is not the foregone conclusion it once was. As experiment has been piled on experiment in this busy field it has become apparent that the problem of the underlying mechanism of thirst is both a complex and knotty one.

The theory that has more or less completely dominated thinking about thirst, until quite recently, is one of great antiquity. It may be traced back to the father of medicine, Hippocrates. It is the analogue of the "local" or peripheral theory of hunger. Albrecht von Haller, the great 18th-century physiologist, wrote in 1747: "Thirst is seated in the tongue, fauces, oesophagus, and stomach . . . which are constantly and naturally moistened by mucous and salival juices, grow dry from a deficiency of those or the like humors, or are irritated by a redundancy of muriatic or alkalescent salts here lodged, there arises a sense much more intolerable than the former [hunger], as thirst is the more dangerous . . ." (262, par. 639). Much the same view was expressed by Ernst Weber a century later. The modern statement is that of W. B. Cannon, who espoused the local theory of thirst in a series of influential publications extending from 1918 to 1934 (106, 107, 108). Cannon says, "The main fact which must be kept in mind is that the thirsty man does not complain of a vague general condition, he complains of a parched and burning throat" (108, p. 255). Cannon believed thirst to be a specific sensation generated in the mouth and pharynx chiefly through the failure of the salivary glands to keep these regions sufficiently hydrated. More than any other tissue in the body, the salivary glands are constituted of water (97 to 99%). Exposed as they are to drying respiratory air currents, they dehydrate readily and create local distress.

The same considerations arise here as were encountered in conjunction with hunger, for thirst, like hunger, is at once the name for a sensory pattern, a drive state (what might be termed appetitive thirst), and a condition of deprivation on the part of the whole organism. In recent years, interest has largely shifted away from thirst as sensation and toward thirst as a motivating force. As animal behavior studies have multiplied, the withholding of water has become one of the most easily manipulated of motivating stimulus situations and the imbibing of water one of the most simply and accurately recorded of responses.

Paralleling the ideas developed for the interpretation of hunger, there have been several competing theories of thirst. These place the stress on water depletion throughout the entire organism and seek a mechanism whereby such water imbalance can be reported to the central nervous system. It has frequently been proposed that osmotic pressure of the blood is the key to thirst. Body cells, surrounded by a fluid having less than the full complement of water and being, therefore, *hypertonic* (having too high a sodium concentration relative to that within the cells), will lose their water to the surrounding fluid and will shrink. If the fluid is *hypotonic* (having too low a sodium concentration) the cell will take on water and will swell in size. The ideal state is one of isotonicity, of course, and it is toward such a balance that all changes in water consumption and elimination tend to go, normally.

No one can doubt that widespread dehydration of body cells must be involved in the stimulation of drinking behavior. Dogs are found to start drinking when their water balance drops as little as 0.5% of body weight. If larger deficits are forced upon them and they then have access, *ad libitum*, to water, they will make up their loss quite precisely. What cells are involved in such nice regulation? What are the avenues of report? Are the specific centers that control drinking and cessation of drinking identifiable, assuming there to be such? Does the parallel with hunger extend so far as to lead us to expect that there may be a "drinking center" and a "drink-terminating center" in the brain?

Not all these questions can be answered with complete assurance as yet, but there are some conclusions and a plethora of conjectures. The fact that osmotic pressure changes are implicated and that such information is somehow relayed to brain centers seems certain. The brain areas acting on the information seem clearly to be sharply localized in the hypothalamus. Lesions made at the base of this body, just behind the pituitary gland, so alter the drinking behavior of animals that they will drink enormous quantities of water without stopping. This, then, appears to locate the inhibitory center for drinking. Contrariwise, removal of the entire anterior hypothalamus has the opposite effect; dogs so operated may quit drinking entirely and have to be given water forcibly to keep them alive. Efforts to localize the excitatory center more precisely have comprised chemical and electrical stimulation as well as selective tissue destruction. Whereas the various relations among nervous centers regulating water utilization are not yet as well understood as are those controlling feeding behavior, there is no reason to doubt that they will come to be. Indeed, one of the large areas for future exploration concerns the somewhat intricate cross-play between hunger and thirst mechanisms. It appears that a hungry but nonthirsty animal may reject water completely but consume it avidly when it is baited with small quantities of meat juice! Such behavior obviously implies a fineness of discrimination the sensory control of which presents a considerable challenge.

14

Vestibular Sensitivity

Equilibrium Mechanisms of the Inner Ear. It was earlier pointed out, in a description of the auditory response system (p. 172), that the bony labyrinth of which the cochlea constitutes one portion also contains two other parts, nonauditory in function. These are the *vestibular sacs* and the *semicircular canals.* In our consideration of audition we set them aside as not germane to the discussion. Now, as we pay attention to the receptor systems involved in internal sensibility, they come to be important to us. Within the vestibule and semicircular canals are initiated many of the sensory processes responsible for muscular tone and postural adjustment. Thoroughgoing injury to the labyrinth has many consequences other than total deafness; flabbiness of the neck, limb, and trunk muscles and disturbed action of the eye muscles are likely to ensue. All these changes, taken together, inevitably mean disordered movements and equilibrium failures.

Although there must be a very intimate coordination between the activities of receptors situated in the semicircular canals and those in the vestibular sacs, the two sets of end organs are somewhat different in construction, and they function in accordance with different principles. One important characteristic they have in common, however. Both participate in neural systems which make little, if any, direct report to the cortex of the brain. The "labyrinthine sense," as it is sometimes called, yields no sensations! That is, it yields none directly in the same way that vision, audition, and the other senses do. It appears to have no "qualities" of its own. After a vigorous swirling about in a rotating chair, for example, observe carefully what the resulting "dizziness" actually feels like. It will be found to have a quite complex pattern of which prominent components are: kinesthetic sensations from the eye muscles, which are making powerful and rapid compensatory adjustments; pressure sensations

401

from the chest, head, and visceral regions; and perhaps a series of pulsating sensations which depend on vascular changes. If the eyes are open there will be elaborate and rapidly changing visual sensations also. Note that all these experiences are accessory and indirectly aroused. There is nothing coming out of the analysis of feelings of dizziness to tell one that the primary source of stimulation is the inner ear.

While the distinction rests on somewhat shaky foundations, the current belief is that the semicircular canals and the organs of the vestibule subserve two somewhat different functions. The canals are thought to be solely responsible for initiating reflex responses to rotary motion imposed on the organism, whereas the vestibular organs, the utricle and the saccule, are believed to respond to changes of head position involving linear motion. There is no denying that the receptor cells, the anatomy and disposition of which are fairly well known in each case, are admirably adapted to this particular division of function. There are, however, some experimental evidences which indicate that the semicircular canals may play at least a secondary role in static positional adjustments and that the utricle may participate in reactions to strong rotary motions. It would perhaps be better to say that both groups of end organs have static and dynamic roles to play. Both the receptors of the canals and those of the sacs serve as tiny accelerometers that monitor angular and linear accelerations of the head in space, reporting with some fidelity both the amount and direction of such movement. The disposition of the two, as we shall see, is such that the canals must be maximally involved when the body pivots about its axis, while it requires tipping or tilting to bring the sacs into a changed relation to gravity and thus alter the linear acceleratory picture.

The manner in which they are constructed tells one a good deal about how the various organs of the nonauditory labyrinth must operate. Let us consider the semicircular canals and the vestibular sacs separately.

The Semicircular Canals.   Lying approximately at right angles to each other, one for each major plane of the body, are the three semicircular canals. Their relations to other parts of the labyrinth and to each other are shown in Figure 14–1. Considering the two labyrinths together (right and left sides of the head), the two lateral canals fall approximately in the same bodily plane, the right anterior and left posterior do the same, and so do the left anterior and right posterior. The six canals thus form a three-coordinate, approximately orthogonal system to which gross bodily motions may be referred; the three "spirit levels" of the body, William James called them. The bony semicircular canals vary from 15 to 22 mm in length, the posterior being the longest and the lateral the shortest. The

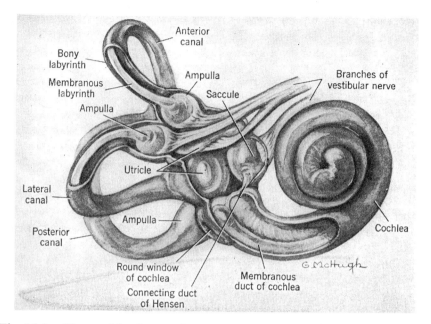

Fig. 14–1. The semicircular canals and their relation to the cochlea. The right labyrinth is shown, large portions of the protecting bone being cut away to reveal the membraneous canals and sacs inside. The three semicircular canals are approximately at right angles to each other.

internal width of the bony canals averages about 0.8 mm. Within the bony labyrinth lies the membranous labyrinth, all parts of which are continuous with each other and with the sacs of the vestibule. Surrounding the entire membranous labyrinth and apparently serving as a lubricant to prevent it from rubbing against its bony surroundings is a watery fluid, *perilymph*. The membranous canal itself contains a liquid, *endolymph*, which plays an important part in stimulation. In response to pressures it either shifts its position or circulates within the canal. If it circulates it flows through tubes which have a "bore" of only about 0.2 mm over most of their length, and a great deal of frictional resistance must have to be overcome.

At one end of each semicircular canal, just as it enters the vestibule, there appears an enlargement. This region is known as the ampulla. It is important because, as is suggested by Figure 14–1, it contains the endings of the vestibular or nonauditory branch of the eighth cranial nerve. The internal structure of the ampulla is remarkable and provides the key to the understanding of how the canals operate. Within each ampulla is a structure, the crista, which houses the terminations of the vestibular nerve. The nerve endings have a not uncommon form, one with which we are familiar from our study of hearing: hair cells (see Figure 14–2). The

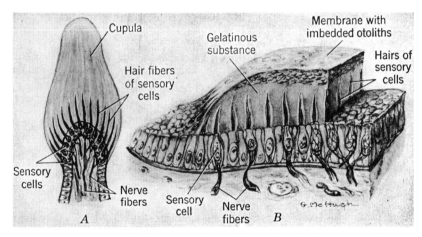

Fig. 14–2. Receptors of the non-auditory labyrinth. *A,* diagram of the crista, showing the hair-cell terminations of the nonauditory branch of the eighth cranial nerve projecting into the cupula, a gelatinous structure. *B,* diagram of the macula, a structure found both in the utricle and the saccule. This similarly houses hair-cell nerve endings.

hair fibers project into a gelatinous mass, the cupula, which extends from one wall of the ampulla to the opposite one. The cupula is fixed at its base (where the hair cells enter) but is free to swing at the distal end. This it does in response to hydraulic pressures created within the endolymph. The immediate stimulus for the discharge of nerve impulses in the hair cells is, therefore, bending of the cupula with consequent distortion of the crista. Though no one has ever actually witnessed it happening, the supposition is that motion of the cupula stretches the hair cells on the side away from the bending and slackens those on the side toward it. Impulses set up in some such fashion in the dendritic endings of the vestibular fibers pass over these fibers to the medulla, where synaptic endings occur in the vestibular nuclei of that organ. The vestibular portion of the eighth nerve (about 19,000 fibers, comprising half the total nerve bundle) contains chiefly large fibers (10μ to 15μ in diameter), though small ones are also present. This means that impulses from the nonauditory labyrinth are, in general, rapidly conducted ones, as might be expected in a system responsible for emergency reflexes.

The ultrastructure of the vestibular epithelium, thanks to the electron microscope, is now becoming better known, and it is already apparent that the fine details of the vestibular nerve endings do not differ greatly from one organ to another. Thus the sensory epithelium of the crista is organized much as are those of the nearby utricle and saccule and, indeed, there are structural resemblances between all these and the hair cells of

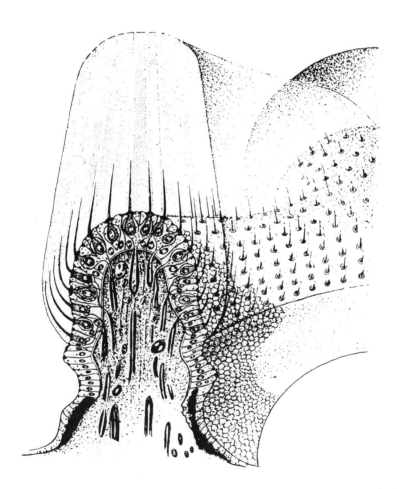

Fig. 14–3. Structure of the crista (semischematic). From Wersäll and Lundquist (*626*).

the cochlea. Perhaps all the hair receptors of the inner ear operate in a basically similar fashion. During appropriate mechanical or other stimulation it seems probable that there are produced shearing movements at the level of the hair attachments which stand in immediate relation to the events that set off nerve impulses (*190*).

The nerve endings of the crista are diagrammed in Figures 14–3 and 14–4. As both indicate, two kinds of terminal cells are to be found. Type

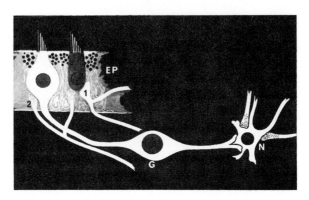

Fig. 14–4. Two types of sensory ending in the crista (schematic). EP=epithelium; G=vestibular ganglion; N=vestibular nuclei. From Engström, Lindeman, and Ades (*190*).

I is flask-shaped and is encompassed by a "nerve chalice." Its neural connections have been described in some detail (*190*) and there is little doubt that it is a generator of sensory impulses. Type I cells are distributed most abundantly at the summit of the crista. Type II endings appear to be structurally more primitive, having a simple cylindrical form without special enclosure but having rather more complicated neural connections. There is evidence that some of the latter may possess efferent fibers; there are known to be such in the vestibular as well as the acoustic nerve (Type 2 in Figure 14–4). Just what they are doing there is still a mystery.

An interesting detail concerns the hairs that project from the cell surfaces of both Type I and Type II receptors. They are "cut on the slant" in all instances, the tallest, the *kinocilium*, being set apart from a collection of 60 to 70 so-called *stereocilia*. Although precise functional particulars are lacking, it seems improbable that so much orderly arrangements is meaningless; the differential microstructure of the hairs must be important for "polarizing" the nerve response. As we shall see, electrophysiological findings tell us that direction of change, as well as amount, is reported with some fidelity by the cristae.

It was said earlier that impulses initiated by the vestibular organs make little direct appeal to the cortex. This is obviously true, since there are no vestibular "feels." However, there is provision in the pathways from the nonauditory labyrinth for projection to the cortex. Andersson and Gernandt (22), using the evoked potential method—stimulating slightly supraliminally the three branches of the cat's vestibular nerve with electric currents and probing the cortex for potentials—found that the vestibular apparatus projects, principally contralaterally to the superior ectosylvian fissure by way of the thalamus. However, they conclude (22, p. 112): ". . . the paucity of cortical projections suggests that these behavioural consequences are largely at the unconscious reflex level." En route to the cortex, at the vestibular nuclei of the brainstem, there are multiple connections, contralaterally, upwards and downwards, so as to involve a whole host of postural and ocular reflexes.

Stimulation of the Vestibular Canals.   The normal or "adequate" stimulus for the receptors of the canals would seem, at first glance, to be bodily motion. But motion, whether straight-line or rotary, can be shown to be insufficient, in itself, to stimulate the cristae. Gently rotate a blindfolded subject in a noiselessly turning chair of the barbershop variety, and it will be found that he perceives motion only when the chair is gaining or losing speed appreciably. If the rate of rotation is held approximately constant he will not feel himself to be turning. It is not motion but change of rate of motion, acceleration or deceleration, that constitutes the adequate stimulus for the semicircular canals.

In the vast majority of normal situations changes in rate of bodily motion are the only stimuli encountered. However, there are other kinds of stimuli, for the most part experimentally or clinically applied only, that initiate ampullar activity. Heat or cold (caloric stimulation) is effective. Syringe the external ear with hot or cold water, and there follows immediately a series of reflex responses of the eye muscles, so-called nystagmic movements, that cause the eyes to sweep slowly in one direction (slow phase) and then snap back to the original position (quick phase). Subjectively such repeated motions are accompanied by dizziness; in the extreme they lead to nausea. Hot water produces nystagmus with the quick phase toward the side of the head stimulated. Cold water does the reverse; it sets up nystagmus with the quick phase towards the opposite side of the head. If both ears are stimulated equally with either cold or warm water, there is a cancellation of effects and no response ensues. The mechanism of coloric stimulation is presumably that of convection currents in the endolymph. One good proof that convection currents are responsible is the finding, in experiments on weightlessness, that people who normally show strong nystagmic eye movements to thermal stimulation of the external ear canal fail to show such responses when receiving uniaural irrigation during the weightless phase of parabolic flight in aircraft (347). Such a consequence could be predicted from the old hypothesis of Bárány, in 1906, viz., that caloric nystagmus results from differences in the specific weight of endolymph at different levels of the horizontal canal (when out of the horizontal position, of course). Obviously, if there is no gravity, there can be no effect of endolymphatic density variations from one part of the canal to another, and there can be created no convection currents based on thermal action.

In the hands of the clinical otologist the caloric irrigation test can be a powerful one for diagnosis. The advantage that thermal stimulation has over rotary acceleration as a means for testing the labyrinthine system lies, of course, in the circumstance that unilateral isolation can be brought about readily. Acceleratory forces obviously do not single out one side of the head, and disturbances of equilibrium and posture are usually based on unilateral defects of canals or sacs or lesions of the cerebellum, cerebrum, or brainstem. Hallpike and his associates, following Bárány, have developed caloric stimulation to a high point of precision (263). With a reclining patient—head propped up by 30 degrees to bring the horizontal canal (the most accessible one to thermal influence) into an approximately vertical position—the ears are separately irrigated with water at either 30° C or 44° C. Appropriate nystagmic movements should be obtained. If a malfunction exists, an imbalance is likely to result. Any directional preponderance to the right or left will reveal the defective canal or pathway. However, there are some complications. Thus, vision would make a great difference in the result as would any voluntary effort on the part of the subject to deviate his eyes. A thermally induced nystagmus that has died down with the eyes open in a lighted room can be reinstated by simply closing the eyes. Also, nystagmus can always be accentuated by an effort to move the eyes in the direction of the rapid component of the jerky eye movements (Alexander's Law).

Another way to excite the semicircular canals is by direct mechanical pressure. There are relatively few situations involving human subjects in which this can reasonably occur. In some cases of deafness due to hardening of middle ear tissues it becomes possible to restore hearing by disengaging it from rigid adhesion within the oval window (the more usual approach) or by making an opening or "window" between the middle and inner ear cavities. Such "fenestration" operations are often attended by the most violent disturbances of equilibrium because of the involvement of the nonauditory parts of the labyrinth. Hydraulically it is all one system, it will be remembered, and temporary difficulties of balance are therefore not surprising when the auditory mechanism is disarranged.

For the fenestration operation to remain permanently successful it is necessary for the artificial window, which is covered over by a tissue flap, to stay open. The bone tends to grow back over the window and undo all that the operation has accomplished. Accordingly, frequent tests are made, mechanical pressure of the index finger being applied at the proper point in the external auditory canal. If there is no occlusion pressure will be transmitted through the hole to the labyrinth, evoking reflex nystagmic responses.

In animal preparations, where the semicircular canals can be laid bare for experimental purposes, direct mechanical (or thermal) stimulation becomes possible. Ewald, in the last century, attained good control with his "pneumatic hammer," a tiny device for mechanically stimulating the canals directly. The hammer consisted of a cylinder, 9.0 mm long and only 1.4 mm in diameter, which contained a movable piston. A small hole being drilled in the wall of a semicircular canal and the foot of the cylinder being securely sealed against the bone, movement of the piston would now apply a mechanical force against the membranous canal and affect the endolymph. In the case of the horizontal canal compression more readily produced movement of the endolymph, while with the two vertical canals decompression was more effective. The index of effectiveness was the turning of the head and eyes by the animal.

Still another agent capable of stimulating the canals, or at least the nerve fibers leading away from them, is electricity. Both direct and alternating currents have been used experimentally, and a few facts have come to light. With direct current somewhat specific responses can be aroused. Thus, if the cathode (negative pole) of the circuit is applied to the left labyrinth of the pigeon a reflex movement of the head to the right will result. Reverse the electrodes, and a left turning of the head is evoked. Whether the site of stimulation is the crista or the vestibular nerve fibers themselves is still uncertain, though suspicion rests strongly on the latter probability. It can be demonstrated that no cupular movement is induced by the current (540). Also, there are many human clinical observations that speak strongly for the vestibular nerve as the essential site of arousal. There are also animal experiments in which extensive tampering with the canals themselves fails to alter the consequences of electrical stimulation. (See 197, pp. 88–89; 141–144.) Nystagmic eye movements can also be produced by direct currents applied to the head. A negative electrode placed on the human mastoid, the positive one being grounded at any convenient bodily locus such as the neck or shoulder, will elicit nystagmus in which the slow phase is away from the side stimulated. Interchange of the electrodes reverses the slow and fast phases.

Alternating currents have been used little in labyrinthine experiments, and as yet there has been worked out no systematic set of relations between the relevant parameters and vestibular sensitivity. A few experiments have tested the effects of slowly alternating faradic currents, and it is apparent that the system responds best to extremely low-frequency stimuli of the order of 1.5 to 2.0 Hz. More current is required, both at higher and lower frequencies of alternation, to evoke a liminal "feeling of motion." Dzendolet (177) recorded objective bodily sway simultaneously with the taking of "sway sensation" thresholds and found that the two indicators are in quite good agreement.

Reactions to Rotation of the Body.   Responses of the semicircular canals have been studied chiefly by means of the rotating chair. The prototype is the Bárány chair, which became well known in World War I as a test for vertigo in prospective aviators. Any heavy rotating base which has relatively noiseless bearings and which can be accelerated and decelerated smoothly may be used. A comfortable chair mounted rigidly on such a base and equipped with a head rest or biting board provides a suitable platform for rotating the body about its vertical axis. It is common practice to arrange it so that the head is inclined forward at an angle of about 30 degrees to bring the horizontal canals to a plane parallel with the floor, that is, to render them really horizontal. This will be accomplished if the head is tipped so that an imaginary line from the corner of the eye to the ear canal opening is horizontal. In fact, it turns out that somewhat greater sensitivity to rotary acceleration is realized if the head is held erect, rather than tilted forward in the customary manner (581). There are other ways of producing rotary accelerations of the body. The torsion swing was introduced by Ernst Mach for this purpose, and there have been devised various rotating platforms on which the subject stands or lies. There are also flight simulators that permit oscillatory motion of the subject's chair.

To measure absolute sensitivity any one of three indicators may be employed: (1) kinesthetic and cutaneous feelings of total bodily motion; (2) nystagmic eye movements; (3) the "oculogyral illusion." The magnitude of the absolute threshold will be a function of the response selected as an indicator, for the three are not equally sensitive. In general, the first and second—perception of bodily motion and observation of nystagmic movements, especially of the slow phase of nystagmus—yield results which are in substantial agreement. Accelerations of the order of 1 degree/sec^2 prove to be liminal, but to cite such an average figure is to fail to recognize the great variability of results from one method of determination to another, for there are several influential factors about which somewhat arbitrary decisions are customarily made in threshold measurements.

Clark (*116*) has reviewed more than a score of studies containing reports of thresholds for feeling of motion generated by angular acceleration. They range from 0.035 degrees/sec^2 to 8.2 degrees/sec^2! In addition to instrumental deficiencies that cause gross inaccuracies, Clark finds the following: (1) considerable variation in the psychophysical method used; this implies, especially, fortuitous adaptation influences; (2) in general, small numbers of subjects; less than a quarter of the experiments employed more than five; (3) lack of precision in the definition of threshold (reaction latency corrected or not, guessing permitted or not, duration of acceleration arbitrary or uncontrolled, etc.); (4) only one general head position (that needed to test the horizontal canals) adopted in nearly all experiments. As a practical consideration related to flight—and many investigators in this field are so oriented—it is interesting that deviations of the horizontal canals are chiefly encountered in yaw; it is the vertically arranged canals that report the much more significant changes of roll and pitch in aircraft. Obviously, for particular situations, one needs a rigorous operational specification of absolute threshold.

The "oculogyral illusion," as it has been called by Graybiel and his associates, who have investigated it extensively (*246*), is a visual effect occurring under angular acceleration of the body in a human centrifuge. It refers to the apparent motion of an isolated visual object (six radial lines of dim light forming a star pattern and viewed against darkness) which is rigidly fixed in space relative to the head of the subject. The observed motion following angular acceleration is in the direction of turn. Shortly after the body has attained a uniform angular velocity there is experienced no further visual motion. Deceleration reverses the apparent direction of visual movement. After stopping, once the seen motion has subsided, it may revive itself but this time it appears to be in the opposite direction (the same as that in response to initial acceleration). The visual effects are presumably correlated exactly with nystagmic responses and, as such, are delicate indicators of labyrinthine stimulation. As compared with threshold accelerations approximating 1 degree/sec^2, obtained by the two cruder methods, the oculogyral illusion may begin to appear with accelerations or decelerations of as little as 0.12 degree/sec^2. There are obvious reasons why the OGY (as current scientific slang has it) should display the high sensitivity it does. Besides generating supplementary information to that provided by the proprioceptive cues and thus enriching the total feeling pattern, it seems probable that the availability of a visual target may enhance overall vigilance in the observational situation. After all, we are more accustomed to "looking" than to "feeling," even in the semidarkness.

Direct study of the eyes' responses to rotatory acceleration and deceleration reveals the nystagmic sequences to be quite elaborate. They are particularly complex if vision is allowed to intervene. Then there occur interactions, especially those of inhibition, between voluntary eye movements and ocular reflexes aroused by action of the canals. If, however, vision is excluded by dark surroundings or by the use of a blindfold, pure labyrinthine nystagmus can be studied. Since the effects of acceleration and deceleration are identical in character (though opposite in direction), observation can be facilitated by bringing the chair to a steady velocity (conventionally, as in the classical Bárány test, 180 degrees/sec), continuing at that speed until all effects of acceleration have subsided, and then decelerating to a fairly rapid stop. Nystagmic movements, with the slow sweep in the direction of rotation, will be observed throughout the period of slowing down and coming to a stop. The slow phase of nystagmus increases in velocity for slightly longer than the duration of deceleration, then very gradually declines in speed, the repetitive sweeps continuing on for about a half minute. Up to this point what has occurred is "primary rotation nystagmus." The total response is not over, however, for with the subsidence of the primary phase there begins, without noticeable interruption, a series of eye movements in the opposite direction. This is *secondary* or *inverse nystagmus*. Its speed develops gradually for well over a minute, attaining a velocity at the peak of perhaps 5 degrees/sec, then shows a very gradual decline for the next several minutes. Altogether, the entire eye movement sequence, with its primary and secondary nystagmic phases, may occupy as much as a 10-min period. The protracted secondary phase is largely missing, of course, if vision is permitted. Fixational efforts easily overcome the relatively weak movements of inverse nystagmus. While for a given individual, under constant experimental conditions, the duration of the primary phase, that of the inverse phase, and the speed attained at the height of inverse nystagmus are likely to be reproducible quantities, there are large and perhaps important individual differences in all these response characteristics.

In addition to eye movements a number of reflex responses of the neck, limbs, and trunk are evoked by rotation. A blindfold subject, spun in a smoothly rotating chair, may show certain of these reactions. During the initial acceleration the head may make slow sweeping motions in the direction opposite to that of rotation, with frequent quick returns in the opposite direction (just as the eyes do in nystagmus). If the spinning is somewhat vigorous a sudden cessation of whirling brings forth compensatory movements of the head, arms, and legs, all responses that tend to prevent the subject from falling over. If, after rapid rotation to the left for a dozen or so turns, the subject is abruptly stopped and is instructed to get out of the chair and stand erect with his arms straight out in front of him he will stand with his head and arms to the left, and right arm up, and the left down, a stance which has been called "the position of the discus thrower." If, under this post-rotatory influence, he changes the position of his head radically he will be in serious danger of falling. In fact, quite apart from the accessory reactions produced, any gross change in head position following strong stimulation of the canals elicits the "falling reaction."

But responses involving adjustments of this magnitude are the result of somewhat intense stimulation. A more common sequence of events would run more nearly as follows. After having instructed the blindfolded subject to raise his right hand whenever he feels himself moving to the right and his left hand to signal left movement, begin with very slow rotation and gradually step up the speed. Once an acceleration of 1–2 degrees/sec² has been reached, the appropriate hand will go up, reporting correctly the direction of rotation. If now a constant speed is maintained the hand will go down and, assuming no accessory cues to the detection of motion to be given (sounds, air currents on the face, etc.), the subject will be unaware of his continued turning. Quite high rotational speeds may go undetected provided the acceleration used in reaching them is subliminal. If brakes are then silently applied, rapidly slowing the chair down, the opposite hand will go up. The sensation is that of turning in the reverse direction and is a direct consequence of supraliminal deceleration. This feeling may last for some time after the subject comes to a halt.

The classical inquiry into cupular performance, the stock-in-trade of otologists for a half century following Bárány's introduction of the turning test (1906–1907), involved relatively rapid rotation (10 turns in 20 sec) and sudden stopping. The difficulty with this procedure, of course, is that one cannot unscramble the consequences of initial acceleration from those of subsequent deceleration. One does not know whether the acceleratory force has subsided or what abrupt braking may have introduced in the response system. The afternystagmus observed in the Bárány test of presumed normals, while averaging about 40 sec in duration, was known to last twice that long in some people. An improvement was introduced when the subject was brought up to speed (180 degrees/sec) subliminally, that is, so gradually as not to permit the detection of his own motion. But there is obviously nothing sacred about this particular velocity, and it remained for van Egmond (*183*) to introduce a systematic procedure that sampled cupular function following rapid decelerations from a number of peak velocities. The van Egmond technique he called *cupulometry* and the graphic representation of the results a *cupulogram*.

Figures 14–5 and 14–6 present two cupulograms, one illustrating the fact that the subject's own report of movement may not coincide with

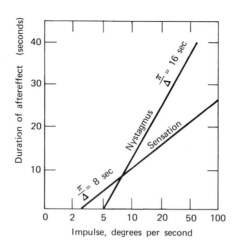

Fig. 14–5. Comparison of cupulograms, from normal subjects, for sensation and nystagmus. From Howard and Templeton *(312)* after Groen. By kind permission of Dr. Groen and the Editorial Secretary, *Acta Otolaryngologica.*

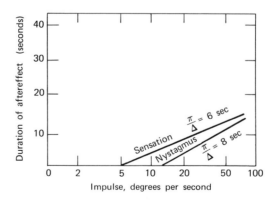

Fig. 14–6. Unusually low values for duration of the aftereffect of rotation. Mean values for 18 experienced aviators are plotted. From Howard and Templeton *(312)* after Groen. By kind permission of Dr. Groen and the Editorial Secretary, *Acta Otolaryngologica.*

observations of his ocular nystagmus, and the other that cupular indications may be altered by influences not present in the cupula. In obtaining
the cupulogram the rotation of the subject, always subliminal, is continued until one or another of a considerable range of speeds has been
attained. After continuous motion at a uniform velocity (the "impulse"
of the cupulogram's abscissa), to dispel any possible effects of the slow
initial acceleration, the subject is brought to a rapid stop (in less than
2 sec). If, now, the observed vestibular indicator, whether it be duration
of nystagmic eye movements, the oculogyral illusion, or sensations of continuing bodily motion, is plotted against the common logarithm of the
impulse, the resulting graph may approximate to a straight line, as in the
illustrations. Curvilinear cupulograms, it is held, are associated with
pathology or functional irregularities. Whatever its meaning, one has
here, as in the audiogram, a single representation of a whole range of
cupular functioning and, as such, it is a valuable device.

A novel attack on cupulometry, generally confirmatory of the work of
the Dutch group, has been made by Békésy (53). In addition to devising
a continuous, "up-and-down" procedure for tracking threshold, one which
performs a service comparable to that of the Békésy audiometer in hearing, it has been possible to bring under measurement the differential
threshold for the feeling of motion generated by horizontal canal stimulation. This was accomplished by requiring an observer, who was slowly
being oscillated back and forth around his vertical head axis by means of
a sinusoidal drive, to adjust the amplitude of movement (and thus the
acceleratory stimulus) until it was just perceptibly greater or smaller in
one direction of rotation than the other. The j.n.d. of amplitude, ΔA,

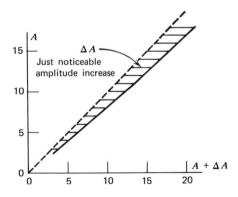

Fig. 14–7.   The j.n.d. of amplitude of oscillatory motion, ΔA, as a function of
amplitude, A. From Békésy (53). Copyright 1955, American Medical Association.

as Figure 14-7 shows, increases with the absolute amplitude, over this range at least.

One of the interesting findings in the Békésy study has to do with the "baseline" of feeling from which motion thresholds are measured. Simply sitting motionless in the dark, the chair in a fixed position, most observers reported brief periods of spontaneous and somewhat erratic movement. Not uncommonly there would be felt sudden rotation, amounting to perhaps 3–4 degrees, in one direction or the other. Another "illusory" effect concerns combined feelings of rotation and "swing", that is, apparent horizontal displacement, even though the motion imparted to the body was strictly in the rotary dimension and was symmetrical in extent in speed. There were even occasional reports of upward or downward displacements. If sensations of motion consequent upon stimulation of the vestibular system seem a little erratic, it could be that they arise from an unstable background body of feeling. Such patterns of feeling in the absence of a suitable acceleratory stimulus are not uncommon in vestibular experiments. They have been given the name, *gyroautokinesis*, and have been compared with analogous appearances in vision, audition, and touch (*118*). False information of this kind can be quite disturbing. Clark even had one observer, considerably practiced in judgments of rotation, who reported on one occasion that he felt as if he were rotating in both directions at once!

Vestibular Sensitivity and Adaptation.   In trying to arrive at a conception of the basic mode of operation of the cupula we have considered three different absolute thresholds, that for feeling of motion, that for nystagmic eye movements, and that for the oculogyral illusion. We have not dealt with high intensity stimulation nor with sustained excitation except to note some of the qualitative phenomena produced by them. Does the vestibular sense adapt and, if so, what are the consequences?

If the response of the cupula to a constantly applied acceleration (or an increasing or decreasing acceleration) meets the expectations prompted by the "heavily damped pendulum" hypothesis, something should be learned by systematically varying acceleration rate and noting what happens to one or more of the available indicators of vestibular sensitivity. In addition to those encountered thus far (sensations of motion, eye movements, OGY), at least three other kinds of data are available: (1) latency of response measures, (2) estimates of the magnitude of sensations of motion, and (3) judgments of angular velocity. Let us consider each in turn.

If response latency, the time between the beginning of rotation and the first indication of cupular response, such as the OGY, is plotted against the amount of angular acceleration imparted to the observer, such a curve as that displayed in Figure 14–8 results. The solid line in this illustration is a theoretical one; it was derived mathematically from the assumption that the cupula behaves like a damped torsion pendulum. Each of the data points represents the averaged reports of 15 observers,

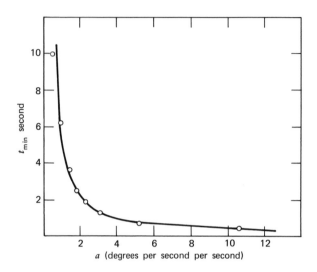

Fig. 14–8. Response latency, t_{min}, as determined by amount of angular acceleration, a. The curve is a theoretical one, derived from the assumption that the cupula behaves like a torsion pendulum. The points are empirical. From Guedry *(252).* Courtesy of Academic Press, Inc.

each making five determinations of threshold. Apparently there is little wrong with the basic assumption, at least so far as its relevance to the initiation of the response goes.

If steady acceleration is maintained over a relatively long period, the feeling of motion will at first be considerably augmented, but will then fall off in a somewhat precipitous manner. Clark and Stewart *(118)* rotated observers for two minutes around a vertical axis in a space vehicle simulator. Three linear rates of acceleration (0.5 degrees/sec²; 1.0 degree/sec²; and 1.5 degrees/sec²) were employed. The magnitude estimates of speed increased for a period of 30 to 40 sec, then declined and hit zero well in advance of the leveling off to a steady velocity. The greater the acceleration rate, the higher the speed estimates, as expected, but reasonably faithful following by the cupula of the stimulus lasted only for the first third of the period. See Figure 14–9. The secondary (reverse) effect

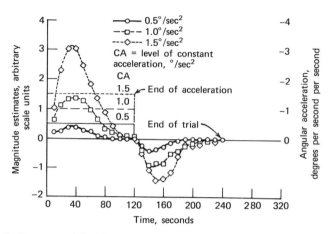

Fig. 14–9. Judgments of bodily motion, by magnitude estimation method, for 10 observers undergoing three different steady accelerations. Estimates in the direction of the accelerated motion, +; in the opposite direction, −. From Clark and Stewart (*118*). Copyright 1968 by the American Psychological Association, and reproduced by permission.

during the constant velocity phase is also related to the vigor of the initial stimulation, as Figure 14–9 shows. The same experiment contained within its apparatus arrangements provision for stepping up velocity at accelerations that were themselves accelerated, so-called *ramp accelerations*. Such second-order accelerations ranged from 0.030 degrees/sec³ (maintained for two minutes) to 0.006 degrees/sec³ (for three-minute durations). Under these circumstances, felt motion held up longer during the speeding-up process, but the magnitude estimates were not at all closely related to the stimulus and, altogether, the effect seems to have been quite complex. There was considerable "waxing and waning" in the individual records, and averaging did not really smooth out the function linking observed motion with the magnitude of the ramp acceleration. See Figure 14–10.

Experiments have been performed in which the observer is first familiarized with the "feel" of rotation through a fixed angle of turn (45 or 90 degrees, say), then is required, under various amounts of acceleration, to signal whenever he judges the requisite amount of turning to have occurred. Experienced angular speed may then be plotted against duration of the constant acceleration. The method relies, of course, on the ability of the observer to keep the standard in mind over extended periods of time, and the difficulty of doing this renders the technique less reliable than one might wish. Nevertheless, results having consider-

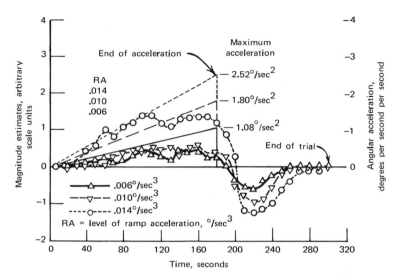

Fig. 14–10. Estimates of bodily motion during and following "ramp accelerations" (second-order accelerations, in which acceleration is itself accelerated). + = in direction of physical motion; − = in the opposite direction. From Clark and Stewart *(118)*. Copyright 1968 by the American Psychological Association, and reproduced by permission.

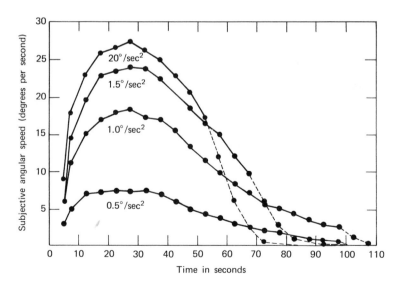

Fig. 14–11. Judged speed during prolonged constant acceleration. Solid lines, during acceleration; dashed lines, postaccelerative. From Guedry *(252)*. Courtesy of Academic Press, Inc.

able consistency have been derived from this procedure. Figure 14–11 shows Guedry's results for four accelerations ranging from 0.5 degrees/sec^2 to 2.0 degrees/sec^2. As the curves reveal, judged angular velocity increased up to its felt maximum in about 30 sec but, even though positive acceleration was kept up (until the dotted portions of the curves), there was a decline in judged speed.

Obviously, findings such as those cited above, both those coming from magnitude estimates of speed and those involving estimations of angular velocity, speak for a serious departure from "torsion pendulum theory" or perhaps for an additional principle entering to modify seriously the neural effects of such a mechanism. Whatever the interpretation, it is clear that the central fact is that sustained stimulation seems to result in an orderly decrease in sensitivity. Wherever we have encountered this phenomenon before—and we shall meet it again in the chemical senses—we have recognized it as adaptation. Apparently the vestibular sense is no exception to the general rule that adaptation is a completely ubiquitous phenomenon.

The question of what the seat of adaptation is can hardly be said to have been settled as yet. There are many reasons why one would picture the process as being essentially peripheral, perhaps at the base of the cupula. Guedry (252, p. 83) lists the following hypotheses about "mechanisms within the sensory detectors": histological changes in the cupula and endolymph, alterations in cupular "stiffness," plastic flow within the cupula, a modulating influence by efferent fibers—there are known to be a few in the vestibular nerve as in some other sensory bundles—and changes in viscosity of the endolymph. But certain evidence that any of these is at work is lacking; "hypotheses" may be too complimentary a word for the guesses thus far advanced. Moreover, there are some difficulties with a peripheral explanation. Why does ocular nystagmus not show a parallel trend? It is presumably initiated by the very afferent fibers that should be reflecting sensory adaptation.

Perhaps, then, adaptation is central, at least on the proximal side of the vestibular nuclei that participate in the reflexes of nystagmus. But direct proof for this is equally lacking. Here again we have to conclude, as we have so often in these pages, that "experiment will ultimately tell us."

Mechanism of Ampullar Action. Direct observation of labyrinthine events is not at all easy to arrange. In vertebrates the structures concerned are quite inaccessible, and in most of the lower forms they are extremely small. In view of the difficulties it is not surprising that until quite recently the mechanism of stimulation was less a subject of experiment than of speculation. Interestingly enough, however, as subsequent events proved, much of the early theorizing was basically sound. In the 1870s the fundamental theory was laid down, it being the joint product of the thinking of the Germans, Mach and Breuer, and the Englishman, Crum Brown. Today we speak of the Mach-Breuer-Brown theory of labyrinthine functioning.

The theory holds that stimulation of the crista comes about through inertia of the endolymph. The semicircular canals, being set approximately in the three dimensions of space, must be affected by all motions of the head. As a canal accelerates or decelerates in rotary motion the endolymph lags behind its containing tube. The back thrust thus created exerts a pressure against the cupula, bending it and stimulating the nerve endings of the crista. As turning continues, the endolymph, subject to the frictional influence of its enclosing walls, takes up the motion of its canal, and stimulation subsides. The cupula is no longer moving relative to the hair cells and imposing a strain on them. If an abrupt braking of the canal's motion occurs, the endolymph, through its own inertia, flows on for a time, and the cupula is bent in the opposite direction.

There are difficulties with this theory, some of which were seen from the beginning. Thus Ernst Mach, the physicist, considered it somewhat improbable that viscosity would permit the flow of endolymph through a tube having a diameter no greater than a fraction of a millimeter. Breuer believed it had to be that way, however. Brown thought it unlikely that a single canal could signal movement in one direction, then reverse its message. What about the principle of nerve specificity? Accordingly, he modified the theory to let a given canal on one side of the head always report movement in a specific direction. Its mate on the other side, silent during the first movement, was to come into play when the direction of rotation was reversed. This amendment to the theory, though ingenious, was most certainly wrong. Experiments involving destruction of semicircular canals in pigeons and rabbits demonstrated that the receptors of a single ampulla must function for motion in both directions (*176*, pp. 212–213).

Crucial evidence verifying the Mach-Breuer-Brown theory was a long time in coming, and the ideas involved remained the subject of controversy for nearly 60 years. Then, in 1931, came the dramatic experiments of Steinhausen (*540*). These, by demonstrating unambiguously the appropriate movements of the cupula in response to positive and negative rotary accelerations and to mechanical and caloric stimulation, proved the essential correctness of the early guesses. The success of Steinhausen's work depended on the judicious selection of an experimental animal and the invention of a novel technique. He made his observations on the pike, which has relatively large and accessible semicircular canals. By cutting away the covering cartilage he was able to render visible a portion of a canal with its ampulla. Injection into the canal of small quantities of dye made visible the gelatinous cupula, which could then be photographed. A small drop of oil inserted into the canal facilitated observation of the movements of the endolymph. Figure 14–12 shows a typical

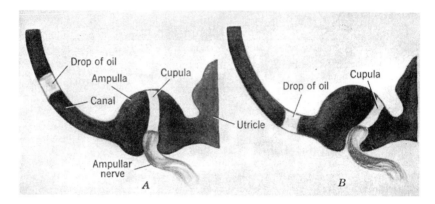

Fig. 14–12. The effect of angular acceleration on the position of the cupula. The displacement of the endolymph was revealed by an injected drop of oil. The cupula was rendered visible by dyeing it with china white. *A*, the cupula in its normal position before rotation of the preparation. *B*, shift of endolymph and consequent change in position of the cupula as a result of rotary acceleration. After Dohlman (*168*). Reproduced from *Proc. roy. Soc. Med.*, 1935, **28**, 1374, by permission of the Honorary Editors and Professor Gosta Dohlman.

response to angular acceleration. Displacement of endolymph with resulting hydrodynamic pressure on the cupula has resulted in extreme tipping of that body with, no doubt, mechanical distortion and excitation of the hair endings of the vestibular nerve. Steinhausen's experiments on the pike and Dohlman's subsequent ones on the cod (*169*) make it clear that, in these forms at least, the cupula completely fills up the lumen of the ampulla. "Streaming" of endolymph can hardly occur if this is the case. Until we learn whether the same situation obtains in higher forms perhaps we do well to think of endolymph as only temporarily displacing the free end of the cupula by hydrodynamic pressure rather than "flowing past" it. However, some circulation of endolymph is demanded by the facts of caloric stimulation; convection currents require a fluid medium.

What happens in the sensory nerve fibers leading away from the ampullae? Records of action potentials in single fibers of the vestibular nerve, while being stimulated by angular accelerations, have been obtained by Löwenstein and Sand (394) in 1940 and, more recently, by Gernandt (229). The former investigators picked up discharges from nerve fibers leading away from the horizontal ampulla of the skate. While still unstimulated, the typical fiber had a "spontaneous" discharge rate of about 5 per second. At angular accelerations of the order of 3 degrees/sec² threshold was reached, this being signalled by *either* an increase in impulse frequency (when rotation was toward the side of the head from which the recording was taken) or a decrease (when rotation was toward the contralateral side). For a given amount of angular acceleration the increase (or decrease) was always the same, impulse frequency being related in a linear fashion to degree of acceleration. (See Figure 14–13.) The maximum impulse frequency is attained promptly, coincidentally with completion of the initial acceleration. If, now, *speed* is maintained at a constant level, impulse frequency falls off until it has reached the normal "spontaneous" rate of 5 per second after about 20 to 30 sec. The cupula does not remain

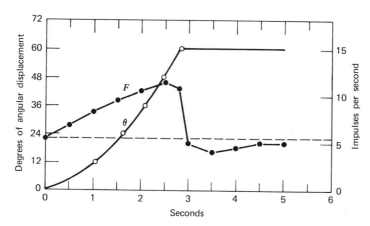

Fig. 14–13. Vestibular action-potential frequency as a function of acceleration. The line labeled θ shows the amount of angular displacement from the initial position of rest and is to be referred to the left axis. Impulse frequency at each half-second interval is shown on curve *F*, which uses the axis on the right. Acceleration was about 15 degrees/sec², and rotation increased in velocity up to a total turn of 60 degrees. At this point motion abruptly ceased. Note the increase in discharge frequency with increasing stimulation and the subsequent precipitous decline. Rotation in the opposite direction produced a corresponding reduction in impulse frequency below that of the "spontaneous" discharge of 5 per second. From Löwenstein and Sand (394). By permission of Cambridge University Press and the authors.

in its extreme position during continuous whirling but, acting like a very slow and heavily damped pendulum, gradually resumes its normal position of rest. The frequent recurrence of the figure, 30 sec (or thereabouts) as the subsidence period for many vestibular effects suggests that we are dealing with an elastic pendulum, the cupula, which has a natural period of that magnitude. If displaced only slightly it would, of course, not require as much time to regain equilibrium. Only the most extreme positive or negative acceleration could produce an aftereffect lasting a full half-minute. This explanation serves quite adequately to account for *primary* postrotational effects. The phenomenon of inverse nystagmus and its corollary, inversion of movement in the oculogyral illusion, are not accommodated by it, of course. These effects would seem to demand that the "pendulum" overshoot and describe at least one more movement in the direction of the original (acceleratory) displacement before finally coming to rest.

The experiments of Gernandt are revealing in that they show in the vestibular fibers of a vertebrate, the cat, similar events to those found by Löwenstein and Sand in a much simpler organism. Using a technique very much like that employed by Galambos and Davis (see Chapter 8) in their study of elements of the auditory branch of the eighth cranial nerve, Gernandt plunged a needle electrode, insulated except at the tip, into the vestibular branch leading from the horizontal ampulla. Single elements could be isolated by appropriate manipulation of the electrode. One hundred such responding elements were examined in relation to rotational acceleration of the animal, their frequencies of spike discharge being recorded. Not all fibers responded in the same way; in fact, three different "types" of fibers were found. By far the commonest performance, recorded in 83% of the fibers, was like that in the Löwenstein and Sand study, that is, when the needle was in the left vestibular nerve and rotation of the cat was to the left, an increase in frequency above the level of the resting "spontaneous" frequency occurred. Rotation in the opposite direction either reduced or entirely obliterated the nerve's response. Elements of Type II, accounting for 12% of the sample, gave a reaction to rotation in either direction by increased frequency of discharge. Type III response, met in only 5 of the 100 fibers, involved a more or less complete inhibition of discharge upon accelerating or decelerating the animal. Normally active, fibers of this type go into a "silent period" on being stimulated. That these three varieties of nerve response do not result from artifacts introduced by movement of the experimental animal or other accident is attested by the fact that substitution of caloric simulation for acceleratory motion does not change the result. All three types of nerve response can be aroused in the proper fibers by irrigation of the external auditory canal with cold (20° C) and hot (43° C) water.

This discovery of three characteristically different patterns of response in fibers of the vestibular branch is difficult to interpret as yet. It is reminiscent, of course, of a similar state of affairs in vision, where several different types of discharge sequence are encountered in optic fibers. In both instances the phenomenon is much in need of thoroughly systematic study.

The Vestibular Sacs: Utricle and Saccule.   The portion of the membranous canal housed within the vestibule proper is divisible anatomically into two separate structures, the utricle and the saccule. The importance of the utricle is clearly established; it contains nerve endings necessary to the preservation of normal posture. However, the indispensability of the saccule is less certain, though it also contains nerve endings of the type found in the utricle. In animal preparations destruction of the saccule results in no obvious defect of equilibrium or locomotion.

Endings of the vestibular nerve impinge upon an area, one in the utricle and one in the saccule, known as the *macula*, an oval, flat thickening of the wall of the vestibule (see Figure 14–2). The saccular macula is disposed in a plane approximately at right angles to that of the utricular macula. As in the case of the ampullar endings, the nerve terminations are hair cells embedded in a gelatinous substance. The mode of stimulation of the hair endings seems to be somewhat different in the vestibular sacs, however. The hair cells are more nearly columnar in shape and have suspended above them tiny crystals of calcium carbonate. This granular mass, called the otolith organ, is believed to be so constituted as to "load" the hair cells and cause them to be stimulated by gravitational pull. When the body is speeding up or slowing down in straight-line motion, the inertia of the otoliths brings about a bending of the hair cells with consequent discharge of their attached nerve fibers. The effective forces are presumably those produced by shearing movements at the level of the hair attachments. Tilting of the head in any direction would be expected to produce the same result.

Just as the rotating chair has provided the means of studying responses to positive and negative acceleratory forces, the tilt table is the common laboratory device for investigating the effects of gravitational pull on the vestibule. It has been assumed that all that is needed is a way of tilting the entire body away from the vertical and horizontal to various measured extents. A stout board to which the body may be securely strapped, equipped with a substantial bearing and set up in the manner of a seesaw, with a protractor and plumb line attached, is a familiar accouterment of the psychological laboratory. As a device for measuring thresholds of otolithic action the tilt table is an entirely ineffectual instrument. Cues from the skin and muscles, generated by restraining straps and head holder, tend to mask those initiated by the otoliths and thus yield misleading measures. The fact is that currently there are available no reliable threshold figures for either bodily tilt or linear acceleration that reflect, in an uncontaminated way, solely the operation of the vestibular sacs. Several interesting phenomena of static sensibility can, of course, be studied qualitatively by means of the tilt table.

Cutaneous cues can be minimized, or at least rendered ambiguous, in certain other situations. One of these is the free fall through space—not likely to entice any large number of experimentalists in the immediate future—while another, somewhat more practicable for this purpose, is full water immersion. An ingenious experiment along the latter lines was performed, under U.S. Navy auspices, by J. L. Brown (96). Five strong swimmers served as subjects, individually, in a tank where they could be directed to descend to a horizontal rod positioned at a depth of either 18 or 25 ft. There, in a "curled" position on the rod, the subject was rotated three, four, or five times, and was left in one of four positions: head up, down, inclined forward or backward. Instructions were to point promptly to where the surface was judged to be, to then shake the head and correct the judgment if necessary. There was no breathing equipment, no cues from bubbles (since the swimmer held his breath throughout), vision was excluded by an opaque mask, water temperature gradients were eliminated, and buoyancy was made relatively ineffectual as a cue by the great depth.

With the head back and down 135 degrees the situation proved to be a fair simulation of zero gravity. The greatest errors were made in this position. Such a result would be predicted, of course, from our knowledge of utricular construction. The otoconia are "hanging" on their supports when the head is in this position, not bending away from the vertical as they normally do. Some judgments of initial position were in error by as much as 180 degrees, though nodding the head rarely failed to correct the first impression, and divers almost never experienced difficulty in returning straightway to the surface.

A diffuse pattern of strains and pressures having cutaneous, kinesthetic, and visceral origins constitutes the sensory indicator of vestibular action, the "feel" of bodily position. With the assumption of each new head position stimulation arising in the hair cells of the maculae starts impulses over the vestibular nerve to the medulla and cerebellum. At these lower centers connections are made with motor fibers going to neck, eye, trunk, and limb muscles. In each of these groups there may occur "tonic" reflexes, patterns of muscular tension appropriate to the body position involved. In lower organisms many of these positional reflexes may be identified and catalogued. Thus there occur entirely predictable deviations of the eyes of fishes when they are slowly turned on the long axis of the body. In some of the reptiles, lizards and turtles notably, and birds —the pigeon has been intensively studied in this regard—the head will be held absolutely still (within mechanical limitations) irrespective of the position in which the body is placed. In higher forms the picture becomes complicated, and in the human it is vastly so. As we ascend the animal scale the vestibular apparatus is connected with postural responses more and more complexly. Both the sacs and canals become diminished in importance as control devices for equilibrium. It follows that damage to the labyrinth is a relatively less serious matter in humans than it would be in simpler organisms where there are not the substitute mechanisms available. In congenital deaf-mutes, for example, whose labyrinths may be completely degenerate, postural adjustments are still made effectively in most everyday situations. Only when vision is excluded or when visual cues become ambiguous is equilibrium threatened. Thus some deaf people report that they dare not go under water when swimming since "up" and "down" then get confused and they are in danger of drowning. Deaf-blinds have been studied with respect to their vestibular sensitivity (656) with the not unexpected finding that they are unable to maintain balance more than a second or two when required to stand on one foot. Nine of ten deaf-blind subjects showed no postrotational responses whatever. After whirling in a chair there was no dizziness or nausea, no illusions of movement appeared, and there was not even a hint of nystagmus.

It was said earlier that the classical distinction—canals for rotatory accelerations, sacs for linear accelerations and gravity—is not entirely sound. We noted that canals and sacs have both dynamic and static roles to play. The utricular macula is so constructed as to permit the tiny calcite crystals, the otoconia, to originate shearing forces that trigger nerve impulses supplying information about both linear and angular accelerations as well as constant velocities of rotation. Löwenstein has pointed out (393, p. 79) that, were it not for their greater inertia, the utricular nerve endings might compete with those of the cupula in the reporting of angular accelerations. It is this inertia—the otoconia have a specific gravity well over twice that of the endolymph surrounding them—that renders them relatively "static" or "tonic."

Nevertheless, some quite lively responses ensue when the otolith organs are appropriately stimulated. Ocular nystagmus can be created by sidewise oscillations of the body. In one experiment (448), subjects were oscillated sidewise in a cube that ran on tracks. Cyclic frequencies ranging from 0.2 to 0.8 cps imparted linear accelerations which, at peak, amounted to 18.6 ft/sec^2. This is an acceleratory force of 0.58g. Under these conditions horizontal nystagmus was produced, the rapid phase of the eye movements being in the direction of motion. Although efforts have been made to evoke it, vertical nystagmus apparently cannot be generated this way. A curious fact is that sidewise harmonic motion seems not to arouse notable feelings of tilt, only those of motion, whereas to and fro acceleration does, a phenomenon familiar from the parallel swing (253).

The Nonauditory Labyrinth, Aviation, and Space Travel. If the array of facts and principles concerning the nonauditory labyrinth is less formidable than in some other sense fields—and the judgment of the historian of sensory psychophysiology would be that it is—it can also be said that developments in aviation bid fair to change all this. With commercial, private, and military aircraft flying at ever higher speeds new and somewhat extreme demands are being placed on their occupants. The sheer requirements of survival demand that all available sensory and motor capacities be brought to bear on the problem of adapting to a complex and kaleidoscopic environment. In response to the needs of modern aviation, research on labyrinthine phenomena is presently receiving more nearly adequate attention and support than in an earlier time, when rotational and gravitational forces were of practical concern only to the acrobat, the ballet dancer, and, if he thought about them, the whirling dervish!

In the maintenance of equilibrium and bodily orientation visual, labyrinthine, cutaneous, and organic cues all commonly come into play. Occasionally auditory sensations have a supporting role. In the flying situation it is, of course, vision that usually provides the most precise data of orientation. The pilot sees the cockpit and external objects, especially the nose of his plane and the horizon, in relation to each other. In night flight and in "weather" he has his instruments which visually give accurate, if somewhat indirect, indications of the plane's attitude in space. Ordinarily, then, the pilot's sensory world is mainly visual and yields sufficiently exact and complete information to permit of the nice adjustments required in complicated maneuvers as well as in straight and level flight, takeoffs, and landings.

However, information obtained visually is not always correct, subject as it is to illusory influences, and returns from other sensory systems cannot always be suppressed. The sense data most frequently coming in conflict with the visual are those arising from the operation of the nonauditory labyrinth. In flight the occupant of an airplane may be subject to three sets of acceleratory forces: angular, radial, and linear. Angular accelerations and decelerations are fortunately only briefly and transiently encountered in flying; stimuli appropriate to the semicircular canals are not commonly long sustained. However, as we shall see, they are potential sources of disorientation in the air. Radial acceleration and deceleration (centrifugal and centripetal force) occur more commonly, being involved in any rotation about an axis at some distance from the plane. Thus radial forces exert themselves on the pilot whenever he goes into a turn, climb, or dive. But the most common acceleratory and deceleratory stimuli, in all kinds of flying, are linearly disposed ones. Any change in speed unaccompanied by change in direction involves either a positive or negative linear acceleration and becomes a potential stimulus to the vestibular sacs. If the change in velocity is sufficiently marked it can serve to initiate some very serious errors of perception.

The effects of linear acceleration and deceleration in a plane have been investigated at the Pensacola Naval Air Station (*117*). An observer sat blindfolded in the rear of a two-place training plane, his head held rigidly in place. His job was to give a running account of all perceptions of bodily position, the reports being taken down on a wire recorder and synchronized with an objective record of the plane's performance as revealed by a three-dimensional accelerometer. The pilot put the plane through its paces of speed changes by suitable manipulation of throttle and flaps, but maintained as closely as possible straight and level flight. The observer was, of course, ignorant of the plane's true performance. Uniformly, all observers reported strong perceptions of tilting forward when the plane was rapidly slowed down and of tilting backward when speed was suddenly increased. The frequency with which such reports were made, the estimated angle of tilt, and the duration of the feelings of tilt all proved to be proportional to the strength of the stimulus, that is, to the amount of acceleration or deceleration. The threshold for the perception of tilt was surprisingly small, $0.02g$, or only about 2% of the acceleration that would be imparted by a force equal to that of gravity. This is the value for positive acceleration. For deceleration the threshold is higher, about $0.08g$. In either case the feeling of tilting is elaborated into the judgment that the plane is actually changing altitude, climbing in the case of positive acceleration and diving in the case of negative. An acceleration of about $0.1g$ was interpreted as a climb at a 20–25 degree angle. The feeling lasted somewhat beyond the real accelerative force. A deceleration of the same magnitude was felt as a dive at a 15-degree angle below the horizontal. No such estimates would be given, of course, if visual cues to position and motion had remained in the picture. However, this experiment demonstrates what might happen to spatial orientation if visual information were to be obliterated. The pilot flying in fog, having just reduced his throttle setting, may see from his instruments that he is still flying level but his otoliths may tell him he is in a dive. Among a great many things an aviator must learn is the difficult lesson of coming to disregard the direct evidence of his senses, in such situations as this, and to place his trust in the less direct but sounder evidence offered by his flight instruments.

A study which combines the effects of angular and radial accelerations and which, therefore, involves the functioning of the entire nonauditory labyrinth, has also been conducted at Pensacola (400). With very much the same arrangements as those of the linear acceleration experiment, the reactions of observers to varying degrees of lateral tilting and turning were studied. Six different angles of bank, at a constant altitude, were tried: 10, 18, 30, 40, 50, and 60 degrees. Angular accelerations varied from 0.10 degree/sec² (onset of the 10-degree bank) to 0.80 degree/sec² (recovery from the 60-degree bank). The observer reported on his perceptions of turning and tilting, judging direction and amount, and also estimated the magnitude of the forces in operation. The first fact that becomes apparent, on analysis of the records, is that feelings of tilting and turning are dangerously unreliable indicators of the true state of affairs. At small angles of bank the plane's change of direction and position went unnoticed much of the time. The absolute threshold for the perception of turning falls between the 10- and 18-degree banks, where the acceleratory force is about 0.15 degree/sec². Positive and negative accelerations give about the same value. Within the limits of the study there is no angle of bank which provides absolutely certain information; even the 60-degree tilt was not detected 100% of the time. Even though the existence of the banking movement is appreciated, there may still be an erroneous judgment of the direction of turn. Moreover, perceptions of tilting and turning have their onset only after a considerable lag; the maneuver has already been in effect for 5 or more sec. A great deal can happen in the air in this time.

Estimates of the amount of lateral tilt are markedly in error. Going into the turn, while the degree of tilt was being varied between 10 and 60 degrees, the observers made average estimates ranging between 4.2 and 11.9 degrees. Recovery from the bank, which was performed somewhat more rapidly and thus involved relatively greater accelerations, was accompanied by an even smaller range of estimated angles: 4.1 to 6.8 degrees. The duration of the feelings of turning and tilting was quite out of line with reality. All angles of bank were held for about a minute; on the average the feelings had subsided in about one-third that time. In view of what we have already seen about linear accelerations it is not surprising to find a fore-and-aft tilting component present in this experiment as well. The onset of turn and the turn itself are both accompanied by clear feelings of backward tilt, estimated to be as high as 45 degrees in the case of the 60-degree bank. After recovery from the turn, and after a noticeable lag, the observer may feel himself to be tilted forward somewhat.

The one datum that was accurately estimated throughout the entire experiment was the magnitude of the g force. While the true g was changing from 1.02 (at 10-degree bank) to 2.00 (at 60 degrees) the observers' estimates were, respectively, 1.00 and 1.95. Estimated and real forces coincided closely all along the line. Yet, from the standpoint of manipulating the controls of an airplane, this is one bit of information that is practically useless! At least, if g needs to be known for any purpose it would be better to measure it with an instrument. All the potentially useful data, which might serve to supplement visual information when it is meager, turn out to be grossly illusory. And illusion, apparently confirmed, whether by presupposition or accident, develops into delusion in short order; then it may become a platform for action.

Another way in which the nonauditory labyrinth may alter the perceptual field in flying is through the operation of the oculogyral illusion. We have already seen what the general conditions for the occurrence of this phenomenon are—a relatively dim but structured visual target viewed against darkness. If such a target is observed in the air during a banking maneuver the target appears to move, the induced motions being both those of total displacement in space and of rotation about the center. The rotary movements are always in the direction of the banking motion of the plane and have a maximum extent of 15 degrees. There is a lag of 4 to 6 sec between the beginning of the banking maneuver and the reported target rotation. The effect lasts varying amounts of time depending on stimulus intensity, from less than 10 sec (10-degree bank) to nearly 30 sec (60-degree bank). Total displacement of the target is a little less predictable but occurs, along with rotary motion, at all angles of bank. This form of distortion of the visual field apparently requires special conditions for its occurrence and thus does not constitute a very serious threat to the flyer. In ordinary daylight flying the visual field is too well illuminated and too replete with geometrical detail to be subject to the oculogyral illusion. In most night flying situations runway illumination, signal lights, cockpit illumination, and general ground lighting all aid in its avoidance. A more serious threat to safety in night flight seems to be occasioned by the so-called autokinetic phenomenon. This effect occurs when a single, relatively confined light source is stared at continuously over a period of time. The light appears to move, gliding, wavering, or wandering in an unpredictable manner through space. This phenomenon is not confined to aviation, of course; one can demonstrate it to himself quite readily in a dark room provided with a "point" source of light. But the autokinetic effect has special implications for aviation in that the conditions of its arousal occur not uncommonly in night flying. It has been responsible for many near accidents and probably, in military aviation, for some fatal ones. In formation flying at night the pilot "flying wing" on a squadron leader will attempt to maintain a constant distance between planes by steadily fixating the light on his leader's wing tip. After a prolonged period of this the autokinetic phenomenon may supervene. The light ahead may appear to describe an arc as in a "wingover" or other radical change in flight path; the hapless pilot makes rapid stick and rudder adjustments in an attempt to "follow," then finds himself either in a collision path with another aircraft or in a spin, recovery from which may be impossible. The use of flashing signal lights and higher illumination levels, together with repeated injunctions to pilots to keep their eyes moving about during night flights, have helped to reduce this particular hazard.

Potentially, the greatest threat to safety in flight is offered by the so-called *Coriolis effect*. This occurs whenever one set of semicircular canals has adjusted to a constant angular velocity—the endolymph has caught up with the canal walls, so to speak—and a new head motion in a different geometrical plane is made. Then there occurs at one and the same time a deceleration in the canals originally stimulated and a new acceleration in a different set of canals. The net result of these complex changes is that motion comes to be perceived in a direction in which real motion is not occurring. There are necessarily many different possible reactions, depending upon whether there are conflicting visual and other sensory cues, but if the Coriolis effect is controlling by virtue of a strong head movement and the absence of competitive information there can be nothing but trouble in the outcome. At very high angular velocities the extent of the head movement that will induce the Coriolis phenomenon need not be large.

Another dangerous maneuver, from the standpoint of vestibular cues, occurs in conjunction with spins. Following a spin in which the feel of rotary motion has adapted out, the relaxation into a straight flight path may be accompanied by the feeling of a continuous turn in the opposite direction. If the vestibular information on pulling out of a spin is relied upon exclusively, there will be made "corrective" movements that will put the aviator back into the original direction of spin. Somewhat similar reactions occur in a banked spiral. Here the reactions made in the absence of visual or instrumental information tend to tighten the spiral. Aviators refer to these two situations as the "graveyard spin" and the "graveyard spiral."

Perhaps the commonest disorientation occurring in flying, though one that does not ordinarily imperil life and limb, is known as the "leans." This usually comes about as the result, in straight and level flight, of the subliminal acquisition of a bank. The poor attitude of the airplane having been discovered, perhaps by instrument, a quick correction is made, whereupon the pilot may then adjust his own attitude to the perceived vertical. A posture is adopted which, in reality, is a leaning one. Variants on the theme are, of course, possible.

Since the middle of the century, when the prospect that relatively complete freedom from gravitational influences on the human body first became a real one, there has been almost frantic investigation of the psychological phenomena associated with weightlessness. Would our astronauts become completely disoriented and confused when the otoliths ceased to add their messages to the general stream of bodily information? Would there be a persistent sensation of falling if the ever-present gravitational component of our perceptual framework were to be lacking? Would changes in the overall feeling pattern lead to befuddlement and, perhaps, catastrophic judgment? Affirmative guesses would not be unreasonable; indeed, they were seriously made in the early 1950's by several "experts."

There are, of course, a fair number of situations in which gravitational pull is taken off the otoliths. One of these we have already encountered in the immersion experiments. With head down in a deep tank, lung pressure and buoyancy just balancing each other, there can be little, if any, shearing force exerted on hair cells by otoconia, and there must result what amounts to a "deafferentation" of the otolithic macula. Other relatively transient "diminished g" situations, complete or partial, occur: (a) when riding in a plane caught in a sudden downdraft; (b) in a descent on a roller coaster; (c) in an unhindered "free fall" before a parachute is opened; (d) in a down trip on an express elevator; (e) when buoyantly floating in quiet water at the seashore. Even when poised in midair on leaving a diving board, when falling out of a tree or off a haymow, or jumping up and down on a trampoline, there are brief instants in which the load is off the utricle. But none of these has much to offer by way of experimental control and all induce the weightless condition far too briefly.

Until ballistic and orbital flights became possible, two expedients were adopted to simulate "zero-g," at least some aspects of it. One of these involved the use of air-bearing platforms which, while they cannot remove gravitational influences from the experimental subject, do succeed in inducing an important mechanical effect, that of depriving him of the normal stabilizing effect of friction. The other was the use of high-speed aircraft describing a particular flight path, a so-called Keplerian parabolic trajectory, that will impart an upward acceleration counteracting gravity for an appreciable interval. See Figure 14–14. Weightless periods of from 15 sec to nearly a minute can be induced this way. The chief difficulty associated with the technique is the unfor-

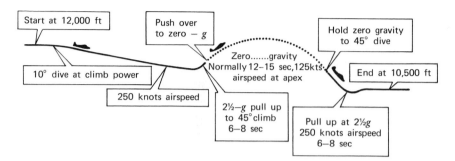

Fig. 14–14. A typical zero-*g* flight maneuver. From Howard and Templeton (*312*) after Hammer.

tunate "pull-up *g*," amounting to 2 to 3 times gravity, that have to initiate and terminate the parabolic path. How much of the "weightless" effect is attributable to these highly unpleasant accelerations and how much to freedom from gravity is not readily ascertained, though the two can usually be separated for experienced observers for whom 2 to 3 *g* may cause no inconvenience.

A tremendous number of parabolic flights have been flown in experiments sponsored by the military since the day, in 1951, when the first Keplerian trajectory was flown for this purpose. By 1958 one Air Force pilot had logged 4000 test maneuvers of this kind. Had there been any seriously incapacitating effects of weightlessness it is to be noted that the logging itself would not have been accomplished! In early trials it was noted that small incoordinations were produced, there being, especially, something of a tendency to overreach with the arms. Allowances were promptly made for these, however, as they also were for overall rotations of the body that accompanied limb movements and for alterations in observed visual position, changed judgments of the weight of objects, etc. The adjustment problem has not proved to be the vexing one it was predicted to be nor have there been the tensions that might have been created by persistent "falling" sensations. The great majority of observers have reported states of well-being and comfort; the feeling is of floating or soaring rather than of falling. Some find the experiments exhilarating.

When, in the preludes to prolonged orbital flight, experiments were carried out, first with animals and then with human observers, on ballistic rockets and space capsules in relatively short orbits, nearly everything that happened was psychologically reassuring (*297*). Not only could the high accelerations of blastoff be sustained but also the basic biological functions of respiration, pulse, and blood pressure returned within a few minutes to a normal range and remained there. The first human to orbit the earth, according to the Russian report, had "no difficulties in the sensory or motor sphere." By and large, this has been the conclusion from all subsequent orbiting adventures by cosmonauts and astronauts. At least, where visual and tactile cues remain, the absence of the customary gravitational load on the otoliths is neither debilitating nor does it impair the normal integrative function in perception.

The nonauditory labyrinth enters into aviation in yet another way; it is concerned with the production of air sickness. This malady, as much the plague of the airways as its relative, seasickness, is of the sea lanes, constitutes for many people a major deterrent to air travel. Air sickness and seasickness are members of a large family of which train sickness, car sickness, and the somewhat rarer illness experienced on roller coasters, during parachute descents, and while riding on camels are others. The feature all these forms of transportation have in common is regularly repeated motion of fairly low frequency. Motion sickness seems never to come from walking, running, or otherwise repeatedly jarring the head in a rapidly recurrent fashion. Marathon runners become exhausted but not nauseated. Nor is motion sickness ever an immediate effect of rhythmic motion; some little time is required for a "buildup" of the reaction.

A comprehensive study of motion sickness was undertaken by Wendt and his colleagues at the University of Rochester (620). They installed a vertical accelerator or "wave machine," a kind of elevator in which it is possible to vary waveform, degree of acceleration, velocity and amplitude of movement, and frequency of wave repetition. These components of motion were combined in various ways to test their relative efficacy as generators of motion sickness. It turns out that sickness rate depends on the frequency with which wave motion is repeated, on waveform, and on total wave energy. As wave frequency is increased sickness rate increases, at first slowly then more rapidly, until a peak rate is reached at about 20 cycles/min. Above this frequency, where each phase of the motion recurs every 3 sec, the stimulus becomes less effective. Rapidly repeated waves result in very little illness. In one experiment more than one-third of the subjects became ill within 20 min when stimulated with a 9-ft wave repeated 13 times a minute, while only 7% became sick in response to a 1-ft wave having a frequency of 32 cycles/min. In another study a motion having an amplitude of 7 ft, occurring at the more moderate frequency of 22 per minute, induced illness in somewhat over half the members of a sizable group of naval officers.

A prime suspect for the role of major causative factor in motion sickness is the disorganization of sensorimotor response that occurs when bodily motions over which we have no control are introduced by our environment. If the whole body is subject to pitching and heaving at unaccustomed rates and if, in addition, vestibular information gets further complicated by the occurrence of head movements, the precise adjustments needed to preserve equilibrium may be quite unpredictable. Feelings of distress may sometimes be obviated by simply holding the head still when seasickness threatens. At the same time, there is no guarantee that such a simple prescription tells the whole story or even really gets at the basic mechanism. It is equally true that some people become deathly ill in "fun houses" at fairs and resorts whenever they enter "phantom swings" or distorted rooms, where nothing at all moves except the visual environment.

It may well be that the vestibular organs, more particularly the otoliths, have a natural periodicity of oscillation determined by their structure. Perhaps, at vibratory periods too slow for the natural resonance of the maculae, sensations might fail to reflect the true state of affairs in bodily motion. Acting on this assumption, Walsh (604) performed the interesting experiment of varying the oscillation period of a horizontal parallel swing. Indeed, he had three different arrangements that would permit prone, supine, and "on-side" positions and swing periods varying from 1 to 12 sec in duration. Whereas amplitudes up to 2 m could be realized, for the determination of purely labyrinthine events uncomplicated by cutaneous and deeper somesthetic cues, it was necessary to limit length of swing so as to restrict accelerations near turning points; otherwise the skin and deep receptors would provide contaminating information. Periods of 3 and 9 sec proved satisfactory; these would yield thresholds, for a well-trained observer, of the order of 3 to 4 cm/sec² (peak accelerations).

The really important finding, however, involved slightly supraliminal stimulation and judgments by eight observers of the direction in which they perceived themselves to be moving at any given instant. At the 1-sec duration of swing, all judgments were substantially correct, but at oscillations ⅓ this speed, or slower, there was a "phase advance." Perception of motion, as indicated by directional finger pointing, was in advance of real motion. Thus the observer regularly anticipated the direction of swing. The first feeling of movement in one direction occurred when the body was actually traveling in the opposite direction. When stationary at a turn the observer felt himself to be moving most rapidly in the direction toward which he was then turning. There was thus a 90-degree phase advance, and the same 90-degree disjunction was also realized at the ⅙-cps rate of swing as well. Suitable tests of reaction time in making the report demonstrated that this was not a phase lag of 270 degrees in indicating direction; that is, there was not a ¾-period delay in report. Although the direct linkage of this "out-of-step" phenomenon with the onset of motion sickness has not been clearly demonstrated, the suspicion is strong that some such incoordination of sensation and movement must be implicated.

There are, of course, notable individual differences in susceptibility to motion illness, yet the presumption is that anyone with an intact vestibular mechanism will become nauseated if the stimulating conditions are severe enough. Both military aviation and naval experience indicate that more than 50% of new personnel are subject to airsickness or seasickness on encountering the rigors of traveling "in weather," yet resistant fliers and sailors with good "sea legs" are developed in quite a short time. In the normal person, habituation to recurrent slow motion occurs with some rapidity. Studies in World War II showed that 10 to 11% of all flying students became airsick at some time during their first 10 flights, but only 1 to 2% were actually eliminated from flight training on these grounds (26, p. 219).

An important step in the screening of military personnel for motion-sickness susceptibility has been taken by the introduction of the so-called Dial Test in the Slow Rotation Room (350). The room, 15 ft in diameter, is ordinarily rotated at 7.5 rpm. The subject is put through a series of head, trunk, and limb movements in which he inspects and sets dials in a predetermined sequence. There are five settings in a group and 20 groups so that the entire performance calls for the completion of 100 settings. The test is really a set of Coriolis sequences, for many aircraft maneuvers are simulated (turns, rolls, wingovers, porpoising movements, etc.) in the course of which are made head movements that combine with the motion imparted by the rotating room to yield complex vestibular stimulation. Instructions are given by a standardized sound tape. The Dial Test, when validated against performance in the air (24 maneuvers in a "Skyraider" aircraft), proves to be a good predictor of airsickness in aerobatics. Anyone who can survive the 100 settings of the Dial Test without feeling squeamish is likely to be able to adjust to an aircraft doing "lazy eights" and "barrel rolls." At least, such a prediction seems to be justified in a general way. Individual differences, as yet unexplained and perhaps inexplicable in the present limited state of knowledge, necessarily prohibit perfect prediction for the individual.

5
The Sense of Smell

Smell and Taste Confusions. Foods and beverages, once taken into the mouth, make at least a dual, usually a triple, appeal. The tissues of the mouth, throat, and nasal cavity are so innervated, and so disposed in relation to one another, that any or all of three sensory systems can go into operation simultaneously in response to the same stimulus. The cutaneous sensibilities of the mouth region are inevitably brought into play. They not only report on texture of foods but contribute the "biting," "burning," or astringent elements of certain of them and the "coolness" or tingle of others. The sense of taste is also obviously involved, end organs in the tongue and palate accounting for a limited but basic repertory of sense qualities. It is, however, olfaction that furnishes the most elaborate of experiences connected with food, for it is the receptor system situated high in the nostrils that supplies the overtones for the fundamental tastes, that adds "aroma," that transforms sheer acceptance of food into appreciation of flavor. Were there no sense of smell there would be no gourmets, only consumers of nutriments.

We are constantly ascribing to taste those sensations that really belong to smell. The confusion is a natural one. Unless one takes the trouble to block off the nostrils and make the test to determine what the tongue by itself can do to identify food flavors, one may never discover how poor the sense of taste is and what a great richness and variety of experience are contributed by smell. The sense of taste, unassisted, is able to detect the sourness of acid, the sweetness of sugar, the bitterness of quinine, and the salt taste of sodium chloride. It fails utterly to encompass the full flavor of meats, fruits, butter, and coffee. These, together with nearly all other foods, depend for their appreciation mainly on their appeal to the sense of smell. Hold the nose and, except for the cues that may be offered to the sense of touch by textural features, a cube of raw potato may be indistinguishable from one of apple. Only the slight sweetness of each comes to register under these conditions. In a similar situation oil of peppermint has only a weakly bitter taste, while making its most forceful impression on cutaneous nerve endings to give a strong feeling of "coolness." With the nose out of action powdered cinnamon yields only a mild sweetness.

The relative sensitivities of the three systems encountered in the mouth and nose region—smell, taste, and feeling—can be assessed by using one of the relatively few substances which serves as a stimulus both to smell and to taste and which, in sufficiently high concentration, also chemically irritates the cutaneous fibers. Such a stimulus is ethyl alcohol. Thresholds of the three kinds of sensation show that smell is evoked with about 1/60,000 the concentration needed to produce a cutaneous ("burning") sensation, while taste results from about $\frac{1}{3}$ the strength necessary for minimal arousal of the skin. Other stimuli would yield somewhat different indices of relative delicacy, but, by and large, they would show olfaction to be considerably ahead of the other two systems in absolute sensitivity. As Parker has said of taste and smell, ". . . the two senses may be said to differ from each other more or less as ordinary scales do from a chemical balance; taste is used in determining the presence of relatively large amounts of substance, smell for only the most minute quantities" (*459*, p. 238).

Physical Properties of Odors.   A wide range of differently constituted materials possesses odor. One property they all have in common, however; they are all *volatile* substances. To stimulate the sense of smell materials must be airborne and in a finely divided state. Solids, unless they pass over readily into the gaseous state at ordinary temperatures, cannot be smelled. Liquids do not become odorous until they vaporize.

Since volatility is a sine qua non for odors, the ease with which substances evaporate should provide an index of their relative stimulating power. If volatility were the only prerequisite the efficacy of a material as an odor stimulus would be given directly by its vapor pressure, since this is a measure of the facility with which molecules escape the parent substance and pervade the surrounding atmosphere. In a general way the relation holds.

Highly odorous liquids, then, are likely to have high vapor pressures; liquids of faint scent are likely to be of low vapor pressure. But there are prominent exceptions. Musk, for example, is one of the most powerful odorants known and is, for this reason, used effectively in the manufacture of perfumes. It is of low volatility, however. The answer in this case seems to be that musk owes its power as a smell stimulus to its favorable chemical composition; only relatively few molecules need be released for this material to be effective. Pure water has a relatively high vapor pressure but is, of course, odorless. Volatility seems to be a necessary but not a sufficient condition for the generation of odor.

Another physical characteristic of possible importance is solubility. The presumption is that odorous materials must be captured by the mucous lining of the nostrils before they can stimulate. This implies that the particles go into solution. If so, they presumably have to be water soluble. Perhaps the odorant must enter the cells containing the actual nerve endings. If so, the odorous material would have to be lipoid soluble as well.

A great many odorous substances are both water soluble and lipoid soluble, and a simple relation between ease of odor production and solubility has not been easy to establish. There are some provocative facts, however. The family of alcohols, which forms a so-called homologous series having the general chemical formula, $C_nH_{(2n+1)}OH$, contains some weakly odorous members, others which have strong odors, and still others that are odorless. The "lower" alcohols (those having few carbon atoms: methyl alcohol, CH_3OH, and ethyl alcohol, C_2H_5OH) have relatively feeble odors. These are readily soluble in water but are practically insoluble in fatty materials. The "higher" alcohols either have no odor at all or, like the lower ones, give only faint odors. Thus, cetyl alcohol, $C_{16}H_{33}OH$, is entirely without odor. In general, the higher alcohols are lipoid soluble but not water soluble. Between the two extremes of the series are a number of compounds which are both water and fat soluble. Butanol, C_4H_9OH, is such an alcohol; it has the powerful odor characteristic of rancid butter. Compounds in the middle of the series are uniformly quite odorous. This would suggest that an odorant, to be effective, has to possess both water and fat solubility. However, as in the case of the attempt to link odor production with volatility, there are exceptions to any such simple rule. One finds, for example, that acetone has low fat solubility but a strong odor. There are other cases which violate the rule and which prevent a straightforward linkage of solubility with odorousness. There remains the possibility, of course, that it is neither water nor fat solubility that is important. The mucous lining of the upper nostrils may have become specially modified, chemically and physically, to do its unique work and may, therefore, be of quite elaborate composition. Some attention has been given to the protein solubility of odorants (*426*, pp. 285–286), with the finding that certain odorants are more readily soluble in protein solutions than in water. This is a promising relation which needs to be investigated with systematic thoroughness, a treatment it has not received as yet.

In addition to volatility and solubility in one or another solvent, odorous materials necessarily possess a large number of other physical properties, some of which may conceivably have something to do with odor production. Many of these properties have been subject to study, and there are some suggestive results, though no sweeping generalities have as yet emerged. Several of the physical characteristics investigated have to do with the manner in which odorous substances absorb, scatter, refract, or otherwise react to light. It was noted long ago that many odorous solutions strongly absorb waves from the infrared portion of the electromagnetic spectrum. Similar absorption in the ultraviolet region of the spectrum has been shown to occur, and this fact has prompted a theory of odor. The interesting transformation of odorous solutions into colloidal suspensoids consequent upon ultraviolet irradiation, the curious fact that the vast majority of odors have refractive indices occupying a very narrow range of values in the neighborhood of 1.5, and the special behavior of odorants with respect to the so-called Raman shift have all been viewed as possible clues to the discovery of the central stimulus property for smell. The last mentioned, the Raman shift, may yet turn out to be important. Many liquids, odorants among them, have the property of so changing monochromatic light shining through them that some of the emergent waves are found to have frequencies both higher and lower than the one received. The difference between the wavelengths of incident and transmitted lights is the Raman shift. The claim is that only substances having shifts between 140 nm and 350 nm are odorous. Much remains to be learned about this relationship. Thus far we only know that the effect occurs with great regularity in odorous solutions, that it presumably is a direct indicator of quite specific intramolecular vibrations, and that many odors which have similar smells also show similar behavior with respect to their Raman spectra.

Odor and Chemical Composition. If there is uncertainty about the physical characteristics necessary in odors there is still more concerning their chemical qualifications. This is not for lack of chemical knowledge about odorous materials. We were perhaps better off in this respect in an earlier time when we knew less chemistry. As matters now stand it is quite impossible to devise any sweeping generalities about the chemical composition of odors. It is found that some compounds of quite different composition smell alike, while others of similar chemical structure are readily distinguished by smell. Even some compounds having identical molecular constituents, differing from each other only with respect to the spatial arrangement of certain of their atoms (stereoisomers), may yield different odors.

This is not to say that no predictions whatever as to odor can be made from a knowledge of chemical composition. Within certain families of substances it is possible to state fairly accurately what the substitution of one radical for another will do or how the addition to or subtraction from the molecule of a particular atom will affect odor. But the rules joining chemistry of odorants with olfactory sensitivity are certainly not uncomplicated, nor are we in possession of any master generalizations linking the two.

By and large, odor stimuli belong to the class of organic rather than inorganic substances. None of the chemical elements which occur free in nature is odorous under usual conditions. If heated to the point of vaporization elementary arsenic yields an odor, one strongly resembling garlic. There are 29 other elements which are also found in the free state; not one of them is capable of exciting smell without first combining with other elements to form compounds. Thus, both hydrogen and sulfur fail to stimulate the nostrils; let them combine to make hydrogen sulfide, and they set up a veritable stench. Of the remaining elements, which are normally to be found only in a combined state, only a few are of olfactory interest. These are the halogen family: chlorine, bromine, iodine, and fluorine; phosphorus, in the yellow form, P_4; and oxygen, as ozone, O_3. The halogens do not occur, at normal temperatures and pressures, in their atomic state. It is the diatomic molecules, Cl_2, Br_2, I_2, and F_2, that excite the sense of smell. The odor of chlorine is familiar from bleaching agents and disinfectants. Bromine and iodine somewhat resemble chlorine, though they are less irritating. Fluorine one handles with great respect, since its chief use (in the form of hydrofluoric acid) is to etch glass! In very dilute solutions it may be smelled, however. Like the other halogens it is an irritant and poisonous. Its odor somewhat resembles that of hypochlorous acid, $HOCl$, to which it is not too distantly related.

The fact that the only seven elements that excite olfaction lie in a somewhat restricted region of the periodic table (the halogens in Group 7, phosphorus and arsenic in Group 5, and oxygen in Group 6) has naturally been of interest to more than one theorist. It would appear that the capacity to function in a high state of valency has something to do with odor production. Yet one is barred from coming to a firm conclusion here by the equally evident fact that other elements in these groups are olfactorily inert.

Another "near generalization" arises from a consideration of the positions of the odorous elements in the so-called *electrochemical series*. The chemical elements may be arranged in sequence, from high to low, depending on the potential difference between the element and an aqueous solution of its salt. The greater the potential difference, the higher the element in the series. Those occupying the top positions, all metals, are able to displace lower elements from their salts. Now it turns out that six of the seven odorous elements occupy six of the last seven places in the series. Arsenic seriously violates the rule by appearing in the middle of the total series, however, and thus prevents the formulation of what might have become an important law of olfactory chemistry.

The key to the mystery of the chemical properties of odors is unlikely to be discovered either within the periodic table of elements or in the electrochemical series. These constructions are too simple. The vast majority of odorants are organic compounds and are relatively complex in constitution. With a few notable exceptions, such as carbon tetra-chloride (CCl_4) and hexachlorethane (C_2Cl_6), organic materials always contain both carbon and hydrogen atoms. In addition, they are likely to contain oxygen. Commonly nitrogen, sulfur, or the halogens are repre-sented in their structure. A wide range of other elements appears in organic compounds, though none other as frequently as those listed above.

Many families of organic compounds have been studied systematically with respect to their odor-producing characteristics. To be sure, there are resemblances of odor pretty clearly traceable to chemical similarities. In general, one expects compounds of phosphorus, bismuth, and arsenic to have odors reminiscent of garlic. Sulfur compounds, by and large, are vile smelling, as are also those of selenium and tellurium. Ethers and esters generally have fragrant odors; the fragrances yielded by many flowers and fruits are due to the esters exuded by them. However, excep-tions to even such rules as these are frequent enough. Thus a prominent sulfur compound, ethyl sulfite, far from having an offensive odor, smells like peppermint. Some of the higher esters, such as refined beeswax, have no odor whatever, owing to their being insoluble and thus incapable of stimulating.

If there are direct and invariable links between chemical makeup and odor we certainly do not know what they are. The whole picture is further confounded by the fact that some organic compounds, certain of the sub-stituted ammonias (amines) among them, change their odor with dilu-tion. Ambergris and civet, both of which are animal secretions, behave in a similar manner, being repulsive in concentrated form but attractive, in fact used as constituents of expensive perfumes, when in great dilution.

The Olfactory Receptors.   The airway of the nostril gives access to the sensitive nerve endings, all but hidden high in a crypt at the top of the nasal cavity. The sensitive region, called the *olfactory cleft*, occupies an area of about 2.5 cm² in each nostril. The two olfactory clefts are separated by the nasal septum.

Figure 15–1 diagrams the nasal passage and suggests some features of

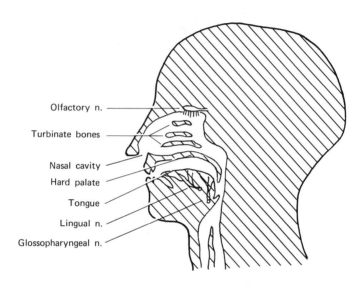

Olfactory n.
Turbinate bones
Nasal cavity
Hard palate
Tongue
Lingual n.
Glossopharyngeal n.

Fig. 15–1.   The nasal passages. From Pfaffmann (*464.*)

the aerodynamics of odor reception. The average volume of the human nasal chamber is 17.1 cc (34.2 cc for the two nostrils combined), and a considerable amount of odor-laden air may thus be in a position to bring about olfactory stimulation. The main movement of air, in ordinary breathing, takes place throughout a high arc in the streamlined nasal cavity, nearly all the inspired current passing through to the pharynx and lungs without affecting the olfactory cleft at all. Such air masses are not rigidly confined to a strictly limited path, however. Both by way of convection and diffusion odorous particles escape the main air stream and find their way to the uppermost reaches of the nasal chamber, where the sensitive olfactory epithelium lies. In mastication of food, motions of the palate and throat create small air movements that send odorous material up to the cleft by way of the rear access provided by the nasopharnyx. Particularly during exhalation, but also during the irregular breathing created by sniffing, swirls of air are generated in the region of the superior turbinate (see Figure 15-1), and "eddy currents" can then transport odorous particles to the sensitive region with some force.

Once having reached the olfactory cleft odorous materials can affect the sensitive receptors. In just what manner, whether by chemical or physical means, we do not know with certainty. But we do know something of the anatomical and physiological features of the presumed receptor cells. The system of nerve endings responsible for smell is, in many respects, the most primitive to be encountered in the body.

The entire patch of tissue which constitutes the surface of the olfactory cleft is known as the *olfactory mucosa* or *olfactory epithelium*. It consists of literally millions of tiny endings of the first cranial (olfactory) nerve, together with an even larger number of columnar or *sustentacular* cells. As their name implies, the latter mainly serve the function of support, though it is the case that the columnar cells are also pigmented and give a brownish yellow appearance to the area. This tends to set the sensitive region off from the neighboring unpigmented epithelium. The nerve terminations, projecting through the supporting cells to the surface, are called *olfactory rods*. The rods are true endings of olfactory nerve fibers. There is no synapse at the level of the epithelial tissues, each rod serving the roles of generator and conductor of nerve impulses. One might regard the olfactory rod as a kind of combined receptor and ganglion cell. Such duality of function is not uncommon in the relatively primitive nervous systems of some of the lower vertebrates. In this case it perhaps reflects the great antiquity of the olfactory system in phylogenetic development.

Much has been learned about the structural details of the olfactory mucosa through studies with the electron microscope. Figure 15–2 reconstructs such information from the rabbit, whose olfactory equipment is far better known than that of the human *(392)*. The rods are about 1μ in diameter, and typically swell to about twice that size at their distal ends. From six to a dozen or more tiny *cilia* arise, sepal-like, from the tip of each rod, and project into the mucous layer which bathes the entire sensitive surface of the olfactory epithelium. The cilia typically extend 1 to 2μ beyond the tip of the rod, but in some nonmammalian preparations they have been seen thinning out to fine processes that stretch out to 100μ or more and lie in a tangled network along the surface. This arrangement suggests that they have a most strategic role to play in initiating neural events. The interesting calculation has been made *(50)* that, if one assumes average observed dimensions for the cilia and their filaments and the best estimates of the number of end organs in the olfactory cleft, there would result an irregular surface of 600 cm² to serve as the adsorption area for odorants. This is an expanse roughly equal to the two pages of print spread before you!

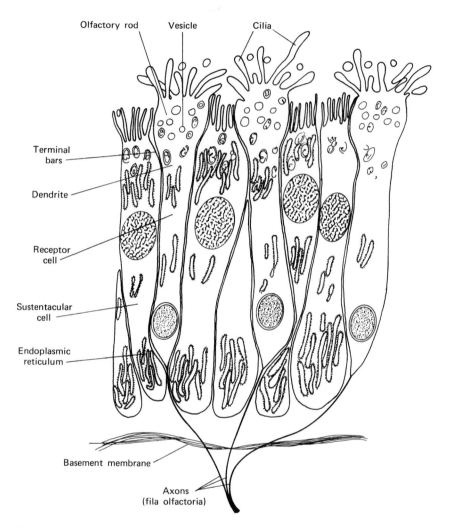

Fig. 15–2. Reconstruction of the olfactory mucosa of the rabbit from electron microscope studies. From T. C. Ruch and H. D. Patton, *Physiology and biophysics*. Philadelphia: Saunders, 1965; after de Lorenzo (*392*).

As the nerve fibers leave the epithelium they are seen to converge into larger and larger bundles. There are no lateral connections to join one part of the sensitive area with another, nor is there any overlap in distribution of fibers. The nerve bundles pass through a number of perforations in the *cribriform plate* of the ethmoid bone, to which the olfactory epithelium is attached, and immediately enter the olfactory bulb, the farthest forward of the brain's extensions. Near the bulb's surface are encountered formations known as *glomeruli*, where the first synapse in the system occurs. In the human olfactory bulb there are perhaps 2000 glomeruli, each receiving many nerve fibers from the olfactory epithelium. A vast network of fibers arises at this point to complicate greatly the picture of nervous conduction. Two types of nerve cells participate, *mitral* cells and *tufted* cells. Dendrites of mitral cells are found in the glomeruli; their cell bodies lie deeper in the bulb. Some of the axons of mitral cells pass directly backwards to form the olfactory tract. Others connect with nearby tufted cells, which in turn send axons back to enter the glomeruli. A circular pathway is thus created, a so-called "reverberatory circuit." The guess is that this kind of arrangement makes for "amplification" of the nerve message, behaving much like a regenerative radio receiver network, and may thus serve to improve the general level of olfactory sensitivity.

In view of this elaborate set of pathways it would be important to know to what extent there is preserved point-to-point transport of impulses from the sensitive epithelium to the beginning of the olfactory tract. Is it possible for olfactory impulses to be organized spatially, as those of all other modalities conceivably are? Adrian (7) has adduced some evidence that there is at least a primitive spatial patterning, some parts of the olfactory tract responding somewhat differentially to different groups of odors. Prompted by this discovery, Clark (120) has carefully followed out the degeneration patterns in the olfactory epithelium of rabbits who had been given localized lesions of the olfactory bulb. Some degree of regional projection was found. Both the anatomical and neurophysical possibilities for spatial organization are apparently present.

We shall not attempt to trace in detail the complicated and as yet little understood pathways from the olfactory bulb back to the cortical smell centers. Considering the relatively minor role that olfaction plays in human life we have a remarkably elaborate olfactory tract. It is, of course, a bequest from our animal ancestors, whose noses were much closer to the ground and for whom olfactory decisions were often life or death affairs. Currently, a many-sided experimental approach is being made in an effort to determine just what parts of the brain are involved in olfaction. The techniques in use are, in general, those found successful in the other sense departments: (a) removal of animals' central nervous tissue in varying amounts and in different locations, with a view to noting the effects on a pre-established discrimination or conditioned response;

(b) stimulation, electrically or chemically, of the motor areas of the brain in an effort to arouse muscular responses associated with olfaction (e.g., chewing and swallowing movements); (c) recording of action potentials at various levels of the central nervous system when the sense organ is being stimulated. The evidences coming from these diverse approaches have then to be put together with those offered by neural anatomy.

Insofar as the various lines of evidence speak with a common voice they point to the critical areas lying deep in the center of the brain mass as the projection zones for smell. Areas that are suspected occupy a nearly closed ring in the lower part of the mesial surface of the rhinencephalon (the "smell brain"). A prominent candidate is the pyriform area, since it readily reveals electrical activity during olfactory stimulation.

Olfactometry. If we raise the question of the minimal stimulus for olfaction, as we did for vision, hearing, and touch, we shall be able to get some answers, though they will not be as satisfactory as for the other senses. Methods are available, however, for determining fairly accurately the threshold amounts of odorous materials. It is even possible to calculate the number of molecules present at threshold concentration. In the case of the strongest odorants the amount that has to be released, to be just detected by the nostrils, is so small that there are no means, chemical or physical, of directly measuring it. The threshold quantity is not indeterminate, however. By starting with a known concentration of the odorous substance and evaporating it into a known volume of air, then repeatedly mixing this with equal parts of air to produce progressive dilutions of $\frac{1}{2}$, $\frac{1}{4}$, $\frac{1}{8}$, etc., a point will be reached where odor sensation will just fail to be elicited. A series of connected containers which will produce such a systematic weakening of an odorant is known as a *dilution osmoscope*.

By this method of measuring the absolute threshold it has been found that the minimum perceptible concentration of vanillin is of the order of 2 ten-millionths of a milligram per cubic meter of air, that of mercaptan (C_2H_5SH) is 0.00004 mg/m^3, while diethyl ether (the anesthetic, $C_2H_5OC_2H_5$) has a threshold concentration of about 1.0 mg/m^3 of air. In the case of mercaptan, it has been calculated that there need be only 1 molecule per 50 trillion molecules of air for this foul odor to be detected. Of course, it should be pointed out that we are talking of molecules, and a "sniff" of 20 cc volume, at the same threshold concentration, could be expected to contain about 10 trillion molecules of mercaptan (*426*, p. 79).

Most studies involving the determination of smell thresholds have made use of the *olfactometer*, an instrument designed by the Dutch physiologist, Zwaardemaker. It is illustrated in Figure 15–3. In its simplest form it consists of a glass tube, open at both ends, over which is loosely slipped a hard rubber or plastic tube, the inner surface of the latter being impregnated with an odorous material. A scale etched on the inner tube indicates the position of the outer one and thus the extent of odor-bearing surface exposed to the stream of air created by the subject's inhalation. The olfactometer exists in two forms, single

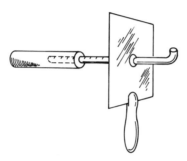

Fig. 15–3. The Zwaardemaker (single) olfactometer. A hard rubber cylinder, impregnated with odorous material, fits loosely on one end of a glass tube, the other end of which enters the nostril. Variations in odor strength are obtained by changing the cylinder's position. From Pfaffmann (*464*).

and double, for stimulation of one nostril (*monorhinic*) or for two simultaneously (*dirhinic*, same odor in both nostrils; *dichorhinic*, different odors). As standardized by Zwaardemaker, the odor cylinder has an inner diameter of 0.8 cm, a length of 10 cm, and a volume of 50 cc. The instrument's scale may be calibrated in smell units, "olfacties," one olfactie being the number of centimeters exposed when threshold is reached. Instead of relying upon a "standard sniff" to deliver the odorous particles, some experimenters have attached a small continuous-flow pump to the instrument, and air moving at 100 cc/sec has been blown through the system for an exposure period of ⅓ sec.

It is this difficulty of insuring that a constant amount of odorous material will be conveyed to the olfactory cleft in successive exposures that led to the substitution of another olfactometric technique for the one devised by Zwaardemaker. Elsberg and Levy (*187*) developed the so-called "blast injection" method of odor stimulation (Figure 15–4). In this procedure an odorous liquid is poured into a 500-cc bottle. An outlet tube leads to the nostrils; an inlet tube is attached to a hypodermic syringe. A pinchcock on the outlet is kept closed while a few cubic

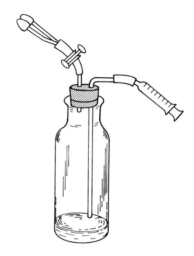

Fig. 15–4. Apparatus used in the blast injection technique of Elsberg and Levy (*187*). An odorous solution is contained in a 500-cc bottle. A known small pressure is created with a hypodermic syringe (seen on the right), and the release of a stopcock sends a "blast" of saturated vapor through the nosepieces. From Pfaffmann (*464*).

cm of air is forced into the bottle, using the syringe as a pump. With the nose piece in place the pinchcock is suddenly removed, releasing a "blast" of odorous vapor into the nostrils. In successive trials the air pressure is varied to find the threshold, which then may be specified in terms of syringe graduations, that is, amounts of excess air pressure in cubic centimeters. As in the case of the olfactometer, a continuous stream of air may be supplied, of course, by attaching the inlet to a compressed air tank or rotary pump. When so modified, the technique is called the "stream injection" method.

The blast injection technique, though fairly widely used for both experimental and clinical purposes, possesses a serious inherent fault. Pressure variations, as well as causing differing amounts of odor-laden air to be "blasted" up to the olfactory cleft, make a differential appeal to the cutaneous receptors of the nostrils. In threshold determinations, therefore, air pressure, rather than odor intensity, may provide the cue. This seems to be the source of the difficulty in Wenzel's (*621*) attempted measurement of the differential threshold for one of the alcohols, even though she improved the original Elsberg technique notably by arranging for uniform pressure to be exerted throughout the duration of a given exposure.

Another serious difficulty inheres in the blast injection technique, that is, the unnatural and unpleasant onslaught of vapor unaccompanied by a breathing effort. Under these conditions it is quite impossible for the observer to adjust his internal mouth and throat muscles so as to admit the proper amount of odorous air. It would obviously be better to permit the observer in an olfactory experiment to breathe naturally. This has been accomplished in several systems in which pure air is mixed with a known amount of odorant and the mixture is delivered in an uncontaminated fashion at a predetermined rate of flow. This is what is done in the apparatus devised by Wenzel (622) and that designed by Stone, Ough, and Pangborn (561), among others. Air, previously filtered to remove all possible impurities, is admitted to a chamber, a plexiglass box, enclosing the head. The bottom of the box is closed off with plio-film after the head is in place. Positive air pressure carrying the odorant prevents contaminants from entering the chamber. The odorous air is made so by bubbling it through an odorous liquid which, if its vapor pressure at a fixed temperature can be ascertained, can also be specified rather accurately as to the number of molecules per unit of time that is borne by the air stream.

The chief advantage of such a "free smelling" situation is, of course, the naturalness, the simulation of normal smelling conditions accomplished, thus minimizing familiarization and training trials. There is adequate control of the immediate environment around the head, especially if the added precaution is taken to cover the hair and face with plastic materials to preclude their adding their own scents to the air entering the nostrils. Such a procedure permits the use of a variety of psychophysical methods, since there is prompt removal of the odorant (owing to the rapidly moving air stream) after a given exposure. Altogether, the avoidance of the artificiality associated with tubes in the nostrils, air blasts, etc., points to this method as vastly superior to earlier ones.

The most elaborate of all attempts to measure olfactory sensitivity is found in the "olfactorium" (205), an instrument consisting of a glass double chamber of 250 ft³ capacity. In the inventors' view the taking of olfactory thresholds in an ordinary room is like attempting to perform audiometric measurements on a busy street corner. In the use of the olfactorium the experimental subject first bathes to eliminate residual body odors, then slips into a plastic envelope before entering the inner glass chamber, a "completely controlled odor environment." Pure air or odor-bearing air of predetermined composition, temperature, humidity, and pressure can be introduced at different places and by different methods to the cabinet. This much preparation for odor stimulation may seem like the ultimate in experimental precautions, but it is probably the case that the low reliability attending measurements in olfaction are due, more often than not, to failure to effect the obvious controls of important variables.

Actually, all the methods for ascertaining olfactory thresholds thus far mentioned represent crude attempts at quantification. One of the persistent problems where chemical stimuli are concerned, is that we have no ready way of stating stimulating power of odors (or taste solutions) in energetic terms. With all other classes of stimuli we can convert intensity measures into ergs or some other unit of energy transfer, and there have been times in our consideration of vision, audition, and cutaneous pressure when we found it useful to do so. In the case of odorants the suggestion has been made by Mullins (437) that a step toward the eventual specification of chemical stimulus energies is to calculate the amount of thermodynamic activity at the site of stimulation, not simply to state the amount or concentration of odorous material waiting outside the nostrils to be transported, by sniffing or blasting, to the mucosa. One of the consequences of Mullins' having computed odorous activity (roughly, the ratio between the partial pressure of the gaseous odorant and the vapor pressure of the pure odorant in liquid form) under a variety of flow conditions, was the discovery that a certain minimum rate of flow has to be maintained if stable thresholds are to be obtained. The same insistence on flow rate to the sensitive membrane is found also in the animal experiments of Beidler (50).

But if complete specification of the olfactory stimulus has not yet arrived, there can be little complaint with recent technological advances in providing precise indications of stimulus purity and of stimulus concentration. The preparative gas chromatograph, now in use by the most careful experimenters in this field, pretty much obviates both problems. Contaminants are common in odorants, especially those coming from complex organic families, and steps have to be taken to insure that a desired odorous solution does not, in fact, contain unwanted components. Moreover, once purified, one normally wishes to vary concentration in some systematic manner. The preparative chromatograph performs both functions, revealing multiple components if present and controlling with great accuracy for stimulus concentration. An excellent illustration of the instrument's use for these dual purposes is found in the "quality-coding" studies of O'Connell and Mozell on single receptor cells of the frog (450).

To what extent is it possible to picture, more intimately, the detailed happenings in the olfactory cleft during stimulation? A study reminiscent of the parallel one in vision (286) has been made by two Dutch investigators, and their calculations lead to interesting conclusions (*591*). If one is to know the quantity of odorous material effective at the epithelium (N), the following enter into consideration: (a) the number of molecules (N_o) entering the nostril under optimal conditions of measuring the absolute threshold; (b) the fraction (f_1) of inhaled air that passes through the 1–2 mm "slit" from the nasal cavity to the mucosal region; (c) the relative amount of odorant (f_2) that gets "trapped," that is, adheres to the mucous walls of the nostril; (d) the proportion of molecules (f_3) that escape adsorption in passing through the mucosal cleft. Obviously, now, the number of effective molecules at the point of stimulation of nerve endings will be given by the relation,

$$N = N_o\ f_1 f_2 f_3$$

N_o will vary with a number of conditions, but the "optimal" ones are being assumed. Experiments with a model of the nasal cavity (see Figure 15–5) lead to the conclusion that, for normal breathing, only 5 to 10%

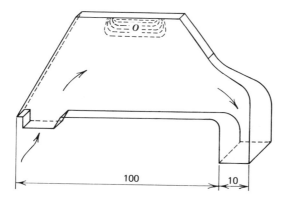

Fig. 15–5. Model of the human olfactory "slit." O=olfactory epithelium, 2.5 cm² in area. From de Vries and Stuiver (*591*) after Stuiver.

of the total flow must pass through the olfactory slit; for higher flow rates (sniffing) it must not exceed 20%. The fraction, f_1, cannot be more than 0.2, then. Calculations of f_2 and f_3, taking a number of factors into consideration, lead to the rough value, 0.5, for each; the number of imponderables being what it is, these are approximations.

The net result is that something like 2% of the inhaled molecules become effective at the mucosa; 98% of the odorant gets absorbed in mucus, avoids the olfactory cleft by joining the respiratory stream, or passes by the sensitive epithelium without affecting sense cells. Careful psychophysical experiments with several odorants, especially the strong mercaptans, yielded curves that connected intensity (molecules per cubic centimeter) with probability of sensing, so-called "frequency of smelling" curves. From the slopes of these, together with the foregoing analysis of probable effectiveness at the mucosa, the conclusion is forced that each of about 40 sense cells must adsorb a single molecule to produce a liminal sensation. Like the eye and ear, the nose is tuned to a point pretty close to the limit.

Differential Olfactory Sensitivity.   The question of ΔI, and the further one of Weber's fraction, $\Delta I/I$, may be raised for smell as for the other sense modalities. Experimental determinations of ΔI, made by several different investigators and covering a span of well over half a century, are in fair agreement. If absolute smell sensitivity is high, differential sensitivity is not; values of ΔI, for several different odorous substances, prove to be uniformly large. According to the results obtained by Zigler and Holway (*662*), who used a modification of Zwaardemaker's olfactometer to measure ΔI for India rubber, the Weber fraction varies systematically with absolute intensity. Thus $\Delta I/I$ has a value close to 1.0 when I is at the low level of 10 olfacties. At 400 olfacties, the highest intensity used, the Weber fraction diminishes to about 0.2.

Other determinations falling in this region are those of Stone and his colleagues whose measurements of ΔI in two experiments (*560, 561*) permitted the bringing together of data on three different odorants: 2-octanone, n-heptyl alcohol, and 2-heptanone. The average Weber fraction for the three was 0.20. In the instance of 2-heptanone (amyl methyl ketone) absolute threshold proved to be in the neighborhood of 0.0009 mg per liter of air inspired—a free breathing system was used—and the differential threshold was measured at several concentrations, varying roughly from 3.5 to 12.5 times the threshold value. Weber fractions were fairly constant over this somewhat restricted range, and averaged out at 0.23.

The Olfactory Qualities.   It has been seen that chemical composition seems not to serve as an entirely adequate basis for the classification of odors. What happens if we rely on direct observation of smell sensations? Many attempts have been made to classify odors on the basis of their resemblances and differences. Odor systems abound. One of the oldest of them, dating from the middle of the eighteenth century, was devised by the Swedish botanist, Linnaeus. It was his odor system, developed primarily as an aid in the classification of plants, that was amplified slightly by Zwaardemaker to give the frequently repeated ninefold arrangement of odor qualities: ethereal (fruits, wines); aromatic (spices, camphor); fragrant (flowers, vanilla); ambrosiac (musk, sandalwood); alliaceous (garlic, chlorine); empyreumatic (roasted coffee, creosote); hircine (goaty odors, rancid fat); foul (bedbugs, French marigolds); and nauseous (feces, carrion flowers). There are some obvious difficulties with this grouping of odors. Among the thousands of specific smells that have to be accommodated by the nine categories there are doubtless many hundreds that could not reasonably be pressed into so simple a scheme. Moreover, it is quite possible to find odors in two different categories of Zwaardemaker's listing that have more resemblance to each other than they do to their fellows in the same odor class. Of course, these are the common difficulties of classification systems, particularly where distinctions are difficult and the number of classificatory rubrics is limited.

Another attempt at odor classification is that of Henning, who has given us the analytic scheme represented by the smell prism (Figure 15–6). The triangular prism is intended to be a hollow one with a multi-

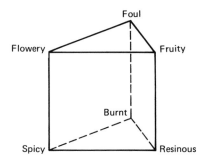

Fig. 15–6. Henning's smell prism. The figure is a hollow one with the six "primaries" occupying the corners and all surfaces being the loci of odors which bear resemblances to several primaries.

tude of discrete odors occupying each of the surfaces. The "primary" qualities are found at the corners: flowery, fruity, foul, spicy, resinous, and burnt. Like all such models of sensory qualities Henning's smell prism is partly based on experimental findings, partly on purely rational considerations. And, like many such geometrical constructions, the figure has a number of unwanted implications inherent in it. Any odor appearing on a line bounding one of the prism faces should have a dual reference. It should resemble both the qualities terminating the line on which it stands. Thus, the odor of thyme should equally resemble "spicy" and "flowery," since it stands on the edge midway between these two corners. Similarly, sassafras is equally "spicy" and "resinous," acetone is equally "resinous" and "fruity," and oil of roses is equally "fruity" and "flowery." Odors standing on one of the square faces of the prism should have a quadruple reference but should most strongly resemble the qualities at the nearest corners. In the same way, odors along diagonal lines that bisect a prism face should have four reference points, since they are at the same time on a face of the prism. An odor lying at the center of a face should equally resemble all the four primaries from which it is equidistant.

There has been, in the main, quite general failure to establish the validity of Henning's smell prism through experimental check. Large individual differences in reaction are encountered, and analytical judgments of odors possess less reliability than could be desired, even where observers have had some training. Difficulties of this sort are found—an observer will report that menthol, say, has an equal resemblance to "resinous" and "flowery" yet deny that it is either "spicy" or "fruity." Moreover, the position his analysis gives it is the center of the flowery-fruity-resinous-spicy face of the prism, and this is already occupied by the odor of arbor vitae. And menthol does not smell like arbor vitae!

The triangular prism, with its limitation to six fundamental odors, seems not to do justice to the complexities of odor sensation. Woodworth, who has made a careful evaluation of Henning's system (650, pp. 482–492), believed that much of the difficulty arises from the nonolfactory components in odor reception. Many odorants stimulate the cutaneous endings in the walls of the nostrils, the resulting sensation being reported over the trigeminal nerve as well as the olfactory. Many other scented materials make a separate appeal to taste. The result is a complex perception, smell plus sweet, sour, cold, warm, or pain—and mixtures of these—which prevents the formation of a simple, reliable judgment concerning the odor component.

If it appears impossible to force all smell sensations into Zwaardemaker's ninefold arrangement or Henning's sixfold one it is perhaps not surprising that another odor system, which attempts to get along with but four categories, should have some difficulty establishing itself (131). The Crocker-Henderson system posits four fundamental odors: fragrant, acid, burnt, and caprylic (goaty). Three of these are familiar from other odor classifications, but "acid" is a term more commonly associated with taste than with smell. Each of the four fundamental qualities is supposed to occur in most complex scents but with varying intensity from substance to substance. The presence of each is presumably detectable in the complex, and not only may it be analyzed out with a little practice but a numerical rating may be given to it, based on relative sensory intensity. The scale selected is a nine point one, 0–8 inclusive. Thus phenylethyl alcohol is said to be fragrant in degree 7, acid in degree 4, burnt in degree 2, and caprylic in degree 3. Phenylethyl alcohol may thus be designated in numerical code: 7423. In the same way a 20% solution of acetic acid is mildly fragrant and goaty, intensely acid, and not at all burnt. Its symbol is 3803. Methyl salicylate stands at the top of the scale of fragrance (8453), while toluene is near the bottom of it (2424). Damask rose has few objectionable qualities (6523). Anisole, with the designation 2577, seems best to be described as having a somewhat sour, quite burnt and goaty odor.

The scheme is an ingenious one, and there are some obvious advantages in specifying odors by numerical code. The test of the Crocker-Henderson system, however, would seem to lie in its adequacy to yield reproducible and unvarying analyses of odorants. Thus far there seems not to have been an entirely unobjectionable evaluation of the system in this regard. One should be forthcoming, for the basic standards of the system have been made commercially available, and there is only required the properly designed experiment to make the rendering of a verdict possible.

Other attempts at systematizing odor sensations have been made, none of them with conspicuous success. It has been supposed that some central principles of smell organization might come from the application of the mathematical technique of factor analysis, and several sets of data involving olfactory judgments have been treated in this way. Thus Hsü (313) has factor analyzed the ratings made of 31 odors with respect to the dimension of pleasantness-unpleasantness. Three clusters of odorants appeared in the analysis, one group characterized by chemical unsaturation (a benzene-ketone group), another having oxygen uniformly present in the molecule (a "plant" group of odors), and a third possessing nitrogen (an "animal" group). Statistical interrelations were sufficiently intimate to prevent a high degree of discreteness in the groupings. One would certainly do as well, in devising a classificatory system, to sort out smells on the basis of the chemical structure of their stimuli, and, to be sure, we have already seen what comes of that. Moreover, affective ratings of odors would hardly seem to be the stuff of which to fabricate an odor system.

Odors can be appreciated in so many nuances of quality and intensity, at least when they are compared directly one with another, that there is a widespread supposition that we must carry about with us a most elaborate set of classificatory concepts where smells are concerned. But, in other sense departments having the capacity for fine discriminations it has invariably been found that attempts to make absolute identifications, to put labels on isolated samples from a continuum, lead to the use of quite restricted numbers of categories. The ability to make distinctions seems, in general, to be limited by "the magical number seven, plus or minus two" (420). Odor qualities are considerably easier to categorize than are intensities, according to the experiments of Engen and Pfaffmann (188, 189), but the number of either that can be correctly recognized and labeled is not impressive. The practiced observer, whether he be asked to identify a large number of odors, either qualitatively similar to each other or drawn from a highly heterogeneous population, is able to classify correctly into only about 16 categories. Confusions abound, and the larger the population to be sorted out, the more errors there are. In the same way, the observer is able to utilize only about four gross steps of intensity; finer gradations cannot be handled. Moreover, if quality and intensity are simultaneously varied in the samples, accuracy does not exceed that for quality alone. As the information theorist would conclude, the human can transmit about four bits of odor information.

Adaptation. In common with all other sensory systems in the body the olfactory sense displays the phenomenon of adaptation. In the absence of any odor stimulation there is a gain in sensitivity, reminiscent of dark adaptation in vision. Also, like the analogous phenomenon of visual light adaptation, there is a decline in sensitivity with continuous odor stimulation. The latter effect, also known as smell fatigue or smell exhaustion, is responsible for some quite abrupt reductions in acuity, changes which on occasion come to be of very real practical concern. Miners long ago recognized the principle, at least implicitly, in their use of canaries and mice for the early detection of the presence of methane, the odorous impurities of which, because of the operation of adaptation, might go unnoticed by human nostrils.

The high levels of sensitivity obtainable through complete removal of olfactory stimuli have not often been studied. Entirely odorfree surroundings were provided, however, by the *camera inodorata* of Komuro (368), one of Zwaardemaker's students, and it was possible to measure sensitivity to a number of odorants under the contrasting conditions of (a) prior exposure to the purest of air, and (b) previous adaptation to the air of the laboratory. Threshold measurements to nine organic reagents were made with the olfactometer. Reductions in threshold values, from the contaminated to the pure air situation, ranged from 9% in the case of pyridine to 39% for artificial musk. The average drop in threshold was of the order of 25%. Apparently we go about partially odor-adapted most of the time.

Sensitivity changes of the opposite variety, reductions attendant upon continued exposure, are not as readily dismissed. Two sets of at least partially juxtaposed facts are encountered on raising the question of the principal phenomena of adaptation. On the one hand, there is the common observation that adaptation in the direction of sensitivity reduction, total or incomplete, occurs with great rapidity in most instances. Enter a room containing a strange odor, sniff several times in an effort to identify it, and it may be found that the smell fades so precipitously as to foil the recognition attempt completely. Adaptation, when judged by the blunting of sensation, appears to be a rapid and thoroughgoing process. On the other hand, the facts gleaned from olfactory electrophysiology do not lead to the same conclusion. Electrical responses in the rabbit (see Figure 15–7) indicate that there is a more or less sustained plateau, after

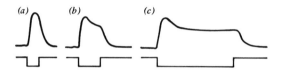

Fig. 15–7. Olfactory adaptation. Potentials from the rabbit's mucosa in response to a steady stream of odorous air *(a)* 0.5 sec; *(b)* 1.0 sec; *(c)* 3.0 sec. All three responses are initially of the order of 2 mV. From Ottoson *(455)*.

an initial reduction, in the potential taken off the mucosa when a continuous stream of odor-laden air is passed over it. If the stimulus is of medium or weak intensity the drop may be less than 50% of the initial response. If the odorant is a very strong one, adaptation may eventually go to completion, but low or moderate intensities apparently never do.

The neural and the human observational facts are thus at odds. Is there a way of reconciling them? Adrian, who originally pictured all adaptation as reflecting purely receptor events, has come to the conclusion that, at least for olfaction, the essential reduction occurring in adaptation must have its site in a less peripheral location. He pictures there to be a competition between the receptor signals and the intrinsic activity of cells in the olfactory bulb *(6)*. Both of these have access to the central pathways of which the mitral cells are the starting point. In the absence of mucosal stimulation the mitral axons produce a continuous self-generated activity that may be broken in on by any supraliminal receptor stimulation. The "message" having been delivered, there is a suppression of the incoming impulses by the rhythmic activity of the bulb. Adaptation has occurred. Much as an attentional shift causes a central switching, adaptation reflects a cutting off of the outside signal.

The mechanism Adrian has suggested leaves much to be explained. Why, if this is the order of events, should adaptation have the regular and reproducible time course it always displays? Why should other central factors not influence it markedly? No, it is possible that adaptation has an essentially central seat rather than the peripheral one we have always imagined, but that it represents a perpetual struggle, a two-way switching between periphery and brain, seems hardly credible.

The neurophysiological evidences, at least thus far along the research road, having failed to prove crucial, what is there to be learned about adaptation from experimental suppressions and extinctions of smell? Perhaps the most rewarding of such studies have been those in which odorants have been pitted against each other with respect to their adapting power. The experiments of Moncrieff (427) are especially revealing. He selected a group of odorants with quite dissimilar smells: acetone, isopropanol, n-butanol, diacetone alcohol, "cellosolve," and methanol. Each was then paired with every other, making a total of 15 comparisons. For every pair there was determined: (1) threshold concentration for each member of the pair, A and B; (2) threshold for A and B after self-adaptation; (3) threshold for B after adaptation to A, and for A after adaptation to B. In every instance self-adaptation produced more suppression (higher threshold concentration for the next sniff) than did heterogeneous adaptation. At the same time, no odorant left any other unaffected; always adaptation to A altered sensitivity to B. An interesting outcome was that A might affect B more than B did A, or vice versa. Whereas radically different compounds chemically affect each other in this way, it is necessary to compare those of closely similar chemical composition to get really high levels of adaptive interaction. Thus amyl and butyl acetate, which have very similar odors, have strong influences on each other; adaptation to one results in great heightening of the other's absolute threshold.

By suitably combining all adaptation data from any pair of odorants it is possible to construct a "coefficient of likeness" which varies on a scale of 0 (no adaptive interaction) to 1.00 (maximum influence of one on the other in adaptation). In the experiment described above, Moncrieff found coefficients ranging from 0.04 (the relatively weak interaction between acetone and diacetone alcohol) to 0.89 (the highly similar amyl and butyl acetate). Of the many pairings, similar and dissimilar, none fell higher or lower. Those compounds selected for their dissimilarity yielded coefficients of 0.20 or under. Those picked because they are confused in identification fell near the middle of the scale. Thus alpha- and beta-ionone (smell of violets) gave a likeness coefficient of 0.45, benzaldehyde and nitrobenzene (almond odor) one of 0.40. Apparently most odorants can be expected to alter to some degree sensitivity to all others. This suggests that some portion of the receptive mechanism is used by all odors, perhaps in the adsorptive process, while individuality in quality is guaranteed by the nonoverlapping features of the multitude of stimulation patterns. As Moncrieff has concluded (*427*, p. 315): "adaptation might provide a means of classifying them [odorants] into a very large number (probably thousands) of classes. The same finding makes it very unlikely that there is a small number of fundamental smells, although it does not exclude the possibility that there may be a small number of types of olfactory receptors."

Adaptation rate, in whatever sense department it is investigated, proves to be a function of stimulus intensity. Some experiments performed by Zwaardemaker show that the sense of smell is not exceptional in this regard. Figure 15–8 reveals the progressive raising of the absolute thresh-

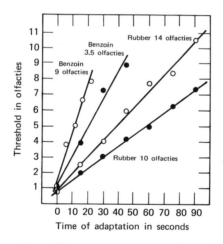

Fig. 15–8. Olfactory adaptation to two concentrations of benzoin and India rubber. Thresholds are progressively raised as adaptation proceeds. The rate of adaptation is faster for benzoin than for rubber. In each case there is more rapid adaptation to the stronger stimulus. After Zwaardemaker (*663*).

old to two different concentrations of benzoin and of India rubber as the time of exposure is increased. In the case of benzoin, to which adaptation is the more rapid, a concentration measuring 9 olfacties with the olfactometer produces a nearly fourfold heightening of the absolute threshold in 5 sec, a change requiring about three times as long with the lower concentration of 3.5 olfacties. Similarly, in the case of the more slowly adapting India rubber, a stimulus having a strength of 14 olfacties brings about the same fourfold threshold increase in a half-minute, whereas the 10-olfactie stimulus requires 45 sec to effect a change of this magnitude.

It is apparent from the straight-line relationships shown in Figure 15–8 that the adaptation process in these cases has not as yet been brought to completion. Either there should be a leveling off of thresholds at some high point on the olfactie scale, adaptation having brought about a new equilibrium with the olfactory environment, or thresholds should become infinitely high. As a matter of fact, the latter should occur because, unlike visual and auditory sensations, which adapt down to a lowered brightness or loudness level but which never reduce themselves to zero intensity so long as the adapting stimulus remains unchanged, odor sensations normally adapt out completely upon prolonged stimulation. This is at once a blessing, in the case of the tannery worker, and a hazard, in the case of those whose "best friends will not even tell them"!

Several other phenomena connected with adaptation appear to be important, but much more work will have to be done on them before their full import can be known. Thus, certain odors undergo qualitative changes along with the intensive one caused by continuous exposure. A case in point is that of nitrobenzol, which has a "bitter almond" odor when first smelled but takes on a quality more nearly resembling that of tar as adaptation proceeds. If the qualitative changes produced by adaptation were charted for all odorants we should be in possession of a powerful set of facts.

Odor Mixture.   The fact that we are as yet quite ignorant of even the simplest relations between different odors is abundantly evident from the current uncertainties regarding their classification. Many thousands of different scents can be discriminated; just how many is not known. And with each passing day the organic chemist is adding new ones. It is quite possible, however, that only a few *elementary* odors are needed to account for the whole range of possible smells. The situation may be much as it is in color, where three primaries are sufficient to synthesize the total gamut of visible hues. Were we as certain of the facts of odor mixture as we are the facts of color mixture, we should be able to approach with confidence such problems as those of odor specification and flavor analysis. As matters now stand our information along these lines is at best characterized as sketchy.

In a general way the procedures available for the mixture of odorous stimuli are analogous to those used in color mixture. Just as one may produce composite colors by superposing on a reflecting screen two different spectral samples, then observing the single result of their union at the retina, "composite" odors may be arrived at by physically mixing two odorous liquids or vapors in a container and sniffing the combined product. There is this difference, however. The spectral samples will lose their identities in the new fusion. Orange may "resemble" both red and yellow, but one does not first see red, then yellow, in the blend. Odors, unless they bear a close qualitative resemblance to each other to begin with, are unlikely to mix with this degree of intimacy. The possible results of the simple mixture of two dissimilar odorous stimuli seem to be: (1) a composite which yields a unitary impression, the new odor resembling both the original constituents; (2) a loosely organized blend in which the originals are successively perceived, each being momentarily present to the exclusion of the other; (3) a fusion, somewhat like a musical chord, where the "partials" can be attended to separately but a unified *Gestalt* is never lost; (4) complete masking of one of the two originals so that only the other survives the combining process; and, more doubtfully, (5) neutralization of each by the other so that the net result is total cancellation of odor.

This last possibility, odor neutralization or "compensation," has been the subject of controversy. Zwaardemaker found it to occur with a number of opposed odors (e.g., cedarwood and India rubber; balsam and beeswax), but Henning regarded the effect to be a sheer myth. It should be said straightway that the bringing together of odorous materials to permit their possible chemical interaction is not at all concerned here. Such "mixture" only produces stimulus alteration, of course. Usually the result of such a change is quite predictable from a knowledge of the component qualities and concentrations. In the case of compensatory mixtures what we are interested in is the result of simultaneous arousal of two antagonistic olfactory processes which may interfere with each other and tend to obliterate sensation. To settle the question it would seem to be necessary to keep the two opposed odorants apart, letting each stimulate a separate receptive area. This can be done, of course, with a double olfactometer and dichorhinic stimulation, since the nasal septum insulates the two clefts from each other. The procedure is analogous to binocular color mixing where blue, presented to one eye, cancels out complementary yellow, presented to the other, to give gray.

Dichorhinic mixing has been performed with many odorants and by many experimenters, but there seems not to be much agreement on the facts. Zwaardemaker regularly combined different odors, always of low intensity, to produce odorlessness. He cautioned that complete neutralization can come about only by the most careful selection of stimuli and graduation of their strengths. Even then the zero point may be only fleetingly observed. Complete neutralization in a three-component mixture he reported to be more difficult of achievement. He obtained it only once in the exploration of 252 mixtures, then by combining terpineol, ethyl bisulfide, and guaiacol (*664*, p. 502). Henning, who also experimented extensively with odor mixtures, denied the possibility of complete neutralization. In dichorhinic smelling, which he regarded to be unnatural and therefore untrustworthy as a technique, there could be unions of two odors which he called "coincidence smells," blends having a unitary character but in which the components could be held apart by straining attention. There could also be "duality smells," where the two odors seemed to have separate but simultaneous existences, each being clearly localized in its own nostril. However, complete abolition of odor through cancellation he thought occurred only through chemical interaction, never through true "physiological mixing."

The resolution of this question lies in the future. Meanwhile, it is possible that Henning was looking for an effect having far greater stability than odor neutralization is supposed to have. It is certainly the case that mixtures tending toward cancellation occur commonly enough. In medical practice Peruvian balsam may be used to neutralize the odor of iodoform. Carbolic acid is often used to counteract objectionable biological odors. Florists know that some flowers, more desirable for their appearance than their fragrance, may be rendered olfactorily inoffensive by adding other odorous flowers or leaves to the bouquet containing them. Within the chemical industry there is a well-developed effort to "engineer" odors. Thus, because many people find sponge rubber, increasingly being used in upholstery and bedding, to have an objectionable scent about it, there is used in its manufacture a "reodorant" which makes the product more generally acceptable. All this may be "masking" rather than "mixing." If so, a separation of the principles should come out of properly designed quantitative experiments; further qualitative ones are unlikely to decide the issue.

One interesting and instructive consequence of dirhinic stimulation has been studied by Békésy with the aid of methods that are characteristically ingenious (*57*). He arranged for separate tubes to carry the same odorant to the two nostrils but in different time and intensity relations. When very short time differentials were employed, the odorant being conducted to one nostril only 0.5 msec or less than to the other, there was a localization shift, the odor seeming to move out of a previously established median position toward the nostril receiving the prior stimulation. Concomitantly, there was a sharpening up of the overall olfactory pattern, a volumic shrinkage in lateral spread. Alterations in intensity of the order of 10%, without simultaneous temporal changes, produced the same result. These findings are, of course, strictly comparable to those encountered in hearing, where localization shifts from the median plane of the head can be induced by either time or intensity differences in diotic stimulation, the temporal factor being the more potent. The curious thing about the times involved, both in smell and hearing, is that the temporal offsets of less than a millisecond, which seem to be entirely efficacious in controlling localization, are but a small fraction of the time taken in the growth of sensation following stimulus onset. This is not a matter of milliseconds, but of whole seconds. Figure 15–9, taken from Békésy's

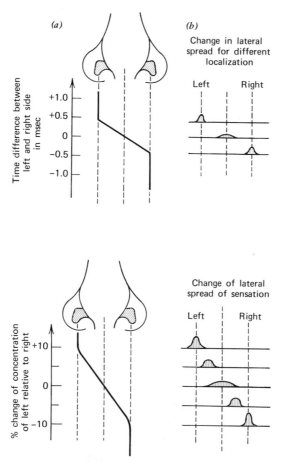

Fig. 15–9. Lateralization of olfactory sensation by introduction of a small time difference (above) and by an intensive shift (below). From Georg von Békésy. Olfactory analogue to directional hearing. *J. Appl. Physiol.* 19: 369–373, 1964.

description of his olfactory localization experiments, shows the time and intensity relations influencing the lateralization phenomenon.

The fact that the dirhinic relations suggested above are those actually operative in the localization of smells by sniffing in a free situation is further shown by experiments in which a single source of odor, a perforated hollow ball 3 cm in diameter, was moved in an arc of 8 cm radius before the observer's nose. Periodically the stream of air passing through the ball was odor-laden and the subject was required to indicate the direction from which the scent of lavender (or benzol, or eucalyptus, or clove) was coming. The least discriminable change in angular displacement of the ball proved to be of the order of 7 to 10 degrees. As the source moved further to the side, the change of direction was perceived with about this accuracy until an angle of 65 degrees with the median plane had been reached. Beyond this the subject could detect no changes. Considering the small spatial separation of the two nostrils, it would appear that time differences of the magnitude of 0.1 msec must be effective in mediating the localization function.

Whether the localizing process is under the control of purely odorous components may reasonably be doubted. Few odorants, perhaps none, are entirely devoid of cutaneous appeal. Schneider and Schmidt (511), repeating and extending the Békésy experiments, looked for the trigeminal component as an essential cue in "olfactory" localization. With nitrogen as a diluent, three odorants (coffee, n-butane, and ammonia) were delivered, both unilaterally and bilaterally, through tubes to the noses of seven observers. Sniffing experiments, both with the head fixed and freely rotated, were also conducted, the odorants being sprayed through perforated balls 8 cm from the nostrils. By and large, success in localization followed the "irritation" sequence, ammonia being most, coffee least readily localized. The authors, while concurring generally in the Békésy findings, concluded, much as von Skramlik had many years ago (530) that only odors which produce accessory trigeminal sensations can be well localized.

The Electrophysiology of Smell.   The changes occurring in the olfactory nerve when odors stimulate the receptor cells have been studied, but they are not known as intimately as are analogous events in other sense departments, vision and audition in particular. However, in common with other sensory pathways the olfactory nerve has been the beneficiary of a very considerable amount of intensive research in recent years. The same methods, in general, that have proved efficacious for the second and eighth cranial nerves have been applied to the first. There are some special difficulties, the chief of which are the small size and inaccessibility of receptor units and the relative fragility of the nerve bundles associated with them. Single fiber analysis is difficult to attain; even small strands teased out of larger conduits contain many tiny threadlike fibrils. These, being thin and unmyelinated, conduct at very slow rates, 0.2 m/sec or less.

Nevertheless, some things have been learned through application of electrophysiological techniques. Just as the eye has its electroretinogram and the ear its cochlear response, the nose has electrical changes that may be obtained directly from the olfactory epithelium itself. An electrode contacting the nasal mucosa records a sizable negative deflection when an odorant flows over the sensitive patch (Figure 15–10). This response

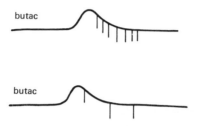

Fig. 15–10. Two successive responses of the olfactory mucosa to butyric acid. The upward (negative) deflection is the electro-olfactogram (EOG), the spikes discharges of fibers. The oscilloscope recording the changes had a 10-sec sweep. From Gesteland, Lettvin, Pitts, and Rojas (*230*).

has been termed by Ottoson (*454*) the electro-olfactogram, EOG, and by others the Ottoson potential. It was the discoverer's belief that this potential is the initial event in the discharge of olfactory nerve impulses, i.e., that it is a generator potential. However, since the successful recording of spikes from single neural units of the olfactory epithelium, which has been accomplished by tiny electrodes of the order of 1 μ in diameter, it has become apparent that the large EOG potential does not stand in a sufficiently intimate relation to the rapid spikes to be their initiator. Moreover, it has been shown (*524*) that responses of nerve twigs go on unimpeded when the Ottoson potential is much reduced or even eliminated by removal of the mucosa with filter paper.

At the same time, the EOG may turn out to be a useful indicator of events in the nasal epithelium, much as the ERG is an overall reporter of electrical imbalances in the eye. For one thing, its amplitude appears to be a function of stimulus strength, and it may well be that systematic recording of its waveform and latency will help to sort out the many variables entering into the stimulation and adaptation processes.

The spikes recorded from axons of single receptor cells in the sensitive area appear to differ from those found in other sensory systems in no important way save that they typically occupy a very low frequency range, 1 to 5 discharges per second. It is rare for them to go as high as 20 per second. The spikes are positive with respect to the EOG. Their bursts in response to an odor absorbed (or adsorbed?) by the overlying mucus characteristically last from one to four seconds and, whether as a result of rapid adaptation or some other precipitous blocking action, leave the receptor unit in a somewhat impaired state of stimulability. A fresh puff of the odorant is met with lowered discharge frequency (see Figure 15–10).

There is a growing body of evidence supporting the idea that there may be some quality differentiation right at the periphery, within the olfactory epithelium. An experiment of Mozell (*431*), in which simultaneous records were taken from two widely separated branches of the frog's olfactory nerve, yielded results that suggest different spatiotemporal patterns of discharge for different odors. Limonene, for example, may appeal to one area of the mucosa more than another, while geraniol, for example, stimulates more strongly a second region; moreover, the difference in latency of response between the two areas is not constant across stimuli. Incoming odors are apparently subject to a time-space encoding.

Such an outcome is not too surprising in view of (1) the histological finding that there is a certain amount of neural correspondence between mucosal areas and general regions of the olfactory bulb (See Clark, above) and (2) Adrian's discovery that there are functional differences between certain bulbar regions.

Adrian's experiments are fundamental (*7, 8*). His first studies, dating back to 1938 (*10*), were on the olfactory stalk of fish. These were soon extended to several kinds of mammals. Recording was by means of thin wire electrodes, insulated except at the tips, which were pushed into the olfactory bulb far enough (1.5–2.5 mm) to contact neural elements, presumably mitral cells. Two kinds of waves were found: "intrinsic" waves, bulbar spontaneous activity, and "induced" waves, those traceable to the action of externally imposed chemical stimuli. Bursts of action potentials accompanied each inspiration of odor-laden air, provided the right odorants were used and in sufficient concentration. In general, the materials effective for human noses proved also to arouse olfactory reactions in cats, rabbits, and hedgehogs. Thus odorless air, carbon monoxide, and carbon dioxide were without effect. Compounds such as hydrogen sulfide, benzene, and acetylene produced trains of impulses. Some interesting species differences appeared. The rabbit gave the best potentials to fruity and aromatic smells, while the cat, unresponsive to floral odors, was especially sensitive to decaying animal material. The hedgehog is characterized by great olfactory versatility, a great range of substances evoking action potentials. Catfish responded strongly to foul materials, the most efficacious of Adrian's stimuli having been a kind of purée of decayed alligator head!

Records of electrical activity taken from electrodes embedded in the olfactory bulb necessarily represent the summed effect of many primary neurones. At best the projection involved is of a fairly general region of the olfactory epithelium, and the end organs contributing to the recorded potentials must be somewhat sparsely distributed throughout that region. It is a matter of considerable interest and no little theoretical importance, therefore, to find that some differences of discharge pattern can be detected by comparing the records taken from different portions of the olfactory bulb.

Adrian originally found three gross areas in the cat, an anterior one most responsive to banana oil and its chemical relatives, a posteroventral one responding strongly to coal gas and other hydrocarbons, and a postero-dorsal region appealed to especially by decayed meat and fish. Tri-methylamine, which has a fishy odor to the human, was especially effective. Subsequently, charting the rabbit's olfactory bulb (8) and inferring the sensitivity of the mucosa from what happens in mitral cells, he was able to differentiate five groups of receptors: (a) those set into action by aro-matic compounds (benzene, toluene); (b) those responsive to esters of fatty acids (amyl and ethyl acetate); (c) those giving their best response to par-affin hydrocarbons (pentane and its relatives); (d) those especially sensitive to the terpenes (cedar oil, limonene); and (e) those appealed to by certain sulfur-containing compounds, such as hydrogen sulfide and mercaptan. Specificity of response was found to be a highly stable phenomenon in that much the same "quality differentiation" would be realized in a given neural unit over a period of several hours. This was especially the case when odorants were kept at a low level of concentration.

But locus of a receptor need not be the only factor at work in what may be a quite complex coding process in the delivery of odor information. Adrian himself drew attention to two other probable determinants. One concerns differential action of the odorant on the olfactory epithelium. The mucosa is far from being uniformly constituted, and we must sup-pose that heavy oils and ethereal substances may distribute themselves quite differently in the folds and hollows of the irregular surface. The other factor is time. It would seem probable that the arousal process might well be characterized by differential latencies and action times, especially as between those substances soluble in water and those requir-ing a lipoidal solvent. There are doubtless other, less obvious factors at work.

The general relations unearthed by Adrian have been confirmed by others (434), who have also shown some of the limitations connected with this kind of research. One of these concerns the crucial role of anesthetics. More than a few investigations in neurophysiology have had their conclusions hemmed in by the restrictions imposed by the anesthetic used to immobilize an experimental animal or to permit the surgery necessary to the implantation of electrodes. Figure 15–11 shows three records of

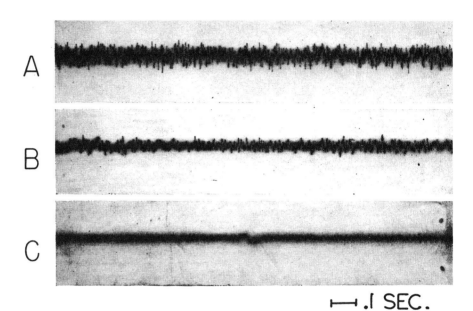

⊢—⊣ .I SEC.

Fig. 15–11. Spontaneous spikes from deep in the olfactory bulb of the rabbit. (A) light urethane anesthesia; (B) after addition of two grams of the anesthetic; (C) after two more grams. From Mozell and Pfaffmann (434).

spontaneous electrical activity deep in the olfactory lobe of the rabbit. The first record, A, reveals quite large spikes; this was the situation under light urethane anesthesia. After the administration of two additional grams of urethane the reduced spike amplitude, shown in B, prevailed. Finally, adding two more grams (C) resulted in still more suppression of the spikes. This is obviously not an area for dilettantes; one has to know much about the management of his experimental preparations.

Little has been accomplished as yet in the matter of direct recording from human olfactory pathways. The areas involved, unlike some in other sense departments, are highly inaccessible in the course of most human brain surgery. An outstanding exception is the set of results reported by Sem-Jacobsen and his collaborators at the Mayo Clinic (*515*). Simultaneous records from the two olfactory bulbs, in a single human case, revealed trains of rhythmic waves, varying between 25 and 39 Hz, in response to tincture of valerian and benzene. Room air yielded no response. Spontaneous waves of the kind found in the rabbit were lacking as was also any evidence of spikes. It is interesting that the two bulbs were not synchronized in their response nor did they discharge at the same amplitude. Whether these differences between human and subhuman records are of any significance will not be clear until much more is done on the human olfactory system. The role of the anesthetic is critical here, as elsewhere, and that of stimulus concentration cannot be overlooked. Also, evidence is accumulating that the role of efferent impulses, creating inhibitory effects especially, must not be neglected. The part played by such centrifugal messages may not be the same in all species, but enough is known about the anatomy of efferent pathways, which in the lateral olfactory tract run down at least to the level of the glomeruli while others connect one bulb with another, to suggest that interactions and balances may be achieved quite complexly. The central nervous system yields up its secrets grudgingly.

Theories of Smell Sensitivity.   Where facts are sparse, guesses are likely to abound. Lack of a sufficiently extensive body of established fact prevents the formation of a consistent and inclusive theory of smell. In its place there has accumulated a multiplicity of ideas, few of which can be dignified with the name "theory" or even "hypothesis." Moncrieff (*426*, p. 314) catalogues 22 separate attempts at providing an odor theory, the earliest dating from 1870. Approximately half of them look to one or another chemical feature of odorants as the basic principle. Most of the remainder emphasize intramolecular vibrations and make of odors sources of wave motion which may arouse the olfactory epithelium to action.

The test of a theory, as we have had occasion to note several times previously while evaluating theories in other sense departments, is provided by (1) its ability to accommodate all relevant existing facts, or at least the better established of them, and (2) its fruitfulness in suggesting new hypotheses, in the experimental verification of which new facts will emerge. Theories of smell which meet these standards adequately are nonexistent. Most of the possible candidates fall down on the first requirement. Not being broadly conceived, they are restricted to consideration of but a single chemical or physical property of odors. Other equally significant facts arise to embarrass them. Nearly all theoretical constructions in this field fail also to meet the second specification of acceptable theories, that they generate experimentally testable hypotheses. In this regard, however, one should not be too critical, for the failure may not be one of thought or ingenuity. The familiar barriers to olfactory research, difficulties of stimulus control and inaccessibility of receptors, may be more to blame.

The theoretical ideas thus far advanced are broadly classifiable into three categories, based on central emphasis: (1) those employing the notion of direct radiation from the odorous source; (2) those positing chemical reactivity as a necessary step in reception; and (3) those involving a radiation mechanism within the nostrils, once the odorous vapor has come into proximity with the olfactory epithelium.

The first of these need not detain us long; several simple considerations defeat it. The facts that odors travel with the wind, are not transmitted through transparent solids or reflected from mirrors, have their strength altered by temperature changes—to mention only a few—all speak against odor as a form of wave motion or corpuscular streaming from the source of scent to the nose.

What of the second class of theoretical constructions, those postulating the occurrence of chemical reactions between particles of the odorant and the tissues in the olfactory cleft? This type of theory has to be taken more seriously. That many of the changes characteristic of chemical reactions actually occur in the course of odor reception cannot be denied. The general facts concerning volatility and solubility we have already reviewed. It is a natural assumption that odor particles, having arrived at the cleft in vaporous form, enter into chemical combination with the substances there, whether aqueous or lipoid, protein or enzyme. A specific hypothesis based on the last-mentioned possibility is that of Kistiakowsky (363). He speculates that the olfactory nerve response may be set off by a system of reactions that are catalyzed by enzymes, as yet unidentified but present in the olfactory epithelium in a number related to that of "the number of basic smells." An odorant is pictured as inhibiting the action of one or more of the enzymes. This in turn causes shifts in the concentrations of the basic smell substances. Such changed concentrations are sufficient to set off appropriate impulses in the first cranial nerve. Kistiakowsky's hypothesis is in harmony with several salient features of the olfactory process and possesses, in addition, the real merit of being relatively simple in conception. The most important argument that can be urged against it applies with equal force to all other chemical hypotheses of odor stimulation, that is, it is difficult to picture a reaction based on sheer chemical change that observes the time schedule found in odor reception. Smell sensations are initiated practically coincidentally with the movement of odor-laden air in the nostrils. Moreover, in most instances there appears to be no perceptible lag in bringing the response to an abrupt termination. The sensation does not appreciably outlast the stimulus, so far as can be judged. How the slate can thus be wiped clean in the twinkling of an eye is not clear. Perhaps, if all the facts were known, we should find that there are greater delays than there appear to be. Perhaps the time relations are not inconsistent with the operation of substances as dilute as the olfactory enzymes need to be. Perhaps a "gradient" of absorption, regulated primarily by the velocity with which odor-laden air strikes the sensitive epithelium, is a necessary condition. Data on the rapidity with which successive odors can replace each other in sensation would be vital to such a hypothesis. Only more intimate studies of events transpiring at the cleft can provide the necessary answers.

A theory of olfaction also falling in the "chemical reactivity" (or, at least, "physicochemical reactivity") class is one based on stereochemical properties of odorants. The first faint glimmerings of this idea must clearly be attributed to the Epicurean poet, Lucretius (first century B.C.). It seems odd that it should only now be contending in the lists. Lucretius put it this way (395):

> . . . seeds [atoms] are kept
> Commixed in things in divers modes. . . .
> Since seeds do differ, divers too must be
> The interstices and paths (which we do call
> The apertures) in all the members, even
> In mouth and palate too. Thus some must be
> More small or yet more large, three-cornered some
> And others squared, and many others round,
> And certain of them many-angled too
> In many modes. For, as the combination
> And motion of their divers shapes demand,
> The shapes of apertures must be diverse
> And paths must vary according to their walls
> That bound them . . . .

Lucretius borrowed the atomic theory of the constitution of things from Democritus, selecting it from among other theories of the universe because of his confidence in the veracity of sense impressions. The senses required "blows" from moving atoms to set them off, and the atoms must systematically differ in kind according as they are capable of arousing one sensation or another (395):

> . . . simple 'tis to see that whatsoever
> Can touch the senses pleasingly are made
> Of smooth and rounded elements, whilst those

Which seem the bitter and the sharp, are held
Entwined by elements more crook'd, and so
Are wont to tear their ways into our senses,
And rend our body as they enter in . . . .

. . . Some, too, there are which justly are supposed
To be nor smooth nor altogether hooked,
With bended barbs, but slightly angled-out,
To tickle rather than to wound the sense—
And of which sort is the salt tartar of wine
And flavours of the gummed elecampane.

[One must not] suppose
That same-shaped atoms through men's nostrils pierce
When foul cadavers burn, as when the stage
Is with Cilician saffron sprinkled fresh,
And the altar exhales Panchaean scent; . . . .

Lucretius was setting forth, not too inexactly, modern steric theory. Several modern exponents have brought it to a relatively high state of development. One such, J. E. Amoore, states the theory this way (18):

". . . certain definite molecular properties characterize all compounds with the same primary odour, and distinguish them from all compounds with different primary odours. Thus the camphoraceous odour is exhibited by spherical molecules about 7Å in diameter, the musky odour by disk-shaped molecules about 10Å across, the floral odour by kite-shaped molecules, the pepperminty odour by wedge-shaped molecules with a polar group near the point of the wedge, ethereal odours by very small or thin molecules, pungent odours by electrophilic molecules and putrid odours by nucleophilic molecules."

The dimensions and shapes of receptor sites that might accommodate these various classes of molecules were determined by making crude models with coins of various sizes. Properly stacked these yielded projections of the molecules which, when transferred by pantograph to a drawing surface, provided the desired shapes and sizes. Figure 15–12 shows outlines of the hypothesized sites, together with their main dimensions in Ångstrom units. The supposition is that molecules must "fit" their sites to the extent of having their surfaces largely in contact with the "complementary" depressions which they are to "fill." Others have been more demanding with their requirements in this respect, and there has been some talk of "lock and key" fits as being necessary; the sites must be as elaborate as the complex molecules they are to accommodate.

A variation on the stereochemical theory has been suggested by Beets

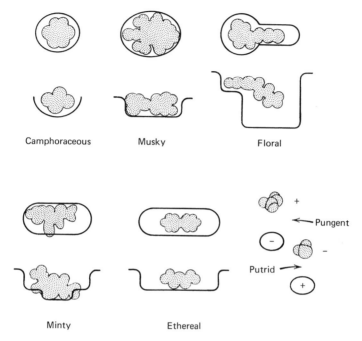

Camphoraceous   Musky   Floral

Minty   Ethereal   Pungent   Putrid

Fig. 15–12. The sites hypothesized to accommodate the seven classes of odorants in Amoore's stereochemical theory. Sizes may be judged by the following illustrations: The camphoraceous site has a depth of 4 Ångstrom units ($\text{Å} = 10^{-10}$ m) and a lesser axis of the oval of 7.5 Å. The musky site has a length of 11.5 Å and a lesser width of 9 Å. Several of the dimensions are in doubt. After Amoore (*19*).

(*47*). His concern was with providing a mechanism whereby it would be possible to take care of the fact that compounds having the same overall molecular structure nevertheless possessed different odors, sometimes radically different ones. The solution of the problem Beets sees as demanding the assumption that, in the interaction between the odorant molecule and the receptor site, variations are introduced by virtue of the particular orientation the molecule assumes in relation to the site to which it is adsorbed. "The orientations of all molecules at the receptor surface are statistically distributed around one or some energetically favorable ones and form a pattern, the shape of which is entirely determined by the nature, position, and steric environment of the functional group or groups in the molecule" (*47*, p. 41). An odorant owes its quality not only to landing in its proper site but to the attitude it assumes in the landing!

Moncrieff, who has done so much to bring order into olfactory psychophysiology, especially its relation to the chemical characteristics of stimuli, also strongly favors a stereochemical theory (428). With the aid of only a few assumptions concerning the essential roles of volatility and adsorption in stimulation, together with the basic postulate of site-filling molecules, he has been able to put together a reasonable account of: quality differentiation, absolute sensitivity level, time relations in stimulation, the adaptation phenomenon, limitations of response of chemically powerful odorants, and the odorlessness of certain gases. This goes further than most theories in charting the possible interrelations.

It is doubtless too early to attempt an evaluation of the stereochemical theory—even despite its embryonic existence for two millennia—for it seems clear that much more will have to be done along olfactometric lines before an assessment would carry conviction. Meanwhile the theory is beginning to perform the service of generating some of the necessary work, and the work, moreover, cuts interestingly across disciplines.

The third type of hypothesis—that postulating vibrational interchange between odorous vapors in the nostrils and the sensitive tissue surface—exists in several different forms. Here belong Dyson's theory of the Raman shift, already alluded to, and Heyninx' belief that the molecules of odorous materials vibrate with a period equal to that of the ultraviolet light they absorb. Here also belongs the hypothesis, revived and elaborated by Miles and Beck (41), that odors are appreciated by way of their infrared absorbing characteristics. It has been known since the researches of Faraday that odorous substances strongly absorb energy from the infrared portion of the electromagnetic spectrum, waves varying roughly from 1μ to 100μ in length. The human body is, of course, an infrared radiator. At normal body temperature waves ranging from 4μ to 20μ, with a peak intensity at about 9μ, are emitted. This being the case, so the theory goes, an odorous vapor in the nostrils can be expected to absorb infrared radiation in accordance with its own unique absorption spectrum, thus producing a transient local cooling of hair cells in the olfactory epithelium. A pattern of receptor elements, thrown out of dynamic equilibrium, discharges its fibers and reports the presence of the absorbent odorous substance.

Several serious objections to the infrared radiation theory have been offered. There are optical isomers of certain substances, limonene, for example, that have precisely the same pattern of infrared absorption but which can be distinguished from each other on the basis of smell. The d-limonene form smells like freshly crushed lemon rind, while l-limonene resembles a moldy lemon. Another pair of isomers, hence with identical infrared lines, are d-carvone and l-carvone. The dextro-member is variously described as like dill or caraway, while the levo-form smells like spearmint. The reverse situation is also known; compounds having considerably different infrared spectra may smell alike. A case in point is butanol and butyldeuteroxide (47). It is possible that the infrared absorption hypothesis can extricate itself from such embarrassments. Meanwhile, it is not apparent that the human nose is designed to do the work of an infrared spectrometer, which is substantially what this provocative but unconvincing theory demands. Simply on thermodynamic grounds, there would have to be a sizable temperature difference between the odorant and the nasal mucosa. Such differences, when they do exist, must be relatively slight.

Moreover, there is direct empirical evidence demonstrating the failure of the mucosal area to yield an electrical response in the presence of an odorant when a thin film of plastic material overlay the tissue (454). The plastic "filter" transmitted freely in the infrared region. Upon its removal the mucosal electrode displayed prompt activity.

A more recent theory, one that does not fall readily into any of the broad classes outlined above, is that of Davies and Taylor (145). Taking as a model the phenomenon of hemolysis (the process whereby hemoglobin is liberated from red blood cells by the action of saponin or other such poisonous agents) and the additional fact that many odorants are known strongly to accelerate this action, it is postulated that normally an odorous particle produces cytolysis (actual penetration of the wall of an olfactory nerve cell) when it adheres to the mucous lining of the cleft. Such "puncturing" occurs in the dwell time of the molecule (or perhaps several, conjointly) on the lipid membrane during adsorption. Whereas its "stay" may be only a fraction of a microsecond, it is estimated that something of the order of a millisecond may be required for the tissue to "heal," for the tiny hole to be obliterated entirely. During this time the normal balance between potassium ions (inside the cell) and sodium ions (outside) is disrupted, there is an ionic flow in both directions, and the cell discharges a train of impulses. The theory is obviously not lacking in ingenuity and has the further attraction that it may be amenable to test by known methods of physical chemistry.

Finally, among the more recently espoused ideas, one must seriously consider the hypothesis, recurring over the years, that differential sensitivity to odors may be largely, if not exclusively, a matter of how odor molecules spread themselves across the olfactory mucosa. Factors favorable and unfavorable to migration of odorant particles could produce spatiotemporal patterns of stimulation. Whatever materials are present in the mucosal "bed" could act differentially on odorants coming within their compass, "catching" some and rejecting others, binding to themselves migrant molecules in accordance with chemical affinities and perhaps fortuitous concentrations. In short, the nasal epithelium may act much like a gas chromatograph.

Much has been made of this possibility by Mozell (432, 433) who has also performed suggestive experiments in the light of it. In a chromatograph a stationary substance capable of absorbing or adsorbing a considerable range of other chemicals serves as a column or bed over which a solution containing an unknown gas or vapor is passed. Components of the latter are sorbed on the former, and the distances passed over in doing so become an analytic indicator of the material's composition. What is more natural than that this simple physical principle should be applied to the functioning of the mucosa? If odorous molecules were to be caught in transit in accordance with their sorption proclivities and retained in a given position long enough to excite olfactory receptor cells, the nose would really be operating much like a chromatograph. Each distinctive odor, perhaps each distinctive concentration of it, would have its own spatiotemporal gradient of excitation based on its dwell time and place in the mucosa, the analog of the chromatographic column.

Is there empirical evidence that the olfactory system actually functions in such a way? Mozell has adduced convincing evidence that it does (433). In the frog it is possible to sample activity in two separate regions, one near the external naris and therefore contacted early in the flow of odorous materials over the odor pathway, the other near the internal naris, encountered somewhat later. The first region is reported over the most medial olfactory nerve branches (MB), the second over the most lateral branches (LB) in the frog's olfactory sac. Impulses in the two branches being separately integrated and recorded, a simple ratio, LB/MB, now provides a measure of the gradient of activity across the mucosal sheet for each odorant presented to the external naris. The smaller LB/MB is, the more sharply activity falls off as an odor passes through the system; the larger the ratio, the less the differential between early and late olfactory activity.

The LB/MB ratio proved to be susceptible to quite accurate and reliable measurement. The fact that such a ratio exists might mean either that there are topographical regions of the mucosa responding well or badly to a particular odorant or that the chromatographic principle is at work, and sorption is going on differentially as odor molecules migrate across the mucosal sheet. A crucial experiment is to reverse the odor flow, allowing the lateral branch to come into play sooner than the medial branch. This was done for 16 different odorant chemicals, mostly organic compounds having quite distinctive odors for humans, two different flow rates, and four different partial pressures. In all instances, reversal of flow not only changed the relative latencies of response in the two nerve branches but also reversed the LB/MB ratios, reversed them in the sense that reciprocals of former values were now obtained. Apparently, it is not that there are local sensitivities to particular odorants; rather, there are differing facilities with which different odorants can migrate across the mucosa. The principle seems doubly sure when it is found that analysis in a commercial chromatograph of the same chemicals produces results that compare closely with those obtained with the frog's external-internal nares "chromatograph."

When it is recalled how much surface is available in the olfactory cleft for sorption of odorants—it has been estimated at perhaps as much as 600 cm²—there would seem to be almost infinite possibilities of patterning provided by the chromatographic theory. It will not only bear watching; it seems a new and helpful note in olfactory theory.

6
The Sense of Taste

Taste is the "poor relation" of the family of senses. It is poor in having only a restricted set of qualities to contribute to the sum of human experience. It is also relatively poor as an object of productive scientific inquiry. The two things are not unrelated. Gustatory phenomena do not loom large in the world of human affairs, not so large as the number of gourmets and gourmands in it would seem to imply, and few scientists have been attracted to their intensive study. However, fully as intriguing mysteries exist here as in other sense fields, as we shall see.

The Stimuli for Taste. To be tasted a substance must normally be soluble in water. This means that taste stimuli can initially be in solid, liquid, gaseous, or vaporous form, provided only that they will go into solution to some extent upon coming into contact with saliva. Their efficacy as taste stimuli then depends on a number of variables, among them solubility, concentration, ionization capacity, temperature, and their basic chemical composition. It is this last factor that has received the most attention. There is general agreement that there are but four basic taste qualities: salt, sour, bitter, and sweet. Curiosity as to the chemical foundation for these differences is natural.

Stimuli for the salty taste are best exemplified by table salt, NaCl. In fact, this is a common taste standard, all other substances being judged for the salty taste by comparison with it. NaCl, upon going into watery solution, immediately becomes ionized (NaCl $\rightarrow$ Na$^+$ + Cl$^-$). Both the anion, Cl$^-$, and the cation, Na$^+$, have some responsibility for the salty taste, as can be judged by observing the effects of joining Cl$^-$ with other cations and Na$^+$ with other anions. KCl, NH$_4$Cl, LiCl, ZnCl$_2$, and CaCl$_2$ all taste salty but not exactly alike, as would be the case if only the anion were responsible. Perhaps certain of these compounds make

an appeal to other basic tastes, bitter or sweet, and thus acquire individuality of pattern through taste mixture or blending. One of this group,
$ZnCl_2$, is an astringent and thus arouses a cutaneous component. A series
of compounds made up of sodium joined with various anions is found to
produce different strengths of the salty taste. The series goes like this, in
order of diminishing strength: Na_2SO_4, NaCl, NaBr, NaI, $NaHCO_3$,
$NaNO_3$. Since the sodium cation is common to all these salts it must be
concluded that the various anions are responsible for the differential
stimulating capacities displayed. Conspicuously salty cations, in addition
to the commonly encountered Na and K, are Li, Mg, and NH_3. Anions
are commonly the halides (Cl, Br, I, F), sulfates, nitrates, carbonates,
and tartrates. One other generality about salty-tasting compounds seems
possible, that is, all of them are of relatively low molecular weight. As
salts get heavier there is a tendency for their taste to change from salty
to bitter. Thus the chlorides, in general, are salty tasting, but cesium
chloride, CsCl, which has a very high molecular weight, is bitter. Other
heavy halides, CsI, KI, RbI, and RbBr, are also bitter tasting. Unfortunately, the generality concerning molecular weight may not be inverted,
for it is not true that salts with light molecules are invariably salty tasting.
Salts of beryllium (atomic weight, 9.02) are sweet; until recently beryllium
was called *glucinum*, "the sweet element."

The attempt to generate simple principles about the stimulus for the
salty taste is further embarrassed by the circumstance that a given salt
may not yield the same quality at all concentrations (*178*). At slightly
supraliminal values, NaCl tastes sweet to many people. KCl, sweet at
threshold, passes through a bitter phase as concentration in increased and
becomes salty only when a strength nearly ten times the liminal value has
been reached. Then, at higher levels, its taste becomes complex, mainly
salty but with bitter and sour overtones. Indeed, one authority, von
Skramlik (*531*), believes all strong salt solutions to possess inherent complexities of this kind and has written a general equation reminiscent of
the color formula in vision:

$$N = xA + yB + zC + vD$$

where A, B, C, and D are sodium chloride (salt), quinine sulfate (bitter),
fructose (sweet), and potassium tartrate (sour) respectively, x, y, z, and v
are their molar concentrations, and N is the molar concentration of the
salt being matched.

The sour taste, like the salty one, results from ionic action. Here it is
possible to be quite specific. The ions concerned are always the cations
resulting from acid dissociation, that is, hydrogen ions. That the hydrogen

ion is the essential agent in the production of the sour taste is shown by the fact that all mineral or *inorganic* acids, such as HCl, H_2SO_4, or HNO_3, taste alike provided they are sampled in equal concentrations. To be sure, the same general statement cannot be made about weak *organic* acids such as acetic, tartaric, and citric. These have distinctive tastes, and they are, moreover, more sour than they should be if hydrogen-ion concentration were the sole principle at work. It is probable that the complex molecular structures found in the organic acids have an influence on more than a single basic taste mechanism and that their "flavor" really depends on gustatory blending. Much of the difficulty in arriving at a single, simple correlate for the sour taste seems to have come from the failure of experimenters to eliminate the chemical interactions between sour stimuli and saliva, the latter serving as a buffer solution in the ensuing stimulation of the gustatory receptors. Minimizing the effect of saliva by first clearing the tongue surface, then confining the acid stimulus to a mechanically isolated area of the tongue which saliva cannot invade, results in uniform threshold values for all acids of equal chemical combining capacity (*465*, p. 1149).

Salty and sour tastes are, then, essentially ionic; they are generated only after molecular dissociation has taken place. The stimuli for the remaining taste qualities, bitter and sweet, may also be ionic, though usually they are not. The most potent bitter materials are the alkaloids brucine, strychnine, and nicotine. A slightly less powerful alkaloid, quinine, is commonly used in taste experiments. These substances operate in the undissociated, molecular form. This is not to say that bitter tastes cannot be aroused by ionic solutions. On the contrary, in appropriate combination, ions of magnesium, silver, ferric iron, cesium, rubidium, and iodine all call forth the bitter taste.

Stimuli for sweetness exist in a profusion of forms and come from many different chemical families. Certain of the soluble lead and beryllium salts ionize to yield the sweet taste. Compounds containing the hydroxyl anion, $-OH^-$, are frequently sweet. The sweetest substances, however, have complex organic molecules which do not ionize. This is true of most of the sugars and of a host of compounds synthesized for use in the confectionery industry. Of recent years there have been concocted many new sweetening agents, some of them several thousand times as sweet as cane sugar. For the most part they are complex aromatics, all containing prominent nitro groups in their structure.

There is a suggestive relationship in the fact that many bitter and sweet stimuli have similar chemical and physical properties. Sweet materials, upon undergoing only a very slight chemical modification, merely an architectural rearrangement of atoms in the case of certain stereoisomers, may have their taste transformed to bitter. It is especially notable that a considerable number of sweet compounds falling in chemically related or "homologous" series tend to become bitter as the series is ascended. The effort to disclose generalities concerning chemical and physical properies of taste stimuli recalls the similar attempt in connection with smell. "Laws" of gustatory stimulation are as difficult to come by as are olfactory ones. If there are any altogether simple principles governing the relation between physicochemical composition and sensation quality they have until now eluded scientific detection. Perhaps when there has been sufficiently extensive and systematic study of all the variables that could conceivably enter to complicate matters we shall be able to cut through to master principles. The view has been with us since the turn of the century (310) that individual cations and anions, in simple salts, contribute their own separate qualities to the total taste. Now, it appears, things are somewhat more devious than that. Perhaps one ion in a salt, at a given concentration, is primarily responsible for the main quality yielded by that salt, but it seems equally clear that the other ion usually modifies the overall effect (179).

The stimuli thus far considered are the normal or "adequate" ones for taste. Two forms of unusual or nonadequate stimulation are known. One involves, somewhat surprisingly, chemical stimulation by way of the blood stream; the other is what has come to be called "electric taste." The arousal of taste by substances transported by the blood has not been studied in any systematic way but has occasionally been reported as a kind of curiosity. The phenomenon is entailed in one of the techniques used by the physiologist to measure "circulation time" of the blood. Thus, if either saccharin or calcium gluconate is injected into a vein at the elbow there ensues, in a matter of a dozen seconds or less, the arousal of a sweet taste.

In a few instances both smell and taste seem to have been aroused by a common agent in the blood (42). Thus patients taking the arsenical, Neosalvarsan, have reported tasting and smelling the substance only a few seconds after receiving it intravenously in the forearm. The average latency was somewhat under 8 sec, approximately the time required for the blood stream to transport it to the head region. Neither nasal obstructions nor cocainization of the olfactory epithelium diminished the sensation. Competition with the nasally presented odors of menthol and benzene produced no alteration, not even mixture. That the locus of action was not a cortical brain center is attested by the fact that patients having peripheral impairments, such as atrophy of the mucosa, were unable to appreciate the blood-borne material. The results were not confined to one substance; camphor and oil of turpentine had the same effect.

Other investigators have reported that the intensely bitter substance, sodium dehydrocholate, and the peanutlike tasting "Vitamin B_4" can be detected by "taste" only a few seconds after being injected into the arm.

There is good evidence that hematogenic smell does not just "happen" when odorous materials are present in the blood stream and circulate to or near the olfactory epithelium. There may be required a mechanical assist. It has been reported (75) that subjects getting injections of essence of citral or peppermint, 1 cc being introduced to the cubital vein of the arm, could not smell the material so long as the breath was being held. The moment breathing was resumed the smell came out strongly. Also, if pure nitrogen were blasted into the nostril through a small polyethylene tube (the breath still being held), the odor was appreciated with a 12-sec latency from the beginning of injection. Since, so far as is known, direct mechanical stimulation of the olfactory epithelium fails to excite that tissue olfactorily, there is something of a mystery here. This is conceivably a very significant phenomenon, whatever its eventual explanation, for it suggests the possibility that the taste and smell mechanisms may be subject to a more or less uniform adaptation to the blood stream that nourishes them. Active stimulation would then have to be pictured as "breaking through" or being superposed on this constant background. The situation is reminiscent of the parallel one in vision, where "brain gray" may be thought of as the invariable uniform field on which colors put in their appearance.

The case of "electric taste" is a little less remarkable. Electric currents may be employed to arouse gustatory sensations, just as they may be used for nonadequate stimulation in all other senses, though the phenomena produced in this way are not as yet well understood. Direct and alternating currents give different results. With direct currents varying effects are created, depending on the direction of flow. With alternating currents the taste aroused is dependent upon frequency of alternation. In both cases current strength is an important variable. With steady direct current as a source, a sour taste is evoked if the anode is applied to the tongue. Reversal of the current brings about a change to a "soapy" taste having a burning quality about it. When prolonged direct current is the stimulus, the situation is really quite complex. In addition to stimulating nerve endings (probably directly), the current produces electrolysis of the saliva, and the resulting dissociation products enter the picture as chemical stimuli. Some simplification can be achieved by using nonpolarizable electrodes and restricting the electrical stimulus to very short pulses. The results then seem to depend on the area of tongue exposed, that is, electrode diameter, and pulse repetition rate. Békésy (58) restricted his pulses to a duration of 0.5 msec, his gold electrode to an area of 50 mm², and varied pulse frequency from 1 to 500 per second. The predominant taste was salty at low repetition rates, sour at medium rates, and bitter at the highest frequencies. If, now, electrode diameter was reduced to 3 mm, the salty taste dropped out, and if a further reduction of the gold tip to 0.3 mm diam was made, there was evoked only a single taste (sour, sweet, salty, or bitter) at all frequencies. The quality of the taste depended exclusively on electrode location.

With low-frequency alternating currents, of the order of 50 Hz, and large electrodes, the sensation qualitatively resembles the anodal taste with the steady current, i.e., sour is evoked. Raise the frequency to the neighborhood of 1000 Hz, however, and the taste becomes predominantly bitter. Frequencies midway between these give somewhat anomalous results.

At one time there appeared to be some basis for the belief that electric taste could yield a "critical fusion point" with rapidly repeated stimulation, like CFF in vision. As part of a systematic program of investigating all sense channels with such stimuli, Allen and Weinberg (14) delivered square-wave pulses to the tongue, speeding up the pulse repetition rate until the subject reported perceiving the sour taste as smooth and continuous rather than interrupted. Time relations in gustatory sensation being what they are—relatively long rise times and ponderous subsidences—it would seem remarkable if variations in the sour taste followed with any fidelity the rapid electrical fluctuations of the kind employed in the Allen and Weinberg experiments (125 to 350 pulses per second, pps). But such were reported, and the conclusion coming out of these experiments was a mischief-maker in the literature of the chemical senses for many years. Eventually, others (336, 470) repeated the work, with suitable improvements, and discovered the basis for the apparent "flicker." It turned out that the electrical stimulus was appealing to more than one sense channel, pressure (and pain, at high intensities) as well as taste. The lower threshold belongs to taste and, even though the current is pulsed, a steady gustatory sensation is evoked. At somewhat higher levels, pressure and eventually pain are brought forth, and these yield a tingling, vibratory pattern. The relations between the two sets of thresholds are displayed in Figure 16-1. As has been demonstrated in other work (104), something like a gustatory critical fusion point may in fact be found but, as might be predicted, it occurs at very low repetition rates, under 10 pps, as befits a system that is essentially sluggish in its response.

Receptors and Neural Pathways for Taste.   Consideration of the receptor mechanism responsible for taste begins with the tongue and its papillae,

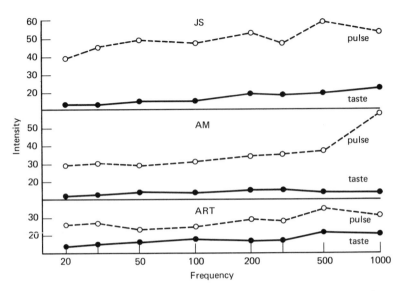

Fig. 16–1. Taste and somesthetic (electric pulses) thresholds compared over a wide frequency range. From Pierrel *(470)*. Copyright 1955 by the American Psychological Association, and reproduced by permission.

though taste sensitivity is by no means confined to the tongue. Regions responsive to taste stimuli exist on the palate, in the pharynx, on the tonsils and epiglottis and, in some people at least, on the mucosa of the lips and cheeks, the underside of the tongue, and the floor of the mouth *(86)*. The areas of greatest responsiveness—and those most investigated by reason of relative ease of access—are the tip, sides, and rear of the dorsal tongue surface. A region surrounding and including the middle of the tongue's upper surface is quite devoid of taste sensitivity. The receptor organs, *taste buds* (see Figure 16–2), comprise a group of individual gustatory cells, from a few to two dozen or more of them forming an ovoid cluster. Each of the gustatory cells terminates distally in a gustatory pore, the direct route of access to taste solutions.

There is good evidence that the individual components of the taste bud, the gustatory cells, have a short life history. Proof that taste cells are constantly being renewed comes from some ingenious experiments in which the poisonous material, colchicine, was injected into the tongues of rats and rabbits *(51, 392)*. This toxic material has the property of slowing down or preventing cell division. Its injection also prevents taste cells from responding, causing a fairly prompt weakening and,

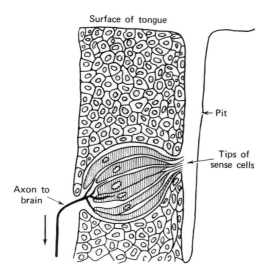

Surface of tongue

← Pit

Tips of
sense cells

Axon to
brain

Fig. 16–2. A taste bud. The individual cells comprising the "bud" are of two kinds, *gustatory* cells, spindle-shaped terminations of the nerve fibers subserving taste, and *sustentacular,* or supporting cells. The tips of the sense cells protrude beyond the surrounding epithelium and are presumably stimulated through direct contact with taste solutions. From PSYCHOLOGY, fourth edition by Robert S. Woodworth. Copyright, 1921, 1929, 1934, 1940, by Holt, Rinehart and Winston, Inc. Reprinted by permission of Holt, Rinehart and Winston, Inc.

after 8 to 10 hr, a complete disappearance of impulses from the affected cells. This, by itself, would not constitute conclusive evidence, for colchicine might simply be acting as an anesthetic, but a further step, that of "tagging" the dividing cells with a radioactive material and observing the result, shows that taste cells have a life of only a few days. The rejuvenation process consists in moving newly formed cells from the outside margins of the bud toward the center. Such turnover implies, of course, that taste cells are "passed along" from one nerve cell to another. If there is any specificity in the system it must either belong to the nerve or, if it resides in the receptor cell, must change almost hourly in a most remarkable way (*150*).

Whereas taste buds are distributed fairly generally over much of the tongue's dorsal surface, they are most numerous in aggregates associated with papillae, visible protuberances on the tongue's surface. Four clearly different forms of papillae are to be found: *fungiform, foliate, circumvallate,* and *filiform.* All but the filiform papillae contain taste buds. Fungiform papillae, mushroomlike in appearance as the name implies, are found scattered somewhat irregularly over the sides and fore-part of the upper tongue surface. Foliate papillae derive from a series of grooves or folds in the midlateral border of the tongue. The circum-vallate papillae, most readily identifiable of all, form a "chevron" near the back of the tongue, the apex toward the throat. Each of these some-

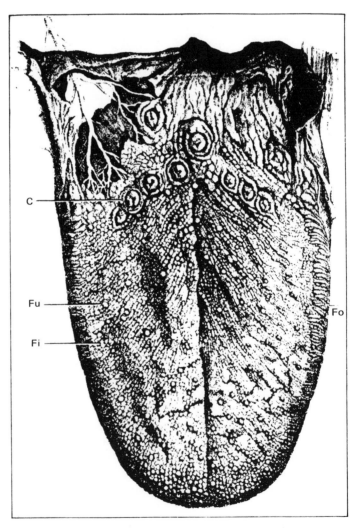

Fig. 16–3. The tongue's papillae: C, circumvallate; Fu, fungiform; Fi, filiform; Fo, foliate. From Warren and Carmichael (*608*) after Wenzel.

what massive but low eminences is surrounded by a kind of "trench" or "moat" which forms a container for taste solutions. Taste pores, *microvilli*, open into the moat.

Papillae of this type have been most carefully studied histologically. Data assembled from examination of well over 50,000 taste buds from a total of several hundred circumvallate papillae (*25*) reveal that there are somewhat over 200 taste buds opening into the trench of the average papilla. There are many more in some; 865 were counted in one exceptional case. At birth there is apparently a full complement of taste buds on the sides of the papilla, but the far wall (beyond the moat) has few, if any, buds. The number on the papillae themselves remains fairly constant from early childhood until middle age. Meanwhile the trench wall becomes populated with buds. With the beginning of the atrophic changes of late maturity both groups of taste buds, those on the papilla and those on the wall, show a diminution in number. A typical count in old age shows less than a hundred buds to each circumvallate papilla, the far wall included. The papillae themselves, moreover, tend to become shrunken and wrinkled, and the surrounding trenches get filled up with squamous epithelial material. If there are sensitivity differences in taste correlated with age variations an anatomical basis for them would appear to be possible.

Details of the structure of the gustatory receptor cell have, in recent years, been made evident through the use of the electron microscope. In the connective tissue at the base of a taste bud there are to be found myelinated sensory fibers having diameters of 1 to 6μ. These lose their protective sheath and project into the taste cells proper as fine fibrils (0.05 to 1.0μ). A single parent fiber may send fibrils into several sense cells and a single cell may derive its nerve supply from several fibers. This kind of overlap is especially characteristic of the older cells near the heart of the bud; the newer ones at the edge are more simply connected (*392*, p. 12).

The tongue and mouth region are innervated by no fewer than four cranial nerves, each of them of the mixed sensorimotor type. Two of these, the seventh (facial) and ninth (glossopharyngeal), are of undoubted importance for taste. Another, the tenth (vagus), is involved to the extent of supplying fibers for the taste buds of the pharynx and larynx. The remaining one is the fifth (trigeminal), which, it is now generally believed, is concerned in its sensory aspect exclusively with cutaneous functions. It is, of course, the trigeminal nerve that supplies the feeling patterns that complicate both olfactory and gustatory perceptions. In fact, current literature has come to speak of "the trigeminal component" in taste and smell.

The pathway to the brain from the anterior two-thirds of the tongue is over the *chorda tympani* branch of the facial nerve. This nerve trunk runs a devious course from the tongue to the medulla of the brain, at one point looping over the ossicles of the middle ear and passing near the eardrum, from which it derives its name. Taste cells of the posterior third of the tongue receive their nerve supply from the glossopharyngeal nerve, which likewise runs to the medulla and joins fibers of the facial nerve to form a well-defined bulbar center. From the medulla, through the optic thalamus, to the cortical projection areas the pathways conducting gustatory impulses seem to parallel those conveying cutaneous impulses from the face, mouth, and tongue. Apposite centers are involved at every stage in the ascent to the highest levels of the central nervous system, and the final projection areas in the cortex also border on each other if, indeed, the two are not completely interspersed. It is difficult to arrive at firm generalities with respect to the ascending pathways for taste in the face of current onslaughts by way of electrophysiological and anatomical researches. There prove to be important species differences (*64*). In the rat and squirrel monkey, taste pathways are apparently present only on the ipsilateral side of the thalamus and there they are slightly spatially separated from the cutaneous modalities of the tongue. Yet human cortical lesions show taste to be bilaterally represented, and taste, touch, and temperature impulses appear to be completely intermingled in the somatic sensory tongue area of the cat. If there is a separate gustatory projection area in the human cortex it is presumably bilaterally present and is situated near the lower end of the postcentral gyrus, just above the fissure of Sylvius. The gustatory projection takes its place next to an orderly succession of somatic centers, the most proximal of which are those for the pharynx, mouth, and tongue. A chain of three neurones has carried the impulses from the tongue to the cortex.

There would be reasons for supposing that gustatory and olfactory centers might lie in close association with each other, intimacy of functional connection between the two senses being what it is. In fact, the close liaison between smell and taste has more than once led to the mistaken belief that the central projection for taste must be in the rhinencephalon. Several lines of evidence combine to show that this is not the case. One set of facts which speak against such an association comes from study of cerebral injuries. Börnstein (*86*) examined twelve patients with sensory disturbances brought about by gunshot wounds involving the parietal lobe of the brain. In each case displaying gustatory impairment there had been destruction of tissue at the base of the postcentral gyrus. Also, there is the testimony of patients whose brains were laid bare under local anesthetic and stimulated electrically in an effort to define the limits of an area invaded by tumor or to reproduce the "warning" symptoms of epileptic attacks to which they were subject, and thus locate the focus of the difficulty causing them (462). Taste sensations could be aroused in this way only in a few instances but then always by stimulation of the parietal cortex, at the lower end of the central fissure. Even though the entire cortex was explored point by point, no other region ever gave a suggestion of gustatory sensation. The close association of smell and taste would seem to have nothing to do with proximity of brain centers but to stem from the accident of the peripheral placement of these two senses and the fact that both respond to chemical stimuli.

Absolute Taste Sensitivity. After all that has been learned concerning absolute sensitivity in the other sense departments it would be surprising indeed to discover that taste thresholds are fixed and immutable, that they are independent of a number of conditions surrounding their measurement. They are not, of course. A number of stimulus and receptor variables have to be taken into account, as do certain factors underlying individual differences in reactivity of the organism. There are at least these variables: the substance used as stimulus, its concentration, its locus of action and the total tongue area involved, stimulus rate of application and overall duration, prior state of adaptation, chemical condition of the saliva and perhaps of the blood, stimulus temperature, presence of any hormonal or dietary deficiencies, the particular species concerned and its genetic constitution. The list is by no means exhaustive, nor are the items in it entirely independent of each other. Thus, prior state of adaptation is conditioned by chemical condition of saliva and blood and these in turn by hormonal and dietary deficiencies. Other dependencies suggest themselves. A catalogue of parameters in psychophysiological experiments is never simple and, moreover, always needs to be cross-indexed.

One of the important and interesting variables is temperature of the stimulus. As a practical matter it has long been known that the taste of food is partially determined by its temperature. Good cooks salt foods when they are neither too hot nor too cold. In making iced tea the sourness of added lemon is not apparent until the tea has cooled down. Confectioners know that candy made for use in the tropics must not be over-sweetened lest it taste insipid.

The relation between temperature and taste sensitivity is not a simple one. Not all substances are affected alike by temperature changes. Measurements of gustatory thresholds for sodium chloride, hydrochloric acid, quinine, and dulcin, as made by Hahn (259) are presented in Figure 16-4. The salt threshold increases steadily with a rise in temperature of the testing solution from 17° C to 42° C. Sensitivity to the bitter stimulus,

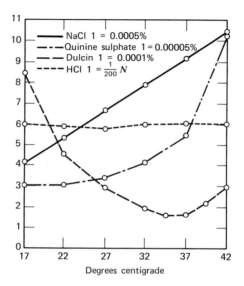

Fig. 16–4. The effect of temperature on taste sensitivity. The four curves, for four different substances, have been made comparable by assigning different ordinate values to them, as noted in the key. Sensitivity to NaCl and quinine declines with increasing temperature and that to HCl is uninfluenced, while dulcin gives an optimal response in the neighborhood of 35° C. From Hahn (*259*).

quinine sulfate, shows a generally similar trend, but the function connecting threshold with temperature, rather than being linear, is a positively accelerated curve. Thresholds for sweet are at a minimum in the neighborhood of 35° C and increase if either warmer or cooler solutions are used. Sensitivity to HCl, the sour stimulus, is unaffected by temperature changes, at least in this concentration of the acid and over this temperature range. A number of other sweet stimuli used in the Hahn experiments gave curves midway between the inflected function for dulcin and the level line for hydrochloric acid. These varied results go some distance in discouraging any oversimplified interpretation of the taste mechanism. The stimulation process must consist of something more than a simple chemical reaction. Nearly all chemical processes are speeded up and made more effective when temperature is raised. In these threshold measurements only sweet solutions seem to behave as if they were entering into a chemical reaction, and even they do not do so in an entirely uniform manner.

A second and important variable affecting threshold determinations has to do with the particular area of the receptive surface used in making the measurements. Not all parts of the tongue's surface are equally responsive to all stimuli. In general, bitter solutions are most readily appreciated near the back of the tongue and sweet stimuli affect the tip of the tongue most strongly, while acids are most easily sensed along the edges about midway back from the tip. Except for the prominent zone on the tongue's top surface, where no taste sensations at all can be aroused, it is possible to evoke the salty taste pretty generally over the entire upper surface and edges, sensitivity being slightly better towards the front. The relative sensitivities of different portions of the tongue's edge to the four basic tastes are shown in Figure 16–5, which is derived from the early but

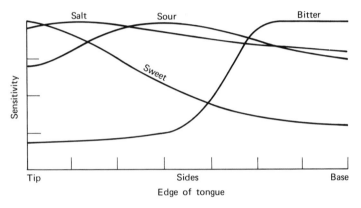

Fig. 16–5. Variations in gustatory sensitivity along the edge of the tongue. A plot of Hänig's data *(265)* by Boring *(84)*. The sensitivity scale is one of threshold reciprocals. Figure reproduced by permission of Appleton-Century-Crofts, Inc., New York.

careful explorations of Hänig *(265)*. Whether or not individual papillae contain cells responsive to only a single kind of stimulus is still a somewhat unsettled point. However, strong evidence has been adduced from explorations of the tongue with carefully manipulated electrical and chemical stimuli *(58, 59)* that individual papillae are specialized in their function and that all gustatory cells belonging to a particular papilla yield the same taste quality when aroused. Both the modern electrical and chemical evidences are compelling, especially when contrasted with those coming from less exact experiments of an earlier time. The classical experiment, performed by systematic exploration of the tongue with a finely pointed camel's hair brush bearing a taste solution, typically finds the great majority of papillae responsive to more than one kind of taste stimulus. Thus Kiesow *(360)*, charting the sensitivities of 35 papillae, found 18 responsive to acid (3 exclusively so), 26 sensitive to sugar solution (7 exclusively), 18 responsive to salt (3 exclusively), and 13 sensitive to a bitter solution. There were none responding solely to the bitter stimulus. This kind of experiment has been repeated many times, always with similar results. It would seem from such data that the vast majority of papillae can mediate more than one sense quality. That those located near the base of the tongue are "biased" in the direction of bitter while those near the tip place the emphasis on sweet would appear to be evidenced not only by topographic studies but also by the tongue's response to several organic compounds falling in the "bittersweet" category. A single chemically pure (if somewhat complex) substance, para-brombenzoic-sulfinide, tastes bitter to the back of the tongue and sweet to the tip. Magnesium sulfate (Epsom salts) also has a dual taste, bitter at the back and salty near the front of the tongue.

The extraordinarily precise experiments of Békésy have led to quite different results and to radically altered conclusions. He has made a "micro-approach" to taste papillae, stimulating them under optical magnifications of 20 to 30 diameters and with correspondingly tiny stimuli. For electrical stimulation he employs direct current (anodal) pulses of 0.5 msec duration applied through gold electrodes only 0.1 to 0.3 mm in diameter. For chemical stimulation he pulls papillae gently out of place with a suction tube and applies miniscule droplets of taste solution directly to the viscous walls of these structures, where fluids in such small quantities readily adhere. Both sets of experiments speak with a common voice, and their message is one of specificity. A single papilla may have many receptive cells but they are not a mixed population; whatever may be the current strength or pulse frequency or whatever the stimulus concentration, only a single quality is aroused. There are, to be sure, instances in which the salty taste, say, can be evoked from one side of a papilla's collar and sour from the opposite side, but careful investigation reveals these to be two different structures joined together. Indeed, as many as three papillae may be so fused near the edge of the tongue or on the palate.

Some extremely interesting anatomical observations have come out of the same experiments (58, p. 1108). Papillae responsive to acids and those receptive to salts appear to be structured somewhat differently from those mediating bitter and those yielding the sweet taste. The sour-salt type is more rounded in shape and has capillaries that form distinguishable subsurface loops. Papillae of the bitter-sweet type are more pointed in contour and have a somewhat deeply disposed vascular supply, for they do not so obviously show local blanching when touched. There are also clear, functional distinctions to be made between the two kinds of papillae. One important characteristic concerns their threshold response to trains of electrical pulses. Figure 16-6 displays this difference. Another functional property is the critical fusion frequency of such a series of direct current pulses. The salt-sour type yields continuous sensation at 3 to 4 pps while a repetition rate of 7 to 10 pps is required to smooth out the bitter and sweet tastes. An observation made long ago (*525*), that

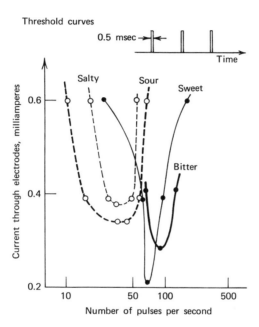

Fig. 16–6.   Responses of taste papillae to trains of electrical pulses. Sweet and bitter papillae respond best at a higher frequency of pulses than do those mediating salty and sour tastes. From Georg von Békésy. Sweetness produced electrically on the tongue and its relation to taste theories. *J. Appl. Physiol.* 19: 1105–1113, 1964.

gymnemic acid has the remarkable property of acting on the tongue to suppress sweet and bitter tastes while leaving sour and salty tastes unaffected, possibly fits in here also.

An especially critical determinant of the taste threshold is the matter of the technique used in applying the stimulus. It makes a difference whether a few drops of test solution are placed on the subject's tongue, the instruction being to identify the taste, or whether two 10-cc samples are presented in successive trials, one of test solution and the other of distilled water, the task being to discriminate between the two by sipping first one and then the other in a leisurely manner. Both of these methods, together with variants of them, were used by Richter and MacLean (*495*) to measure the threshold of the salty taste. Individual differences were large, a common finding in taste experiments, and these tended to obscure certain differences due to method. However, average thresholds for a large group of subjects ranged from a low concentration of 0.016% (water and NaCl discriminated, the two being sampled as frequently and in as large or small amounts as desired) to a high of 0.192% (NaCl being identified without comparison with any other solution, three drops being placed on the extended tongue). Individual thresholds, under the same circumstances, ranged from 0.007% to 0.350%, values which stand in a 1:50 ratio.

There are some other, generally less crucial, factors influencing the measurement of the absolute gustatory threshold. Enough has been said, however, to indicate that it is possible to tabulate sensitivities to taste stimuli only in a very gross way. Table 16-1, adapted from a summary compiled by Pfaffmann (*467*), indicates the order of magnitude of thresholds for some representative stimuli. Although it is not the only way of doing so, the convention is becoming established of reporting threshold (and other) intensities in terms of *molar concentration* (moles), the number of grams of solute divided by its molecular weight, per liter of total solution.

Table 16–1. Absolute Thresholds for Representative Taste Stimuli

	Average threshold (Molar Concentration)	Range
Acid: Hydrochloric acid (HCl)	0.0009	0.00005–0.01
Acid: Formic acid (HCOOH)	0.0018	0.0007–0.0035
Salt: Sodium chloride (NaCl)	0.01[a]	0.001–0.08
Salt: Sodium chloride (NaCl)	0.03[b]	0.003–0.085
Sweet: Sucrose ($C_{12}H_{22}O_{11}$)	0.01[a]	0.005–0.016
Sweet: Sodium saccharin	0.000023	0.00002–0.00004
Bitter: Quinine sulfate [($C_{20}H_{24}N_2O_2$) H_2SO_4]	0.000008	0.0000004–0.000011
Bitter: Caffeine ($C_8H_{10}N_4O_2$)	0.0007	0.0003–0.001

After Pfaffmann, *467*, pp. 507–533, Tables, 2, 4, 6, 8.
[a] Detection threshold.
[b] Recognition threshold.

Differential Taste Sensitivity.   Although relatively large concentrations of stimulus solution are needed to reach the absolute threshold for taste, as compared with those required to arouse smell, the relative size of the increment (ΔI) to produce a just perceptible increase in sensation strength is no larger. That is to say, by and large, the Weber fraction ($\Delta I/I$) for taste is about the same size as that for smell. If we take the values $\frac{1}{2}$ to $\frac{1}{6}$ as the representative ones for the Weber fraction in smell (since these embrace the typical results for the middle span of intensities under a variety of conditions), a similar rough bringing together of the experimental data for taste would show fractions ranging from $\frac{1}{2}$ to $\frac{1}{10}$. But the measure of differential sensitivity, like that of absolute sensitivity, is affected by a number of experimental variables. Its magnitude is partially determined by the taste quality appealed to, whether salt, sour, sweet, or bitter. Moreover, the method of applying the stimulus is critical. Although differential taste sensitivity has been the subject of measurement for nearly a century, there are remarkably few sets of results that may be compared closely with one another. Experimental controls generally have been inadequate and, indeed, not until quite recently have all four taste qualities been explored under strictly comparable conditions and with suitably rigorous procedures. In a comprehensive study conducted by Schutz and Pilgrim at the Quartermaster Food and Container Institute (*514*), solutions were presented in small glasses that provided a 6 ml test sample which the subjects swirled around in their mouths, then made their judgments of taste intensity. Four solutions were used, each at five concentrations. Mean Weber fractions (all solution strengths combined) were: salt (sodium chloride), 0.15; sour (citric acid), 0.25; sweet (sucrose), 0.17; bitter (caffeine) 0.30. For gustation as a whole the value was 0.20, and this fraction, $\frac{1}{5}$, presumably is as representative a value as can be found. Individual differences are of some importance, as Figure 16–7 demonstrates.

As in the other sense departments ΔI is not unaffected by the absolute intensity at which the determinations are carried out, just as it is not uninfluenced by temperature, by the prevailing state of adaptation, by the experimental procedure used in conducting the experiment and, in fact, by the whole host of conditions affecting the absolute threshold itself. The systematic effect of intensive changes has been determined carefully for one of the taste qualities, salt (*311*). The result of plotting the Weber fraction against stimulus intensity, over the range from absolute threshold to the point at which the salty taste gets complicated by the introduction of a painful sting, is shown in Figure 16–8. Discriminability is poor at low intensities and improves up to a level of about 3.0 moles. It should be said that the experiment establishing this function was conducted by the

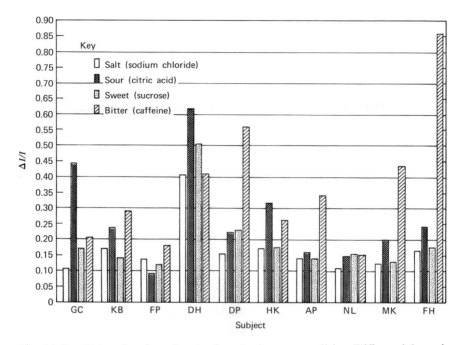

Fig. 16–7. Weber fractions for the four basic taste qualities. Differential sensitivity for each of ten observers. From Schutz and Pilgrim *(514)*. Copyright 1957 by the American Psychological Association, and reproduced by permission.

"single-drop" technique, an estimate of sensation strength being given by the subject after the stimulation of the outstretched tongue by one drop of the test fluid. If the buccal cavity is flooded with test solution and rinsed between samples, as occurred in the Schutz and Pilgrim experiment cited above, the effect of altering intensity is relatively insignificant for bitter, unimportant for sour and sweet except near the absolute threshold, and of consequence for salt only at the two ends of the scale, near the absolute and terminal thresholds.

The question of sensitivity to relatively small changes in intensity is connected with the further one of ability to estimate absolute levels of taste intensity. To what extent is it possible to relate perceived strength of taste sensation to physical concentration of gustatory stimulus? In an earlier day we should be said to be raising the question of the adequacy of Fechner's "psychophysical law"; now we say we are asking whether a "psychological scale" of taste intensity is possible. Lewis *(382;226, pp.*

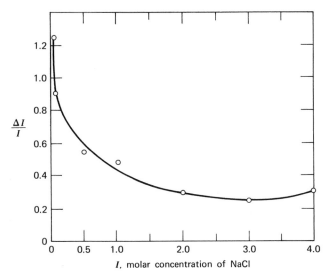

Fig. 16–8. Differential sensitivity to salt as a function of concentration. The Weber fraction, $\Delta I/I$, becomes progressively smaller with an increase in absolute sensitivity, up to a concentration of about 3.0 mole, at which point gustatory sensation begins to be complicated by the arousal of a painful sting from the chemical action of salt. After Holway and Hurvich *(311)*. Courtesy of the *American Journal of Psychology* and Dr. Hurvich.

83–84) found that such a scale could be devised. He had subjects taste a standard solution, then select from a series of graded comparison solutions the one which tasted "half as strong" as the standard. Each of the four basic tastes was represented, the standard solutions being sodium chloride, sucrose, quinine sulfate, and tartaric acid. All were used in several concentrations, and the "halving" procedure was repeated with each. This is the so-called "fractionation" method for devising scales of observational intensity.

Not only was it found possible to construct continuous scales from these data and to relate them to stimulus concentrations, but it was discovered that intensive cross comparisons between different taste qualities could be made. Thus, it turns out to be possible for subjects to select, with satisfactory consistency, a salt solution that tastes just half as strong as a standard sugar solution. In a similar manner quinine and tartaric acid may be related to sugar *(44)*. The strengths of all four basic tastes having thus been specified in terms of a common denominator, sugar, it is but one additional step to select a unit of measurement, define it, and generalize to a "psychological scale of taste strength." The fundamental unit chosen was the "gust," which is defined as the "psychological strength of a 1 per cent sucrose solution." Figure 16-9 shows the way in which obser-

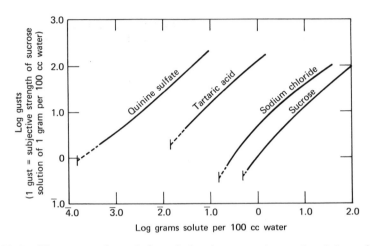

Fig. 16–9. The gust scale and the relation between observational intensity and stimulus strength for each of the four fundamental tastes. From Beebe-Center and Waddell (*44*). By permission of the Journal Press.

vational intensity, in gusts, is related to stimulus concentration for the four fundamental tastes. The gust scale should recall the "dol" scale for pain (see Chapter 11) which, as a matter of fact, has a similar logic underlying its construction.

Another way to go about obtaining a psychological scale, of course, is to adopt the direct frontal attack provided by the "magnitude estimation" method of Stevens (*550*). This we have encountered before in other sensory realms. For taste, as for the other senses, sensation intensity proves to be related to stimulus intensity by a power function; a log-log plot of the two yields a straight line. The slope of the line, that is, the exponent of the power function, varies roughly between 0.8 (saccharin) and 2.2 (sucaryl), with values for salt (NaCl) and sugar (sucrose) near 1.3. Whereas the full significance of the power function slope is not yet apparent and will not be until far more than the presently available information on this fundamental relation is at hand, the slope is obviously a direct index of "dynamic range," the sweep of the scale over which intensitive variations are appreciated. The sweetness of saccharin grows relatively slowly

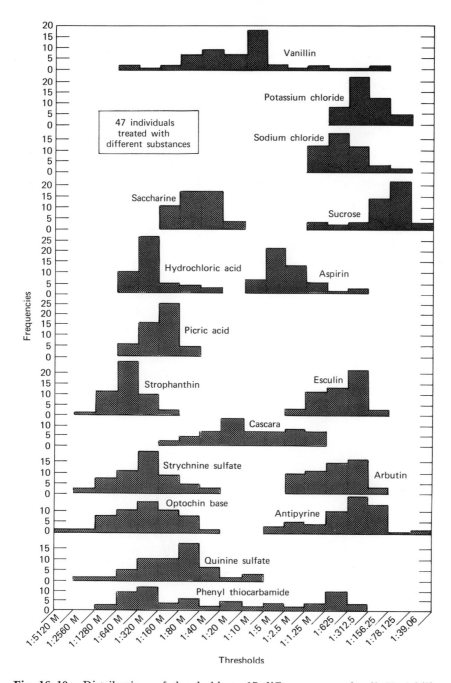

Fig. 16–10. Distributions of thresholds to 17 different taste stimuli. Variability of response is particularly evident in the case of vanillin (top) and PTC (bottom). From Blakeslee and Salmon *(74)*. Courtesy of the National Academy of Sciences.

as concentration is increased, while that of sucaryl leaps ahead rapidly and reaches its tolerable limit earlier in the intensity series.

Individual Differences in Taste Sensitivity: "Taste Blindness."   It was noted earlier that individual differences in taste sensibility are likely to be of some magnitude. Gustatory thresholds are notoriously variable, not only from person to person, but in the same person from time to time. How much of the measured variation is traceable to crudeness of method and how much to constitutional factors has not been established, but it is clear that differences of the size encountered could not result exclusively from faulty techniques. There are displayed in Figure 16–10 distributions of absolute thresholds of 47 subjects to 17 different test solutions. Two of the distributions, those for vanillin (top) and phenyl thiocarbamide (bottom), should especially pique our curiosity. Both show an extraordinarily large spread. The graph for phenyl thiocarbamide (PTC, as it has come to be called) embraces a particularly wide range of values. Moreover, in this distribution the great majority of cases do not cluster about a central value, as they do for vanillin. There is even a suggestion that the PTC curve is bimodal. This becomes a certainty when figures for a larger population are considered. Witness the curve in Figure 16–11, plotted from results of testing several hundred subjects (*123*). This embraces an even larger range of thresholds than does the PTC graph of

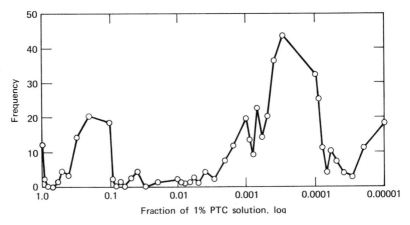

Fig. 16–11.   Variation in sensitivity to PTC (phenylthiocarbamide). The occurrence of two modes in the distribution suggests why there originally seemed to be two gustatory "types": tasters and non-tasters. From the data of Setterfield, Schott, and Snyder (*518*) as charted by Cohen and Ogdon (*123*). By permission of the *Psychological Bulletin* and the American Psychological Association.

Figure 16–10. There seems little doubt that two widely separated groups are involved, one of low, the other of high, sensitivity.

The phenomenon of two typically different reactions to PTC constitutes one of the major mysteries in the realm of human sensibilities. The effect was first noticed in 1931 by Dr. A. L. Fox, a chemist in the du Pont laboratories (206). Some PTC powder, while being transferred to a bottle, escaped into the laboratory air, and another chemist working nearby remarked on the bitter taste. Dr. Fox himself could get no taste whatever from the substance. The two chemists then tried crystals of the material on their tongues and got the same individual results; one was a "taster," the other a "nontaster." This incident precipitated an ever-widening series of investigations, extensive and intensive, on so-called "taste blindness," an effort which has not come to an end as yet. It was soon found that phenyl thiocarbamide is only one of a group of chemically related compounds, all of which behave in this way, though PTC has been the most widely used of the family and there are by now very extensive data on it. The responses of tens of thousands of cases are in the literature (123). The early investigators made the unfortunate mistake of regarding the phenomenon to be an all-or-nothing affair—either people could taste PTC or they couldn't. As soon as the commercially available product had been purified and higher concentrations could be used for testing it was found that the simple dichotomy, "taste blind" versus "taste normal," did not hold. Those who did not have their threshold in the "normal" range (less than 0.01% solution, say) were merely relatively insensitive, but their thresholds could be surpassed with sufficiently high concentrations of the stimulus.

People relatively insensitive to PTC show raised thresholds to only a narrow range of compounds, the ureas containing the $NC = S$ group. To the homologous oxygen compounds ($NC = O$), such as uracil, they give a normal response, as they apparently also do to all sweet, acid, and salty substances. Figure 16–12 compares PTC "tasters" with "nontasters" with respect to various of the urea compounds.

One of the curious effects connected with the tasting of PTC has to do with the influence of saliva. Experiments, more scientific than esthetic, in which the saliva of a "taster" (low PTC threshold) is used by a "nontaster" (high PTC threshold), and vice versa, show that a non-taster cannot improve his sensitivity by substituting a taster's saliva for his own. However, a taster can reduce his sensitivity to PTC by using either water or the saliva of a nontaster in lieu of his own saliva. For a taster to retain his capacity to detect small concentrations of PTC he must have his own saliva at work. This circumstance has led to a certain amount of speculation about the role of saliva in tasting. Obviously it is not to be regarded

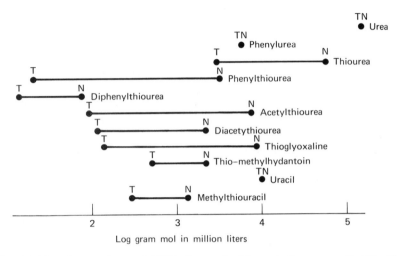

Fig. 16–12. Comparison of PTC "tasters" (T) and "nontasters" (N). Shown are average thresholds for compounds falling within the urea group. From Kalmus and Hubbard *(339)*. Courtesy of Charles C. Thomas, Publisher, Springfield, Illinois.

as merely a source of moisture for putting taste stimuli into solution, though this is certainly one of its functions. The suggestion has been made that salivary constitution is a highly individual matter, and it may be that some people ("nontasters") have a protein or colloid in their saliva that precipitates PTC as an insoluble product. Possibly further research on the biochemistry of saliva will provide the answer.

The Taste Qualities. Throughout our discussion of taste, thus far, there has been somewhat frequent and confident reference to the four basic taste qualities: salt, sour, sweet, and bitter. Without debate a fundamental question seems to have been settled: What are the elementary tastes? There has not always been complete agreement on this subject, though currently there are few who would dissent from the common four-fold classification. The question of the elementary qualities in gustation is an old one *(84,* pp. 452–457), as is the analogous question in each of the other sense modalities. At the end of the sixteenth century there were nine basic tastes: sweet, sour, sharp, pungent, harsh, fatty, bitter, insipid, and salty. By the middle of the eighteenth century there were 11, if one followed Linnaeus (add astringent, viscous, aqueous, and nauseous, but drop pungent and harsh), or 12, if Haller were taken as the authority (add to the original list spirituous, aromatic, urinous, and putrid, but drop fatty). Some of these gradually disappeared, it being shown that they really represented fusions of taste and touch. Others vanished for want of positive evidence to keep them alive. It was doubtless the demonstration, just about as the twentieth century was being ushered in, that salt, sour, sweet, and bitter have their own individual modes of distribution that tended to establish these four (which had always been present in all lists) as the fundamental taste qualities. The appearance of the four in the positions of "primacy," at the corners of Henning's taste tetrahedron (see Figure 16–13), a geometrical figure devised to represent relations between taste qualities, strengthens the case for this analysis.

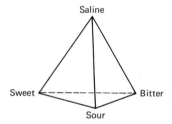

Fig. 16–13. Henning's taste tetrahedron. The figure is a solid, with gustatory sensations analyzable into two primaries located on the edges, into three primaries on the four triangular surfaces, and into four on the interior. After Henning (*295*).

It is interesting that the taste tetrahedron should seem to place the stress on four different kinds of gustatory sensation, with the implication that four separate physiological processes and possibly four different kinds of receptor cells are involved, because Henning viewed taste as one, not as four, senses. It is membership in a common modality that he was trying to emphasize in bringing the four qualities together in a single figure. All tastes are "unitary" in the same sense that visual orange, purple, and blue-green are unitary. While resembling two other qualities they do not break up spontaneously into these components. However, as in vision and olfaction, some gustatory qualities are outstanding and serve as convenient reference points for the description of other, related tastes. Thus, the taste of sodium bicarbonate is most readily described as lying on the line of the taste tetrahedron connecting salt with sour. Potassium bromide lies between salt and bitter. Lead acetate is on the line between sour and sweet. Acetone is the representative of a large number of compounds having both sweet and bitter components and therefore falls on the line connecting these two qualities. Some tastes have more than a dual reference and so occupy positions either on a surface of the tetrahedron, if there are three qualities concerned, or in the interior of the figure, if there are four. Thus, the "metallic" taste simultaneously has resemblances to sweet, bitter, and salt and must, therefore, take up its position on the appropriate triangular face of the tetrahedron.

The only serious contender for status as a primary gustatory quality—over and above the classic quartet of salty, sour, sweet, and bitter—is the taste called "alkaline." This term appears in some old classifications but dropped out following disagreements about its primacy. Some thought the alkaline taste to be compounded of gustatory and cutaneous qualities, while others suggested that smell might also be involved. There are currently few defenders of a "fifth taste."

Most tastes encountered in foods would presumably yield an analysis with all four fundamental taste qualities present in some degree. The entire internal area of the tetrahedron should consist of such collocations of four qualities, each discriminably different locus representing a unique, if complex, taste.

That food products may be subject to just such an analysis is the import of some preliminary work by Beebe-Center (43). He was prompted by very much the same considerations as those that led Crocker and Henderson to their system of odor specification, described in the previous chapter. Four qualitative standards were set up—aqueous solutions of sucrose for sweet, of quinine sulfate for bitter, of tartaric acid for sour, of sodium chloride for salty—and each of these was prepared in nine graded concentrations. The intensitive steps ranged from 1 gust (see above) to 100 gusts in steps of 0.25 log gusts. About 2 j.n.d. are represented by each of the 8 steps on the scale of intensity. The result of analyzing 14 different food products by direct comparison with the taste standards is given in Table 16–2.

There are some surprising emphases in this listing. The most significant one does not immediately meet the eye. It is that nearly all these foods, selected for their flavor, have relatively low ratings on the various taste scales. The intensities of the standards, after all, extended up to 100 gusts. There is only one food on the list, honey, which exceeds the halfway point (50 gusts) on any of the scales of psychological intensity. This circumstance indicates the relative blandness of many foods notable for distinctive "flavor" and points up a conclusion, arrived at much earlier on the basis of other considerations, that flavor is largely a matter of odor, not taste.

Table 16–2. Analysis of Certain Food Products, in Gusts

	Sweet	Bitter	Sour	Salt
Cola drink	11.2	2.2	5.0	1.3
Ale	2.5	28.2	10.0	1.3
Unsweetened grapefruit juice	3.2	2.0	35.5	2.0
Consomme	1.4	1.3	4.5	7.9
Tokay wine	10.0	4.2	4.2	1.8
Riesling wine	1.0	7.5	6.7	1.3
"Root" tonic	4.2	1.3	3.2	1.3
Coffee, unsweetened	1.0	42.3	3.2	1.0
Coffee, 5% sucrose	3.2	23.8	3.2	1.3
Anchovy fillet	1.3	23.8	5.6	10.0
Sweet pickles	3.2	3.2	13.4	3.2
Sour pickles	1.0	1.8	18.0	3.2
Raspberry jam	23.8	1.8	10.0	1.3
Honey	56.4	2.4	1.8	1.3
Means	8.8	10.4	8.9	2.7

Data from J. G. Beebe-Center *(43)*.

Taste Mixtures.   If one can make an analytic dissection, so to speak, of the gustatory components of flavor it should also be possible, knowing the elements, to synthesize complex tastes by suitable mixing of the appropriate solutions. If the four primary taste qualities merely go together in an additive fashion to create various blends, then accurate predictions of the mixture products can be based on the most elementary arithmetic. If, on the other hand, there are mutual interactions, whether of suppression or enhancement, between the four systems of sensitivity, the desired predictions cannot be made without further knowledge of the combining principles at work.

Unfortunately, the current evidence is somewhat equivocal. Few thoroughgoing experiments have been conducted in the area of taste mixture, and those that have been performed differ so radically among themselves as to discourage conclusions of any real degree of generality. However, this much seems certain—there are clear instances of inter-action effects. Whether presented simultaneously to two different parts of the tongue or combined in a single physical mixture, two stimulus solutions, each appealing to a different taste quality, are not likely to function independently of each other.

Both facilitatory and inhibitory phenomena have been reported. Thus

Kiesow, who is responsible for some of the earliest experiments on "taste contrast" (359), found sweet, sour, and salt all to interact with each other in the direction of mutual enhancement. Bitter neither influenced nor was influenced by the others. Kiesow applied his solutions to individual papillae with a pointed brush and either stimulated opposite sides of the tongue simultaneously ("simultaneous contrast") or the same place successively, the first stimulus being washed away before the second was delivered ("successive contrast"). All results are in the form of observed increases in sensation intensity of one taste as a result of the action of another. If a subliminal sugar solution were applied to one side of the tongue the simultaneous presentation of salt to the other side would cause sweet sensitivity to surge upward and make the sugar perceptible. Reversal of the solutions would do the same for salt. Similar results obtained for combinations of sour and salt and, less certainly, for sweet and sour.

Interactions involving gross stimulation of the gustatory receptors, as contrasted with the relatively more "punctiform" approach of Kiesow, are less well understood. Recent experiments fail to agree. On the one hand, Hahn and Ulbrich (260), stimulating an area 1.5 cm in diameter near the tip of the tongue, find small but definite reductions in thresholds to saccharin, for example, as a result of adding to the test solution just subliminal concentrations of quinine sulfate, sodium chloride, or hydrochloric acid. However, exactly the opposite direction of interaction, mutual inhibition, is found by Anderson (21) in some careful experiments conducted by the "sipping" method. Threshold concentrations of sucrose, quinine hydrochloride, or tartaric acid were combined with sodium chloride solutions in measuring the absolute threshold to the latter. Salt thresholds were uniformly raised in the presence of the sweet, bitter, or sour stimulus. Less definite but generally inhibitory relations came out of other pairings of stimuli.

The foregoing results are for stimuli operating in the neighborhood of the absolute threshold. What about the combining of qualitatively different taste solutions of higher concentrations? This is a research area of great interest to those concerned with food processing. Apparently there are some complex relations to be considered. Some acids increase the saltiness of salt, yet salt may reduce the sourness of acids (192). The presence of salt may increase or decrease the sweetness of sugar. Whereas all sugars seem to reduce the sourness of all acids, acids do not uniformly suppress the sweet taste of all sugars. Two of the common acids, hydrochloric and acetic, have little effect on the sweetness of sucrose, while the action of citric acid, one of the least sour-tasting of the acids, is actually to increase the observed sweetness of sucrose. The sweet taste of fructose, contrariwise, is reduced by acetic and some other acids, but not by hydrochloric and citric acids. Obviously, there is yet much to be learned about taste interactions at the levels of intensity encountered in foods and beverages.

Only recently have there been performed experiments that systematically relate each of the four basic tastes to each other at relatively high levels of stimulation (471, 458). One set of these, carried out at the U.S. Army Quartermaster's Food and Container Institute (340), ascertained

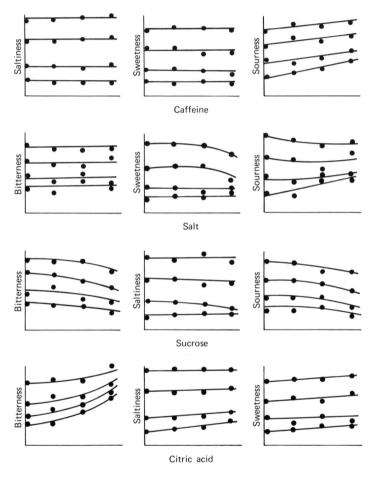

Fig. 16–14.   Taste interactions. Ordinates show four concentration levels of the primary stimulus, while abscissae have four levels of the secondary stimulus. From Pilgrim (471), after Kamen, Pilgrim, Gutman, and Kroll.

the effect on judged intensity of a particular quality (e.g., saltiness) in the presence of one of the other basic tastes (e.g., bitter, represented by caffeine). Primary and secondary solutions were mixed and their tastes therefore had to be held apart attentively. Each taste solution to be judged (primary) existed in four concentrations as did also the additive (secondary) one, thus making 16 combinations of each pair of solutions. In general, the secondary solutions were, by design, weaker than the primary ones.

The family of 12 graphs contained in Figure 16–14 summarizes the results of this extensive investigation. Caffeine has no effect on either saltiness or sweetness, but definitely enhances sourness at all levels. NaCl leaves bitterness unaffected but reduces sweetness at the higher levels and both enhances and impairs sourness, depending on concentration. Sugar reduces both bitterness and sourness (as both coffee drinkers and lemonade makers know) but has little effect on saltiness. The sour reagent,

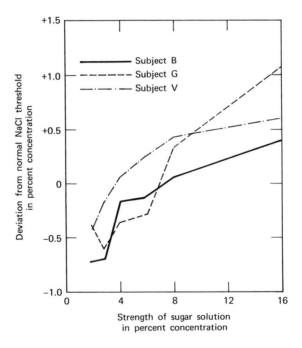

Fig. 16–15. Taste interaction at different intensity levels. The results obtained by Bujas (*103*) in an experiment testing the effect on the threshold for NaCl, applied to one side of the tongue, of simultaneous stimulation of the other side with a sugar solution. Low concentrations of sugar enhance, and high concentrations depress, saline sensitivity.

citric acid, has varying enhancing effects, with a particularly strong influence on bitterness.

A suggestive relationship which, if borne out by more extensive work, might go far toward harmonizing the seemingly diverse results of interaction experiments, was found by Bujas (*103*). He used Hahn's technique of letting taste solutions flow over the tongue, stimulating through a 1.5-cm diameter opening in a U tube. In fact, two such stimulators were used, the areas contacted being 1 cm apart and 3 cm back from the tip of the tongue. Salt and sugar solutions at 32° C were presented, salt to one side of the tongue, sugar to the other. All exposures were uniformly 7 sec in duration. First, sensitivity to salt solution was established, the absolute threshold being measured in one system while water flowed through the other. Then sugar, in one of six concentrations, replaced the water, and the salt threshold was redetermined. As can be seen in Figure 16–15, Bujas found evidence for both enhancement and depression of saline sensitivity through the simultaneous action of a neighboring sweet stimulus. At low concentrations of sugar, intensities not far above threshold strength, the result is like that originally gotten by Kiesow; the effect is a facilitatory one, the salt threshold being lowered. At higher sugar concentrations there is a reversal of effect. Sweetness now interferes with detection of the salt stimulus and the salty taste is "masked." In passing from one phenomenon to the other there must, of course, be a neutral point; there must be some concentration of sugar which neither depresses nor heightens salt sensitivity. It is apparent from these data that fairly high intensities of the sweet stimulus are in effect when neutrality is realized. Bujas' three subjects, showing individual differences in this respect, as in absolute sensitivity itself, gave values of 3.75%, 7.00%, and 8.5% for the neutral concentrations.

A most remarkable set of interactions among the primary taste qualities—and not only these but with two of the basic cutaneous ones as well—has been adduced by Békésy (*56*). Prompted by the suggestive relations inherent in von Kries' duplexity theory of vision (rods versus cones) and the known arrangement of the auditory receptors of the Organ of Corti (outer versus inner hair cells), Békésy raised the question of other possible duplex sensory relations, and devised a set of experiments with the two sides of the upper surface of the tongue as the sites of stimulation. He arranged for thin streams of fluid to be led to the tongue surface through openings in a plastic block stimulator, each of the tiny channels of flow being 4 mm long by 1.5 mm wide, the two slits situated 15 mm apart and parallel to each other. Various stepped concentrations of NaCl, HCl, cane sugar, and quinine solutions, as well as streams of cold and warm water could be presented in carefully timed exposures, singly, two simultaneously, or two in predetermined positive or negative time delay.

One effect of presenting two different tastes to opposite sides of the tongue—over and above the enhancements and suppressions of sensitivity found by others—is that of a change in spatial patterning such that localization shifts may occur. Especially if magnitude is made equal for the two stimuli, whether they are qualitatively alike or not, there is sometimes a tendency for the two sensations to fuse and to be localized along the midline of the tongue. However, when different stimuli were presented in the two lateral slits, such fusion did not necessarily occur. Sometimes there was an interaction between tastes, sometimes not. The general relations coming out of the experiment are represented in Figure 16–16.

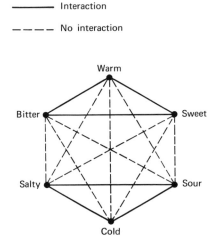

Fig. 16–16. Duplexity theory of taste. Qualities connected by solid lines interact; those joined by dashed lines do not. Four taste qualities, coupled with two from somesthesis, thus form two opposed systems. From Békésy (56). Copyright 1964 by the American Association for the Advancement of Science.

Bitter and sweet interacted; so did salty and sour. But—and this is the most surprising result—warm, a cutaneous, nongustatory quality, fused with sweet and bitter, while cold went along with salty and sour tastes. If this lateralization phenomenon is to be given heavy weight among the considerations deciding primacy of the sense qualities, where does this leave us? With a duplex taste apparatus? And with what kind of relationship between the gustatory and cutaneous realms? Not all phenomena of taste speak for what have been regarded commonly as the four separate and autonomous processes of salty, sour, sweet, and bitter.

Gustatory Adaptation. Taste receptors have their sensitivity automatically reduced by being exposed to a continuous, unvarying stimulus, just as olfactory end organs do under analogous conditions. In fact, the addition of the sense of taste completes the catalogue of sense departments displaying adaptation; this has been found to be an entirely universal phenomenon in the world of sensation.

It was clear, from Kiesow's early experiments (*360*), that individual papillae display the adaptation phenomenon. Application of taste solutions to isolated papillae would, in some instances, eventually make them totally unresponsive. It has not always been equally clear that more general stimulation of the tongue and mouth would result in total abolition of taste sensitivity. This was shown to be the case, however, in a series of experiments by Dallenbach and his students (*1, 339*). Five different concentrations of NaCl (0.84 mole to 3.93 moles) were employed as adapting solutions and the tongue and mouth were continuously irrigated, an entrance tube carrying the solution in at mouth temperature and an exit tube serving as a drain after the fluid had circulated. Typically, the salty taste declined gradually in intensity until it finally disappeared altogether. Adaptation was complete. The time between onset of the stimulus and total cessation of gustatory sensation ("adaptation time") proved to be a function of NaCl concentration. Low intensities gave relatively short adaptation times, less than 20 sec on the average; high intensities took longer to adapt, nearly 2 min for the highest concentration used. Individual differences were marked, and aftereffects were prominent. However, it was demonstrated that the taste sensations persisting after the stimulus flow had been stopped were due to the action of traces of salt lingering in crevices of the tongue and cheeks, in the interstices between the teeth, etc. Similar siphoning into the mouth of solutions of sour (tartaric acid in three strengths: from 0.0022 mole to 0.013 mole), sweet (sucrose in five concentrations: from 0.066 mole to 1.26 moles), and bitter (quinine hydrochloride in three intensities: from 0.000013 mole to 0.000083 mole) led to entirely comparable results for these qualities. In all cases adaptation continued to completion, time to extinction being primarily a function of stimulus intensity. Average adaptation times were, approximately: sour, 1.5 min (weak) to 3.0 min (strong); sweet, 1.0–5.0 min; bitter, 1.5–2.5 min. After-tastes were present in all instances and were traceable to the same general cause as that operating with salt. Sugar could be washed away fairly promptly, but quinine was dislodged only with difficulty.

Whereas these studies tell us much about the nature of gustatory adaptation, they naturally do not inform us as to the exact course of the adaptation process. Extensive experiments by Hahn, employing his familiar U-tube arrangement, provide not only a picture of the course of adaptation but one of the recovery process as well (258). Figure 16–17

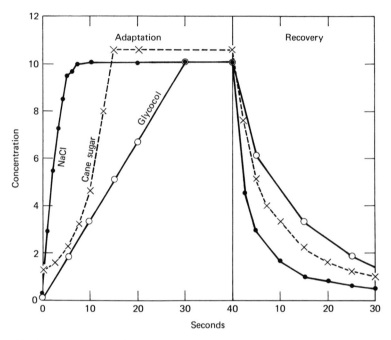

Fig. 16–17. Gustatory adaptation and recovery. Ordinates give threshold concentrations, the units being arbitrary ones with the value 10 representing the adapting concentration. The three substances, salt, sugar, and glycocol, show different courses of adaptation and different rates of recovery. From Pfaffmann (465) after Hahn, Kuckulies, and Taeger, 1938.

charts the rise of the thresholds throughout an adaptation period of 40 sec and their subsequent decline during a 30-sec recovery interval. The sensitivity alterations for a single saline stimulus (5% NaCl solution) and two different sweet stimuli (10% cane sugar and 1% glycocol solutions) are represented. It is apparent that the changes produced by adaptation are prompt and extensive, and also that the course of adaptation is in part dependent on the nature of the substance producing it.

Another important variable, the effect of which is not shown in Figure 16-17 but which entered into Hahn's experiments, is temperature. The effect of warming a 10% sucrose solution from 17° C to 32° C is not only to reduce the absolute threshold, prior to adaptation, but to shift the entire adaptation curve downward so that after 5 sec of continuous stimulation the warmer solution has elevated the threshold only half as much as has the cooler one. Within 15 sec the entire process is complete in both instances, however. The influence of temperature on the rapidity of adaptation is important for us to know about because this effect can only be interpreted to mean that adaptation has a peripheral, rather than a central, locus. The differential effect of temperature must be exerted at the tongue surface, of course. The fact that the influence of temperature is on the adaptation process rather than on the stimulation process itself —and these are two different things—is demonstrated with glycocol. This substance, though tasting sweet, is an organic acid (amino-acetic acid, $CH_2NH_2 \cdot COOH$; also known as "glycine"). As with its distant inorganic relative, HCl, its absolute taste threshold depends not at all on temperature. However, the speed with which adaptation to glycine proceeds is definitely a function of temperature. Hahn has shown (259, p. 934) that adaptation to a 0.1% solution of glycine at 17° C produces about the same elevation of threshold in 20 sec that is brought about by a 22° C solution of the same strength in a whole minute.

Further insight into the nature of gustatory adaptation—and, indeed, into the whole matter of the basic properties of the taste mechanism—may be obtained through experiments designed to test the effects of varying the immediate environment of the tongue. Saliva is far from being composed exclusively of water. It is a weak solution of NaCl, among other things. Prominent ionic components, additionally, are calcium and potassium, and these occur as chlorides, phosphates, sulfates, and carbonates, especially the latter. Several organic constituents have been identified also: proteins, glycoproteins, enzymes, and the substance known as mucin, from which saliva's sticky character derives. There is present much carbon dioxide, both in solution and in combined form, indicating that the products of the salivary glands participate in a host of active chemical changes.

What would happen if the taste receptors did not have access to the chemicals in which they are normally bathed? Would their sensitivity level be significantly affected? Presumably so. The situation would be similar to the one we encountered in olfaction, where removal of the accidental stimuli ordinarily entering the nostrils (the *camera inodorata* of Komuro) greatly lowered the absolute threshold.

The relevant experiment has been performed by McBurney and Pfaffmann (399). Between applications of NaCl test stimuli they adapted the tongue continuously to a stream of distilled water of neutral temperature. Under such treatment the NaCl threshold was greatly altered. As contrasted with an average threshold of .0043 M for normal adaptation to saliva, average for the distilled water situation was .00014 M. Adaptation to saline solutions of various strengths, all of them low (3 steps from .000069 M to .015 M NaCl), resulted in corresponding shifts of threshold to a level just above that of the adapting solution in each case. Measurement of the NaCl concentration present in normal saliva shows the usual threshold to be regulated by the amount of salt bathing the receptors. As salivary changes occur, reflecting a complex series of chemical interactions in the buccal cavity, the sensitivity of taste receptors may be expected to change along with them.

The Electrophysiology of Taste.   Attention to the changes occurring in afferent nerves belonging to other sense modalities has uniformly been found to be profitable. There are also some things to be learned from the fibers carrying gustatory impulses. Experiments have been made on many different animal preparations in an effort to discover the nature of gustatory afferent impulses and their relation to the stimulation process. Except for the stimulus specificities displayed by them, the gustatory fibers behave like all other afferents. Their response is "all or none"; changes in stimulus intensity bring about characteristic changes in discharge frequency in individual fibers and variation in the number of fibers active at any one time; and they display the "equilibration" phenomenon. The latter consists of a high initial impulse rate and a smooth frequency decline in the presence of an unchanging stimulus; this would seem to be the direct correlate of sensory adaptation. All these features can be observed in the oscillographic records displayed in Figure 16–18, taken from Pfaffmann's classical study of single gustatory fibers in the cat.

It is not easy, in the nerves subserving gustatory sensitivity, to get single fiber information. Vision, audition, and olfaction are served by single large cranial nerves (II, VIII, and I). Taste, it will be remembered, is cared for by three different collections of fibers—those in the *chorda tympani* (a branch of VII) in the tongue's anterior part, the glossopharyngeal (IX) in the posterior third, and the vagus (X) in the pharynx and larynx. In general, fibers are not only difficult of access but are more fragile, because they are smaller, than the analogous ones in other nerves, and they are more difficult to "shred out" of a bundle in intact condition. However, the fibers of the chorda tympani become accessible, though mainly collectively, as they pass through a bony canal of the middle ear en route to the brain. Most of our information about the gustatory afferents comes from studies of the chorda tympani.

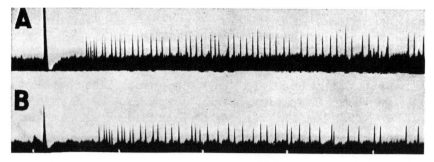

Fig. 16–18. Action potential record from a single nerve fiber in response to acid on the tongue. In *A* the stimulus was 0.5 *N* acetic acid, in *B* 0.01 *N* hydrochloric acid. In each case the first large upward deflection signals the application of the drop of acid. Time marks are 0.1 sec. From Pfaffmann *(463)*. From original of Fig. 4, C. Pfaffmann, *Journal of Cellular and Comparative Physiology,* 1941, 17, 248.

Naturally, animal preparations have yielded the bulk of the data and, with respect to single fiber performance, all of it. However, something is known about functioning in the human; this has come about from taking advantage of ear operations that have necessitated severing the chorda tympani. Zotterman and his colleagues *(160)* have recorded the impulses produced in the cut end of the chorda tympani in 32 otosclerotic patients undergoing surgery in Stockholm. In 17 of the cases there were good records of the nerve's electrical activity during stimulation of the tongue. Figure 16–19 shows several curves displaying the measured relation between NaCl concentration (0.01 to 1.0 M) and the strength of the nerve response. Recording was from the entire bundle, and the "strength" is that of an integrator charge, the voltage accumulated in a condenser circuit over a short standard time span. The initial NaCl response agrees well with absolute threshold determinations ("detection" thresholds, in the neighborhood of 0.01M NaCl). Sugars also give a measurable electrophysiological response, and here also the relative magnitude of the electrical activity reflects the usual order of sweetness of the various sugars. An incidental but not uninteresting finding was that cold water applied to the tongue gave a prompt and vigorous response in the chorda, whereas stimulation with warm water (37° to 43° C) gave none. Also notable was the fact that distilled water at tongue temperature had no effect whatever, a finding quite unlike that in the chicken, dog, and monkey, all of which have what has come to be called a "water taste," since they typically show clear potentials under these conditions.

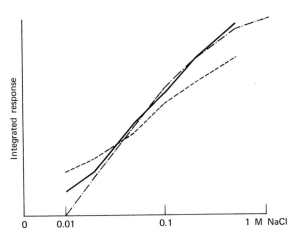

Fig. 16–19. Peak electrical responses in the cut end of the chorda tympani initiated by NaCl of different molarities on the tongue. Records from 17 people undergoing surgery for correction of otosclerosis. From Diamant, Funakoshi, Ström, and Zotterman *(160)*.

This difference between human response and subhuman ones is by now well known in gustatory electrophysiology. Indeed, large species differences in sensitivity and in response magnitude have come to be expected; they tend to make one extremely cautious about sweeping conclusions in this area. The rat, guinea pig, and hamster give relatively strong nerve responses to NaCl and weak ones to KCl; however, the cat, dog, and raccoon have large KCl responses and meager NaCl responses. To sugars the guinea pig and hamster respond quite vigorously, whereas the dog and raccoon yield only moderate potentials, and the cat shows practically no nerve activity at all *(49)*.

It is not only the electrophysiological indications that point up species differences. Experience with animals shows, for example, saccharin to be sweet to the rat, as for man, but unpleasant to the chicken, and a quite indifferent stimulus to most calves. Pigs apparently fall into three classes in their reaction to saccharin. A minority dislike it, rejecting it in a wide range of concentrations, but it is obviously pleasant to some, while still others react in an indifferent manner *(341)*.

One thing is absolutely certain about taste receptors: they are never all alike in their response to stimulation. It is a commonplace that effectiveness of stimulation is found to vary from spot to spot on the tongue, when electrical indications are consulted. At the time the first neural studies were made there was some expectation that receptors especially suited to receive salt, others sweet, others sour, and still others bitter stimuli would make known their presence in the taste buds. At least, it seemed a reasonable guess that the attached nerve fibers would display specificities of this kind. In the first thoroughgoing search, that of Pfaffmann in 1941, there was no such outcome. Single sensory afferents in the chorda tympani proved to be selective to a degree, but their specificities seemed not to coincide with the classical presuppositions. Some fibers of the cat reported the presence of acid, others gave responses to both acid and salty stimuli, while others were set into activity by both acid and quinine. Subsequently, other combinations, including reactions to sweet substances, have appeared. And, as has already been indicated, there are several species in which pure water produces a train of waves in gustatory nerves, while application of NaCl and other salts to the tongue brings about an immediate inhibition of the neural messages set off by water.

Clearly, the story is not a simple one. And of special significance is the finding that nerve specificities of the kind one would assume on the basis of Johannes Müller's ancient doctrine ("salt-reporting" fibers, "sour-reporting" fibers, etc.) show little evidence of being present in the gustatory afferent bundles. One possibility, of course, is that the fibers are quality-specific but that the fibers terminate on two or more sense cells, each of which has its own chemical specificity. Another is that the receptor cells are quite nonspecific in their response to stimulating chemicals and that much of nerve stimulation is thereby "nonadequate" in the classical sense of that term. The latter, of course, does not square with the evidence for specificity adduced by Békésy in the human tongue. But perhaps it shouldn't, species differences being what they are.

Kimura and Beidler (*361*) have performed the delicate experiment of inserting tiny pipette electrodes into individual taste cells in the rat's tongue, and have recorded intracellular electrical changes in response to various chemical stimuli applied to the cell. Several important facts emerged, an indisputable one being that no two taste cells are quite identical in sensitivity. The functions connecting magnitude of electrical potential with stimulus concentration are highly individual. Functions for ten different taste cells are shown in Figure 16–20. Also, it is evident that no single taste quality "owns" the cell; always it is responsive to stimuli normally responsible for two or more different qualities. Some cells have a broad "spectrum" of stimuli to which they will respond, while others are more narrowly tuned. Moreover, the width of that spectrum varies from one concentration to another. It begins to appear that specificity, if it is present in the rat, has to be sought at the molecular level, on particular local sites of the receptor cell's limiting membrane.

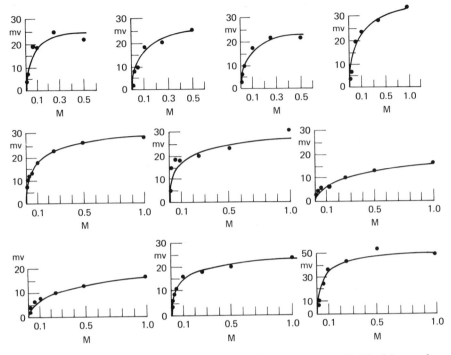

Fig. 16–20. Responses of 10 different taste cells in the rat to NaCl of increasing molarity applied to the tongue. From Beidler (*49*) after Kimura and Beidler. Courtesy of The Wistar Press.

Some highly suggestive evidence that this may be so comes from the remarkable experiment of Oakley (*449*). In the rat he showed that gustatory afferents from both the front of the tongue (seventh nerve branch, the chorda tympani) and the back (ninth, glossopharyngeal) when cut and allowed to regenerate, would form new functioning taste buds. Moreover, since the normal nerves from the two regions may show distinguishably different responses to some stimuli, and regenerated nerves and taste buds do not obviate this difference, he was able to devise a quite crucial experiment. With microsuturing it was possible to bring about cross-regeneration, the chorda being attached to the back, the glossopharyngeal to the front portion of the tongue. Now, recording the summated neural responses from the two regions, direct comparisons could be made among four sets of fibers: the normal chorda and glossopharyngeal responses on one side of the tongue and the transplanted fibers on the other. The results were clear-cut. All responses without exception were characteristic of the tongue region involved. The regenerated chorda tympani fibers attached to the base of the tongue acted like fibers of the ninth nerve; regenerated glossopharyngeal fibers coming from the front of the tongue behaved like fibers belonging to the normal chorda tympani supply.

The situation at the receptor cell being what it is, one would scarcely look for much greater simplicity in the afferent fiber discharged by the cell. Single sensory fibers teased out of the chorda tympani yield records that differ, naturally, from those of the sense cell in showing a train of spaced impulses rather than steady potentials. As elsewhere in the nervous system, frequency signals intensity, and all spikes are of uniform height,

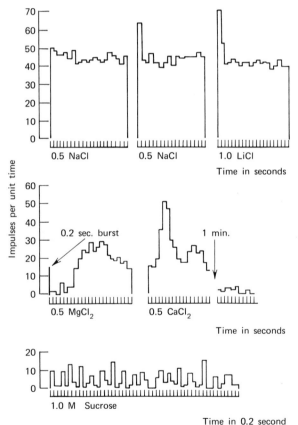

Fig. 16–21. Single-fiber responses in the rat's chorda tympani. Only the two NaCl histograms are from the same fiber. Note time variations. From Fishman *(198)*. Courtesy of The Wistar Press.

as demanded by the all-or-nothing principle. Stimulation of the appropriate tongue region with taste solutions produces the expected discharges. But it is difficult to see much constancy of performance. The variations are both spatial and temporal, and several different impulse sequences are found. As with receptor cells, there are highly individual responses from fiber to fiber for a given stimulus.

Figure 16–21, taken from the single fiber analysis made by Fishman (*198*), shows five different patterns of responding in the chorda tympani of the rat and hamster: (1) an initial high-frequency burst of impulses lasting a second or two, followed by an abrupt decline, then a sustained repetitive discharge lasting as much as three minutes; (2) a steady discharge, much like the first type, but without the initial burst; (3) a burst, lasting one- or two-tenths of a second, followed by "silence," then a gradual rise to a peak and subsequent decline; (4) a gradual rise and decline of impulse frequency; and (5) rhythmic bursts, with clear bunching of impulses and fairly regular intervals between groups.

Nerve potentials may be recorded at higher levels of the afferent path to the cortex, although access becomes more difficult. The chief barrier to getting the whole, intimate story of functioning in the central nervous system, here as elsewhere, is the depressant effect of whatever anesthetic is used in the experiment. Nevertheless, enough comes through at lower centers to suggest that events a little further along the afferent pathway

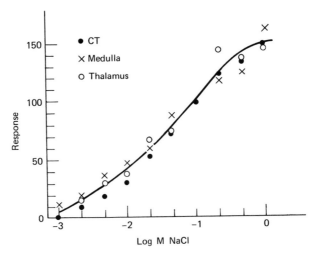

Fig. 16–22. Comparison of responses to NaCl in the rat's chorda tympani nerve, the medulla, and the thalamic gustatory area. From Pfaffmann (*468*). Copyright 1961 by The University of Nebraska Press.

are not too different from those transpiring at the chorda tympani. Figure 16–22 is a composite plot of the relative magnitude of response to NaCl, the three loci of recording being the chorda tympani, the brainstem at the medulla, and the gustatory thalamus (*468*). Surprisingly enough, the message does not change much as it proceeds from the peripheral neurons toward the cortex. Little success has yet attended efforts to record directly from the cortex, but the difficulty is technical and should in time be overcome. Perhaps implanted electrodes in the "waking" brain will supply the desired data.

Theories of Taste Sensitivity. This chapter was introduced with the characterization of taste as the poor relation of the family of senses. Nowhere is its poverty more manifest than in the realm of theory. Gustatory theory, in general, is lacking in ideas and vague in the elaboration of the few it possesses. Only one general principle ever seems to assert itself. It is that tastes are generated through interaction of sapid substances and some material or materials, as yet unidentified, on the sensitive surfaces of the tongue, palate, etc., or perhaps housed in the cellular confines of the papillae. This is the burden of Crozier's hypothesis (*133*, p. 1029) that "the qualitative differentiation of the taste-buds might be due to the fact that there are four separate receptive substances, appropriately segregated in distribution, corresponding to the four conspicuous gustatory qualities." It is the idea underlying the taste theories of Lasareff, Hahn, and others (*426*, p. 125), which postulate chemical reactions yielding decomposition products which, in turn, ionize and stimulate the appropriate papillae.

It is only one step from this type of theory to the assumption that tastes might be generated through interference with one or more enzymes existing in the gustatory tissues. Indeed, there is some good evidence that such enzymes do exist and that they may have their balance disturbed through the action of substances having gustatory properties. El-Baradi and Bourne (*186*) have found two different enzymes to be present in the foliate papillae of the rabbit. These have been identified by histochemical methods as a phosphatase and another, unknown esterase. The reactions of both are strongly inhibited by sapid substances but not the same ones in the two cases. The phosphatase (or possibly, group of related phosphatases) is readily affected by vanillin, capsicum, and infusions of tea; to a lesser extent it responds to the presence of oil of peppermint, oil of aniseed, and coffee infusions. However, sugar, salt, and quinine have no effect on it. On the other hand the unknown esterase, found to be present in high concentration in the taste buds and in smaller amounts in the neighboring epithelial tissue of the tongue, has its histochemical reaction strongly inhibited by quinine but remains unaffected by salt and sugar.

However, the notion that enzymatic action within the taste cell is the transducer mechanism encounters some difficulties. Beidler, who has himself proposed a theory of taste (48), believes the dynamics of the chemical interactions at the receptor surface to indicate that the initial events in response triggering must be those of surface adsorption. The rapidity of events in stimulation suggests that ions of the chemical stimulus are loosely bound to some substance of the taste receptor, perhaps a protein. The behavior of inorganic salts, when these are the stimuli, especially the prepotency commonly shown by the cation in determining what taste will ensue, makes the more elaborate enzyme theory somewhat implausible. Enzymes could, of course, participate in the more intricate events that bring about electrical discharge of the sense cell.

Most theories of sensory functioning, we have consistently seen throughout the parade of senses, are theories of the physiological mechanism responsible for setting receptor organs into action. Pfaffmann has looked beyond the receptor and, whereas it would be inexact to say that he has a theory of taste, he has done some helpful gustatory theorizing (466, 469). In particular, he has recognized the impossibility of retaining end organ specificity and accounting for taste qualities in the classical manner. When single fibers report on all classes of stimuli and when water alone can elicit taste reactions in some species, it is difficult to see how quality differentiation can depend either on types of receptors or types of afferent fibers. Pfaffmann proposes the utilization of the central idea contained in Nafe's pattern theory of feeling (439). Different chemicals evoke different afferent input patterns, and it is the particular combination of fibers involved, together with their temporal and spatial variations of discharge, that yield a single, integrated result that is now "salty," now "bitter." It is interesting to see a principle worked out for one sense channel doing such valiant service in another.

References

1. Abrahams, H., Krakauer, D., & Dallenbach, K. M. Gustatory adaptation to salt. *Amer. J. Psychol.,* 1937, **49,** 462–469.
2. Abramov, I. Further analysis of the responses of LGN cells. *J. opt. Soc. Amer.,* 1968, **58,** 574–579.
3. Adair, E. R., Stevens, J. C., & Marks, L. E. Thermally induced pain, the dol scale, and the psychophysical power law. *Amer. J. Psychol.,* 1968, **81,** 147–164.
4. Ades, H. W. Central auditory mechanisms. In J. Field, H. W. Magoun, & V. E. Hall, (Eds.), *Handbook of physiology, Neurophysiology, I.* Washington, D.C.: American Physiological Society, 1959. Chap. 24 (pp. 585–619).
5. Adrian, E. D. *The basis of sensation.* New York: Norton, 1928.
6. Adrian, E. D. Olfactory adaptation. *J. Physiol., Lond.,* 1951, **112,** 38P.
7. Adrian, E. D. Olfactory discrimination. *Année psychol.,* 1951, **50,** 107–113.
8. Adrian, E. D. The action of the mammalian olfactory organ. *J. Laryngol, Otol.,* 1956, **70,** 1–14.
9. Adrian, E. D., Cattell, McK., & Hoagland, H. Sensory discharges in single cutaneous nerve fibres. *J. Physiol., Lond.,* 1931, **72,** 377–391.
10. Adrian, E. D., & Ludwig, C. Nervous discharges from olfactory organs of fish. *J. Physiol., Lond.,* 1938, **94,** 441–460.
11. Adrian, E. D., & Zotterman, Y. The impulses produced by sensory nerve-endings. Part II. The response of a single end-organ. *J. Physiol., Lond.,* 1926, **61,** 151–171.
12. Akita, M., & Graham, C. H. Maintaining an absolute test hue in the presence of different background colors and luminance ratios. *Vision Res.,* 1966, **6,** 315–323.
13. Allen, F. On reflex visual sensations and color contrast. *J. opt. Soc. Amer.,* 1923, **7,** 913–942.
14. Allen, F., & Weinberg, M. The gustatory sensory reflex. *Quart. J. exp. Psychol.,* 1925, **15,** 377–383.
15. Allers, R., & Halpern, F. Wechselwirkungen gleichzeitiger Erregung mehrere Hautsinne. I. Die Beeinflussung der Tastschwelle durch die Hauttemperatur. *Pflüg. Arch ges. Physiol.,* 1921, **193,** 595–609.
16. Alpern, M. Relation between brightness and color contrast. *J. opt. Soc. Amer.,* 1964, **54,** 1491–1492.

17. Alston, J. H. The spatial condition of the fusion of warmth and cold in heat. *Amer. J. Psychol.*, 1920, **31**, 303–312.

18. Amoore, J. E. The stereochemical theory of olfaction. 2. Elucidation of the stereochemical properties of the olfactory receptor sites. New York: *Proc. Sci. Sect., Toilet Goods Assoc.* Spec. Suppl. to No. 37, 1962.

19. Amoore, J. E. *Molecular basis of odor.* Springfield, Ill.: Thomas, 1970.

20. Anand, B. K., & Brobeck, J. R. Hypothalamic control of food intake in rats and cats. *Yale J. Biol. Med.*, 1951, **24**, 123–140.

21. Anderson, R . J. Taste thresholds in stimulus mixtures. *Microfilm Abstr.*, 1950, **10** (4), 287–288.

22. Andersson, S., & Gernandt, B. E. Cortical projection of vestibular nerve in cat. *Acta oto-laryngol., Stockh.*, Suppl. 116, 1954, 10–18.

23. Andersson, B., & Zotterman, Y. The water taste in the frog. *Acta physiol, scand.*, 1950, **20**, 95–100.

24. Arden, G. B., & Weale, R . A., Nervous mechanisms and dark-adaptation. *J. Physiol., Lond.*, 1954, **125**, 417–426.

25. Arey, L. B., Tremaine, M. J., & Monzingo, F. L. The numerical and topographical relations of taste buds to human circumvallate papillae throughout the life span. *Anat. Rec.*, 1935, **64**, 9–25.

26. Armstrong, H. G. *Aerospace medicine.* Baltimore: Williams & Wilkins, 1961.

27. Aronoff, S., & Dallenbach, K. M. Adaptation of warm spots under continuous and intermittent stimulation. *Amer. J. Psychol.*, 1936, **48**, 485–490.

28. Arthur, R. P., & Shelley, W. B. The peripheral mechanism of itch in man. In G. E. W. Wolstenholme & M. O'Connor (Eds.), *Pain and itch.* Boston: Little, Brown, 1959. Pp. 84–97.

29. Auerbach, E., & Wald, G. The participation of different types of cones in human light and dark adaptation. *Amer. J. Ophthalmol.*, 1955, **39**, 24–40.

30. Baker, H. D. The course of foveal light adaptation measured by the threshold intensity increment. *J. opt. Soc. Amer.*, 1949, **39**, 172–179.

31. Baker, H. D. Initial stages of dark and light adaptation. *J. opt. Soc. Amer.*, 1963, **53**, 98–103.

32. Baker, H. D., & Rushton, W. A. H. The red-sensitive pigment in normal cones. *J. Physiol., Lond.*, 1965, **176**, 56–72.

33. Barlow, H. B. Summation and inhibition in the frog's retina. *J. Physiol., Lond.*, 1953, **119**, 69–88.

34. Bartlett, N. R. Thresholds as dependent on some energy relations and characteristics of the subject. In C. H. Graham (Ed.), *Vision and visual perception.* New York: Wiley, 1965. Chap. 7 (pp. 154–184).

35. Bartley, S. H. *Vision.* New York: Van Nostrand, 1941.

36. Bazett, H. C. Temperature sense in man. In *Temperature, its measurement and control in science and industry.* New York: Reinhold, 1941. Pp. 485–501.

37. Bazett, H. C., & McGlone, B. Studies in sensation: The mode of stimulation of cutaneous sensations of cold and warmth. *Arch. Neurol. Psychiat., Chicago,* 1932, **27**, 1031–1069.

38. Bazett, H. C., McGlone, B., & Brocklehurst, R. J. The temperatures in the tissues which accompany temperature sensations. *J. Physiol., Lond.*, 1930, **69**, 88–112.

38a. Bazett, H. C., McGlone, B., Williams, R. G., & Lufkin, H. M. Sensation. I. Depth, distribution, and probable identification in the prepuce of sensory end-organs concerned in sensations of temperature and touch; thermometric conductivity. *Arch. Neur. Psychiat., Chicago*, 1932, **27**, 489–517.

39. Beasley, W. C. Discriminations based on varying the relative amplitudes of four frequencies in combination. In Valentine's *Readings in experimental psychology*. New York: Harper, 1931. Pp. 350–354.

40. Beasley, W. C. Normal hearing for speech for each decade of life. *Publ. Hlth. Rep., Wash.*, 1938, Hearing Study Ser., No. 5.

41. Beck, L. H. Osmics: olfaction. In Glasser's *Medical physics*, Vol. 11. Chicago: Year Book Publishers, 1950. Pp. 658–664.

42. Bednar, M., & Langfelder, O. Ueber das intravenöse (hämatogene) Riechen. *Mschr. Ohrenheilk.*, 1930, **64**, 1133–1139.

43. Beebe-Center, J. G. Standards for the use of the gust scale. *J. Psychol.*, 1949, **28**, 411–419.

44. Beebe-Center, J. G., & Waddell, D. A general psychological scale of taste. *J. Psychol.*, 1948, **26**, 517–524.

45. Beecher, H. K. *Measurement of subjective responses*. New York: Oxford University Press, 1959.

46. Beecher, H. K., Keats, A. S., Mosteller, F., & Lasagna, L. The effectiveness of oral analgesics (morphine, codeine, acetylsalicylic acid) and the problem of placebo "reactors" and "non-reactors." *J. Pharmacol.*, 1953, **109**, 393–400.

47. Beets, M. J. G. A molecular approach to olfaction. In E. J. Ariens (Ed.), *Molecular pharmacology*, Vol. II. New York: Academic Press, 1964. Pp. 3–51.

48. Beidler, L. M. A theory of taste stimulation. *J. gen. Physiol.*, 1954, 38, 133–139.

49. Beidler, L. M. Biophysical approaches to taste. *Amer. Sci.*, 1961, **49**, 421–431.

50. Beidler, L. M. Gustatory and olfactory receptor stimulation. In. W. Rosenblith (Ed), *Sensory communication*. New York: Wiley, 1961. Chap. 8 (pp. 143–157).

51. Beidler, L. M. Dynamics of taste cells. In Y. Zotterman (Ed.), *Olfaction and taste*. New York: Macmillan, 1963. Pp. 133–145.

52. Békésy, G. von. Ueber die Hörschwelle und Fühlgrenze langsamer sinusförmiger Luftdruckschwankungen. *Ann. d. Phys.*, 1936, **26**, 554–566.

53. Békésy, G. von. Subjective cupulometry. *Arch. Otolaryngol.*, 1955, **61**, 16–28.

54. Békésy, G. von. Synchronism of neural discharges and their demultiplication in pitch perception on the skin and in hearing. *J. acoust. Soc. Amer.*, 1959, **31**, 338–349.

55. Békésy, G. von. *Experiments in hearing*. New York: McGraw-Hill, 1960.

56. Békésy, G. von. Duplexity theory of taste. *Science*, 1964, **145**, 834–835.

57. Békésy, G. von. Olfactory analogue to directional hearing. *J. appl. Physiol.*, 1964, **19**, 369–373.

58. Békésy, G. von. Sweetness produced electrically on the tongue and its relation to taste theories. *J. appl. Physiol.*, 1964, **19**, 1105–1113.

59. Békésy, G. von. Taste theories and the chemical stimulation of single papillae. *J. appl. Physiol.*, 1966, **21**, 1–9.

60. Békésy, G. von. *Sensory inhibition.* Princeton, N. J.: Princeton University Press, 1967.

61. Békésy, G. von, & Rosenblith, W. A. The mechanical properties of the ear. In S. S. Stevens (Ed.), *Handbook of experimental psychology.* New York: Wiley, 1951. Chap. 27 (pp. 1075–1115).

62. Belonoschkin, B. Ueber die Kaltreceptoren der Haut. *Z. Biol.,* 1933, **93**, 487–489.

63. Benjamin, F. B. Release of intercellular potassium as a factor in pain production. In D. R. Kenshalo (Ed.), *The skin senses.* Springfield, Ill.: Thomas, 1968. Chap. 23 (pp. 466–479).

64. Benjamin, R. M. Some thalamic and cortical mechanisms of taste. In Y. Zotterman (Ed), *Olfaction and taste.* New York: Macmillan, 1963. Pp. 309–329.

65. Bentley, M. The synthetic experiment. *Amer. J. Psychol.,* 1900, **11**, 405– 425.

66. Beranek, L. L., Sleeper, H. P., Jr., & Moots, E. E. The design and construction of anechoic sound chambers. *OSRD* Rep. No. 4190, Harvard University, 1945.

67. Berglund, B., Berglund, U., & Ekman, G. Temporal integration of vibrotactile stimulation. *Percept. mot. Skills,* 1967, **25**, 549–560.

68. Berry, W., & Imus, H. Quantitative aspects of the flight of colors. *Amer. J. Psychol.,* 1935, **47**, 449–457.

69. Bigelow, N., Harrison, I., Goodell, H., & Wolff, H. G. Studies on pain: quantitative measurements of two pain sensations of the skin, with reference to the nature of the "hyperalgesia of peripheral neuritis." *J. clin. Invest.,* 1945, **24**, 503–512.

70. Bishop, G. H. Responses to electrical stimulation of single sensory units of skin. *J. Neurophysiol.,* 1943, **6**, 361–382.

71. Bishop, G. H. Relation of pain sensory threshold to form of mechanical stimulator. *J. Neurophysiol.,* 1949, **12**, 51–57.

72. Bishop, G. H. The relation between nerve fiber size and sensory modality: phylogenetic implications of the afferent innervation of the cortex. *J. nerv. ment. Dis.,* 1959, **128**, 89–114.

73. Blackwell, H. R., & Blackwell, O. M. Rod and cone receptor mechanisms in typical and atypical congenital achromatopsia. *Vision Res.,* 1961, **1**, 62–107.

74. Blakeslee, A. F., & Salmon, T. H. Genetics of sensory thresholds: individual taste reactions for different substances. *Proc. nat. Acad. Sci., Wash.,* 1935, **21**, 84–90.

75. Bocca, E., Antonelli, R., & Mosciaro, O. Mechanical co-factors in olfactory stimulation. *Acta oto-laryngol., Stockh.,* 1965, **59**, 243–247.

76. Boeke, J. Nerve endings, motor and sensory. In W. Penfield (Ed.), *Cytology and cellular pathology of the nervous system,* Vol. I. New York: Hoeber, 1932. Pp. 243–315.

77. Borg, G. A. V. Physical performance and perceived exertion. *Stud. psychol. et paedog.,* 1962, **11**, 1–64.

78. Boring, E. G. The sensations of the alimentary canal. *Amer. J. Psychol.,* 1915, **26**, 1–57.

79. Boring, E. G. The thermal sensitivity of the stomach. *Amer. J. Psychol.,* 1915, **26**, 485–494.

80. Boring, E. G. Cutaneous sensation after nerve-division. *Quart. J. exper. Physiol.,* 1916, **10**, 1–95.

81. Boring, E. G. Auditory theory with special reference to intensity, volume, and localization. *Amer. J. Psychol.,* 1926, **37**, 157–188.

82. Boring, E. G. *The physical dimensions of consciousness.* New York: Appleton-Century, 1933.

83. Boring, E. G. The size of the differential limen for pitch. *Amer. J. Psychol.,* 1940, **53**, 450–455.

84. Boring, E. G. *Sensation and perception in the history of experimental psychology.* New York: Appleton-Century, 1942.

85. Boring, E. G., & Stevens, S. S. The nature of tonal brightness. *Proc. nat. Acad. Sci., Wash.,* 1936, **22**, 514–521.

86. Börnstein, W. S. Cortical representation of taste in man and monkey. II. The localization of the cortical taste area in man and a method of measuring impairment of taste in man. *Yale J. Biol. Med.,* 1940, **13**, 133–156.

87. Boyd, I. A., & Roberts, T. D. M. Proprioceptive discharges from the stretch receptors in the knee-joint of the cat. *J. Physiol., Lond.,* 1953, **122**, 38–58.

88. Brecher, G. A. Die untere Hör- und Tongrenze. *Pflüg. Arch. ges. Physiol.,* 1934, **234**, 380–393.

89. Bremer, J. L., & Weatherford, H. L. *A textbook of histology* (6th ed.), Philadelphia: Blakiston, 1944.

90. Brewster, D. On the influence of successive impulses of light upon the retina. *Phil. Mag.,* 1834, Ser. 3, **4**, 241–245.

91. Brindley, G. S. The colour of light of very long wavelength. *J. Physiol., Lond.,* 1955, **130**, 35–44.

92. Brindley, G. S. Human colour vision. *Progr. Biophysics,* 1957, 8, 49–94.

93. Brindley, G. S. Double pain from an electrical stimulus. *J. Physiol., Lond.,* 1962, **162**, 49P–50P.

94. Broca, A., & Sulzer, D. La sensation lumineuse en fonction du temps. *J. Physiol. et de Pathol. gén.,* 1902, **4**, 632–640.

95. Brown, J. E., & Rojas, J . A. Rat retinal ganglion cells: receptive field organization and maintained activity. *J. Neurophysiol.,* 1965, **28**, 1073–1090.

96. Brown, J. L. Orientation to the vertical during water immersion. *Aerospace Med.,* 1961, **32**, 209–217.

97. Brown, J. L. Flicker and intermittent stimulation. In C. H. Graham (Ed.), *Vision and visual perception.* New York: Wiley, 1965. Chap. 10 (pp. 251–320).

98. Brown, J. L., & Mueller, C. G. Brightness discrimination and brightness contrast. In C. H. Graham (Ed.), *Vision and visual perception.* New York: Wiley, 1965. Chap. 9 (pp. 208–250).

99. Brown, K. T. The electroretinogram: Its components and their origins. *Vision Res.,* 1968, **8**, 633–677.

100. Brown, P. K., & Wald, G. Visual pigments in single rods and cones of the human retina. *Science,* 1964, **144**, 45–52.

101. Brown, R. H., & Page, H. E. Pupil dilatation and dark adaptation. *J. exp. Psychol.,* 1939, **25**, 347–360.

102. Brücke, E. Ueber den Nutzeffekt intermittierender Netzhautreizungen. *Sitzber. Akad. Wiss., Wien,* Math-Naturwiss. Kl., 1864, **49**, II, 128–153.

103. Bujas, Z. Quelques remarques sur le contraste et l'inhibition à la suite d'excitations gustatives simultanées. *C.r. Soc. Biol., Paris,* 1934, **116**, 1304–1306.

104. Bujas, Z. Quelques données sur le goût électrique, *Année psychol.*, 1949, **50**, 159–168.

105. Burnham, R. W., Hanes, R. M., & Bartleson, C. J. *Color: a guide to basic facts and concepts.* New York: Wiley, 1963.

106. Cannon, W. B. The physiological basis of thirst. *Proc. roy. Soc. Lond.*, 1918, **90B**, 283–301.

107. Cannon, W. B. *Bodily changes in pain, hunger, fear, and rage* (2nd ed.). New York: Appleton-Century, 1934.

108. Cannon, W. B. Hunger and thirst. In C. A. Murchison (Ed.), *Handbook of general experimental psychology.* Worcester, Mass.: Clark University Press, 1934. Chap. 5 (pp. 247–263).

109. Cannon, W. B., & Washburn, A. L. An explanation of hunger. *Amer. J. Physiol.*, 1912, **29**, 441–454.

110. Carr, H. Head's theory of cutaneous sensitivity. *Psychol. Rev.*, 1916, **23**, 262–268.

111. Catton, W. T. Mechanoreceptor function. *Physiol. Revs.*, 1970, **50**, 297–318.

112. Chapanis, A. The dark adaptation of the color anomalous measured with lights of different hues. *J. gen. Physiol.*, 1947, **30**, 423–437.

113. Chapanis, A. How we see: a summary of basic principles. In *Human factors in undersea warfare.* Washington: National Research Council, 1949. Chap. 1 (pp. 3–60).

114. Chapanis, A., Garner, W. R., & Morgan, C. T. *Applied experimental psychology.* New York: Wiley, 1949.

115. Chapman, L. F., Goodell, H., & Wolff, H. G. Structures and processes involved in the sensation of itch. In W. Montagna (Ed.), *Cutaneous innervation.* New York: Pergamon, 1960. Chap. VIII (pp. 161–188).

116. Clark, B. Thresholds for the perception of angular acceleration in man. *Aerospace Med.*, 1967, **38**, 443–450.

117. Clark, B., & Graybiel, A. Linear acceleration and deceleration as factors influencing nonvisual orientation during flight. *J. Aviat. Med.*, 1949, **20**, 92–101.

118. Clark, B., & Stewart, J. D. Magnitude estimates of rotational velocity during and following prolonged increasing, constant, and zero angular acceleration. *J. exp. Psychol.*, 1968, **78**, 329–339.

119. Clark, M., Luce, D., Abrams, R., Schlosberg, H., & Rome, J. Preliminary experiments on the aural significance of parts of tones of orchestral instruments and on choral tones. *J. Audio Eng. Soc.*, 1963, **11**, 45–54.

120. Clark, W. E. LeG. Inquiries into the anatomical basis of olfactory discrimination. *Proc. roy. Soc. Lond.*, 1957, **146B**, 299–319.

121. Clarke, F. J. J. A study of Troxler's effect. *Optica Acta*, 1960, **7**, 219–236.

122. Cleghorn, T. E., & Darcus, H. D. The sensibility to passive movement of the human elbow joint. *Quart. J. exper. Psychol.*, 1952, **4**, 66–77.

123. Cohen, J., & Ogdon, D. P. Taste blindness to phenyl-thio-carbamide and related compounds. *Psychol. Bull.*, 1949, **46**, 490–498.

124. Collins, W. F., Nulsen, F. E., & Randt, C. T., Relation of peripheral nerve fiber size and sensations in man. *Arch. Neurol.*, 1960, **3**, 381–385.

125. Coltman, J. W. Acoustics of the flute. *Physics Today*, 1968, **21**, 25–32.

126. Cornsweet, T. N. Changes in the appearance of stimuli of very high luminance. *Psychol. Rev.*, 1962, **69**, 257–273.

127. Cornsweet, T. N. *Visual perception.* New York: Academic Press, 1970.
128. Cornsweet, T. N., Fowler, H., Rabedeau, R. G., Whalen, R. E., & Williams, D. R. Changes in the perceived color of very bright stimuli. *Science,* 1958, **128,** 898–899.
129. Crawford, B. H. Visual adaptation in relation to brief conditioning stimuli. *Proc. roy. Soc. Lond.,* 1947, **134B,** 283–300.
130. Creed, R. S., & Ruch, T. C. Regional variations in sensitivity to flicker. *J. Physiol., Lond.,* 1932, **74,** 407–423.
131. Crocker, E. C. *Flavor.* New York: McGraw-Hill, 1945.
132. Crowe, S. J., Guild, S. R., & Polvogt, L. M. Observations on the pathology of high-tone deafness. *Johns Hopkins Hosp. Bull.,* 1934, **54,** 315–379.
133. Crozier, W. J. Chemoreception. In C. A. Murchison (Ed.), *Handbook of general experimental psychology.* Worcester, Mass.: Clark University Press, 1934. Chap. 19 (pp. 987–1036).
134. Culler, E. A. In Symposium on tone localization in the cochlea. *Ann. Otol., etc., St. Louis,* 1935, **44,** 807–813.
135. Culler, E. A., Coakley, J. D., Lowy, K., & Gross, N. A revised frequency-map of the guinea-pig cochlea. *Amer. J. Psychol.,* 1943, **56,** 475–500.
136. Cutolo, F. A preliminary study of the psychology of heat. *Amer. J. Psychol.,* 1918, **29,** 442–448.
137. Dadson, R. S., & King, J. H. A determination of the normal threshold of hearing and its relation to the standardization of audiometers. *J. Laryngol. Otol.,* 1952, **66,** 366–378.
138. Dallenbach, K. M. The temperature spots and end-organs. *Amer. J. Psychol.,* 1927, **39,** 402–427.
139. Dallenbach, K. M. The temperature spots and end-organs. In R. H. Wheeler (Ed.), *Readings in psychology.* New York: Crowell, 1930. Pp. 496–516.
140. Dallenbach, K. M. A method of marking the skin. *Amer. J. Psychol.,* 1931, **43,** 287.
141. Dallenbach, K. M. Pain: history and present status. *Amer. J. Psychol.,* 1939, **52,** 331–347.
142. Dallenbach, K. M. Smell, taste, and somesthesis. In E. G. Boring, H. S. Langfeld, & H. P. Weld (Eds.), *Introduction to psychology.* New York: Wiley, 1939. Chap. 19 (pp. 600–626).
143. Dallos, P., Schoeny, Z. G., Worthington, D. W., & Cheatham, M. A. Cochlear distortion: effect of direct-current polarization. *Science,* 1969, **164,** 449–451.
144. Dartnall, H. J. A. The properties of visual pigments in photoreceptors. In H. Davson (Ed.), *The eye* (Vol. 2). New York: Academic Press, 1962.
145. Davies, J. T., & Taylor, F. H. A theory of quality of odours. *J. Theor. Biol.,* 1965, **8,** 1–7.
146. Davis, H. *Hearing and deafness: a guide for laymen.* New York: Murray Hill, 1947.
147. Davis, H. Psychophysiology of hearing and deafness. In S. S. Stevens (Ed.), *Handbook of experimental psychology.* New York: Wiley, 1951. Chap. 28 (pp. 1116–1142).
148. Davis, H. Biophysics and physiology of the inner ear. *Physiol. Revs.,* 1957, **37,** 1–49.
149. Davis, H. Military standards and medicolegal rules. In H. Davis & S. R. Silverman (Eds.), *Hearing and deafness* (rev. ed.). New York: Holt, Rinehart, & Winston, 1960. Chap. 9 (pp. 242–264).

150. Davis, H. Discussion of L. M. Beidler's "Dynamics of taste cells." In Y. Zotterman (Ed.), *Olfaction and taste*. New York: Macmillan, 1963. Pp. 145–148.

151. Davis, H. Guide for the classification and evaluation of hearing handicap. *Trans. Amer. Acad. Ophthalmol. Otolaryngol.*, 1965 (July-August), 740–751.

152. Davis, R. C., Garafolo, L., & Kveim, K. Conditions associated with gastrointestinal activity. *J. comp. physiol. Psychol.*, 1959, **52**, 466–475.

153. Daw, N. W. Goldfish retina: organization for simultaneous color contrast. *Science*, 1967, **158**, 942–944.

154. Dawson, W. W. The thermal excitation of afferent neurones in the mammalian cornea and iris. In J. D. Hardy (Ed.), *Temperature, its measurement and control in science and industry, Part 3: Biology and Medicine*. New York: Reinhold, 1963. Chap. 20 (pp. 199–210).

155. Dearborn, G. V. N. A case of congenital general pure analgesia. *J. nerv. ment. Dis.*, 1932, **75**, 612–615.

156. Desmedt, J. E. Neurophysiological mechanisms controlling acoustic input. In G. L. Rasmussen & W. F. Windle (Eds.), *Neural mechanisms of the auditory and vestibular systems*. Springfield, Ill.: Thomas, 1960. Chap. 11 (pp. 152–164).

157. Desmedt, J. E. Auditory evoked potentials from cochlea to cortex as influenced by activation of the efferent olivo-cochlear bundle. *J. acoust. Soc. Amer.*, 1962, **34**, 1478–1496.

158. Detwiler, S. R. Some biological aspects of vision. *Sigma Xi Quart.*, 1941, **29**, 112–129 and 142.

159. DeValois, R. L., Abramov, I., & Jacobs, G. H. Analysis of response patterns of the LGN cells. *J. opt. Soc. Amer.*, 1966, **56**, 966–977.

160. Diamant, H., Funakoshi, M., Ström, L., & Zotterman, Y. Electrophysiological studies on human taste nerves. In Y. Zotterman (Ed.), *Olfaction and taste*. New York: Macmillan, 1963. Pp. 193–203.

161. Diamond, A. L. Foveal simultaneous brightness contrast as a function of inducing- and test-field luminances. *J. exp. Psychol.*, 1953, **45**, 304–314.

162. Diamond, A. L. Foveal simultaneous contrast as a function of inducing-field area. *J. exp. Psychol.*, 1955, **50**, 144–152.

163. Dimmick, F. L., & Hubbard, M. R. The spectral location of psychologically unique yellow, green, and blue. *Amer. J. Psychol.*, 1939, **52**, 242–254.

164. Dimmick, F. L., & Hubbard, M. R. The spectral components of psychologically unique red. *Amer. J. Psychol.*, 1939, **52**, 348–353.

165. Dirks, D. D., & Malmquist, C. Shifts in air-conduction thresholds produced by pulsed and continuous contralateral masking. *J. acoust. Soc. Amer.*, 1965, **37**, 631–637.

166. Ditchburn, R. W., & Ginsborg, B. L. Vision with a stabilized retinal image. *Nature (Lond.)*, 1952, **170**, 36–37.

167. Dodt, E., & Zotterman, Y. Mode of action of warm receptors. *Acta physiol. scand.*, 1952, **26**, 345–357.

168. Dohlman, G. Some practical and theoretical points in labyrinthology. *Proc. roy. Soc. Med.*, 1935, **28**, 1371–1380.

169. Dohlman, G. Investigations in the function of the semicircular canals. *Acta oto-laryngol., Stockh.*, Suppl. 51, 1944, 211–219.

170. Donaldson, H. H. On the temperature sense. *Mind*, 1885, **10**, 399–416.

171. Doughty, J. M., & Garner, W. R. Pitch characteristics of short tones. Two kinds of pitch threshold. *J. exp. Psychol.,* 1947, **37**, 351–365.

172. Douglas, W. W., & Ritchie, J. M. Mammalian non-myelinated nerve fibers. *Physiol, Revs.,* 1962, **42**, 297–334.

173. Dowling, J. E. Night blindness. *Sci. Amer.,* 1966, **215**, 78–84.

174. Dowling, J. E. The site of visual adaptation. *Science,* 1967, **155**, 273–279.

175. Dunlap, K. Alleged binocular color mixing. *Amer. J. Psychol.,* 1944, **57**, 559–563.

176. Dusser de Barenne, J. G. The labyrinthine and postural mechanisms. In C. A. Murchison (Ed.), *Handbook of general experimental psychology.* Worcester, Mass.: Clark University Press, 1934. Chap. 4 (pp. 204–246).

177. Dzendolet, E. Sinusoidal electrical stimulation of the human vestibular apparatus. *Percept. mot. Skills,* 1963, **17**, 171–185.

178. Dzendolet, E., & Meiselman, H. L. Gustatory quality changes as a function of solution concentration. *Percept. Psychophys.,* 1967, **2**, 29–33.

179. Dzendolet, E., & Meiselman, H. L. Cation and anion contributions to gustatory quality of simple salts. *Percept. Psychophys.,* 1967, **2**, 601–604.

180. Ebbecke, U. Ueber die Temperaturempfindungen in ihrer Abhängigkeit von der Hautdurchblutung und von den Reflexzentren. *Pflüg. Arch. ges. Physiol.,* 1917, **169**, 395–462.

181. Egan, J. P. The effect of noise in one ear upon the loudness of speech in the other ear. *J. acoust. Soc. Amer.,* 1948, **20**, 58–62.

182. Egan, J. P. Perstimulatory fatigue as measured by heterophonic loudness balances. *J. acoust. Soc. Amer.,* 1955, **27**, 111–120.

183. Egmond, A. A. J. van. The Bárány test compared with cupulometry. *Acta oto-laryngol., Stockh., Suppl.* 78, 1948, 33–39.

184. Eisler, H. Subjective scale of force for a large muscle group. *J. exp. Psychol.,* 1962, **64**, 253–257.

185. Ekman, G., Berglund, B., & Berglund, U. Loudness as a function of the duration of auditory stimulation. *Scand. J. Psychol.,* 1966, **7**, 201–208.

186. El-Baradi, A. F., & Bourne, G. H. Theory of tastes and odors. *Science,* 1951, **113**, 660–661.

187. Elsberg, C. A., & Levy, I. The sense of smell. I. A new and simple method of quantitative olfactometry. *Bull. neurol. Inst. N. Y.,* 1935, **4**, 5–19.

188. Engen, T., & Pfaffmann, C. Absolute judgments of odor intensity. *J. exp. Psychol.,* 1959, **58**, 23–26.

189. Engen, T., & Pfaffmann, C. Absolute judgments of odor quality. *J. exp. Psychol.,* 1960, **59**, 214–219.

190. Engström, H., Lindeman, H. H., & Ades, H. W. Anatomical features of the auricular sensory organs. In *Second Symposium on the Role of the Vestibular Organs in Space Exploration* (NASA SP–115), 1966. Pp. 33–46.

191. Etholm, B. Evoked responses in the inferior colliculus, medial geniculate body, and auditory cortex by single and double clicks in cats. *Acta oto-laryngol., Stockh.,* 1969, **67**, 319–325.

192. Fabian, F. W., & Blum, H. B. Relative taste potency of some basic food constituents and their competitive and compensatory action. *Food Res.,* 1943, **8**, 179–193.

193. Feinberg, G. Light. *Sci. Amer.,* 1968, **219**(3), 50–59.

194. Feindel, W. H., Weddell, G., & Sinclair, D. C. Pain sensibility in deep somatic structures. *J. Neurol. Psychiat.,* 1948, **11**, 113–117.

195. Fick, A. Zur Theorie der Farbenblindheit. *Pflüg. Arch. ges. Physiol.,* 1896, **64,** 313–320.
196. Finck, A. Low-frequency pure tone masking. *J. acoust. Soc. Amer.,* 1961, **33,** 1140–1141.
197. Fischer J., & Wolfson, L. E. The inner ear. New York: Grune and Stratton, 1943.
198. Fishman, I. Y. Single fiber gustatory impulses in rat and hamster. *J. cell. comp. Physiol.,* 1957, **49,** 319–334.
199. FitzGerald, M. J. T. The innervation of the epidermis. In D. R. Kenshalo (Ed.), *The skin senses.* Springfield, Ill.: Thomas, 1968. Chap. 4 (pp. 61–81).
200. Fletcher, H. *Speech and hearing.* New York: Van Nostrand, 1929.
201. Fletcher, H. A space-time pattern theory of hearing. *J. acoust. Soc. Amer.,* 1930, **1,** 311–343.
202. Fletcher, H. The mechanism of hearing as revealed through experiment on the masking effect of thermal noise. *Proc. nat. Acad. Sci., Wash.,* 1938, **24,** 265–274.
203. Fletcher, H., & Munson, W. A. Relation between loudness and masking. *J. acoust. Soc. Amer.,* 1937, **9,** 1–10.
204. Forbes, A., & Gregg, A. Electrical studies in mammalian reflexes. *Amer. J. Physiol.,* 1915, **39,** 172–235.
205. Foster, D., Scofield, E. H., & Dallenbach, K. M. An olfactorium. *Amer. J. Psychol.,* 1950, **63,** 431–440.
206. Fox, A. L. The relationship between chemical constitution and taste. *Proc. nat. Acad. Sci., Wash.,* 1932, **18,** 115–120.
207. Frey, M. von. Ueber die zur ebenmerklichen Erregung des Drucksinns erforderlichen Energiemengen. *Z. Biol.,* 1919, **70,** 333–347.
208. Frey, M. von. Versuche über schmerzerregende Reize. *Z. Biol.,* 1922, **76,** 1–24.
209. Frey, M. von, & Kiesow, F. Ueber die Function der Tastkörperchen. *Z. Psychol.,* 1899, **20,** 126–163.
210. Fulton, J. F. *Physiology of the nervous system* (2nd ed.). New York: Oxford University Press, 1943.
211. Galambos, R. Suppression of auditory nerve activity by stimulation of efferent fibers to the cochlea. *J. Neurophysiol.,* 1956, **19,** 424–437.
212. Galambos, R., & Davis, H. The response of single auditory-nerve fibers to acoustic stimulation. *J. Neurophysiol.,* 1943, **6,** 39–57.
213. Galambos, R., & Davis, H. Action potentials from single auditory-nerve fibers. *Science,* 1948, **108,** 513.
214. Galambos, R., Schwartzkopf, J., & Rupert, A. Microelectrode study of superior olivary nuclei. *Amer. J. Physiol.,* 1959, **197,** 527–536.
215. Galilei, Galileo. Dialogues concerning two new sciences (Trans. Crew, H., & de Salvio, A.). Evanston, Ill.: Northwestern University Press, 1950.
216. Gardner, E. *Fundamentals of neurology.* Philadelphia: Saunders, 1947.
217. Garner, W. R. An informational analysis of absolute judgments of loudness. *J. exp. Psychol.,* 1953, **46,** 373–380.
218. Gatti, A., & Dodge, R. Ueber die Unterschiedsempfindlichkeit bei Reizung eines einzelnen, isolierten Tastorgans. *Arch. ges. Psychol.,* 1929, **69,** 405–425.
219. Geldard, F. A. The measurement of retinal fatigue to achromatic stimulation. I, II. *J. gen. Psychol.,* 1928, **1,** 123–135; 578–590.

220. Geldard, F. A. The description of a case of total color blindness. *J. opt. Soc. Amer.,* 1933, **23,** 256–260.

221. Geldard, F. A. Flicker relations within the fovea. *J. opt. Soc. Amer.,* 1934, **24,** 299–302.

222. Geldard, F. A. The perception of mechanical vibration. I. History of a controversy. *J. gen. psychol.,* 1940, **22,** 243–269.

223. Geldard, F. A. The perception of mechanical vibration. II. The response of pressure receptors. *J. gen. Psychol.,* 1940, **22,** 271–280.

224. Geldard, F. A. The perception of mechanical vibration. III. The frequency function. *J. gen. Psychol.,* 1940, **22,** 281–289.

225. Geldard, F. A. The perception of mechanical vibration. IV. Is there a separate "vibratory sense"? *J. gen. Psychol.,* 1940, **22,** 291–308.

226. Geldard, F . A. Somesthesis and the chemical senses. *Ann. Rev. Psychol.,* 1950, **1,** 71–86.

227. Geldard, F. A. Vision, audition, and beyond. In W. D. Neff (Ed.), *Contributions to sensory physiology,* Vol. 4. New York: Academic Press, 1970. Pp. 1–17.

228. Georgi, A. Effect of wavelength on the relationship between critical flicker frequency and intensity in foveal vision. *J. opt. Soc. Amer.,* 1963, **53,** 480–486.

229. Gernandt, B. E. Response of mammalian vestibular neurons to horizontal rotation and caloric stimulation. *J. Neurophysiol.,* 1949, **12,** 173–185.

230. Gesteland, R. C., Lettvin, J. Y., Pitts, W. H., & Rojas, A. Odor specificities of the frog's olfactory receptors. In Y. Zotterman (Ed.), *Olfaction and taste.* New York: Macmillan, 1963. Pp. 19–34.

231. Gibson, K. S., & Tyndall, E. P. T. The visibility of radiant energy. *Sci. Papers U.S. Bur. Stand.,* 1923, **19,** No. 475.

232. Gibson, R. H. Electrical stimulation of pain and touch. In D. R. Kenshalo, (Ed.), *The skin senses.* Springfield, Ill.: Thomas, 1968. Chap. 11 (pp. 223–261).

233. Gilmer, B. von H. The relation of cold sensitivity to sweat duct distribution and the neurovascular mechanisms of the skin. *J. Psychol.,* 1942, **13,** 307–325.

234. Gilmer, T. E. The integrating power of the eye for short flashes of light. *J. opt. Soc. Amer.,* 1937, **27,** 386–388.

235. Goff, G. D. Differential discrimination of frequency of cutaneous mechanical vibration. *J. exp. Psychol.,* 1967, **74,** 294–299.

236. Goldscheider, A. Untersuchungen über den Muskelsinn. I. Ueber die Bewegungsempfindung. In *Gesammelte Abhandlungen von A. Goldscheider,* Vol. II. Leipzig: Barth, 1898. Pp. 97–200.

237. Goldscheider, A. Untersuchungen über den Muskelsinn. II. Ueber die Empfindung der Schwere und des Widerstandes. In *Gesammelte Abhandlungen von A. Goldscheider,* Vol. II. Leipzig: Barth, 1898. Pp. 201–281.

238. Goldstein, M. H., Hall, J. L., II, & Butterfield, B. O. Single-unit activity in the primary auditory cortex of unanesthetized cats. *J. acoust. Soc. Amer.,* 1968, **43,** 444–455.

239. Graham, C. H. Color theory. In S. Koch (Ed.), *Psychology: a study of a science.* Vol. I. New York: McGraw-Hill, 1959. Pp. 145–287.

240. Graham, C. H. (Ed.) *Vision and visual perception.* New York: Wiley, 1965.

241. Graham, C. H., Sperling, H. G., Hsia, Y., & Coulson, A. H. The determination of some visual functions of a unilaterally color-blind subject: Methods and results. *J. Psychol.,* 1961, **51**, 3–32.

242. Granit, R. The components of the retinal action potential in mammals and their relation to the discharge in the optic nerve. *J. Physiol., Lond.,* 1933, **77**, 207–239.

243. Granit, R. *Sensory mechanisms of the retina.* New York: Oxford University Press, 1947.

244. Granit, R. Retina and optic nerve. In H. Davson (Ed.), *The eye* (Vol. 2). New York: Academic Press, 1962. Chap. 22 (pp. 541–574).

245. Gray, J. A. B., & Malcolm, J. L. The initiation of nerve impulses by mesenteric corpuscles. *Proc. roy. Soc. Lond.,* 1950, **137B**, 96–114.

246. Graybiel, A., Kerr, W. A., & Bartley, S. H. Stimulus thresholds of the semicircular canals as a function of angular acceleration. *Amer. J. Psychol.,* 1948, **61**, 21–36.

247. Greene, L. C., & Hardy, J. D. Adaptation of thermal pain in the skin. *J. appl. Physiol.,* 1962, **17**, 693–696.

248. Gregory, R. L., & Ross, H. E. Arm weight, adaptation, and weight discrimination. *Percept. mot. Skills,* 1967, **24**, 1127–1130.

249. Grindley, G. C. The variation of sensory thresholds with the rate of application of the stimulus. I. The differential threshold for pressure. *Brit. J. Psychol.,* 1936, **27**, 86–95.

250. Grindley, G. C. The variation of sensory thresholds with the rate of application of the stimulus. II. Touch and pain. *Brit. J. Psychol.,* 1936, **27**, 189–195.

251. Grossman, S. P. *A textbook of physiological psychology.* New York: Wiley, 1967.

252. Guedry, F. E. Psychophysiological studies of vestibular function. In W. D. Neff (Ed.), *Contributions to sensory physiology,* Vol. 1. New York: Academic Press, 1965. Pp. 63–135.

253. Guedry, F. E. Influence of linear and angular acceleration on nystagmus. In *Second Symposium on the Role of the Vestibular Organs in Space Exploration* (NASA SP–115), 1966. Pp. 185–198.

254. Guilford, J. P., & Lovewell, E. M. The touch spots and the intensity of the stimulus. *J. gen. Psychol.,* 1936, **15**, 149–159.

255. Guirao, M., & Stevens, S. S. Measurement of auditory density. *J. acoust. Soc. Amer.,* 1964, **36**, 1176–1182.

256. Häggqvist, G. Histophysiologische Studien über die Temperatursinne der Haut des Menschen. *Anat. Anz.,* 1913, **45**, 46–63.

257. Hahn, H. Die physiologische Konstanten und Variablen des Temperatursinnes. *Z. Psychol.,* 1929, **60**, 162–232.

258. Hahn, H. Die Adaptation des Geschmacksinnes. *Z. Sinnesphysiol.,* 1934, **65**, 105–145.

259. Hahn, H. Ueber die Ursache der Geschmacksempfindung. *Klin. Wochschr.,* 1936, **15**, 933–935.

260. Hahn, H., & Ulbrich, L. Eine systematische Untersuchung der Geschmacksschwellen. *Pflüg. Arch. ges. Physiol.,* 1948, **250**, 357–384.

261. Hahn, J. F. Vibrotactile adaptation and recovery measured by two methods. *J. exp. Psychol.,* 1966, **71**, 655–658.

262. Haller, A. von. *First lines of physiology*. London: Johnson, 1966. (Reprint of the 1786 translation of the Latin edition of 1767). 2 vols.

263. Hallpike, C. S. Some types of ocular nystagmus and their neurological mechanisms. *Proc. roy. Soc. Med.*, 1967, **60**, 1043–1054.

264. Hallpike, C. S., & Rawdon-Smith, A. F. The Helmholtz resonance theory of hearing. *Nature, Lond.*, 1934, **133**, 614.

265. Hänig, D. P. Zur Psychophysik des Geschmacksinnes. *Philos. Stud., (Wundt)*, 1901, **17**, 576–623.

266. Harbert, F., Young, I. M., & Wenner, C. H. Auditory flutter fusion and envelope of signal. *J. acoust. Soc. Amer.*, 1968, **44**, 803–806.

267. Hardy, A. C. *Handbook of colorimetry*. Cambridge, Mass.: Technology Press, 1936.

268. Hardy, J. D. Sensitivity of temperature detection in man. In A. V. S. de Reuck, & J. Knight (Eds.), *Touch, heat, and pain*. Boston: Little, Brown, 1966. Pp. 294–296.

269. Hardy, J. D., Stolwijk, J. A. J., Hammel, H. T., & Murgatroyd, D. Skin temperature and cutaneous pain during warm water immersion. *J. appl. Physiol.*, 1965, **20**, 1014–1021.

270. Hardy, J. D., Stolwijk, J. A. J., & Hoffman, D. Pain following step increase in skin temperature. In D. R. Kenshalo (Ed.), *The skin senses*. Springfield, Ill.: Thomas, 1968. Chap. 21 (pp. 444–457).

271. Hardy, J. D., Wolff, H. G., & Goodell, H. Studies on pain; a new method for measuring pain threshold: observations on spatial summation of pain. *J. clin. Invest.*, 1940, **19**, 649–657.

272. Hardy, J. D., Wolff, H. G., & Goodell, H. Studies on pain: discrimination of differences in intensity of a pain stimulus as a basis of a scale of pain intensity. *J. clin. Invest.*, 1947, **26**, 1152–1158.

273. Harris, J. D. Pitch discrimination. *J. acoust. Soc. Amer.*, 1952, **24**, 750–755.

274. Hartline, H. K. The nerve messages in the fibers of the visual pathway. *J. opt. Soc. Amer.*, 1940, **30**, 239–247.

275. Hartline, H. K., & Graham, C. H. Nerve impulses from single receptors in the eye. *J. cell. comp. Physiol.*, 1932, **1**, 277–295.

276. Head, H. *Studies in neurology*. London: Oxford University Press, 1920.

277. Hecht, S. On the binocular fusion of colors and its relation to theories of color vision. *Proc. nat. Acad. Sci., Wash.*, 1928, **14**, 237–240.

278. Hecht, S. The retinal processes concerned with visual acuity and color vision. *Bull. Howe Lab. Ophthalmol.* (Harvard), 1931, No. 4, 1–88.

279. Hecht, S. The interrelations of various aspects of color vision. *J. opt. Soc. Amer.*, 1931, **21**, 615–639.

280. Hecht, S. Vision: II. The nature of the photoreceptor process. In C. A. Murchison (Ed.), *Handbook of general experimental psychology*. Worcester, Mass.: Clark University Press, 1934. Chap. 14 (pp. 704–828).

281. Hecht, S. The instantaneous visual threshold after light adaptation. *Proc. nat. Acad. Sci., Wash.*, 1937, **23**, 227–233.

282. Hecht, S. Rods, cones, and the chemical basis of vision. *Physiol. Revs.*, 1937, **17**, 239–290.

283. Hecht, S., & Mandelbaum, J. Dark adaptation and experimental human vitamin A deficiency. *Amer. J. Physiol.*, 1940, **130**, 651–664.

284. Hecht, S., & Shlaer, S. Intermittent stimulation by light. V. The relation between intensity and critical frequency for different parts of the spectrum. *J. gen. Physiol.*, 1936, **19**, 965–977.

285. Hecht, S., & Shlaer, S. An adaptometer for measuring human dark adaptation. *J. opt. Soc. Amer.*, 1938, **28**, 269–275.

286. Hecht, S., Shlaer, S., & Pirenne, M. H. Energy at the threshold of vision. *Science*, 1941, **93**, 585–587.

287. Hecht, S., & Williams, R. E. The visibility of monochromatic radiation and the absorption spectrum of visual purple. *J. gen. Physiol.*, 1922, **5**, 1–34.

288. Heinbecker, P., Bishop, G. H., & O'Leary, J. L. Pain and touch fibers in peripheral nerves. *Arch. Neurol. Psychiat., Chicago*, 1933, **29**, 771–789.

289. Heiser, F. Stimulus-duration and sensations of warmth. *Amer. J. Psychol.*, 1937, **49**, 58–66.

290. Heiser, F., & McNair, W. K. Stimulus-pressure and thermal sensation. *Amer. J. Psychol.*, 1934, **46**, 580–589.

291. Helmholtz, H. L. F. von. *Physiological optics* (Trans. J. P. C. Southall), Vol. II. Rochester, N. Y.: Optical Society of America, 1924.

292. Helmholtz, H. L. F. von. *Sensations of tone* (Trans. A. J. Ellis) (5th ed.) New York: Longmans, Green, 1930.

293. Helson, H. Current trends and issues in adaptation-level theory. *Amer. Psychologist*, 1964, **19**, 26–38.

294. Henney, K. *Principles of radio* (3rd ed.) New York: Wiley, 1938.

295. Henning, H. Die Qualitätenreihe des Geschmacks. *Z. Psychol.*, 1916, **74**, 203–219.

296. Henning, H. *Der Geruch* (2nd ed.) Leipzig: Barth, 1924.

297. Henry, J. P., Augerson, W. S., Belleville, R. E., Douglas, W. K., Gunzke, M. K., Johnston, R. S., Laughlin, P. C., Mosely, J. D., Rohles, F. H., Voas, R. B., & White, S. C. Effects of weightlessness in ballistic and orbital flight. *Aerospace Med.*, 1962, **33**, 1056–1068.

298. Hensel, H. Temperaturempfindung und intracutane Wärmebewegung. *Pflüg. Arch. ges. Physiol.*, 1950, **252**, 165–215.

299. Hensel, H. Classes of receptor units predominantly related to thermal stimuli. In A. V. S. de Reuck & J. Knight (Eds.), *Touch, heat, and pain*. Boston: Little, Brown, 1966. Pp. 275–290.

300. Hensel, H. Cutaneous warm receptors in primates. *Pflüg. Arch. ges. Physiol.*, 1969, **313**, 150–152.

301. Hensel, H., & Boman, K. Afferent impulses in cutaneous sensory nerves in human subjects. *J. Neurophysiol.*, 1960, **23**, 564–578.

302. Hensel, H., & Huopaniemi, T. Static and dynamic properties of warm fibres in the infraorbital nerve. *Pflüg. Arch. ges. Physiol.*, 1969, **309**, 1–10.

303. Hensel, H., Iggo, A., & Witt, I. A quantitative study of sensitive cutaneous thermoreceptors with C afferent fibres. *J. Physiol., Lond.*, 1960, **153**, 113–126.

304. Hensel, H., Ström, L., & Zotterman, Y. Electrophysiological measurements of depth of thermoreceptors. *J. Neurophysiol.*, 1951, **14**, 423–429.

305. Hensel, H., & Witt, I. Spatial temperature gradient and thermoreceptor stimulation. *J. Physiol., Lond.*, 1959, **148**, 180–187.

306. Hensel, H., & Zotterman, Y. Action potentials of cold fibres and intracutaneous temperature gradient. *J. Neurophysiol.*, 1951, **14**, 377–385.

307. Hensel, H., & Zotterman, Y. Quantitative Beziehungen zwischen der Entladung einzelner Kältefasern und der Temperatur. *Acta Physiol. scand.*, 1951, **23**, 291–319.

308. Hetherington, A. W., & Ranson, S. W. Hypothalamic lesions and adiposity in the rat. *Anat. Rec.*, 1940, **78**, 149–172.

309. Hinchcliffe, R.   The anatomical locus of presbycusis. *J. Speech Hear. Disorders*, 1962, **27**, 301–310.

310. Höber, R., & Kiesow, F.   Ueber den Geschmack von Salzen und Laugen. *Z. physikal. Chemie*, 1898, **27**, 601–616.

311. Holway, A. H., & Hurvich, L. M.   Differential gustatory sensitivity to salt. *Amer. J. Psychol.*, 1937, **49**, 37–48.

312. Howard, I. P., & Templeton, W. B.   *Human spatial orientation.*   New York: Wiley, 1966.

313. Hsü, E. H.   A factorial analysis of olfaction. *Psychometrika*, 1946, **11**, 31–42.

314. Hubel, D. H.   Integrative processes in central visual pathways of the cat. *J. opt. Soc. Amer.*, 1963, **53**, 58–66.

315. Hubel, D. H.   The visual cortex of the brain. *Sci. Amer.*, 1963, **209**, No. 5, 54–62.

316. Hubel, D. H., & Wiesel, T. N.   Receptive fields of single neurones in the cat's striate cortex. *J. Physiol., Lond.*, 1959, **148**, 574–591.

317. Hubel, D. H., & Wiesel, T. N.   Receptive fields of optic nerve fibers in the spider monkey. *J. Physiol., Lond.*, 1960, **154**, 572–580.

318. Hubel, D. H., & Wiesel, T. N.   Receptive fields, binocular interaction and functional architecture in the cat's visual cortex. *J. Physiol., Lond.*, 1962, **160**, 106–154.

319. Hubel, D. H., & Wiesel, T. N.   Receptive fields and functional architecture in two nonstriate visual areas (18 and 19) in the cat. *J. Neurophysiol.*, 1965, **28**, 229–289.

320. Huddart, J.   An account of persons who could not distinguish colours. *Philos. Trans.*, 1777, **67**, 260–265.

321. Hunt, C. C., & McIntyre, A. K.   An analysis of fibre diameter and receptor characteristics of myelinated cutaneous afferent fibres in cat. *J. Physiol., Lond.*, 1960, **153**, 99–112.

322. Hurvich, L. M., & Jameson, D.   The binocular fusion of yellow in relation to color theories. *Science*, 1951, **114**, 199–202.

323. Hurvich, L. M., & Jameson, D.   Introduction to and translation of Ewald Hering's *Outlines of a theory of the light sense.*   Cambridge, Mass.: Harvard University Press, 1964.

324. Hurvich, L. M., & Jameson, D.   *The perception of brightness and darkness.*   Boston: Allyn and Bacon, 1966.

325. Hutchins, C. M.   Founding of a family of fiddles. *Physics Today*, 1967, **20**, 23–37.

326. Iggo, A.   Cutaneous heat and cold receptors with slowly conducting (C) afferent fibres. *Quart. J. exp. Physiol.*, 1959, **44**, 362–370.

327. Iriuchijima, J., & Zotterman, Y.   The specificity of afferent cutaneous C fibres in mammals. *Acta Physiol. scand.*, 1960, **49**, 267–278.

328. Jacobs, G. H., & Wascher, T. C.   Bezold-Brücke hue shift: further measurements. *J. opt. Soc. Amer.*, 1967, **57**, 1155–1156.

329. James, W.   *Principles of psychology.*   New York: Holt, 1890, 2 vols.

330. Jameson, D., & Hurvich, L. M.   Effect of exposure time on perceived color and color contrast. *J. opt. Soc. Amer.*, 1962, **52**, 1326(A).

331. Jameson, D., & Hurvich, L. M.   Theory of brightness and color contrast in human vision. *Vision Res.*, 1964, **4**, 135–154.

332. Jenkins, W. L.   Adaptation in isolated cold spots. *Amer. J. Psychol.*, 1937, **49**, 1–22.

333. Jones, L. A. The fundamental scale of pure hue and retinal sensibility to hue differences. *J. opt. Soc. Amer.,* 1917, **1,** 63–77.
334. Jones, L. A., & Lowry, E. M. Retinal sensibility to saturation differences. *J. opt. Soc. Amer.,* 1926, **13,** 25–34.
335. Jones, M. H. Second pain: fact or artifact. *Science,* 1956, **124,** 442–443.
336. Jones, M. H., & Jones, F. N. The critical frequency of taste. *Science,* 1952, **115,** 355–356.
337. Judd, D. B. Chromaticity sensibility to stimulus differences. *J. opt. Soc. Amer.,* 1932, **22,** 72–108.
338. Judd, D. B. Current views on colour blindness. *Doc. ophthalmol.,* 1949, **3,** 251–288.
339. Kalmus, H., & Hubbard, S. J. *The chemical senses in health and disease.* Springfield, Ill.: Thomas, 1960.
340. Kamen, J. M., Pilgrim, F. J., Gutman, N. J., & Kroll, B. J., Interactions of suprathreshold taste stimuli. QMFCIAF Rep. No. 14–60, Proj. 7–85–15–007.
341. Kare, M. R. Comparative aspects of the sense of taste. In M. R. Kare & B. P. Halpern (Eds.), *Physiological and behavioral aspects of taste.* Chicago: University of Chicago Press, 1961. Chap. 2 (pp. 6–15).
342. Kare, M. R., & Halpern, B. P. (Eds.), *Physiological and behavioral aspects of taste.* Chicago: University of Chicago Press, 1961.
343. Katsuki, Y. Neural mechanism of auditory sensation in cats. In W. A. Rosenblith (Ed.), *Sensory communication.* New York: Wiley, 1961. Chap. 29 (pp. 561–583).
344. Katz, D. The vibratory sense and other lectures. *Univ. Maine Bull.,* 1930, **32,** 90–104.
345. Katz, M. S. Brief flash brightness. *Vision Res.,* 1964, **4,** 361–373.
346. Keele, C. A. Measurement of responses to chemically induced pain. In A. V. S. de Reuck & J. Knight (Eds.), *Touch, heat, and pain.* Boston: Little, Brown, 1966. Pp. 57–72.
347. Kellogg, R. S., & Graybiel, A. Lack of response to thermal stimulation of the semicircular canals in the weightless phase of parabolic flight. *Aerospace Med.,* 1967, **38,** 487–490.
348. Kelly, K. L., & Judd, D. B. *The ISCC–NBS method of designating colors and a dictionary of color names.* Washington: U.S. Government Printing Office, 1955. (National Bureau of Standards Circular No. 553).
349. Kemp, E. H., & Johnson, E. P., Localization of response in the cochlea as determined by electrical recording. *Science,* 1939, **90,** 405.
350. Kennedy, R. S., & Graybiel, A. Validity of tests of canal sickness in predicting susceptibility to airsickness and seasickness. *Aerospace Med.,* 1962, **33,** 935–938.
351. Kenshalo, D. R. Comparison of thermal sensitivity of the forehead, lip, conjunctiva, and cornea. *J. appl. Physiol.,* 1960, **15,** 987–991.
352. Kenshalo, D. R. Improved method for the psychological study of the temperature sense. *Rev. sci. Instrum.,* 1963, **34,** 883–886.
353. Kenshalo, D. R., Decker, T., & Hamilton, A. Comparisons of spatial summation on the forehead, forearm, and back produced by radiant and conducted heat. *J. comp. physiol. Psychol.,* 1967, **63,** 510–515.
354. Kenshalo, D. R., Holmes, C. E., & Wood, P. B. Warm and cool thresholds as a function of rate of stimulus temperature change. *Percept. Psychophys.,* 1968, **3,** 81–84.

355. Kenshalo, D. R., Nafe, J . P., & Dawson, W. W. A new method for the investigation of thermal sensitivity. *J. Psychol.*, 1960, **49**, 29–41.

356. Kenshalo, D. R., & Scott, H. H. Temporal course of thermal adaptation. *Science*, 1966, **151**, 1095–1096.

357. Kiang, N. Y–S. *Discharge patterns of single fibers in the cat's auditory nerve.* Cambridge, Mass.: MIT Press, 1965.

358. Kiang, N. Y–S. Stimulus coding in the auditory nerve and cochlear nucleus. *Acta oto-laryngol., Stockh.*, 1965, **59**, 186–200.

359. Kiesow, F. Beiträge zur physiologischen Psychologie des Geschmachkssinnes (Fortsetzung). *Philos. Stud. (Wundt)*, 1894, **10**, 523–561.

360. Kiesow, F. Contribution á la psycho-physiologie de la cavité buccale. *Arch. ital. Biol.*, 1898, **30**, 377–398.

361. Kimura, K., & Beidler, L. M. Microelectrode study of taste receptors of rat and hamster. *J. cell. comp. Physiol.*, 1961, **58**, 131–140.

362. Kirschmann, A. Ueber die quantitativen Verhältnisse des simultanen Helligkeits- und Farben-Contrastes. *Philos. Stud. (Wundt)*, 1891, **6**, 417–491.

363. Kistiakowsky, G. B. On the theory of odors. *Science*, 1950, **112**, 154–155.

364. Klemmer, E. T., & Frick, F. C. Assimilation of information from dot and matrix patterns. *J. exp. Psychol.*, 1953, **45**, 15–19.

365. Knudsen, V. O. Hearing with the sense of touch. *J. gen. Psychol.*, 1928, **1**, 320–352.

366. Köhler, W. Akustische Untersuchungen. II. *Z. Psychol.*, 1910, **58**, 59–140.

367. Kolbe, H. Die zeitliche Veränderung der Unterschiedsschwelle während der Einwirkung eines stetigen Dauerdruck- oder Dauerlichtreizes. *Z. Sinnesphysiol.*, 1936, **67**, 53–68.

368. Komuro, K. Le minimum perceptible de l'odorat dans une enceinte absolument inodore. *Arch. néerl. Physiol.*, 1921, **6**, 20–24.

369. Krakauer, D., & Dallenbach, K . M. Gustatory adaptation to sweet, sour, and bitter. *Amer. J. Psychol.*, 1937, **49**, 469–475.

370. Kryter, K. D., Ward, W. D., Miller, J. D., & Eldredge, D. H. Hazardous exposure to intermittent and steady-state noise. *J. acoust. Soc. Amer.*, 1966, **39**, 451–464.

371. Kuffler, S. W. Discharge patterns and functional organization of mammalian retina. *J. Neurophysiol.*, 1953, **16**, 37–68.

372. Laidlaw, R. W., & Hamilton, M. A. A study of thresholds in apperception of passive movement among normal control subjects. *Bull. neurol. Inst. N.Y.*, 1937, **6**, 268–273.

373. Landgren, S. The response of thalamic and cortical neurons to electrical and physiological stimulation of the cat's tongue. In W. A. Rosenblith (Ed.), *Sensory communication.* New York: Wiley, 1961. Chap. 23 (pp. 437–453).

374. Lanier, L. H. An experimental study of cutaneous innervation. *Proc. Assoc. Res. nerv. ment. Dis.*, 1934, **15**, 437–456.

375. Lashley, K. S. The problem of cerebral organization in vision. In H. Klüver, (Ed.), *Biological symposia*, Vol. VII. Lancaster, Pa.: Jacques Cattell Press, 1942.

376. Laurens, H., & Hamilton, W. F. The sensibility of the eye to differences in wave-length. *Amer. J. Physiol.*, 1923, **65**, 547–568.

377. Leibowitz, H., Mote, F. A., & Thurlow, W. R. Simultaneous contrast as a function of separation between test and inducing fields. *J. exp. Psychol.*, 1953, **46**, 453–456.

378. Lele, P. P., & Weddell, G. The relationship between neurohistology and corneal sensibility. *Brain,* 1956, **79,** 119–154.
379. Lele, P. P., Weddell, G., & Williams, C. M. Relationship between heat transfer, skin temperature, and cutaneous sensibility. *J. Physiol., Lond.,* 1954, **126,** 206–234.
380. Lettvin, J. Y., Maturana, H. R., McCulloch, W. S., & Pitts, W. H. What the frog's eye tells the frog's brain. *Proc. I.R.E.,* 1959, **47,** 1940–1951.
381. Levine, H. A., & Dallenbach, K. M. Adaptation of cold spots under continuous and intermittent stimulation. *Amer. J. Psychol.,* 1936, **48,** 490–497.
382. Lewis, D. R. Psychological scales of taste. *J. Psychol.,* 1948, **26,** 437–446.
383. Lewis, T. *The blood vessels of the human skin and their responses.* London: Shaw, 1927.
384. Lewis, T. *Pain.* New York: Macmillan, 1942.
385. Lickley, J. D. *The nervous system.* New York: Longmans, Green, 1931.
386. Licklider, J. C. R. Basic correlates of the auditory stimulus. In S. S. Stevens (Ed.), *Handbook of experimental psychology.* New York: Wiley, 1951. Chap. 25 (pp. 985–1039).
387. Licklider, J. C. R. Three auditory theories. In S. Koch (Ed.), *Psychology: a study of a science.* Vol. I. New York: McGraw-Hill, 1959. Pp. 41–144.
388. Licklider, J. C. R., & Miller, G. A. The perception of speech. In S. S. Stevens (Ed.), *Handbook of experimental psychology.* New York: Wiley, 1951. Chap. 26 (pp. 1040–1074).
389. Lindahl, O. Experimental skin pain induced by injection of water-soluble substances in humans. *Acta physiol. scand., Suppl.* 179, 1961, **51,** 1–90.
390. Locke, J. *Essay concerning human understanding.* Book II, Chap. viii, par. 21, (1690).
391. Loewenstein, W. R. The generation of electric activity in a nerve ending. *Ann. N. Y. Acad. Sci.,* 1959, **81,** 367–387.
392. Lorenzo, A. J. D. de. Studies on the ultrastructure and histophysiology of cell membranes, nerve fibers and synaptic junctions in chemoreceptors. In Y. Zotterman (Ed.), *Olfaction and taste.* New York: Macmillan, 1963. Pp. 5–17.
393. Löwenstein, O. The functional significance of the ultrastructure of the vestibular end organs. In *Second Symposium on the Role of the Vestibular Organs in Space Exploration.* Washington: NASA SP–115, 1966. Pp. 73–90.
394. Löwenstein, O., & Sand, A. The mechanism of the semicircular canal. A study of the responses of single-fibre preparations to angular accelerations and to rotation at constant speed. *Proc. roy. Soc. Lond.,* 1940, **129B,** 256–275.
395. Lucretius [Titus Lucretius Carus] *De Rerum Natura.* Translated into English verse – *Of the Nature of Things* – by William Ellery Leonard. New York: The Heritage Club, 1957.
396. Luft, E. Ueber die Unterschiedsempfindlichkeit für Tonhöhen. *Philos. Stud. (Wundt),* 1888, **4,** 511–540.
397. Lythgoe, R. J., & Tansley, K. The relation of the critical frequency of flicker to the adaptation of the eye. *Proc. roy. Soc. Lond.,* 1929, **105B,** 60–92.

398. MacAdam, D. L. Color science and color photography. *Physics Today,* 1967, **20,** 27–39.

399. McBurney, D. H., & Pfaffmann, C. Gustatory adaptation to saliva and sodium chloride. *J. exp. Psychol.,* 1963, **65,** 523–529.

400. MacCorquodale, K. Effects of angular acceleration and centrifugal force on nonvisual space orientation during flight. *J. aviat. Med.,* 1948, **19,** 146–157.

401. McDougall, W. The sensations excited by a single momentary stimulation of the eye. *Brit. J. Psychol.,* 1904, **1,** 78–113.

402. McMurray, G. A. Experimental study of a case of insensitivity to pain. *Arch. Neurol. Psychiat., Chicago,* 1950, **64,** 650–667.

403. Marks, L. E., & Stevens, J. C. Perceived warmth and skin temperature as functions of the duration and level of thermal stimulation. *Percept. Psychophys.,* 1968, **4,** 220–228.

404. Marks, W. B., Dobelle, W. H., & MacNichol, E. F., Jr. Visual pigments of single primate cones. *Science,* 1964, **143,** 1181–1183.

405. Maruhashi, J., Mizuguchi, K., & Tasaki, I. Action currents in single afferent nerve fibres elicited by stimulation of the skin of the toad and the cat. *J. Physiol., Lond.,* 1952, **117,** 129–151.

406. Matthews, B. H. C. The response of a muscle spindle during active contraction of a muscle. *J. Physiol., Lond.,* 1931, **72,** 153–174.

407. Matthews, B. H. C. Nerve endings in mammalian muscle. *J. Physiol., Lond.,* 1933, **78,** 1–53.

408. Maxwell, J. C. On the theory of three primary colours. In *The scientific papers of James Clerk Maxwell,* Vol. I. Cambridge: Cambridge University Press, 1890. Paper XXII (pp. 445–450).

409. Melzack, R., & Casey, K. L. Sensory, motivational, and central control determinants of pain. In D. R. Kenshalo (Ed.), *The skin senses.* Springfield, Ill.: Thomas, 1968. Chap. 20 (pp. 423–443).

410. Melzack, R., Rose, G., & McGinty, D. Skin sensitivity to thermal stimuli. *Exp. Neurol.,* 1962, **6,** 300–314.

411. Melzack, R., & Schecter, B. Itch and vibration. *Science,* 1965, **147,** 1047–1048.

412. Melzack, R., & Wall, P. D. Pain mechanisms: a new theory. *Science,* 1965, **150,** 971–979.

413. Mendelson, M., & Loewenstein, W. R. Mechanisms of receptor adaptation. *Science,* 1964, **144,** 554–555.

414. Mettler, F. A., Finch, G., Girden, E., & Culler, E. Acoustic value of the several components of the auditory pathway. *Brain,* 1934, **57,** 475–483.

415. Meyer, M. F. The hydraulic principles governing the function of the cochlea. *J. gen. Psychol.,* 1928, **1,** 239–265.

416. Meyer, M. F. *How we hear: how tones make music.* Boston: Branford, 1950.

417. Michael, C. R. Receptive fields of single optic nerve fibers in a mammal with an all-cone retina. I. Contrast-sensitive units. *J. Neurophysiol.,* 1968, **31,** 249–256.

418. Millen, J. W. Observations on the innervation of blood vessels. *J. Anat., Lond.,* 1948, **82,** 68–80.

419. Miller, D. C. *Anecdotal history of the science of sound.* New York: Macmillan, 1935.

420. Miller, G. A. The magical number seven, plus or minus two: Some limitations on our capacity for processing information. *Psychol. Rev.*, 1956, **63**, 81–97.

421. Miller, G. A., & Taylor, W. G. The perception of repeated bursts of noise. *J. acoust. Soc. Amer.*, 1948, **20**, 171–182.

422. Miller, M. R., Ralston, H. J. III, & Kasahara, M. The pattern of cutaneous innervation of the human hand, foot, and breast. In W. Montagna (Ed.), *Cutaneous innervation* (Advances in biology of skin, Vol. 1). New York: Pergamon, 1960. Chap. I (pp. 1–47).

423. Miller, W. H., Ratliff, F., & Hartline, H. K. How cells receive stimuli. *Sci. Amer.*, 1961, **205**, 223–238.

424. Milner, P. M. *Physiological psychology.* New York: Holt, Rinehart, & Winston, 1970.

425. Møller, A. R. Acoustic reflex in man. *J. acoust. Soc. Amer.*, 1962, **34**, 1524–1534.

426. Moncrieff, R. W. *The chemical senses.* New York: Wiley, 1944.

427. Moncrieff, R. W. Olfactory adaptation and odour likeness. *J. Physiol., Lond.*, 1956, **133**, 301–316.

428. Moncrieff, R. W. *The chemical senses* (Rev. ed.). Cleveland, O.: Chemical Rubber Co., 1967.

429. Moreland, J. D., & Cruz, A. Colour perception with the peripheral retina. *Optica Acta*, 1959, **6**, 117–151.

430. Mote, F. A., & Riopelle, A. J. The effect of varying the intensity and duration of pre-exposure upon subsequent dark adaptation in the human eye. *J. comp. physiol. Psychol.*, 1953, **46**, 49–55.

431. Mozell, M . M. Olfactory discrimination: electrophysiological spatiotemporal basis. *Science*, 1964, **143**, 1336–1337.

432. Mozell, M. M. The spatiotemporal analysis of odorants at the level of the olfactory receptor sheet. *J. gen. Physiol.*, 1966, **50**, 25–41.

433. Mozell, M. M. Evidence for a chromatographic model of olfaction. *J. gen. Physiol.*, 1970, **55**, 46–63.

434. Mozell, M. M., & Pfaffmann, C. The afferent neural processes in odor perception. *Ann. N.Y. Acad. Sci.*, 1954, **58**, 96–108.

435. Mueller, C. G., & Lloyd, V. V. Stereoscopic acuity for various levels of illumination. *Proc. nat. Acad. Sci., Wash.*, 1948, **34**, 223–227.

436. Mueller, E. E., Loeffel, R., & Mead, S. Skin impedance in relation to pain threshold testing by electrical means. *J. appl. Physiol.*, 1953, **5**, 746–752.

437. Mullins, L. J. Olfaction. *Ann. N. Y. Acad. Sci.*, 1955, **62**, 247–276.

438. Murray, E. Binocular fusion and the locus of "yellow." *Amer. J. Psychol.*, 1939, **52**, 117–121.

439. Nafe, J. P., The pressure, pain, and temperature senses. In C. A. Murchison (Ed.), *Handbook of general experimental psychology.* Worcester, Mass.: Clark University Press, 1934. Chap. 20 (pp. 1037–1087).

440. Nafe, J. P., & Kenshalo, D. R. Stimulation and neural response. *Amer. J. Psychol.*, 1958, **71**, 199–208.

441. Nafe, J. P., & Wagoner, K. S. The insensitivity of the cornea to heat and pain derived from high temperatures. *Amer. J. Psychol.*, 1937, **49**, 631–635.

442. Nafe, J. P., &. Wagoner, K. S. The nature of pressure adaptation. *J. gen. Psychol.*, 1941, **25**, 323–351.

443. Neisser, U. Temperature thresholds for cutaneous pain. *J. appl. Physiol.*, 1959, **14**, 368–372.

444. Newby, H. A. *Audiology* (2nd ed.) New York: Appleton-Century-Crofts, 1964.

445. Newhall, S. M., Nickerson, D., & Judd, D. B. Final report of the OSA subcommittee on the spacing of the Munsell colors. *J. opt. Soc. Amer.*, 1943, **33**, 385–422.

446. Newman, E. B., Stevens, S. S., & Davis, H. Factors in the production of aural harmonics and combination tones. *J. acoust. Soc. Amer.*, 1937, **9**, 107–118.

447. Nickerson, D., & Newhall, S. M. A psychological color solid. *J. opt. Soc. Amer.*, 1943, **33**, 419–422.

448. Niven, J. I., Hixson, W. C., & Correia, M. J. Elicitation of horizontal nystagmus by periodic linear acceleration. *Acta oto-laryngol., Stockh.*, 1966, **62**, 429–441.

449. Oakley, B. Altered taste responses from cross-regenerated taste nerves in the rat. In T. Hayashi (Ed.), *Olfaction and taste, II*. Oxford: Pergamon, 1967. Pp. 535–547.

450. O'Connell, R. J., & Mozell, M. M. Quantitative stimulation of frog olfactory receptors. *J. Neurophysiol.*, 1969, **32**, 51–63.

451. Ogden, R. M. *Hearing*. New York: Harcourt, Brace, 1924.

452. Ogle, K. N., & Reiher, L. Stereoscopic depth perception from after-images. *Vision Res.*, 1962, **2**, 439–447.

453. Østerberg, G. Topography of the layer of rods and cones in the human retina. *Acta ophthalmol., Kbh., Suppl.* 6, 1935, 1–106.

454. Ottoson, D. Analysis of the electrical activity of the olfactory epithelium. *Acta physiol. scand., Suppl* 122, 1956, **35**, 7–83.

455. Ottoson, D. Generation and transmission of signals in the olfactory system. In Y. Zotterman (Ed.), *Olfaction and taste*. New York: Macmillan, 1963. Pp. 35–44.

456. Ough, C. S., & Stone, H. An olfactometer for rapid and critical odor measurement. *J. Food Sci.*, 1961, **26**, 452–456.

457. Palva, T., & Kärjä, J. Suprathreshold auditory adaptation. *J. acoust. Soc. Amer.*, 1969, **45**, 1018–1021.

458. Pangborn, R. M. Taste interrelationships. *Food Res.*, 1960, **25**, 245–256.

459. Parker, G. H., & Stabler, E. M. On certain distinctions between taste and smell. *Amer. J. Physiol.*, 1913, **32**, 230–240.

460. Pattle, R. E., & Weddell, G. Observations on electrical stimulation of pain fibres in an exposed human sensory nerve. *J. Neurophysiol.*, 1948, **11**, 93–98.

461. Pendleton, C. R. The cold receptor. *Amer. J. Psychol.*, 1928, **40**, 353–371.

462. Penfield, W., & Boldrey, E. Somatic motor and sensory representation in the cerebral cortex of man as studied by electrical stimulation. *Brain*, 1937, **60**, 389–443.

463. Pfaffmann, C. Gustatory afferent impulses. *J. cell. comp. Physiol.*, 1941, **17**, 243–258.

464. Pfaffmann, C. Studying the senses of taste and smell. In T. G. Andrews (Ed.), *Methods of psychology*. New York: Wiley, 1948. Chap. 10 (pp. 268–288).

465. Pfaffmann, C. Taste and smell. In S. S. Stevens (Ed.), *Handbook of experimental psychology*. New York: Wiley, 1951. Chap. 29 (pp. 1143–1171).

466. Pfaffmann, C. The afferent code for sensory quality. *Amer. Psychologist,* 1959, **14,** 226–232.

467. Pfaffmann, C. The sense of taste. In J. Field, H. W. Magoun & V. E. Hall (Eds.), *Handbook of physiology, Neurophysiology, I.* Washington, D. C.: American Physiological Society, 1959. Chap. 20 (pp. 507–533).

468. Pfaffmann, C. The sensory and motivating properties of the sense of taste. In M. R. Jones (Ed.), *Nebraska symposium on motivation.* Lincoln, Neb.: University of Nebraska Press, 1961. Pp. 71–110.

469. Pfaffmann, C. Sensory processes and their relation to behavior: studies on the sense of taste as a model S–R system. In S. Koch (Ed.), *Psychology: a study of a science,* Vol. 4. New York: McGraw-Hill, 1962. Pp. 380–416.

470. Pierrel, R. Taste effects resulting from intermittent electrical stimulation of the tongue. *J. exp. Psychol.,* 1955, **49,** 374–380.

471. Pilgrim, F. J. Interactions of suprathreshold taste stimuli. In M. R. Kare & B. P. Halpern (Eds.), *Physiological and behavioral aspects of taste.* Chicago: University of Chicago Press, 1961. Chap. 4 (pp. 66–78).

472. Pirenne, M. H. Physiological mechanisms of vision and the quantum nature of light. *Biol. Rev.,* 1956, **31,** 194–241.

473. Plomp, R. Rate of decay of auditory sensation. *J. acoust. Soc. Amer.,* 1964, **36,** 277–282.

474. Plomp, R. Beats of mistuned consonances. *J. acoust. Soc. Amer.,* 1967, **42,** 462–474.

475. Plomp, R., & Levelt, J. M. Tonal consonance and critical bandwidth. *J. acoust. Soc. Amer.,* 1965, **38,** 548–560.

476. Poggio, G. F., & Mountcastle, V. B. A study of the functional contributions of the lemniscal and spinothalamic systems to somatic sensibility. Central nervous mechanisms in pain. *Bull. Johns Hopk. Hosp.,* 1960, **106,** 266–316.

477. Pollack, I. The information of elementary auditory displays. *J. acoust. Soc. Amer.,* 1952, **24,** 745–749.

478. Polyak, S. L. *The retina.* Chicago: University of Chicago Press, 1941.

479. Prentice, W. C. H. New observations of 'binocular yellow.' *J. exp. Psychol.,* 1948, **38,** 284–288.

480. Priest, I. G. Note on the relation between the frequencies of complementary hues. *J. opt. Soc. Amer.,* 1920, **4,** 402–404.

481. Priest, I. G., & Brickwedde, F. G. The minimum perceptible colorimetric purity as a function of dominant wavelength with sunlight as a neutral standard. *J. opt. Soc. Amer.,* 1926, **13,** 306–307.

482. Pritchard, R . M. Stabilized images on the retina. *Sci. Amer.,* 1961, **204,** 72–78.

483. Purdy, D. M. Spectral hue as a function of intensity. *Amer. J. Psychol.,* 1931, **43,** 541–559.

484. Purdy, D. M. The Bezold-Brücke phenomenon and contours for constant hue. *Amer. J. Psychol.,* 1937, **49,** 313–315.

485. Quilliam, T. A. Unit design and array patterns in receptor organs. In A. V. S. de Reuck & J. Knight (Eds.), *Touch, heat, and pain.* Boston: Little, Brown, 1966. Pp. 86–112.

486. Rahm, W. E., Jr., Strother, W. F., & Gulick, W. L. The stability of the cochlear response through time. *Ann. Otol. Rhinol. Larnygol.,* 1958, **67,** 972–977.

487. Ramón y Cajal, S. *Histology* (Trans. M. Fernán-Núñez). Baltimore: William Wood, 1933.

488. Rasmussen, G. L. The olivary peduncle and other fiber projections of the superior olivary complex. *J. comp. Neurol.*, 1946, 84, 141–219.

489. Rasmussen, T., & Penfield, W. Further studies of the sensory and motor cerebral cortex of man. *Fed. Proc.*, 1947, 6, 452–460.

490. Ratliff, F. *Mach bands: quantitative studies on neural networks in the retina.* San Francisco: Holden-Day, 1965.

491. Ratliff, F., & Riggs, L. A. Involuntary motions of the eye during monocular fixation. *J. exp. Psychol.*, 1950, 40, 687–701.

492. Reeves, P. Rate of pupillary dilation and contraction. *Psychol. Rev.*, 1918, 25, 330–340.

493. Rein, H. Ueber die Topographie der Warmempfindung. *Z. Biol.*, 1925, 82, 513–535.

494. Rich, G. J. A study of tonal attributes. *Amer. J. Psychol.*, 1919, 30, 121–164.

495. Richter, C. P., & MacLean, A. Salt taste threshold of humans. *Amer. J. Physiol.*, 1939, 126, 1–6.

496. Riesz, R. R. Differential intensity sensitivity of the ear for pure tones. *Phys. Rev.*, 1928, 31, 867–875.

497. Riggs, L. A. Electrophysiology of vision. In C. H. Graham (Ed.), *Vision and visual perception.* New York: Wiley, 1965. Chap. 5 (pp. 81–131).

498. Riggs, L. A. The "looks" of Helmholtz. *Percept. Psychophys.*, 1967, 2, 1–13.

499. Riggs, L. A., Johnson, E. P., & Schick, A. M. L. Electrical responses of the human eye to changes in wavelength of the stimulating light. *J. opt. Soc. Amer.*, 1966, 56, 1621–1627.

500. Riggs, L. A., Ratliff, F., Cornsweet, J. C., & Cornsweet, T. N. The disappearance of steadily fixated visual test objects. *J. opt. Soc. Amer.*, 1953, 43, 495–501.

501. Rivers, W. H. R. *Instinct and the unconscious.* Cambridge: Cambridge University Press, 1920.

502. Robertis, E. de, & Lasansky, A. Ultrastructure and chemical organization of photoreceptors. In G. K. Smelser (Ed.), *The structure of the eye.* New York: Academic Press, 1961. Pp. 29–49.

503. Roehrig, W. C. The influence of the portion of the retina stimulated on the critical flicker-fusion threshold. *J. Psychol.*, 1959, 48, 57–63.

504. Rose, J. E., Brugge, J. F., Anderson, D. J., & Hind, J. E. Phase-locked response to low-frequency tones in single auditory nerve fibers of the squirrel monkey. *J. Neurophysiol.*, 1967, 30, 769–793.

505. Rose, J. E., & Mountcastle, V. B. Touch and kinesthesis. In J. Field, H. W. Magoun, & V. E. Hall (Eds.), *Handbook of physiology, Neurophysiology, I.* Washington, D. C.: American Physiological Society, 1959. Chap. 17 (pp. 387–429).

506. Rosenblith, W. A., Miller, G. A., Egan, J. P., Hirsh, I. J., & Thomas, G. J. An auditory afterimage? *Science*, 1947, 106, 333–335.

507. Rosenthal, S. R. Histamine as possible chemical mediator for cutaneous pain. Dual pain response to histamine. *Proc. Soc. exp. Biol. (N. Y.)*, 1950, 74, 167–170.

508. Rosenzweig, M. R. Cortical correlates of auditory localization and of related perceptual phenomena. *J. comp. physiol. Psychol.*, 1954, 47, 269–276.

509. Rushton, W. A. H. Visual pigments in man. *Sci. Amer.*, 1962, **207**, 120–132.

510. Scharf, B. Complex sounds and critical bands. *Psychol. Bull.*, 1961, **58**, 205–217.

511. Schneider, R. A., & Schmidt, C. E. Dependency of olfactory localization on non-olfactory cues. *Physiol. Behav.*, 1967, **2**, 305–309.

512. Schouten, J. F., Ritsma, R. J., & Lopes-Cardozo, B. Pitch of the residue. *J. acoust. Soc. Amer.*, 1962, **34**, 1418–1424.

513. Schumacher, G. A., Goodell, H., Hardy, J. D., & Wolff, H. G. Uniformity of the pain threshold in man. *Science*, 1940, **92**, 110.

514. Schutz, H. G., & Pilgrim, F. J. Differential sensitivity in gustation. *J. exp. Psychol.*, 1957, **54**, 41–48.

515. Sem-Jacobsen, C. W., Petersen, M. C., Dodge, H. W., Jr., Jacks, Q. D., & Lazarte, J. A. Electric activity of the olfactory bulb in man. *Amer. J. med. Sci.*, 1956, **232**, 243–251.

516. Senders, V. L. The physiological basis of visual acuity. *Psychol. Bull.*, 1948, **45**, 465–490.

517. Sergeev, K. K. The receptor function of the cornea. *Sechenov physiol. J. U.S.S.R.*, 1958, **44**, 97–100.

518. Setterfield, W., Schott, R. G., & Snyder, L. H. Studies in human inheritance. XV. The bimodality of the threshold curve for the taste of phenyl-thio-carbamide. *Ohio J. Sci.*, 1936, **36**, 231–235.

519. Shelden, C. H. Depolarization in the treatment of trigeminal neuralgia. In R. S. Knighton & P. R. Dumke (Eds.), *Pain*. Boston: Little, Brown, 1966. Chap. 28 (pp. 373–386).

520. Sherrick, C. E. Variables affecting sensitivity of the human skin to mechanical vibration. *J. exp. Psychol.*, 1953, **45**, 273–282.

521. Sherrick, C. E. Observations relating to some common psychophysical functions as applied to the skin. In G. R. Hawkes (Ed.), Symposium on cutaneous sensitivity. *U. S. Army Med. Res. Lab. Rep.*, No. 424, 1960. Pp. 147–158

522. Sherrick, C. E., & Albernaz, P. L. Auditory threshold shifts produced by simultaneously pulsed contralateral stimuli. *J. acoust. Soc. Amer.*, 1961, **33**, 1381–1385.

523. Sherrington, C. S. *The integrative action of the nervous system.* London: Constable, 1906.

524. Shibuya, T. Dissociation of olfactory neural response and mucosal potential. *Science*, 1964, **143**, 1338–1340.

525. Shore, L. E. A contribution to our knowledge of taste sensations. *J. Physiol., Lond.*, 1892, **13**, 191–217.

526. Shower, E. G., & Biddulph, R. Differential pitch sensitivity of the ear. *J. acoust. Soc. Amer.*, 1931, **3**, 275–287.

527. Sinclair, D. C. *Cutaneous sensation.* New York: Oxford University Press, 1967.

528. Sinclair, D. C., & Stokes, B. A. R. The production and characteristics of "second pain." *Brain*, 1964, **87**, 609–618.

529. Sivian, L. J., & White, S. D. On minimum audible sound fields. *J. acoust. Soc. Amer.*, 1933, **4**, 288–321.

530. Skramlik, E. von. Ueber die Lokalisation der Empfindung bei den niederen Sinnen. *Z. Sinnesphysiol.*, 1926, **56**, 69–140.

531. Skramlik, E. von. *Handbuck der Physiologie der niederen Sinne.* 1. Die Physiologie der Geruchs- und Geschmackssinnes. Berlin: Junk, 1926.
532. Skramlik, E. von. Psychophysiologie der Tastsinne. *Arch. ges. Psychol.,* Ergänzungsbd. **4,** 1937.
533. Sloan, L. L. Congenital achromatopsia: A report of 19 cases. *J. opt. Soc. Amer.,* 1954, **44,** 117–128.
534. Sloan, L. L., & Wollach, L. A case of unilateral deuteranopia. *J. opt. Soc. Amer.,* 1948, **38,** 502–509.
535. Small, A. M., Jr. Auditory adaptation. In J. Jerger (Ed.), *Modern developments in audiology.* New York: Academic Press, 1963. Chap. 8 (pp. 287–336).
536. Smith, F. O. An experimental study of retinal sensitivity and discrimination for purple under different degrees of intensity of stimulation. *J. exp. Psychol.,* 1925, **8,** 381–397.
537. Southall, J. P. C. *Introduction to physiological optics.* New York: Oxford University Press, 1937.
538. Speidel, C. C. Adjustments of nerve endings. *Harvey Lectures,* 1941, **36,** 126–158.
539. Steindler, O. Die Farbenempfindlichkeit des normalen und farbenblinden Auges. *Sitzungsber. Akad. Wiss., Wien,* 1906, **115,** 39–62.
540. Steinhausen, W. Ueber den experimentellen Nachweis der Ablenkung der Cupula terminalis in der intakten Bogengangsampulle des Labyrinths bei der thermischen und adäquaten rotatorischen Reizung. *Z. Hals- Nas.-Ohrenheilk.,* 1931, **29,** 211–216.
541. Sternbach, R. A. Congenital insensitivity to pain: a critique. *Psychol. Bull.,* 1963, **60,** 252–264.
541a. Sternbach, R. A. *Pain, a psychophysiological analysis.* New York: Academic Press, 1968.
542. Stevens, J. C., & Cain, W. S. Effort in isometric muscular contractions related to force level and duration. *Percept. Psychophys.,* 1970, **8,** 240–244.
543. Stevens, J. C., & Mack, J. D. Scales of apparent force. *J. exp. Psychol.,* 1959, **58,** 405–413.
544. Stevens, J. C., & Rubin, L. L. Psychophysical scales of apparent heaviness and the size-weight illusion. *Percept. Psychophys.,* 1970, **8,** 225–230.
545. Stevens, J. C., & Stevens, S. S. Warmth and cold: dynamics of sensory intensity. *J. exp. Psychol.,* 1960, **60,** 183–192.
546. Stevens, S. S. The attributes of tones. *Proc. nat. Acad. Sci., Wash.,* 1934, **20,** 457–459.
547. Stevens, S. S. The relation of pitch to intensity. *J. acoust. Soc. Amer.,* 1937, **8,** 191–195.
548. Stevens, S. S. Machines cannot fight alone. *Amer. Sci.,* 1946, **34,** 389–400.
549. Stevens, S. S. The psychophysics of sensory function. *Amer. Sci.,* 1960, **48,** 226–253.
550. Stevens, S. S. To honor Fechner and repeal his law. *Science,* 1961, **133,** 80–86.
551. Stevens, S. S. The surprising simplicity of sensory metrics. *Amer. Psychologist,* 1962, **17,** 29–39.
552. Stevens, S. S. Intensity functions in sensory systems. *Int. J. Neurol.,* 1967, **6,** 202–209.

553. Stevens, S. S., & Davis, H. *Hearing.* New York: Wiley, 1938.

554. Stevens, S. S., Davis, H., & Lurie, M. H. The localization of pitch perception on the basilar membrane. *J. gen. Psychol.,* 1935, **13,** 297–315.

555. Stevens, S. S., & Galanter, E. H. Ratio scales and category scales for a dozen perceptual continua. *J. exp. Psychol.,* 1957, **54,** 377–411.

556. Stevens, S. S., & Guirao, M. Scaling of apparent viscosity. *Science,* 1964, **144,** 1157–1158.

557. Stevens, S. S., Guirao, M., & Slawson, A. W. Loudness, a product of volume times density. *J. exp. Psychol.,* 1965, **69,** 503–510.

558. Stevens, S. S., & Harris, J. R. The scaling of subjective roughness and smoothness. *J. exp. Psychol.,* 1962, **64,** 489–494.

559. Stevens, S. S., & Stone, G. Finger span: ratio scale, category scale, and jnd scale. *J. exp. Psychol.,* 1959, **57,** 91–95.

560. Stone, H. Determinants of odor difference limens for three compounds. *J. exp. Psychol.,* 1963, **66,** 466–473.

561. Stone, H., Ough, C. S., & Pangborn, R. M. Determination of odor difference thresholds. *J. Food Sci.,* 1962, **27,** 197–202.

562. Strughold, H. Ueber die Dichte und Schwellen der Schmerzpunkte der Epidermis in der verschiedenen Körperregionen. *Z. Biol.,* 1924, **80,** 367–380.

563. Strughold, H., & Karbe, M. Vitale Färbung des Auges und experimentelle Untersuchung der gefärbten Nervenelemente. *Z. Biol.,* 1925, **83,** 297–308.

563a. Strughold, H., & Porz, R. Die Dichte der Kaltpunkte auf der Haut des menschlichen Körpers. *Z. Biol.,* 1931, **91,** 563–571.

564. Svaetichin, G., & MacNichol, E. F. Retinal mechanisms for chromatic and achromatic vision. *Ann. N. Y. Acad. Sci.,* 1958, **74,** 385–404.

565. Sweet, W. H. Pain. In J. Field, H. W. Magoun., & V. E. Hall (Eds.), *Handbook of physiology, Neurophysiology, I.,* Washington, D. C.: American Physiological Society, 1959. Chap. 19 (pp. 459–506).

566. Talbot, W. H., Darian-Smith, I., Kornhuber, H. H., & Mountcastle, V. B. The sense of flutter-vibration: Comparison of the human capacity with response patterns of mechanoreceptive afferents from the monkey hand. *J. Neurophysiol.,* 1968, **31,** 301–334.

567. Tasaki, I. Afferent impulses in auditory nerve fibers and the mechanism of impulse initiation in the cochlea. In G. L. Rasmussen & W. F. Windle (Eds.), *Neural mechanisms of the auditory and vestibular systems.* Springfield, Ill.: Thomas, 1960. Chap. 3 (pp. 40–47).

568. Terrace, H. S., & Stevens, S. S. The quantification of tonal volume. *Amer. J. Psychol.,* 1962, **75,** 596–604.

569. Terzuolo, P., & Adey, W. R. Sensorimotor cortical activities. In J. Field, H. W. Magoun & V. E. Hall (Eds.), *Handbook of physiology, Neurophysiology, II.* Washington, D. C.: American Physiological Society, 1959. Chap. 33 (pp. 797–835).

570. Thomas, G. J. Equal-volume judgments of tones. *Amer. J. Psychol.,* 1949, **62,** 182–201.

571. Thomas, W. G., & Preslar, M. J. A calibration study of one hundred audiometers currently employed in hearing conservation programs. *J. acoust. Soc. Amer.,* 1967, **42,** 1148.

572. Thompson, R. F. *Foundations of physiological psychology.* New York: Harper & Row, 1967.

573. Thurlow, W. R. Binaural interaction and the perception of pitch. *J. exp. Psychol.,* 1943, **32,** 13–36.

574. Tice, F. G. Individual differences in fusion frequency correlated with other visual processes. Unpublished Ph.D. dissertation. University of Virginia, 1941.

575. Titchener, E. B. Psychology: science or technology? *Pop. Sci. Mo.,* 1914, **84,** 39–51.

576. Tomita, T. Electrical activity in the vertebrate retina. *J. opt. Soc. Amer.,* 1963, **53,** 49–57.

577. Tonndorf, J., & Khanna, S. M. Some properties of sound transmission in the middle and outer ears of cats. *J. acoust. Soc. Amer.,* 1967, **41,** 513–521.

578. Tonndorf, J., & Khanna, S. M. Submicroscopic displacement amplitudes of the tympanic membrane (cat) measured by a laser interferometer. *J. acoust. Soc. Amer.,* 1968, **44,** 1546–1554.

579. Tonndorf, J., & Khanna, S. M. The role of the tympanic membrane in middle ear transmission. *Ann. Otol. Rhinol. Laryngol.,* 1970, **79,** 743–753.

580. Tower, S. S. Pain: definition and properties of the unit for sensory reception. *Res. Publ. Assoc. nerv. ment. Dis.,* 1943, **23,** 16–43.

581. Travis, R. C. The effect of varying the position of the head on voluntary response to vestibular stimulation. *J. exp. Psychol.,* 1938, **23,** 295–303.

582. Troland, L. T. The psychophysiology of auditory qualities and attributes. *J. gen. Psychol.,* 1929, **2,** 28–58.

583. Troland, L. T. The Hering theory in modern form. Par. 332 in *The principles of psychophysiology,* Vol. II. New York: Van Nostrand, 1930.

584. Tyrrell, H. V. J., Taylor, D. A., & Williams, C. M. The 'Seebeck effect' in a purely ionic system. *Nature, Lond.,* 1956, **176,** 668–669.

585. Vendrik, A. J. H., & Vos, J. J. Comparison of the stimulation of the warmth sense organ by microwave and infrared. *J. appl. Physiol.,* 1958, **13,** 435–444.

586. Verriest, G. Further studies on acquired deficiency of color discrimination. *J. opt. Soc. Amer.,* 1963, **53,** 185–195.

587. Verrillo, R. T. Effect of contactor area on the vibrotactile threshold. *J. acoust. Soc. Amer.,* 1963, **35,** 1962–1966.

588. Verrillo, R. T. Effect of spatial parameters on the vibrotactile threshold. *J. exp. Psychol.,* 1966, **71,** 570–575.

589. Verrillo, R. T. A duplex mechanism of mechanoreception. In D. R. Kenshalo (Ed.), *The skin senses.* Springfield, Ill.: Thomas, 1968. Chap. 7 (pp. 139–159).

590. Verrillo, R. T., Fraioli, A. J., & Smith, R. L. Sensation magnitude of vibrotactile stimuli. *Percept. Psychophys.,* 1969, **6,** 366–372.

591. Vries, H. de, & Stuiver, M. The absolute sensitivity of the human sense of smell. In W. A. Rosenblith (Ed.), *Communication processes.* New York: Wiley, 1961. Chap. 9 (pp. 159–167).

592. Wagner, H. G., MacNichol, E. F., Jr., & Wolbarsht, M. L. The response properties of single ganglion cells in the goldfish retina. *J. gen. Physiol.,* 1960, **43,** 45–62.

593. Wald, G. The photochemistry of vision. *Doc. ophthalmol.,* 1949, **3,** 94–137.

594. Wald, G. General discussion of retinal structure in relation to the visual process. In G. K. Smelser (Ed.), *The structure of the eye.* New York: Academic Press, 1961. Pp. 101–115.

595. Wald, G. Blue-blindness in the normal fovea. *J. opt. Soc. Amer.,* 1967, **57,** 1289–1303.

596. Wald, G., & Brown, P. K. Human color vision and color blindness. *Cold Spring Harbor Symp. on Quant. Biol.,* 1965, **30**, 345–361.

597. Wald, G., & Clark, A. B. Visual adaptation and the chemistry of the rods. *J. gen. Physiol.,* 1937, **21**, 93–105.

598. Wall, P. D. Cord cells responding to touch, damage, and temperature of skin. *J. Neurophysiol.,* 1960, **23**, 197–210.

599. Wall, P. D., & Sweet, W. H. Temporary abolition of pain in man. *Science,* 1967, **155**, 108–109.

600. Wallace, S. R. Studies in binocular interdependence. I. Binocular relations in macular adaptation. *J. gen. Psychol.,* 1937, **17**, 307–322.

601. Wallace, S. R. Studies in binocular interdependence. II. Some qualitative phenomena. *J. gen. Psychol.,* 1938, **19**, 169–177.

602. Wallace, S. R. Studies in binocular interdependence. III. An active principle. *J. gen. Psychol.,* 1939, **20**, 33–45.

603. Walls, G. L. Factors in human visual resolution. *J. opt. Soc. Amer.,* 1943, **33**, 487–505.

604. Walsh, E. G. The perception of rhythmically repeated linear motion in the horizontal plane. *Brit. J. Psychol.,* 1962, **53**, 439–445.

605. Walshe, F. M. R. The anatomy and physiology of cutaneous sensibility: a critical review. *Brain,* 1942, **65**, 48–112.

606. Wangensteen, O. H., & Carlson, A. J. Hunger sensations in a patient after total gastrectomy. *Proc. Soc. exp. Biol., N.Y.,* 1931, **28**, 545–547.

607. Ward, W. D. Auditory fatigue and masking. In J. Jerger (Ed.), *Modern developments in audiology.* New York: Academic Press, 1963. Chap. 7 (pp. 240–286).

608. Warren, H. C., & Carmichael, L. *Elements of human psychology.* Boston: Houghton Mifflin, 1930.

609. Waterston, D. Observations on sensation: the sensory functions of the skin for touch and pain. *J. Physiol., Lond.,* 1933, **77**, 251–257.

610. Weddell, G. The multiple innervation of sensory spots in the skin. *J. Anat., Lond.,* 1941, **75**, 441–446.

611. Weddell, G. The anatomy of pain sensibility. *J. Anat., Lond.,* 1947, **81**, 374.

612. Weddell, G. Studies related to the mechanism of common sensibility. In W. Montagna (Ed.), *Cutaneous innervation* (Advances in biology of skin, Vol. 1). New York: Pergamon, 1960. Chap. VII (pp. 112–160).

613. Weddell, G., Sinclair, D. C., & Feindel, W. H. An anatomical basis for alterations in quality of pain sensibility. *J. Neurophysiol.,* 1948, **11**, 99–109.

614. Wegel, R. L., & Lane, C. E. The auditory masking of one pure tone by another and its probable relation to the dynamics of the inner ear. *Phys. Rev.,* 1924, **23**, 266–285.

615. Weinberg, M., & Allen, F. On the critical frequency of pulsation of tones. *Phil. Mag.,* 1924, **47**, 50–62.

616. Weiss, A. D. Auditory perception in relation to age. In J. E. Birren et al., *Human aging.* Washington, D.C., 1963. PHS Publ. No. 986. Chap. 9 (pp. 111–140).

617. Weitz. J. Vibratory sensitivity as affected by local anesthesia. *J. exp. Psychol.,* 1939, **25**, 48–64.

618. Weitz, J. Vibratory sensitivity as a function of skin temperature. *J. exp. Psychol.,* 1941, **28**, 21–36.

619. Weitzman, D. O., & Kinney, J. S. Appearance of color for small, brief, spectral stimuli, in the central fovea. *J. opt. Soc. Amer.*, 1967, **57**, 665–670.

620. Wendt, G. R. Vestibular functions. In S. S. Stevens (Ed.), *Handbook of experimental psychology.* New York: Wiley, 1951. Chap. 31 (pp. 1191–1223).

621. Wenzel, B. M. Differential sensitivity in olfaction. *J. exp. Psychol.*, 1949, **39**, 129–143.

622. Wenzel, B. M. Olfactometric method utilizing natural breathing in an odor-free environment. *Science*, 1955, **121**, 802–803.

623. Werner, G., & Mountcastle, V. B. Neural activity in mechanoreceptive cutaneous afferents: stimulus-response relations, Weber functions, and information transmission. *J. Neurophysiol.*, 1965, **28**, 359–397.

624. Werner, G., & Mountcastle, V. B. Quantitative relations between mechanical stimuli to the skin and neural responses evoked by them. In D. R. Kenshalo (Ed.), *The skin senses.* Springfield, Ill.: Thomas, 1968. Chap. 6 (pp. 112–138).

625. Wersäll, R. The tympanic muscles and their reflexes. *Acta oto-laryngol., Stockh., Suppl.* 139, 1958, 1–112.

626. Wersäll, J., and Lundquist, Per-G. Morphological polarization of the mechano-receptors of the vestibular and acoustic systems. In *Second Symposium on the Role of the Vestibular Organs in Space Exploration* (NASA SP–115), 1966, 57–72.

627. Westheimer, G. The Maxwellian view. *Vision Res.*, 1966, **6**, 669–682.

628. Wever, E. G. *Theory of hearing.* New York: Wiley, 1949.

629. Wever, E. G. Development of traveling-wave theories. *J. acoust. Soc. Amer.*, 1962, **9**, 1319–1324.

630. Wever, E. G. Electrical potentials of the cochlea. *Physiol. Revs.*, 1966, **46**, 102–127.

631. Wever, E. G., & Bray, C. W. Present possibilities for auditory theory. *Psychol. Rev.*, 1930, **37**, 365–380.

632. Wever, E. G., & Bray, C. W. The perception of low tones and the resonance-volley theory. *J. Psychol.*, 1937, **3**, 101–114.

633. Wever, E. G., & Bray, C. W. Distortion in the ear as shown by the electrical responses of the cochlea. *J. acoust. Soc. Amer.*, 1938, **9**, 227–233.

634. Wever, E. G., Bray, C. W., & Lawrence, M. A quantitative study of combination tones. *J. exp. Psychol.*, 1940, **27**, 469–496.

635. Wever, E. G., & Lawrence, M. The patterns of response in the cochlea. *J. acoust. Soc. Amer.*, 1949, **21**, 127–134.

636. Wever, E. G., & Lawrence, M. The place principle in auditory theory. *Proc. nat. Acad. Sci.*, 1952, **38**, 133–138.

637. Wever, E. G., & Lawrence M. Auditory theory: an experimental study of the place principle. *Bull. N.Y. Acad. Med.*, 1953, **29**, 159–163.

638. Wever, E. G., & Lawrence, M. *Physiological acoustics.* Princeton, N. J.: Princeton University Press, 1954.

639. Whitfield, I. C., & Evans, E. F. Responses of auditory cortical neurons to stimuli of changing frequency. *J. Neurophysiol.*, 1965, **28**, 655–672.

640. Wilska, A. Eine Methode zur Bestimmung der Hörschwellenamplituden des Trommelfells bei verschiedenen Frequenzen. *Skand. Arch. Physiol.*, 1935, **72**, 161–165.

641. Wilska, A.   On the vibrational sensitivity in different regions of the body surface. *Acta physiol. scand.*, 1954, **31**, 285–289.

642. Wilson, M. H., & Brocklebank, R. W.   Complementary hues of afterimages. *J. opt. Soc. Amer.*, 1955, **45**, 293–299.

643. Wing, M. E.   The response of the otolith organs to tilt. *Acta oto-laryng., Stockh.*, 1963, **56**, 537–545.

644. Wingfield, R. C.   An experimental study of the apparent persistence of auditory sensation. *J. gen. Psychol.*, 1936, **14**, 136–157.

645. Winkelmann, R. K.   *Nerve endings in normal and pathologic skin.*   Springfield, Ill.:   Thomas, 1960.

646. Winkelmann, R. K.   Similarities in cutaneous nerve end-organs.   In W. Montagna (Ed.), *Cutaneous innervation.*   (Advances in biology of skin, Vol. 1).   New York: Pergamon, 1960.   Chap. II (pp. 48–62).

647. Wolf, H.   Exakte Messungen über die zur Erregung des Drucksinnes erforderlichen Reizgrössen.   Inaugural dissertation, Jena, 1937.

648. Wolff, H. G., & Wolf, S.   *Pain.*   Springfield, Ill.:   Thomas, 1948.

649. Wood, A. G.   A quantitative account of the course of auditory fatigue.   Unpublished Master's thesis. University of Virginia, 1930.

650. Woodworth, R. S.   *Experimental psychology.*   New York: Holt, 1938.

651. Woodworth, R. S.   *Psychology* (4th ed.).   New York: Holt, 1940.

652. Woollard, H. H., Weddell, G., & Harpman, J. A.   Observations on the neurohistological basis of cutaneous pain. *J. Anat., Lond.*, 1940, **74**, 413–440.

653. Woolsey, C. N.   Organization of cortical auditory system.   In W. A. Rosenblith, (Ed.), *Sensory communication.*   New York: Wiley, 1961.   Chap. 14 (pp. 235–257).

654. Woolsey, C. N., Marshall, W. H., & Bard, P.   Representation of cutaneous tactile sensibility in the cerebral cortex of the monkey as indicated by evoked potentials. *Johns Hopkins Hosp. Bull.*, 1942, **70**, 399–441.

655. Woolsey, C. N., & Walzl, E. M.   Topical projection of nerve fibers from local regions of the cochlea to the cerebral cortex of the cat. *Johns Hopkins Hosp. Bull.*, 1942, **71**, 315–344.

656. Worchel, P., & Dallenbach, K. M.   The vestibular sensitivity of deaf-blind subjects. *Amer. J. Psychol.*, 1948, **61**, 94–99.

657. Wright, W. D.   A re-determination of the trichromatic coefficients of the spectral colours. *Trans. opt. Soc., Lond.*, 1928–1929, **30**, 141–164.

658. Wright, W. D.   *The measurement of colour.*   New York: Macmillan, 1958.

659. Wright, W. D.   A new look at 37 years of research. *Vision Res.*, 1964, **4**, 63–74.

660. Wyszecki, G., & Stiles, W. S.   *Color science: Concepts and methods, quantitative data and formulas.*   New York: Wiley, 1967.

661. Zigler, M. J.   Pressure adaptation time: a function of intensity and extensity. *Amer. J. Psychol.*, 1932, **44**, 709–720.

662. Zigler, M. J., & Holway, A. H.   Differential sensitivity as determined by amount of olfactory substance. *J. gen. Psychol.*, 1935, **12**, 372–382.

663. Zwaardemaker, H.   *L'odorat.*   Paris: Doin, 1925.

664. Zwaardemaker, H.   An intellectual history of a physiologist with psychological aspirations.   In C. A. Murchison (Ed.), *A history of psychology in autobiography,* Vol. I.   Worcester, Mass.:   Clark University Press, 1930.   Pp. 491–516.

665. Zwicker, E.   "Negative afterimage" in hearing. *J. acoust. Soc. Amer.*, 1964, **36**, 2413–2415.

666. Zwicker, E., Flottorp, G., & Stevens, S. S.   Critical band width in loudness
     summation. *J. acoust. Soc. Amer.,* 1957, **29,** 548–557.
667. Zwislocki, J. J., Damianopoulos, E. N., Buining, E., & Glantz, J.   Central
     masking: Some steady-state and transient effects. *Percept. Psychophys.,*
     1967, **2,** 59–64.

Index of Names

557

Index of Subjects

567